EFFECTS *of* POISONOUS PLANTS *on* LIVESTOCK

ACADEMIC PRESS RAPID MANUSCRIPT REPRODUCTION

Proceedings of a Joint United States–Australian Symposium on Poisonous Plants at Utah State University, Logan, Utah, June 19–24, 1977.

EFFECTS *of* POISONOUS PLANTS *on* LIVESTOCK

Edited by

RICHARD F. KEELER

Poisonous Plant Research Laboratory
Agricultural Research Service
United States Department of Agriculture
Logan, Utah

KENT R. VAN KAMPEN

Department of Animal, Dairy, and Veterinary Sciences
Utah State University
Logan, Utah

LYNN F. JAMES

Poisonous Plant Research Laboratory
Agricultural Research Service
United States Department of Agriculture
Logan, Utah

ACADEMIC PRESS New York San Francisco London 1978

A Subsidiary of Harcourt Brace Jovanovich, Publishers

The United States–Australian Symposium on Poisonous Plants was held under the auspices of the United States–Australian Agreement for Scientific and Technical Cooperation for Joint Meetings. Financial and physical facility support were generously provided by the National Science Foundation, the Australian Department of Science, the Agricultural Research Service of the United States Department of Agriculture, and by Utah State University.

ACADEMIC PRESS, INC.
111 Fifth Avenue, New York, New York 10003

United Kingdom Edition published by
ACADEMIC PRESS, INC. (LONDON) LTD.
24/28 Oval Road, London NW1 7DX

Library of Congress Cataloging in Publication Data

Joint United States-Australian Symposium on Poisonous Plants, Utah State University, 1977.
Effects of poisonous plants on livestock.

"Held under the auspices of the United States-Australian Agreement for Scientific and Technical Cooperation for Joint Meetings."
1. Stock poisoning plants—Congresses. 2. Stock poisoning plants—UnitedStates—Congresses. 3. Stock poisoning plants—Australia—Congresses. I. Keeler, Richard F. II. Van Kampen, Kent R. III. James, Lynn F. IV. Title.
SF757.5.J64 1977 636.089'59'52 77-25330
ISBN 0-12-403250-8

PRINTED IN THE UNITED STATES OF AMERICA

Contents

III. SIMPLE PHYTOTOXINS

IV. PLANT HEPATOTOXINS

V. PLANT CARDIO/PULMONARY TOXINS

VIII. OTHER TOXICITIES

List of Participants

Numbers in parentheses indicate the pages on which the authors' contributions begin.

HELEN ACLAND, University of Pennsylvania, Kennett Square, Pennsylvania 19348

A.F. ALEXANDER (285), Department of Veterinary Pathology, College of Veterinary Medicine, Colorado State University, Fort Collins, Colorado 80523

J.G. ALLEN (241), Department of Agriculture, Western Australia, Perth, Western Australia, Australia

MILTON J. ALLISON (101), National Animal Disease Center, Agricultural Research Service, USDA, Ames, Iowa 50010

CHARLES K. ANDERSON, Veterinary Research Laboratory, Montana State University, Bozeman, Montana 59715

E. MURL BAILEY, JR., College of Veterinary Medicine, Texas Agricultural Experiment Station, Texas A & M University, College Station, Texas 77840

J.M. BENSON (273), Department of Environmental Toxicology, University of California, Davis, Davis, California 95616

JAMES P. BLAISDELL, USDA Forest Service, Intermtn. Forest and Range Experimental Station, Ogden, Utah 84403

J.T. BLAKE, Animal, Dairy, and Veterinary Sciences, Utah State University —UMC 56, Logan, Utah 84322

CHARLES H. BRIDGES, Texas Agricultural Experiment Station, College of Veterinary Medicine, Texas A & M University, College Station, Texas 77840

GARY W. BRIDGES, Veterinary Phys. and Pharm., College of Veterinary Medicine, Texas A & M University, College Station, Texas 77840

DENNIS BROWN (409), Poisonous Plant Research Laboratory, Agricultural Research Service, USDA, Logan, Utah 84321

DONALD R. BUHLER, Department of Agricultural Chemistry, Oregon State University, Corvallis, Oregon 97331

J.W. CALL (587), Animal, Dairy, and Veterinary Sciences, Utah State University—UMC 56, Logan, Utah 84322

JAMES R. CARLSON (251, 261), Department of Animal Science, Washington State University, Pullman, Washington 99163

ARTHUR A. CASE, College of Veterinary Medicine, Department of Veterinary Medicine and Surgery, University of Missouri–Columbia, Columbia, Missouri 65201

PETER CHEEKE, Department of Animal Science, Oregon State University, Corvallis, Oregon 97331

P.A. COCKRUM (565), CSIRO, Animal Health Research Laboratory, Private Bag, Parkville, Victoria 3052, Australia

ERIC E. CONN (301), Department of Biochemistry and Biophysics, University of California, Davis, California 95616

D.R. CORDY (327), Department of Pathology, School of Veterinary Medicine, University of California, Davis, California 95616

R.I. COX (451), Ian Clunies Ross Animal Research Laboratory, Prospect, CSIRO Division of Animal Production, Blacktown NSW 2148, Australia

E.H. CRONIN (521), Poisonous Plant Research Laboratory, Agricultural Research Service, USDA, Logan, Utah 84321

M. WARD CROWE (419), Department of Veterinary Science, University of Kentucky, Lexington, Kentucky 40504

C.C.J. CULVENOR (189, 349, 565), CSIRO Division of Animal Health, PHI Parkville, Melbourne, Victoria 3052, Australia

EARL O. DICKINSON (251, 261), Department of Veterinary Science, University of Nebraska, Lincoln, Nebraska 68583

JOHN O. DICKINSON (201), College of Veterinary Medicine, Washington State University, Wagner Hall, Pullman, Washington 99164

ALAN R. DOSTER (311), Pathology Department, College of Veterinary Medicine, University of Georgia, Athens, Georgia 30602

EARL L. DRAKE, Department of Veterinary Science, University of Nevada, Reno, Nevada 89511

DON D. DWYER (13), Department of Range Science, Utah State University —UMC 52, Logan, Utah 84322

GARY R. EVANS, Soil Conservation Service, USDA, Washington, D.C. 20013

SELWYN L. EVERIST (47, 93), Consultant Botanist, 13 Sunset Avenue, Bongaree, Bribie Island, Queensland 4507, Australia

MURRAY E. FOWLER, College of Veterinary Medicine, University of California, Davis, California 95616

HARRY JAMES FOX, Bureau of Land Management, Division of Range, U.S. Department of the Interior, Washington, D.C. 20240

J.L. FRAHN (349, 565), CSIRO, Animal Health Research Laboratory, Private Bag, Parkville, Victoria 3052, Australia

JOHN E. GARST (311), Biochemistry Department, Vanderbilt University, Nashville, Tennessee 37232

ROBERT T. GEMMELL (229), Department of Anatomy, University of Queensland, St. Lucia, Brisbane, Queensland 4067, Australia

EDWIN R. GOODE, JR., Agricultural Research Service, USDA, Beltsville, Maryland 20705

W.J. HARTLEY (363, 391), Department of Veterinary Medicine, University of Sydney, Camden, NSW 2570, Australia

ERNEST HASKELL, Agricultural Research Service, USDA, Berkeley, California 94705

STEPHEN L. HATCH, Department of Animal and Range Science, New Mexico State University, Las Cruces, New Mexico 88001

TREVOR J. HEATH (229), Faculty of Veterinary Science, University of Queensland, St. Lucia, Brisbane, Queensland 4067, Australia

M.P. HEGARTY (575), CSIRO, Division of Tropical Crops and Pastures, Cunningham Laboratory, St. Lucia, Queensland 4067, Australia

WERNER HERZ (487), Department of Chemistry, Florida State University, Tallahassee, Florida 32306

A. HOLIAN (217), Department of Biochemistry and Biophysics, School of Medicine, University of Pennsylvania, Philadelphia, Pennsylvania 19174

S.K. HOLIAN (217), Department of Biochemistry and Biophysics, School of Medicine, University of Pennsylvania, Philadelphia, Pennsylvania 19174

P.T. HOOPER (161, 337), Arid Zone Research Institute, Alice Springs, NT 5750, Australia

J. HRDLICKA (241), Veterinary School, University of Queensland, St. Lucia, Brisbane, Queensland 4067, Australia

M.W. HULL (217), Veterinary Research Laboratory, Montana State University, Bozeman, Montana 59715

J.C. HURLEY (217), Department of Chemistry, Eastern Montana College, Billings, Montana 59101

G. WAYNE IVIE (475), Veterinary Toxicology and Entomology Research Laboratory, Agricultural Research Service, USDA, College Station, Texas 77840

M.V. JAGO (349), CSIRO, Animal Health Research Laboratory, Private Bag, Parkville, Victoria 3052, Australia

LYNN F. JAMES (3, 135, 139, 379, 465, 587), Poisonous Plant Research Laboratory, Agricultural Research Service, USDA, Logan, Utah 84321

P.W. JENNINGS (217), Department of Chemistry, Montana State University, Bozeman, Montana 59715

A. EARL JOHNSON (209, 273), Poisonous Plant Research Laboratory, Agricultural Research Service, USDA, Logan, Utah 84321

JOHN D. JONES, Agriculture Canada, Food Research Institute, Central Experimental Farm, Ottawa, Ontario K1A OC6, Canada

RICHARD F. KEELER (273, 397), Poisonous Plant Research Laboratory, Agricultural Research Service, USDA, Logan, Utah 84321

W.R. KELLY (293), Department of Veterinary Pathology, University of Queensland, St. Lucia, Brisbane, Queensland 4067, Australia

BRUCE W. KENNEDY, Nutrition and Avian Sciences Department, University of California, Davis, California 95616

ROBERT R. KING (201), College of Veterinary Medicine, Washington State University, Pullman, Washington 99163

JOHN M. KINGSBURY (81), Plant Science Building, Cornell University, Ithaca, New York 14850

G.W. LANIGAN (349), CSIRO, Animal Health Research Laboratory, Private Bag, Parkville, Victoria 3052, Australia

J.S. LEE (241), School of Veterinary Medicine, University of South Korea, Suewon, South Korea

P. LEE (217), Department of Industrial Engineering, Montana State University, Bozeman, Montana 59715

H.W. LEIPOLD (429), Department of Pathology, College of Veterinary Medicine, Kansas State University, Manhattan, Kansas 66506

ROBERT D. LINNABARY (311), Pathology Department, Vanderbilt University, Nashville, Tennessee 37232

TRAVIS LITTLEDIKE, National Animal Disease Center, Agricultural Research Service, USDA, Ames, Iowa 50010

T. McEWAN (147), Department of Primary Industries, Animal Research Institute, Fairfield Road—Yeerongpilly, Brisbane, Queensland 4105, Australia

M.D. McGAVIN, Department of Pathobiology, College of Veterinary Medicine, University of Tennessee, Knoxville, Tennessee 37901

WALTER MAJAK, Agriculture Canada, Range Research Station, Kamloops, British Columbia V2B 8A9, Canada

A.R. MATTOCKS (177), Medical Research Council Laboratories, Carshalton, Surrey SM5 4EF, England

GENE W. MILLER (35), Department of Biology, Utah State University, Logan, Utah 84322

RUSSELL J. MOLYNEUX, Western Regional Research Center, Agricultural Research Service, USDA, Albany, California 94710

P.H. MORTIMER (353), Research Division, New Zealand Department of Agriculture, Ruakura Agricultural Research Center, Hamilton, New Zealand

DANIEL J. MUCHIRI, Agency of International Development, Veterinary Physiology and Pharmacology, Texas A & M University, College Station, Texas 77843

STEVEN S. NICHOLSON, Louisiana State University, Cooperative Extension Service and School of Veterinary Medicine, Baton Rouge, Louisiana 70815

D. B. NIELSEN (521), Poisonous Plant Research Laboratory, Agricultural Research Service, USDA, Logan, Utah 84321

FREDERICK W. OEHME (67), Comparative Toxicology Laboratory, Kansas State University, Manhattan, Kansas 66506

JOHN D. OLSEN (535), Poisonous Plant Research Laboratory, Agricultural Research Service, USDA, Logan, Utah 84321

ARLAND E. OLSON (35), Animal, Dairy, and Veterinary Sciences, Utah State University, Logan, Utah 84322

O.E. OLSON (121), Chemistry Department, South Dakota State University, Brookings, South Dakota 57006

R.J. PANCIERA (499, 555), Department of Pathology, College of Veterinary Medicine, Oklahoma State University, Stillwater, Oklahoma 74074

MICHAEL A. PASS (229), Faculty of Veterinary Science, University of Queensland, St. Lucia, Queensland 4067, Australia

HOWARD B. PETERSON (35), Department of Agriculture and Irrigation Engineering, Utah State University, Logan, Utah 84322

R.D. PLOWMAN, Agricultural Research Service, USDA, Utah State University—UMC 48, Logan, Utah 84322

J.A.S. PRIBANIC (217), Chemistry Department, Montana State University, Bozeman, Montana 59715

JOHN C. REAGER, Texas Veterinary Medical Diagnostic Laboratory, College Station, Texas 77840

S.K. REEDER (217), Sunkist Growers, Inc., Ontario, California 91761

GUY E. REYNOLDS, School of Veterinary Medicine, Oregon State University, Corvallis, Oregon 97331

R.W. RHEES (465), Zoology Department, Brigham Young University, Provo, Utah 84601

J.D. ROBBINS, Agricultural Research Service, USDA, Richard B. Russell Agricultural Research Center, Athens, Georgia 30605

J.E. ROBBINS (217), Chemistry Station, Montana State University, Bozeman, Montana 59715

JOSEPH L. SCHUSTER (23), Department of Range Science, Texas A & M University, College Station, Texas 77843

ALAN A. SEAWRIGHT (229, 241, 293), Veterinary School, University of Queensland, St. Lucia, Brisbane, Queensland 4067, Australia

H.J. SEGALL, Department of Physiological Sciences, School of Veterinary Medicine, University of California, Davis, California 95616

J.N. SEIBER (273), Department of Environmental Toxicology, University of California, Davis, California 95616

LLOYD A. SELBY (441), College of Veterinary Medicine, University of Missouri, Columbia, Missouri 65201

WARREN C. SHAW, Agricultural Research Service, USDA, Beltsville, Maryland 20705

J.L. SHUPE (35), Animal, Dairy, and Veterinary Sciences, Utah State University—UMC 48, Logan, Utah 84322

ROBERT SIMMONS, 521 North 7th East, Boise, Idaho 83702

C.S. SISODIA, W.C.V.M., University of Saskatchewan, Saskatoon, Saskatchewan S7N OWO, Canada

HARRY E. SMALLEY, Veterinary Toxicology and Entomology Research Laboratory, Agricultural Research Service, USDA, College Station, Texas 77840

L.W. SMITH (565), CSIRO, Animal Health Research Laboratory, Private Bag, Parkville, Victoria 3052, Australia

ROBERT E. STEGER, Texas Agricultural Extension Service, San Angelo, Texas 76901

FRANK R. STERMITZ (371), Department of Chemistry, Colorado State University, Ft. Collins, Colorado 60523

HARVEY L. TOOKEY (507), Northern Regional Research Laboratory, Agricultural Research Service, USDA, Peoria, Illinois 61604

CECIL H. VANETTEN (507), Northern Regional Research Laboratory, Agricultural Research Service, USDA, Peoria, Illinois 61604

KENT R. VAN KAMPEN (135, 465), Animal, Dairy, and Veterinary Sciences, Utah State University—UMC 48, Logan, Utah 84322

R.H. WASSERMAN (545), Department of Physical Biology, New York State College of Veterinary Medicine, Cornell University, Ithaca, New York 14853

J.H. WHITTEM (7, 57), Embassy of Australia, Washington, D.C. 20036

AGEE M. WIGGINS, School of Veterinary Medicine, Auburn University, Auburn, Alabama 36830

M. COBURN WILLIAMS (379), Poisonous Plant Research Laboratory, Agricultural Research Service, USDA, Logan, Utah 84321

BENJAMIN J. WILSON (311), Environmental Toxicology Center, School of Medicine, Vanderbilt University, Nashville, Tennessee 37215

DAVID G. WILSON, Bureau of Land Management (D-330), Denver Federal Center, Denver, Colorado 80225

GAROLD S. YOST (371), School of Pharmacy, University of California, San Francisco, California 94143

Preface

The effects of plants on livestock have been a concern since man became aware that some plants were poisonous. However, concerted effort to study these effects awaited organized application of the scientific method and, more particularly, development of certain physical and biological sciences. By the beginning of the twentieth century, studies were well underway in both the United States and Australia. Research in these two countries on the effects of poisonous plants on livestock has been in the forefront since that time. It has been stimulated by the nature of pastoral practices in the two countries, where much of the land has not been suited to uses other than livestock grazing. Research began with the identification of hazardous plants, and then progressed to studies of the gross and microscopic effects of the plants on animals and to studies on biochemical mechanisms of action once identification of toxins was achieved. Recently, efforts have centered on elucidation of structural, configurational, and conformational aspects of toxins using analogs and on more precise definition of pathologic effects. The driving force throughout has been the hope that one could utilize the body of knowledge to reduce morbidity and mortality of livestock in the field.

This volume is the outcome of a U.S.–Australian symposium on the effects of poisonous plants on domestic livestock. The symposium was held at Utah State University in Logan, Utah, on June 19–24, 1977. The material in each chapter was presented at the symposium generally by the senior author. In a few instances, the papers were read by a colleague, as noted in the table of contents. In addition to the contributions that make up the chapters of this volume, a number of movies and informal papers were presented at the symposium. They are not published here, but were significant contributions to the success of the symposium. They were the following:

Movies

Perennial Ryegrass Staggers, P. H. Mortimer
Phalaris Staggers, W. J. Hartley
Bermuda Grass Tremors, S. S. Nicholson
Cycad Poisoning, P. T. Hooper
Lathyrism in the Horse, M. E. Fowler
Yellow Wood Poisoning in Cattle and Sheep, A. A. Seawright
Pimelea Poisoning (St. George Disease), A. A. Seawright
Macrozamia Poisoning in Cattle, A. A. Seawright

Nigropallidal Encephalomalacia, M. E. Fowler
Taxus Poisoning in a Horse, J. M. Kingsbury
Birdsville Disease, P. T. Hooper
CNS Problems in a Horse, M. E. Fowler
Lantana Poisoning, A. A. Seawright
Locoweed Poisoning, L. F. James

Informal Papers

Poisoning by White Heads (*Sphenosciadium capitellatum*) in Horses and Cattle, M. E. Fowler

Predicting Timber Milkvetch Toxicity on Rangelands in British Columbia, W. Majak

A Possible Case of Phytotoxicity of Mediterranean People after Consumption of the European Migratory Quail, B. W. Kennedy

Research on the Toxicity of Endophytic Fungi of Pasture Grasses, J. D. Robbins

Rapid Isolation of Pyrrolizidine Alkaloids Derived from *Amsinckia intermedia* and *Senecio vulgaris*, H. J. Segall and C. W. Qualls

A Probe into the Toxicodynamics of Delphinine and Aconitine, C. S. Sisodia

Brief Note on "Bent Leg" in Lambs (*Trachymene* Poisoning) in Australia, A. A. Seawright

The responsibility for the scientific content of each chapter in this volume rests with the individual authors. Any opinions, findings, and conclusions or recommendations expressed in this publication are those of the authors and do not necessarily reflect the views of the National Science Foundation, the U.S. Department of Agriculture, the Australian Department of Science, or any other organization.

Acknowledgments

We express our appreciation to all individuals who directly contributed to the success of the symposium and this volume. Several individuals helped make the symposium a pleasant experience for participants. They include Utah State University President Glen L. Taggart, who welcomed the group to the University, Dr. Wayne Ringer and Ms. Nickie McCabe of the Conference and Institute Division of Utah State University, who provided local arrangements, and Dr. Edwin R. Goode, Jr., USDA, ARS, Washington, D.C., who helped set the stage for the week with appropriate introduction remarks. The editors express appreciation to the authors for the excellent contributions and timely cooperation in publication of this volume.

In coordinating arrangements between the two countries, Mr. Selwyn Everist served as Australian Coordinator, Dr. Lynn F. James as U.S. Coordinator, and Dr. J. H. Whittem, Scientific Attache, Australian Embassy, Washington, provided liaison between both groups and made initial contacts with the National Science Foundation and with the Australian Department of Science. The editors were aided as a local organizing committee with Dr. Lynn James as Chairman, by Dr. James L. Shupe of Utah State University and Dr. R. D. Plowman, Area Director of the Idaho–Montana–Utah Area of USDA-ARS.

Mr. Arthur Holmgren, Curator, and Ms. Leila Shultz, Assistant Curator, Intermountain Herbarium, graciously gave of their time to function as tour guides on a one-day tour of desert and mountain rangelands, providing registrants with a firsthand acquaintance with poisonous plants indigenous to the area.

Finally, this volume would not have been possible without the tireless help of Ms. Laverna Taylor, who typed each manuscript in its final form in a most expert and efficient way, as well as participating in proofing and correspondence, Ms. Norma Thorne, who typed much of the correspondence related to the volume and symposium, and Ms. Louise Dunning, who assisted with proofing, assembly of manuscripts, copy work, and mailings.

I. INTRODUCTORY REMARKS

Chairman: R. D. Plowman

OVERVIEW OF POISONOUS PLANT PROBLEMS IN THE UNITED STATES

Lynn F. James
Poisonous Plant Research Laboratory, Agricultural Research Service
U.S. Department of Agriculture

I. OVERVIEW

Poisonous plants are a principal cause of economic loss to the livestock industry in the western United States (1,2). The estimated loss amounts to 51 million dollars annually in the United States (3); of this, 23 million dollars is lost in the 11 western States (4). However, these figures are estimates because we have no good reporting system by which to substantiate them. These estimates were derived by use of a mortality figure of 3-5% annually (2), which has been accepted as being a good estimate by most people working in the area of poisonous plants, and I can accept this figure as representative for direct losses. However, in my opinion , these estimations fall short of the actual dollar loss because in evaluating losses, we tend to count animals that die and the obvious visible losses and leave out the more subtle losses such as effect on weight gains, management losses, and forage losses. In some years, these losses may surpass the more obvious losses in amount. The National Academy of Science calculates that 8.7% of the nutritionally sick animals in western United States were sick as a result of eating poisonous plants (5). This percentage is in addition to the 5% mortality loss but does not include many other associated losses. Unfortunately, notice is taken only of the large death losses that occur because of grazing certain plants such as halogeton, larkspur, lupine, and locoweed. Lesser death losses are often ignored because they are difficult to assess. The total impact of poisonous plants on the livestock economy is indeed difficult to estimate.

Many poisonous plants grow on our ranges and pastures, and their importance varies from year to year, depending on many factors. For example, the pattern of moisture or the amount of moisture received has a profound effect on the likelihood that a given poisonous plant will be a problem at a given time. If moisture comes in one pattern, the more palatable grasses or forage may be available before the poisonous plant is available, and critical amounts of poisonous plants are not grazed. If moisture comes in a different pattern or there is a lack of moisture, poisonous plants may become available first and appear more succulent, and large amounts may be grazed. Another difficulty is that of determining the cause of death and of recognizing the many other effects on livestock of poisonous plants.

Direct losses from poisonous plants--death, chronic illness and debilitation, photosensitization, abortions, and birth defects, to enumerate a few--are difficult in themselves to assess; but even more difficult to enumerate are many significant indirect losses resulting from increased costs and problems in grazing ranges and pastures infested with poisonous plants. These indirect costs and problems include fencing, decreased forage production and utilization, altered grazing programs, loss of forage, and in some instances, supplemental feeding programs. A true picture of the total impact of poisonous plants on the economy must include all these losses.

In addition to recognizing the losses due to poisonous plants, we should mention briefly some of the causes for these losses. Overgrazing of pastures and ranges is probably the greatest factor in causing losses from poisonous plants. The rangelands are located in the regions of the United States of lower precipitation and are subjected to periodic droughts. These drought periods favor the growth of many of the poisonous plants and decrease production of the more desirable plants. Decreased production leads to increased poisonous plant problems during these periods.

Under certain conditions, poor management can become a prominent factor in livestock poisoning. These conditions usually involve trailing, trucking, herding procedures, watering, or salting of animals.

Lack of education or awareness of livestockmen, range managers, and those who administer State and Federal rangelands is an important factor in livestock poisoning. Livestockmen especially must be aware of the potential poisonous plant problems on their ranges and pastures and have some knowledge of how to cope with them from a managerial point of view.

The economic losses of livestock due to poisonous plants is serious. Many of these losses are preventable. Approximately 75% of the land area of the western United States is rangeland. The forage on range areas can best be used by ruminant animals; i.e., sheep, cattle, and some wildlife. The least energy-dependent means of producing red meat is through foraging native range plants that require little fossil fuel production costs, and the forage resource is renewed each year without tillage, fertilization, or mechanical harvesting. Because grazing rangelands provides a most efficient means of converting solar energy into chemical energy (food), we must use this resource wisely. Poisonous plants are a serious impediment to the wise use of grazing lands in the United States and the world.

Poisonous plants are a principal cause of economic loss to the livestock industry in western United States. Although various estimates of the amount of these losses have been made, it is highly unlikely that their true dollar value is understood. The difficulty in arriving at a good estimate is due to the many and varied effects of poisonous plants on livestock along with attendant losses.

II. REFERENCES

1. Marsh, H., "Newson's Sheep Diseases," 2nd Ed., p. 342. Williams & Wilkens Co., Baltimore, Maryland, 1958.
2. Stoddart, L. A., and Smith A. D., "Range Management," 1st Ed., pp. 430-473. McGraw Hill Book Co., New York, 1943.
3. Keeler, R. F., "Toxins and Teratogens of the Lily and Nightshade Families," Society of Economics and Botany Symposium on Poisonous Plants, Miami, Florida, June 12, 1977.
4. Schmitz, E. M., Freeman, B. N., and Reed, R. E., "Livestock Poisoning Plants of Arizona," p. 6. University of Arizona Press, 1968.
5. Anonymous, "Prenatal and Postnatal Mortality in Cattle," p. 58. National Academy of Science Publication 1685, 1968.

POISONOUS PLANT PROBLEMS IN AUSTRALIA

J. H. Whittem
Embassy of Australia

I. OVERVIEW

In the early stages of planning the program for this conference, it seemed to some of us that it would be useful to set the stage for the week's proceedings by presentation of general papers on the economic importance and epidemiology of intoxication of plant origin in the U.S.A. and in Australia. Then we came around to the view that anything so general would be superfluous, even perhaps insulting, to this audience of specialists, which should not need to be reminded of the economic justification for its work. The pendulum had swung back a little, though, by the time the program was finalized, and I found myself committed to present a short overview of the Australian scene.

Everist, in the opening sentence of his very fine book (1), said:

> "No published estimates are available of the effects of plant poisoning on livestock industries of Australia but the aggregate of losses from this cause must run into millions of dollars each year."

In Australia no serious attempt has been made by local, state or federal authorities to collect the raw data for morbidity or mortality studies. In modern Australia this is a job for the new epidemiological service of the Australian Bureau of Animal Health, utilizing computer techniques.

The difficulties of collecting reliable data on plant poisoning, at least in Australia, are many, and I mention the more important of them here in the hope of eliciting American comment and experience. In this area, the concept of "garbage in, garbage out" applies to electronic data storage to a very great extent due to the innate uncertainties in the input.

In the first place, mortalities due to plant poisoning usually occur in more remote pastoral situations. Then, timely and efficient autopsies are seldom performed, unless there is a particular and active interest on the part of field workers in the affected area and research workers or pathologists at the regional diagnostic or research laboratory.

Further to complicate the problem, many intoxications produce no pathognomonic lesions or recognizable biochemical changes, and many plant genera and species contain similar or identical toxic principles.

Again, diagnosis may be hampered by the time-consuming techniques required for identification of plant fragments in the alimentary canal, or worse, a diagnosis may not be reached due to non-application of these procedures.

Feeding trials to confirm suspicion of plant poisoning are seldom carried out due to lack of interest or opportunity, or lack of suitable (i.e. toxic) plant material in sufficient quantity.

Finally, appropriate internationally recognized codes for machine recording of poisoning by the many Australian poisonous plant species would have to be devised and adopted.

Nevertheless, I believe that the Australian Bureau of Animal Health should be encouraged to expand its area of interest to include collection and publication of data relating to morbidity and mortality from poisonous plants, and the most effective ways and means of so doing constitute a legitimate, modern area of research.

However, in spite of the absence of exact epidemiological information and lack of economic assessment of the consequences of plant poisoning in Australia, there has been much interest in the subject at both the research and publication level for more than half a century. The phytotoxicologists's bookshelf contains Chippendale and Murray (2), Everist (*loc cit*), Gardner and Bennetts (3), and Hurst (4) as general references, and Bull, Culvenor, and Dick (5) as a special volume. His reprint collection contains papers by virtually all the great Australian veterinary pathologists, and by many of the better known veterinary administrators and academics.

What is the anatomy of this research effort, and what led to Australian excellence in the area? Historically, scientific interest in poisonous plants has followed expansion of pastoral or grazing interests in the "inland" in Australia as it followed them in the "West" in the U.S.A. with the objective of providing a basis of knowledge to improve the empirical procedures developed by managers, shepherds, cowboys and stockmen in the pre-scientific days. The probable truth that the consequent research has tended to provide more Ph.D. theses than practical solutions to herdsmen's problems is irrelevant at this point of the discussion though perhaps worth some consideration at a later stage of the meeting when we examine our research objectives.

Thus, early research tended to be local in origin, carried out regionally at State Agricultural Experiment Stations, or their Australian equivalent and at government and academic veterinary research laboratories. Much Australian work on Birdsville Disease (6), Kimberley Horse Disease (7), Georgina River Poisoning (8), *Gastrolobium* Poisoning (9) and Lupinosis (10), falls into this category.

Sometimes a disease syndrome was perceived to be of wider extent or greater importance, or multifocal in distribution, and so came to be regarded as a national problem. Then a committee might be set up to consider the evidence, examine the results and to stimulate and finance further research. One such Australian case was "toxemic jaundice" - an enzootic syndrome in sheep on the riverine plain of the inland southeast of New South Wales and Victoria. After many years of painstaking observations and experiments the syndrome was shown to be compounded of chronic copper poisoning and pyrrolizidine alkaloidosis due to ingestion of *Heliotropium europeum* - a free seeding weed which provides virtually the only green growth after summer rainstorms in this predominantly winter rainfall area (11).

There is no doubt that the formation of the "Toxemic Jaundice Committee," comprising senior officers of CSIRO Division of Animal Health and the New South Wales Department of Agriculture, produced a significant acceleration in solution of the field problem, and also led directly to international studies of pyrrolizidine alkaloidosis which are still progressing a quarter of a century later.

I will conclude this overview by drawing your attention to the broad outlines of recent and current Australian research topics, but will reserve until a later more philosophic paper, my own comments on how some of these came to be chosen, or funded, or even fashionable.

Quick perusal of issues of the Australian Veterinary Journal over the last few years reveals papers dealing with the following genera of poisonous plants; *Pimelea* (12-15), *Macrozamia* (16), *Pennisetum* (17), *Solanum* (18), *Cupressus* (19), *Xanthorrhoea* (20), *Leucaena* (21), *Lolium* (22), *Swainsona* (23), *Trachymene* (24), and *Wedelia* (25).

This list includes native herbage, shrubs and trees as well as "improved" or introduced grasses and shrubs. These papers deal with the problems of plant poisoning at all levels from "letters to the editor" speculating on phytotoxins responsible for bony dystrophies or congenital defects in lambs to research papers dealing with the chemical structure of the toxin of *Pimelea*.

Indeed, at this meeting, the Australian workers will present papers dealing with a number of plant genera including *Lantana, Myoporum, Pimelea, Cycas, Lolium, Swainsona, Phalaris, Trachemene, and Lupinus;* while more general topics will include pyrrolizidine alkaloidosis, phytoestrogens, comparative neuropathology, and taxonomic aspects of toxigenicity.

So we have some fascinating and important problems in Australia and I hope that I have whetted your appetites for a week of good scientific presentations in this stimulating atmosphere in the intermountain zone where so many other phytotoxins abound, and where the Australian contributors have much to see and learn that will be novel and useful to them.

II. REFERENCES

1. Everist, S. L., "Poisonous Plants of Australia," Angus and Robertson, Sydney, 1974.
2. Chippendale, G. C., and Murray, R. M., "Poisonous Plants of the Northern Territory," Northern Territory Administration, 1963.
3. Gardner, C. A., and Bennetts, H. W., "The Toxic Plants of Western Australia," Western Australian Newspapers Ltd., Perth, 1956.

4. Hurst, E., "The Poison Plants of New South Wales," New South Wales Poison Plants Committee, Sydney, 1942.
5. Bull, L. B., Culvenor, C. C. J., and Dick, A. T., "The Pyrrolizidine Alkaloids," North Holland Publishing Co., Amsterdam, 1968.
6. Rose, A. L., Banks, A. W., and McConnell, J. D., *Aust. Vet. J.* 27, 189 (1951).
7. Rose, A. L., Gardner, C. A., McConnell, J. D., and Bull, L. B. *Aust. Vet. J.* 33, 25 (1957).
8. Whittem, J. H., and Murray, L. R., *Aust. Vet. J.* 39, 168 (1963).
9. McEwan, T., *Queensl. J. Agric. Sci.* 21, 11 (1964).
10. Gardiner, R. M., "Advances in Veterinary Science," Vol. 11, p. 85. Academic Press, New York, 1967.
11. Bull, L. B., Dick, A. T., Keast, J. C., and Edgar, G., *Aust. J. Agric. Res.* 7, 281 (1956).
12. McClure, T. J., and Farrow, B. R., *Aust. Vet. J.* 47, 100 (1971).
13. Clark, I. A., *Aust. Vet. J.* 47, 123 (1971).
14. Roberts, H. B., and Healy, P. J., *Aust. Vet. J.* 47, 123 (1971).
15. Roberts, H. B., McClure, T. J., Ritchie, E., Taylor, W. C., and Freeman, P. W., *Aust. Vet. J.* 51, 325 (1975).
16. Gabbedy, B. J., Meyer, E. P., and Dickson, J., *Aust. Vet. J.* 51, 303 (1975).
17. Gabbedy, B. J., Gwynn, R., Hopkinson, W. I., Kay, B. E., and Wood, P. M., *Aust. Vet. J.* 50, 369 (1974).
18. McMenimon, N. P., *Aust. Vet. J.* 52, 432 (1976).
19. Mason, R. W., *Aust. Vet. J.* 50, 419 (1974).
20. Munday, B. L., Mason, R. W., and Hartley, W. J., *Aust. Vet. J.* 52, 92 (1976).
21. Falvey, L., *Aust. Vet. J.* 52, 243 (1976).
22. Berry, P. H., and Wise, J. L., *Aust. Vet. J.* 51, 525 (1975).
23. Hartley, W. J., and Gibson, A. J., *Aust. Vet. J.* 47, 300 (1971).
24. Clark, L., Carlisle, C. H., and Beasley, P. S., *Aust. Vet. J.* 51, 4 (1975).
25. Oelrichs, P. B., and Muller, W. A., *Toxicon* 10, 63 (1972).

II. GENERAL TOPICS

Chairman: C. C. J. Culvenor

IMPACT OF POISONOUS PLANTS ON WESTERN U.S. GRAZING SYSTEMS AND LIVESTOCK OPERATIONS

by
Don D. Dwyer
Range Science Department, Utah State University

I. ABSTRACT

The history of range livestock production is replete with documentation of animals lost to poisonous plants. Death loss is easy to measure. The insidious economic losses of physical malformations, abortions, and simply reduced growth and production from otherwise healthy animals is not so easy to quantify. Today, more than a century since the first published reports of livestock losses from plant poisoning, ranchers are little better off than they were then as far as management recommendations to deal with poisonous plants on rangelands. The many complex physiological interactions occurring between the poisonous plants and the animals that graze them make it a very difficult problem to understand, except that animals die, get very sick, abort, or produce obviously deformed offspring as a result of consuming poisonous plants. Researchers must seek more answers to basic questions regarding the synergism that exists among the animal, the poisonous plant, and the environmental conditions surrounding the two. This research should include studies on aspects of animal behavior and how it relates to plant selection during grazing.

II. INTRODUCTION

Toxic plants have had a detrimental effect on range livestock since before 1850, when livestock production became a business enterprise (1). Losses exceeding a hundred animals on a single occasion have been documented. In Texas, a man named Kendall wrote to his friend Randall in 1860 (2) saying:

> "You may have heard that Shaeffer (R. W. Shaeffer, who established the famous Shaeffer Ranch in Jim Wells County) had extremely bad luck with his last inportation of sheep; he left some 120 head down by Yorktown, and in a few days some 70 died--poisoned outright by eating some weed, or else pannicked (sic) to death by drinking bad water... A man named Chase, with some 80 odd fine bucks from Vermont, lost 60 near the same place a month before."

Kendall also noted that "two young men from Vermont, Fisk and Chase, arrived... with 104 fine merino bucks; they halted near Goliad to rest and recruit the animals; the latter got hold of some kind of poison wild pea or bean vines and 70 died in a week"

(2). These references point out that one of the very earliest problems in grazing livestock was poisonous plants. At that time the ranchers were unsure which plant or plants were the cause, much less their names.

Even today, more than a century later, untold economic losses occur each year through death, physical malformations, abortions, photosensitization, and simply, reduced growth and production in grazing animals. In 1968 nearly 9% of the nutritionally sick animals in the western United States were sick because they had consumed poisonous plants (3). It is impossible to assign a precise economic value to these losses for the rancher, the livestock industry, or the consumer. Few knowledgeable persons, though, would dispute that it is a large figure.

The direct waste through animal death can often be significantly reduced by careful management, but very probably death is the smallest component of the total value. The insidious losses of reduced weight gain, abortion, and general unthriftiness have perhaps the greatest economic impact and these are very difficult to identify, much less correct.

III. KINDS OF LIVESTOCK OPERATIONS IN THE WEST

Generally speaking the 11 western states have three kinds of range livestock enterprises - cow-calf, ewe-lamb, and cow-calf and ewe-lamb combined. Some cow-calf operators may retain yearlings for later sale if market and forage conditions are favorable to do so. All of these ranching operations depend primarily on native forages for feed for the animals. In north latitudes where snow cover prevents grazing, hay is fed for as much as four to five months but most ranchers depend on rangelands from 11 to 12 months for feed for their livestock.

Often livestock will graze on different kinds of ranges during the year. For example in Utah and Nevada, sheep will graze on sagebrush-grass foothill range in the spring, on high elevation mountain range in the summer, on sagebrush-grass range again in the fall, and in the winter they will graze on desert saltbush range (4). Cattle can be managed similarly, being moved from one kind of range to another. In the southwestern United States, livestock often graze the same range year-round. When livestock spend so much of their time on open range, the chance of encountering poisonous plants is greatly enhanced.

IV. GENERAL CHARACTERISTICS OF WESTERN RANGELANDS

Typically rangelands of the western United States are characterized by rough topography, low and erratic precipitation, and poorly developed soils (5). The amount of grazeable forage produced for livestock is almost always low by agronomic standards usually requiring 2 to 8 hectares per animal unit month of grazing. Some ranges produce so little forage that 12 hectares per animal unit month of grazing are needed (5).

The areas grazed are very extensive. Fenced pastures as large as 2000 hectares are not unusual, with distances to water of up to 10 km. On less arid ranges these extremes would be reduced somewhat. Still, the physical conditions under which range livestock production is carried out in the western United States are rather harsh, and they contribute to the problems associated with plant poisoning.

Further complicating range livestock operations is the complex pattern of land ownership in the West. Nearly half of the western 11 states is publicly owned and managed by federal agencies. In Utah, for example, 66% of the area is public land most of which is managed by the Forest Service and the Bureau of Land Management (5). In addition there is land owned by the state of Utah leaving less than 30% in private ownership. This, of course, means that plans for ranch operation and management must be coordinated and planned with as many as three other landlords, each having sets of rules and regulations they are required to follow.

V. IMPACT OF POISONOUS PLANTS ON RANGE LIVESTOCK PRODUCTION AND MANAGEMENT

The forage on arid and semi-arid rangelands is the major agricultural crop they produce. This forage is shared among the various herbivores grazing the range, but primarily among the cattle, sheep, and wild ungulates. Despite the need for all the forage possible, many ranges cannot be properly and fully utilized because poisonous plants grow on them (6). Their mere presence often prevents implementation of grazing programs by a livestock operator.

In view of the large numbers of poisonous plant species that occur in the United States (7), those identified as really troublesome on western rangelands are relatively few. James and Johnson (6) discussed or mentioned 36 species in their work treating major plant toxicities of the western United States. The classic range management text (5) lists 38. These lists can be further reduced when attention is focused on a specific ranch unit. In this case only rarely would more than four or five plant species dangerous to livestock be found.

For the western United States, the major poisonous plants causing the greatest direct affect on the range livestock industry can be included in the following genera:

Common name	Genus	Susceptible animal (5)
Bitterweed and Rubberweed	*Actinea*	Sheep
Death camas	*Zygadenus*	All, especially sheep
Halogeton	*Halogeton*	All, mostly sheep
Larkspur	*Delphinium*	Cattle
Loco	*Astragalus*	All

Common name	Genus	Susceptible animal (5)
Lupine	*Lupinus*	Sheep
Milkweed	*Asclepias*	All, mostly sheep

This is a rather small list and it is recognized that some might quarrel with it, choosing to add a genus or two but still the list would not be large regardless of who might develop it. For a given ranch, however, it does not matter that the list of important poisonous plant genera is short or long, since it requires relatively few plants of only one species to do a great deal of economic damage.

Sagebrush (*Artemisia*) and juniper (*Juniperus*) are generally not considered serious poisonous plant problems, yet Johnson *et al.* (8) found that when sheep were fed 3/4 lb of big sagebrush for 1, 2, or 3 days it could be lethal. Evidence also was accumulated that juniper caused abortion in sheep. These kinds of data give reason to suspect that certain plant species rather than the obvious ones in the list above are contributing to unexplained death loss, low birth rates, and reduced weight gains on range livestock.

Past research on the obvious offenders has helped the rancher better cope with certain poisonous plant problems (9,10,11). There is little doubt that cases where several hundred sheep are killed at one time from grazing a poisonous plant will be rare events in the future. But for the range livestock producer to avoid such losses often entails considerable economic cost. Most death losses from poisonous plants can be minimized only through preventive measures and these measures often cost money.

Generally, removing poisonous plants does not increase forage production. Consequently, the extent of livestock loss dictates how much money is expendable for controlling toxic plants. Few antidotes to plant toxins are available, but most losses can be prevented with the following management practices (6,12):

- Make sure that animals have an adequate supply of good-quality feed. Most poisonous plants are relatively unpalatable, so animals seldom consume enough to cause poisoning, except when they are hungry. They may need supplemental feed in the early spring, when the quality of native grass is low, to keep them from consuming evergreen or early-growing poisonous plants.
- Provide livestock with an adequate supply of salt and minerals at all times. Animals on deprived diets may seek out poisonous plants with high salt or high phosphorus content.
- Feed animals before placing them on a range containing poisonous plants. This applies to animals being trailed, after hauling, or being worked. Avoid trailing hungry animals through or holding animals on dense stands of poisonous plants.
- Do not move livestock to fresh pasture where poisonous plants are growing abundantly. Livestock may be poisoned when grazing unfamiliar range, even though animals accustomed to the area are not poisoned.
- Remove animals from pastures that are treated with herbicides to control the poisonous species or other noxious plants.

Some plants become more palatable and/or more poisonous after treatment with herbicides.

• Put livestock on pastures at the proper season, when the desirable plants are at the proper stage of growth, not when poisonous plants are most dangerous. Fencing may be necessary to keep livestock off areas infested with poisonous plants during critical periods, or the plants may need to be removed from some pastures.

• Prevent the introduction of noxious plants. Before putting strange animals into an area, hold them in dry-lot for 24 hours or longer to permit foreign seeds to pass through the animal.

It must be recognized the above seven "rules" have evolved with experience that has accumulated since the first livestock were poisoned by plants. Some points are obvious. Others are unproven scientifically but intuitively are logical. These management rules have been quoted in the literature in some form or fashion since the first ones appeared in the classic publication of C. D. Marsh, "Stock Poisoning Plants of the Range" in 1919 (13).

The following examples will illustrate how ranch management and operation is affected by the presence of poisonous plants.

A. Kind and Class of Livestock

Sheep are more susceptible than cattle to certain poisonous plant species and vice versa (5). This means there are certain ranges in the western United States that can be grazed only by sheep or only by cattle because of the poisonous plant species they contain; or grazing time has to be adjusted so as to avoid the period of danger.

Since sheep are largely managed by herders, if the herders are aware of the poisonous plants on the range, the sheep can be guided to avoid the poisonous plants. Cattle are rarely herded and thus cannot be directed away from poisonous plants except at the extra cost of herding.

B. Seasonal vs Year-long Grazing

Much of the 11 western states is grazed on a seasonal basis as contrasted to grazing the full year on the same range. This means the livestock are either hauled by truck or trailed from one range to another. Livestock graze differently on a new range, frequently selecting plants they normally would not (14). Poisonous plants are often included in the new diet of the transported animals. To reduce this possibility, the livestock must be fed hay in drylot so they are not hungry when turned onto the range. Hungry animals are more apt than full ones to graze poisonous plants. On range grazed year-long this radical change in diet does not occur. The diet changes slowly as natural seasonal variations progress.

C. Low Quantity and Quality of Natural Forage

Poisonous plants have a serious impact on livestock operations when forage quantity and quality are limiting. During periods of drought, prolonged over-grazing, or years of excessive grazing utilization, animals are more susceptible to plant poisoning because desirable forage is insufficient. Livestock tend to graze more poisonous plants under these conditions than when there is adequate desirable forage (15).

Poisonous plants such as larkspur (16) undergo early spring growth ahead of the main forage species. Animals that have consumed dry range forage or hay all winter often choose to graze the green, succulent poisonous plants in the spring. This is probably a result of the low nutritional status of the animal at the time.

D. Large Pastures

Except for closely herded flocks of sheep, livestock graze over extensive areas of range. Free roaming cattle are not seen frequently by the rancher. The large grazing areas comprise a variety of vegetative types and conditions which often provide good habitats for poisonous plants. It is quite possible for animals to be killed or seriously debilitated by poisonous plants and the owner not be aware of the problem. When the situation is discovered the evidence of the cause may be gone and some other factor given as the cause of the difficulty.

E. Land Ownership

There are conditions when the offending poisonous plants could be economically controlled with herbicide but the fact the land is not owned by the operator prevents the treatment. The complicated land ownership pattern and the regulations restricting use of chemicals on public rangeland often prohibit the rancher from controlling the population of poisonous plants when all other conditions make it possible to do so.

Grazing poisonous plants can occasionally be avoided by utilizing a rotation system of grazing to prevent animals from being in the pasture containing the poisonous plants when they are dangerous. However, such a grazing system might not be possible to implement since regulations often preclude the additional fencing that would be required of the system on public lands.

VI. POISONOUS PLANTS: CONFUSION AND FRUSTRATION

For the range livestock producer there is much confusion and frustration associated with managing livestock operations with poisonous plant problems. Symptoms of poisoning, while well-defined for many plant species in the laboratory under forced feeding conditions, do not usually follow the classic description under range conditions (12). Some poisonous plants can be grazed without any trouble most of the time but be extremely toxic at certain times. Poisoning may occur on lush pastures at one time and under drought at another. Several species of poisonous plants may have the same or a very similar poisonous principle and thus cause similar symptoms. A single species can be poisonous in several ways, so that the symptoms vary, depending on the toxic ingredient most active at the particular time.

Livestock losses from poisonous plants are related commonly to poor livestock management or low range condition, though exceptions to this are very frequent. Some poisonous plants are considered unpalatable yet under defined conditions they may be grazed with relish.

From an ecological point of view the relation of kinds and amounts of poisonous plants varies with the grazing history of the particular land area. As range condition declines, poisonous plants increase, and thus the incidence of animal poisonings is augmented. Except for a few poisonous plants that have been introduced, halogeton being a good example (17), most poisonous plants are native to western ecosystems. They respond to overgrazing by increasing in abundance making them more available to the animals. Since plant poisonings have been more common on poor condition rangeland than on good or excellent rangelands, one assumes that animals do not prefer to graze poisonous plants when given choices that include adequate palatable grass. For the most part this is true, but it is substantiated largely by intuition and deductive reasoning.

Much poisonous plant research is not reproducible in the field because the symptoms and lethal dose were determined mostly by force feeding animals in confinement. It is virtually impossible to duplicate the vast array of diet combinations possible when a free ranging animal is given access to 30 or 40 plant species which include perhaps two or three species of poisonous plants. Nutritional status and age of the grazing animal together with synergistic effects of plants grazed, no doubt, add to the endless confusion surrounding plant poisonings under range conditions.

VII. INFORMATION NEEDED ON POISONOUS PLANTS AS RELATED TO RANGE LIVESTOCK PRODUCTION

There is much we need to know about poisonous plants and their impact on the man-animal-plant system in order to produce livestock on rangelands effectively and efficiently. We are long past the time we can pass off poisonous plants as a symptom of an overgrazed range. Livestock producers require more information to deal with poisonous plant problems than six or eight "management rules" to avoid poisoning. These rules have had value historically when the best rule to follow was to keep the animals away from poisonous plants or to try to prevent the livestock from eating them when they were hungry enough to do so.

The problems now are far more subtle than outright death and its prevention, since most poisonous plants have been identified and their period of danger established. But the questions of abortion, malformed offspring, and general unthrifty conditions of otherwise healthy livestock are not so easily handled. These questions have to do with the effects of various combinations of plants consumed during specific nutritional conditions of the animals. They are related to why healthy livestock choose to eat plants that do them harm, even kill them, and to the animal behavioral mechanisms associated with plant selection. Information is essential that will tell us <u>why</u> animals graze the plants they graze. In this answer may lie the solution to preventing them from selecting plants that injure or kill them.

The many complex physiological interactions occurring between the plants and the animals that graze them make it very difficult to know much very specific except for the obvious effects of plant poisoning; that is to say, that animals die, get very sick, or produce obviously deformed offspring as a result of consuming toxic plants. Much of the research the past three or four decades has been spent identifying plants that are poisonous to livestock, defining the poisonous principles, establishing the period of toxicity, and describing symptoms of poisoning.

It is time for scientists to develop some creative approaches to poisonous plant research. Studies are needed of the interactions involved among the plants making up the diet of grazing animals, and between those plant combinations and the animals themselves. James *et al.* (18), for example, found interactions between *Halogeton glomeratus* consumption and water consumption by sheep; the studies indicated that when thirsty sheep are permitted to drink, ingestion of *Halogeton* increases dramatically thus resulting in poisoning. By having knowledge of this kind of interaction, the livestock producer has management options other than simply avoiding *Halogeton* infested areas with his sheep.

The main recommendation forthcoming after more than three decades of poisonous plant research is the same as it was at the beginning--manage to keep the animals from consuming the offending plants. Poisonous plants are too numerous and widespread to eliminate, so further research must show the livestock producer how to better live with them and describe the conditions under which the least damage is done.

In summary, virtually every aspect of livestock production under range conditions is impacted by poisonous plants. Research has not provided many solutions to the real world problems of managing range livestock on a range with poisonous plants, outside of those recommendations given by Marsh in 1919 (13). We do know more about how and why an animal died and that insidious losses exist and will continue. Researchers must seek more answers to basic questions regarding the synergism that exists among the animal, the poisonous plant, and the environmental conditions surrounding the two. This research should include studies on aspects of animal behavior and how this relates to plant selection during grazing.

VIII. REFERENCES

1. Pammel, L. H., "A Manual of Poisonous Plants," The Torch Press, Cedar Rapids, Iowa, 1911.
2. Brown, H. J. (Ed.), "Letters from a Texas Sheep Ranch," University of Illinois Press, Urbana, 1959.
3. National Academy of Science, "Prenatal and Postnatal Mortality in Cattle," *Nat. Acad. Sci. Publ. No.* 1685, Wash., D.C., 1968.
4. Cook, C. W., "Development and Use of Foothill Ranges in Utah," *Utah Agric. Exp. Stn. Bull.* 461, 1966.
5. Stoddart, L. A., Smith, A. D., and Box, T. W., "Range Management," McGraw-Hill, New York, 1975.
6. James, L. F., and Johnson, A. E., *J. Range Manage.* 29, 356-363 (1976).
7. Kingsbury, J. M., "Poisonous Plants of the United States and Canada," Prentice-Hall, Inc., Englewood Cliffs, N. J., 1964.
8. Johnson, A. E., James, L. F., and Spillett, J., *J. Range Manage.* 29, 278-285 (1976).
9. Binns, W., James, L. F., and Johnson, A. E., *J. Range Manage.* 24, 110-113 (1971).
10. Cronin, E. H., Nielsen, D. B., and Madsen, N. *J. Range Manage.* 29, 364-367 (1976).
11. James, L. F., and Cronin, E. H., *J. Range Manage.* 27, 424-426 (1974).
12. Herbel, C. H., Steger, R., and Gould, W. L., "Managing Semidesert Ranges of the Southwest," *N. M. State Coop. Ext. Circ.* 456, 1974.
13. Marsh, C. D., "Stock-Poisoning Plants of the Range," *USDA Bull.* 575, U.S. Government Printing Office, Wash, D.C., 1919.
14. Schmutz, E. M., Freeman, B. N., and Reed, R. E., "Livestock-Poisoning Plants of Arizona," University of Arizona Press, Tucson, Arizona, 1968.
15. Sperry, O. E., Dollahite, J. W., Morrow, J., and Hoffman, G. O. "Texas Range Plants Poisonous to Livestock," *Tex. Agric. Exp. Stn. Bull.* 796, 1955.
16. Cronin. E. H., *J. Range Manage.* 24, 258-263 (1971).
17. Frischknecht, N. C., *J. Range Manage.* 21, 8-12 (1968).
18. James, L. F., Butcher, J. E., and Van Kampen, K. R., *J. Range Manage.* 23, 123-127 (1970).

POISONOUS PLANT MANAGEMENT PROBLEMS AND CONTROL MEASURES ON U.S. RANGELANDS

Joseph L. Schuster
Texas A&M University

I. ABSTRACT

Poisonous plants create significant management problems on U.S. rangelands. Their presence, even in small amounts can require changes in grazing management, livestock handling and range improvement practices. Grazing management aimed at preventing poisoning has as its objectives reduction of toxic species populations and improvement of desirable vegetation. Guidelines for reducing livestock losses to poisonous plants include: know the plants and their toxic principles; through good range management maintain range in condition least conducive to high poisonous plant populations; practice proper mineral and nutrient supplementation; avoid grazing areas where poisonous plants are abundant; use livestock not poisoned by plants present; avoid turning hungry animals onto ranges containing poisonous plants; and control poisonous plant populations when feasible. Chemical, mechanical, and other control methods are available for most poisonous species.

II. INTRODUCTION

The economic impact of livestock poisoning by plants in the United States is enormous. Monetary losses from plant poisoning were estimated to be over $17 million for cattle and $6 million for sheep annually during the 1951-60 period by the Agricultural Research Service (1). It is estimated that poisonous plants kill from 3 to 5 percent of the cattle, sheep and horses on western ranges (2). These estimates are for death losses and do not include losses due to reduced reproduction, lack of weight gain, and birth defects. It has been estimated that 8.7 percent of the nutritionally sick animals in western United States are sick as a result of eating poisonous plants (3). In dollars and cents, the losses in reproduction and gain of animals that are poisoned but not killed probably exceed the death loss (4). Estimates of economic loss from poisonous plants should also include cost associated with the problems related to the grazing management of ranges infested with poisonous plants. In Texas alone total losses have been estimated to be between 50 and 100 million dollars annually (5).

Poisonous plants constitute one of the most significant management problems on western and southwestern ranges. Kingsbury (6) in an extensive review of poisonous plants in the U.S. and

Canada reported on over 1,000 species that are toxic to livestock in some way. In the southwest, Sperry *et al.* (5) described 80 poisonous range species in Texas; Gay and Dwyer (4) listed 100 poisonous species for New Mexico; and Schmutz *et al.* (7) named 300 species as being poisonous in Arizona. Of the Arizona plants, 30 were believed to cause major livestock losses, 36 to be of secondary importance, and over 145 rarely problems on rangelands.

Poisonous plant problems are more prevalent in western than in eastern states. Livestock losses during settlement of the United States were also greatest in the western states because settlers recognized many of the eastern species as being poisonous and acted accordingly, but did not recognize some of the species that are poisonous in the west (6). Generally, poisonous plants are not overly abundant in climax vegetation, and good range management will minimize their threat (8). However, with few exceptions such as halogeton (*Halogeton glomeratus*), poison hemlock (*Conium maculatum*), and St. Johnswort (*Hypericum perforatum*), poisonous plants are native components of western range ecosystems. Some are of only limited distribution, but cause significant livestock losses where they occur. Others are widely distributed, but cause problems only where locally abundant.

III. MANAGEMENT PROBLEMS

The presence of poisonous plants, even in small amounts, can create serious management problems for the livestock producer. To prevent livestock losses, forage may have to be left ungrazed, grazing systems may have to be altered, and additional improvements such as fencing and plant control measures may be required. Various plant, animal, and climatic interactions bring about unique problems.

Some researchers contend that poisonous plants are generally not consumed by livestock in harmful amounts unless forced to do so by hunger or by accident. Certain species, however, either because of their succulance, taste, or addictive properties are sought out by livestock. For example, locoweeds (*Astragalus spp.*) are not especially palatable to livestock, but when locoweed is green and other forage dry, livestock will eat it. The initial grazing may be due to the early growth habit of locoweed making it the only green plant available in early spring on much of its range. Once the animals begin eating it they become addicted and will seek out locoweed - even dried and blackened year-old stems (9). Prevention of further poisoning requires removal of the animals to locoweed free range.

Examples of species which are grazed readily by livestock are the larkspurs (*Delphinium spp.*). Since they are readily grazed by cattle, prevention of poisoning where larkspur is present in appreciable amounts is difficult. Fortunately, as with many other poisonous plants with non-cumulative effects, cattle may utilize small amounts of larkspur over prolonged periods without apparent effect (10). Sheep, being less affected by larkspur than cattle, have been used to graze larkspur infested areas (7).

Herbicidal applications have been known to increase both palatability of plants, and content of the toxin. For example, Williams and Cronin (11,12) found that treated plants of tall larkspur (*Delphinium barbeyi*) increased in palatability and in alkaloid content following applications of phenoxy herbicides. Williams (13) found, however, that the concentration of miserotoxin contained in timber milkvetch (*Astragalus miser*) decreased after treatment with 2,4,5-T (2,4,5-trichlorophenoxy acetic acid) or silvex [2-(2,4,5-trichlorophenoxy) propionic acid]. After four weeks treated plants contained only 1/3 as much as the controls. Therefore, post treatment grazing is an important consideration following applications of herbicides (14).

Another problem in managing ranges infested with poisonous plants is that manifestations of intoxication are not always immediately apparent. The effect on the animal and on the developing fetus of pregnant animals may be chronic as with locoism in sheep. Intoxication of the mother and fetus is parallel, illustrating the dangers of allowing pregnant sheep, cattle, or horses to graze locoweed-infested ranges. By the time intoxication becomes apparent, considerable damage has been done to both the mother and developing offspring (15).

Some species such as locoweeds and halogeton maintain their toxicity throughout their green growth period and even after maturity and senescence (9). James *et al.*, (16) observed poisoning in sheep grazing dried year-old *Astragalus pubentissimus*, and cattle grazing dried year-old *A. lentiginosus*. Others, such as tall larkspur, lose some of their toxicity with maturity (12). Knowledge of these characteristics must be known for proper grazing management.

Hungry animals such as those being trailed and bedded down overnight are less selective in their grazing, especially after watering. After their thirst has been quenched, they graze less selectively, and on ranges where halogeton or other toxic plants are present in abundance, may consume enough poisonous plants in a short period to become intoxicated (17).

Animals reared in poisonous plant infested ranges often learn to avoid the poisonous species through experience. However, livestock brought in from non-infested areas are often poisoned by plants such as burroweed (*Haplopappus tenuisectus*) or locoweed even though animals accustomed to grazing the area are not poisoned. This creates management problems when outside livestock are the only source of replacement.

IV. MANAGEMENT PRACTICES

In the early days of the livestock industry, losses from plant poisoning were considered unavoidable. These beliefs have been gradually modified. Experience and research have demonstrated that many losses can be avoided or at least reduced through proper management practices. Only occasionally will unpredictable and unavoidable losses occur under good management.

A. Prevention and Livestock Poisoning

One of the most effective means of reducing livestock losses from poisonous plants on rangelands is grazing management - management both to improve forage conditions and to reduce infestations of poisonous plants. With all practices the goal should be to keep animals from consuming lethal amounts of poisonous plants. The reduction of the population of the toxic species and improvement of desirable vegetation are the major objectives.

In lieu of good range management practices or where poisonous plant infested areas are unavoidable, certain livestock-management practices will help reduce livestock losses from poisonous plants. General rules, to follow when poisonous plants are a problem, have been given by several authorities (2,4,7,8,10,18). These are summarized as follows:

1. Learn identification and toxic principles of poisonous plants on range.
2. Use good grazing management to maintain range in condition least conducive to high poisonous plant populations.
3. Adjust stocking rates so that animals have ample forage plants in relation to poisonous plants.
4. Supplement salt, minerals, and nutrients as needed.
5. Avoid grazing areas where poisonous plants are abundant. Fencing off such areas or herding may be necessary.
6. Use a class of livestock not generally poisoned by the plants present.
7. Avoid turning hungry animals onto ranges containing poisonous plants. Hungry animals are less selective. The hazard is too high while trailing or after shipping.
8. Provide adequate water at all times to prevent non-selective grazing following water deprivation and subsequent watering.
9. Reduce poisonous plant populations with mechanical, chemical, or other control methods.

The ability to identify poisonous plants and to know their poisonous principles is basic to grazing management of ranges infested by these plants. The manager should know, for example, that plants such as mountain mahogany (*Cercocarpus montanus*), arrowgrass (*Triglochin spp.*), catclaw (*Acacia greggii*) and chokecherry (*Prunus spp.*), although valuable forage species, under certain conditions (frost and drought) accumulate enough hydrocyanic acid to be highly toxic. Certain species such as snakeweed (*Gutierrezia spp.*) and princes plume (*Stanleya spp.*) are selenium accumulators and present problems on high selenium soils. The poisoning by some species such as halogeton, bitterweed, and shinnery oak (*Quercus havardii*) is not cumulative; whereas others such as jimmyweed (*Isicoma wrightii*) and sneezeweed (*Helenium hoopesii*) have cumulative effects. Prevention of poisoning and treatment of affected animals requires different practices for these species. Table 1 gives the distribution, toxic principles, and livestock affected for 33 poisonous species found on western U.S. ranges.

Grazing management, which enhances the better forage species, is cited most often as the surest and most economical means of preventing livestock losses to poisonous plants. This is especially true where the poisonous species are annuals or weak perennials and do not normally hold dominant positions in the climax plant community. Where poisonous plants can be held to minor components of the forage they seldom present problems.

Where forage is adequate, animals normally vary their diets and seldom consume enough poisonous plants to cause poisoning. Notable exceptions would be palatable species such as larkspur. Additionally, competition from vigorous forage species as maintained by proper grazing management tends to prevent the invasion of poisonous plants. As the relative abundance of poisonous plants declines so does the possibility of livestock poisoning.

Grazing management systems such as the deferred-rotation system developed by Merrill (26) bring about improved forage conditions and reduced losses from plant poisoning. Not one loss of cattle, sheep, or goats has been attributed to bitterweed (*Hymenoxys odorata*) poisoning in the original four-pasture deferred-rotation system, developed on the Experiment Station near Sonora, Texas, in an area where bitterweed poisoning is common. Although it has not been as successful in a similar study at the Texas Agricultural Experiment Station at Barnhart, (96 kilometers away), losses have been reduced drastically, compared with continuous grazing at excessive rates. The newer short duration grazing system in effect both at Sonora and Barnhart also appears to enhance vegetative composition so that bitterweed is crowded out and presents no significant problem for livestock grazing.[1]

The grazing systems at Barnhart and Sonora also utilize a combination of cattle, sheep, and goats as the livestock species. According to Merrill,[1] this combination of livestock stops spot grazing by sheep. The cattle graze the rougher forage more or less evenly, and the sheep graze behind the cattle. This combination prevents spot grazing which often results in invasion by bitterweed. There have been no losses of sheep to bitterweed during the 28-year study of the four-pasture deferred-rotation systems when grazing was at a moderate rate with a combination of cattle, sheep, and goats. Merrill attributes this to an adequate diet both quantitatively and qualitatively, and reduced occurrence of bitterweed under good range condition.

Dietary supplementation has been purported to be effective in prevention of livestock losses to plant poisoning. For example, dicalcium phosphate was once recommended to prevent halogeton

[1]L. B. Merrill, personal communication, 1977.

TABLE 1

Common Toxic Plants of Southwestern and Western United States[1]

Name	Distribution	Toxic principle	Livestock affected	Control[2]
Apocynum cannabinum Indian hemp	Throughout U.S.	Glycosides	All, especially sheep	2,4-D
Asclepias spp. Milkweed	Throughout U.S.	Glycosides	All, especially sheep	2,4,5-T; amitrole; 2,3,6TBA; picloram
Astragalus spp. *Oxytropis spp.* Locoweeds	Western U.S.	Selenium; Locoine	All	Grubbing; 2,4-D
Baileya multiradiata Desert Baileya	Southwestern U.S. and Mexico	Unknown	Sheep and goats	2,4-D
Cicuta spp. Water hemlock	Wet habitats throughout U.S.	Cicutoxin	All, and humans	Grubbing; a,4-D; 2,4,5-T
Conium maculatum Poison hemlock	Introduced throughout U.S.	Alkaloids	All, and humans	Silvex
Cymopterus watsonii Spring parsley	Intermountain States	Photosensitizing compounds	Sheep and cattle	None satisfactory
Delphinium spp. Larkspur	Throughout U.S.	Alkaloids	All, but mostly cattle	2,4,5-T; silvex
Drymaria spp. Inkweed	Southwestern U.S. and Mexico	Alkaloids	All, expecially cattle	Grubbing; 2,4-D
Gutierrezia sarothrae Snakeweed	Western U.S.	Saponin	Sheep and cattle	Grubbing; mowing; picloram; 2,4-D

Halogeton glomeratus Halogeton	Introduced; Intermountain States	Oxalates	All, but mostly sheep	2,4-D
Helenium hoopesii Orange sneezeweed	Western U.S.	Dugaldin; Lactones	Mostly sheep; cattle less	2,4-D
Hymenoxys odorata Bitterweed	Southwestern U.S. and Mexico	Hymenoxon	Sheep	2,4-D; picloram; hand pulling
Hymenoxys richardsonii Pinque	Western U.S. and Canada	Unknown	All, especially sheep	2,4-D; picloram
Hypericum perforatum St. Johnswort	Introduced; throughout U.S.	Hypercin	All, but goats least	2,4-D; Klamath beetle
Isocoma wrightii Jimmyweed	Southwestern U.S. and Mexico	Tremetol	All	Grubbing; 2,4-D; picloram
Lupinus spp. Lupine	Throughout U.S. and Canada	Alkaloids	All, also deer	2,4-D; 2,4,5-T
Oxytenia acerosa Copperweed	Southwestern U.S. and Mexico	Alkaloid	All, especially cattle	Grubbing
Prunus virginiana Chokecherry	Western U.S.	Hydrocyanic acid	All, especially sheep	2,4,5-T; dicamba; picloram
Psilostrophe spp. Paperflowers	Southwestern U.S. and Mexico	Unknown	Sheep primarily; cattle suspected	None practical
Pteridium aquilinum Bracken fern	Throughout U.S.	Thiaminase-horses; Unknown-cattle	All, especially cattle and horses	Cultivation; mowing; amitrole

Table 1 *(continued)*

Name	Distribution	Toxic principle	Livestock affected	Control[2]
Quercus havardii *Quercus gambelii* Shinnery and scrub oak	Southwestern and central western U.S.	Tannins	All, especially cattle	Silvex; 2,4,5-T; picloram
Sarcobatus vermiculatus Greasewood	Western U.S. and Mexico	Oxalates	All, but mostly sheep	2,4-D; picloram; 2,4,5-T
Senecio longilobus Threadleaf groundsel	Southwestern U.S. and Mexico	Alkaloids	All, cattle and horses most	Hand pulling or grubbing; 2,4-D
Solanum spp. Nightshades	Throughout U.S.	Glycoalkaloids	All	Grubbing; 2,4-D 2,4,5-T; picloram
Tetradymia canescens *Tetradymia glabrata* Horsebursh	Western U.S.	Photosenitizing compounds	Sheep	None practical
Triglochin maritima *Triglochin palustris* Arrowgrass	Western U.S.; Canada; Mexico	Hydrocyanic acid	All	None practical
Veratrum californicum Veratrum	Pacific coast; northern Rocky Mountain States	Alkaloids	All	Silvex
Zigadenus spp. Deathcamas	Western U.S.	Alkaloids	All, especially sheep	2,4-D

[1]Sources: (2,4,6,7,8,18,19,20,21,22,23,24).
[2]Herbicide terminology follows that recommended by Weed Science Society of America (25).

poisoning (and poisoning by other oxalate producing plants) on the basis of experiments where sheep survived lethal doses of halogeton when it was force fed simultaneously with enough dicalcium phosphate to combine with the oxalate in halogeton. Subsequent experimentation has found that the amount required to prevent intoxication is larger than can be practically used under range conditions (17). The high level of calcium necessary to prevent poisoning can be maintained only a short time after the calcium is consumed (10).

The value of supplemental feeding appears to lie in its affect on general animal health and on increased grazing selectivity rather than on antitoxin effects. Salt, minerals, and nutrients should be supplied as needed. Where addiction occurs as in locoweed poisoning, prevention of poisoning lies almost exclusively in preventing animals from grazing areas infested with locoweed, especially during periods such as early spring when animals graze the plant heavily. James and Van Kampen (27) found that protein and mineral supplements were of no value in preventing locoweed poisoning or birth defects due to locoweed poisoning. In fact, they found evidence that protein reinforces the action of the locoweed toxin.

Fencing and herding is often used to prevent livestock poisoning. On bitterweed infested areas of Texas it is recommended that the worst bitterweed areas be fenced, and that bitterweed should be controlled in at least one pasture (28). Most bitterweed poisoning occurs during winter and spring. Therefore the bitterweed free pasture is used to carry the sheep during the danger period. This also results in deferment of the bitterweed infested pastures which ultimately results in better range condition with less bitterweed and more valuable forage. Another practice, in the absence of a bitterweed-free pasture, is to concentrate all sheep on one pasture. Such overstocking will reduce the bitterweed population without lethal amounts consumed by the large numbers of sheep. Daily observation is required. Animals that become intoxicated should be removed.

For physiological, metabolic, or grazing preference reasons different kinds of livestock often vary in their degree of susceptibility to some poisonous plant species. Knowledge of this variation can be used to reduce livestock losses. Because sheep are less susceptible to larkspur toxicity, grazing of sheep on heavily infested larkspur sites can be recommended (7). Cattle and horses are not as susceptible to bitterweed or western sneezeweed (*Helenium hoopesii*) as are sheep. Changing from sheep to cattle in situations where these two species exist is warranted in many cases.

James and Cronin (17) presented 11 management practices that minimize deaths in sheep from halogeton poisoning. These practices appear sound for livestock management in halogeton-infested areas as well as with other species for which the toxins are degraded by rumen bacteria and which do not have cumulative effects. The first six practices deal with proper grazing and livestock management which enhance or maintain good range condition. They urge grazing with the right kind and amount of livestock during the proper season, and the use of a grazing plan. The last five practices deal with livestock management to prevent losses when halogeton is present as follows:

1. Limited grazing of halogeton to allow sheep time to adapt to grazing oxalate-containing plants. This allows time for the rumen flora to adapt to the oxalate.
2. Introduce animals to halogeton-infested areas gradually. Even after a short absence (2 or 3 days) from halogeton areas, they should not graze in dense stands.
3. Do not unload animals from truck into halogeton unless both supplemental feed and water are available.
4. Never allow hungry animals to graze in large, dense patches of halogeton often found around old bedgrounds, along trails or roads, and around watering places.
5. Do not trail thirsty sheep into watering places surrounded by halogeton without supplementing them with other food. Thirst inhibits grazing; sheep will not graze until they have been watered. Even small quantities of supplemental food will increase the variety of plants grazed.

B. Poisonous Plant Control

Grazing management is effective in poisonous plant control if the species in question are not climax constituents, and are abundant only in lower stages of succession. If, however, the species is a perennial and an abundant constituent of the climax plant community, range condition improvement may, in fact, increase its relative abundance. This has been a general observation and not confirmed through research.[2]

If grazing management fails to reduce poisonous plant populations to manageable numbers, control measures may be necessary. These include mechanical, chemical, and biological measures as well as the use of fire. Such treatments are generally expensive, and in many cases not practical except on small areas such as holding pens, traps, and around watering places. Quite often, however, control is necessary if forage in a pasture infested with a poisonous plant is to be used. Often it is not a case of whether the rancher can afford to control, but rather whether he can afford not to control and stay in the livestock business.

The recommended control treatment for the most common poisonous plants of the southwestern and western United States are given in Table 1. For some species such as spring parsley (*Cymopterus watsonii*), arrowgrass (*Triglochin spp.*), and horsebrush (*Tetradymia spp.*) no satisfactory control recommendations were found. These are examples of species which require proper grazing and livestock

---

[2]Personal communication with Dr. R. E. Steger, Range Specialist, Texas Agricultural Extension Service, San Angelo, Texas.

management techniques. Certainly, these and any other species can be controlled by some mechanical or cultural treatment. Recommended treatments were reported only where research has proven them successful and where experience has proven them practical.

The herbicides used most commonly for range plant control are 2,4-D (2-4-dichlorophenoxyacetic acid), 2,4,5-T, silvex, picloram (4-amino-3,4,6-trichloropicolinic acid), dicamba (3,6-dicloro-O-anisic acid), amitrole (3-amino-s-triazole), and a promising new chemical, tebuthiuron [N(5-1,1-1,3,4-thiadizol-2 yl)-N,N^1 dimethylurea] which is in the process of being cleared for range use. The most widely used herbicide for the herbaceous species is 2,4-D. Silvex and 2,4,5-T are generally recommended for woody species, while picloram, dicamba, and tebuthiuron are used for either herbaceous or woody species.

Applications should be made with the recommended herbicide, at the most susceptible plant growth stage, and with the recommended form and rate of the herbicide. Most species of poisonous plants are susceptible to one or more herbicides, but only the most commonly recommended were named in Table 1. Others are effective, but since local conditions, management practices, soils, and application equipment affect the chemical used, no specific recommendations are made.

Chemical treatments as well as mechanical treatments such as mowing, grubbing, hand pulling, may be economically feasible around heavily used areas such as bedgrounds, holding pens, waterholes, and corrals. Disturbance associated with these areas generally opens up the sod and allows invasion of noxious species. Spot treatment around these areas is generally recommended even when it is not practical to control the plants in larger pastures.

Seldom is one method completely successful. They must often be repeated, and in many cases, combinations of methods, in a control system in conjunction with good grazing practice, is the key to success.

Management, following control, is often as important as the control. Defer the controlled area from grazing for 90 days or longer to avoid grazing toxic plants, and to allow better forage species to regain vigor. Good forage species must replace poisonous plants for benefits of poisonous plant control to be lasting. A good grazing system, which encompasses periodic deferments and proper stocking, will assure lasting success of poisonous plant control treatments.

V. REFERENCES

1. Agricultural Research Service, "Losses in Agriculture," *U.S. Dep. Agric. Handb.* 291, Washington, D.C., 1965.
2. Agricultural Research Service, "Twenty-two Plants Poisonous to Livestock in the Western States," *U.S. Dep. Agric. Bull.* 327, Washington, D.C., 1968.

3. National Academy of Science, "Prenatal and Postnatal Mortality in Cattle," *N. A. S. Publ.* 1685, Washington, D.C., 1968.
4. Gay, C. W., and Dwyer, D. D., "Poisonous Range Plants," *Coop. Ext. Serv. Cir.* 391, New Mexico State University, Las Cruces, New Mexico, 1967.
5. Sperry, O. E., Dollahite, J. W., Hoffman, G. O., and Camp, B. J., "Texas Plants Poisonous to Livestock," *Tex. Agric. Ext. Bull.* B-1028, College Station, Texas, 1964.
6. Kingsbury, J. M., "Poisonous Plants of the U.S. and Canada," Prentice-Hall, Englewood Cliffs, N. J., 1964.
7. Schmutz, E. M., Freeman, B. N., and Reed, R. E., "Livestock Poisoning Plants of Arizona," University of Arizona Press, Tucson, Arizona, 1968.
8. Stoddart, L. A., Smith, A. D., and Box, T. W., "Range Management," 3rd ed., McGraw-Hill Book Co., New York, 1975.
9. James, L. F., *Clin. Toxicol.* 5:567 (1972).
10. James, L. F., and Johnson, A. E., *J. Range Manage.* 29, 359 (1976).
11. Williams, M. C., and Cronin, E. H., *Weeds* 11, 317 (1963).
12. Williams, M. C., and Cronin, E. H., *J. Range Manage.* 19, 274 (1966).
13. Williams, M. C., *J. Range Manage.* 23, 400 (1970).
14. Cronin, E. H., Nielson, D. B., and Madson, N., *J. Range Manage.* 29, 364 (1976).
15. James, L. F., *Can. J. Comp. Med.* 40, 380 (1976).
16. James, L. F., Bennett, K. L., Parker, K. G., Keeler, R. F., Binns, W., and Lindsay, B., *J. Range Manage.* 21, 360 (1968).
17. James, L. F., and Cronin, E. H., *J. Range Manage.* 27, 424 (1974).
18. Steger, R. E., "Poisonous Range Plants of New Mexico," *Coop. Ext. Serv. Bull.* 400 B-1, Las Cruces, New Mexico, 1970.
19. Bovey, R. W., "Response of Selected Woody Plants in the United States to Herbicides," *U.S. Dep. Agric. Handb.* 493, Washington, D.C., 1977.
20. Cronin, E. H., *J. Range Manage.* 24, 258 (1971).
21. Gesink, R. W., Alley, H. P., and Lee, G. A., *J. Range Manage.* 26, 139 (1973).
22. Johnson, A. E., *Can. J. Comp. Med.* 38, 406 (1974).
23. Kim, H. L., Rowe, L. D., and Camp, B. J., *Res. Commun. Chem. Path. Pharmacol.* 11, 647 (1975).
24. Murphy, A. H., *J. Range Manage.* 8, 76 (1955).
25. Weed Science Society of America, Terminology Committee, *Weeds* 12, 328 (1964).
26. Merrill, L. B., *J. Range Manage.* 7, 152 (1954).

INORGANIC TOXICANTS AND POISONOUS PLANTS

J. L. Shupe, Howard B. Peterson, Arland E. Olson,
and Gene W. Miller
Utah State University

I. ABSTRACT

Poisonous vegetation and inorganic toxicants have caused death losses in animals throughout history. Livestock and wildlife are exposed to a multitude of both naturally occurring and induced toxic agents. The major sources of these toxic agents for livestock and wildlife are poisonous vegetation, industrial wastes, heavy metals, rodenticides, insecticides, fungicides, herbicides, feed additives, fertilizers, and biotoxins. With increasing industrialization there is an increase in the number and complexity of toxicologic problems in livestock and wildlife. These problems are seldom induced by one toxic substance alone, but are usually the result of a combination of toxicants from multiple sources. The potential additive or synergistic influence of such combinations is of major concern. Overgrazing by animals is usually conducive to increased adverse effects of poisonous plants, inorganic toxicants, or combinations thereof. These facts are important in both the diagnosis of toxicologic problems and in the management of land, water, and animals in prevention and treatment.

II. INTRODUCTION

Since about 1918, there has been a marked expansion of certain types of industrialization into agricultural, rangeland, and wildlife habitat areas. The use of chemicals, such as herbicides, pesticides, and fertilizers to enhance agricultural production has also added another dimension to the complexity of environmental changes. With this expansion and the new changes has come a significant increase in the number and type of toxic hazards to which livestock and wildlife are exposed. The current impetus to locate, develop, and utilize geothermal energy sources will very likely increase water-associated environmental hazards that previously existed with limited numbers of springs and geysers. There are also natural pollutants from such sources as erosion, dust storms, volcanoes, and forest fires. Toxic substances from these and other sources can seriously complicate the clinical aspects and proper diagnosis of livestock losses where poisonous plants are present and/or suspected. Figure 1 illustrates many possible routes whereby animals may encounter inorganic toxicants alone or in combinations and/or with poisonous plants. Careful consideration of these many possible interactions should be given whenever planning research or making diagnostic investigations.

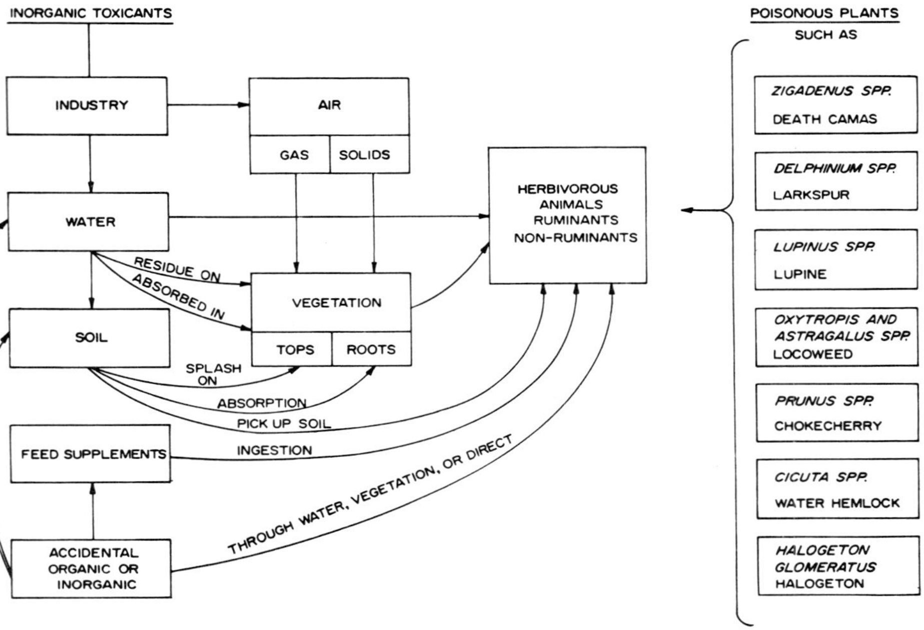

Fig. 1. *Diagramatic presentation of possible routes of inorganic and poisonous plant toxicants to animals.*

III. POISONOUS PLANTS

We are at a loss to adequately define poisonous plants. For our discussion, however, four generalized groupings are suggested.

a. Poisonous plants, those that synthesize organic toxicants.
b. Accumulator plants, those that accumulate significant amounts of elements such as heavy metals, selenium, fluorides, or nitrates.
c. Polluted plants, those contaminated with toxic substances such as heavy metals, fluorides, herbicides, or pesticides. Most of these toxicants are on the vegetation rather than metabolized within.
d. Conditionally toxic plants, those that are usually safe under normal conditions, but can become hazardous under certain conditions. Some such plants include sudan grass, sorghum, alfalfa, and clovers.

IV. DIAGNOSTIC FACTORS

Whether a toxic response takes place depends on a number of variables and interactions. Evaluation of observed problems is especially difficult when more than one toxin is involved, since effects may be additive, synergistic, or alleviating.

In a disease of unknown etiology, poisoning should be considered possible. Three relevant categories are: (a) exposure to known poisons; (b) exposure to unknown substances that may be poisonous; and (c) diseases of undetermined etiology in which poisoning must be considered part of the differential diagnosis.

It has been well documented that certain plants induce toxic effects or death under specified circumstances. It is also known that poisonous plants cause heavy losses of range animals in some areas. Estimates of losses vary and are usually influenced by a number of factors. In addition to actual death losses there could be and are many missed and undiagnosed sublethal and subclinical cases attributable to poisonous plants. Many cases could be properly diagnosed if the competence of essential disciplines are utilized when and where necessary. Vegetation that induces bloat in ruminants causes heavy death losses annually. Certain types of vegetation and management practices are associated with heavy, annual death losses of cattle in the intermountain area.

In localized areas where poisonous plants have been incriminated as causing heavy losses in animals, other etiological factors have also sometimes been diagnosed as causing losses. These factors have included industrial inorganic toxicants, agricultural chemicals, research chemicals, radiation, and infectious and nutritional diseases. Differential diagnosis in such situations necessitates the utilization of pathologic, chemical, microbiologic, and serologic disciplines to support epidemiologic studies and clinical findings.

Inorganic materials can be toxic or hazardous or produce less than maximum performance in animals that ingest excessive amounts. An effective evaluation of inorganic toxicosis in animals requires information on: (a) clinical signs, lesions and bodily retention of the elements(s); (b) level, form, and distribution of the element and/or elements in water, soils, and mineral deposits; (c) uptake and distribution of the element and/or elements by vegetation (plants); and (d) potential for absorption and retention of the element(s) by humans when consuming animal products.

V. LEAD TOXICOSIS

Mining, processing, and commercial uses of lead have been extensive for a long time. The low solubility of lead in the aqueous phase of natural systems is manifested in many ways directly relevant to the understanding of the behavior of lead in the environment. The element is not readily transferred from soils to vegetation. The concentration of lead in natural bodies of water is extremely low in proportion to the concentration in the sediments of lakes and streams.

Lead is one of the most frequent causes of poisoning in animals (1). The major concern today is with chronic effects of long-term exposure (2,3).

Certain interactions of lead occur with other mineral elements. Large amounts of dietary zinc appear to prevent the development of clinical signs of lead toxicosis in horses (4). Low dietary calcium and phosphorus has been correlated with greater concentrations of lead in young growing horses (5).

A. Case Study

In 1954, a request was made to investigate the death of eight horses in an area where poisonous plants had been identified. The owner of the dead animals informed us that they had lost animals in the same area for years and that their neighbors had also lost animals. The losses occurred in the spring of the year when pasture forage was limited. The affected animals also had access to a range area containing some death camas (*Zigadenus paniculatus*). There was evidence that a limited amount of the plants had been eaten. The owner was informed that the deaths were probably due to ingestion of death camas. We now feel that this was an improper diagnosis.

Since 1954, animal losses have continued to occur in the same geographic area. From 1970 to 1974 a study was conducted to ascertain (if possible) the cause of these continued death losses. The detailed epidemiological survey included ambient air, soil, vegetation, and animal studies. The vegetation work indicated exposure to plants containing excessive levels of a number of elements (Table 1), that the degree of exposure to poisonous plants was insufficient to induce death losses, and that the signs, lesions, and chemical analyses of tissues from the animals did not support the 1954 diagnosis of poisonous plant toxicosis.

TABLE 1

Summary of Vegetation Analysis Data for a Two-Year Period

Station No.[1]	Values are ug/g (ppm) dry weight basis							
	Pb	Zn	Cu	Cd	Mo	As	Se	F
1	116.5	77.4	267.4	2.9	55.4	46.2	1.9	26.6
2	104.9	109.4	379.4	3.4	79.1	93.7	3.3	47.4
3	38.4	52.5	113.6	1.4	22.7	12.4	2.0	24.7
13	282.6	141.4	47.9	5.0	6.1	4.5	1.6	14.7
18[2]	4.8	20.2	17.5	0.6	2.0	0.6	1.7	8.2

[1]Different sample stations near industrial area.
[2]Cache Valley Station included for control.

Livestock in and adjacent to the problem area were studied. Clinical signs, gross and histopathologic findings, and chemical analyses were obtained and correlated. Excessive levels of lead were found in the kidneys, liver, stomach and fecal contents, bone, and hair. Acid-fast intranuclear inclusions were found in the epithelial cells of the kidneys (6).

VI. FLUORIDE TOXICOSIS

Fluorine is universally present in varying amounts in soils, water, atmosphere, vegetation, and animal tissues. Because of its extreme chemical reactivity, it is found in nature in its combined (fluoride) form.

Livestock and people normally ingest variable amounts of fluoride. No adverse effects are known to accompany normal, low-level fluoride ingestion. In fact, fluorides ingested in proper amounts for each species at proper ages are beneficial on tooth and bone structure. Fluoride is now considered by some researchers as an essential nutrient (7). However, amounts greater than the optimal levels induce fluoride toxicosis (8). The principal sources of excessive fluoride for animals are vegetation, water, and occasionally undefluorinated mineral supplements (9). The amounts of fluoride obtained from the atmosphere via the lungs and from pharmaceutical products is usually negligible.

Fluorides may be present in the effluent, dust, or waste products of certain mining, smelting, refining, processing, or manufacturing operations, and occurs in geothermal waters (which are used increasingly for watering animals) (10). Fluoride toxicosis, therefore, has been and will continued to be an important toxicologic problem in animals unless proper preventive and control measures are used (11).

A. Case Study 1

In 1950 a serious problem was observed in many cattle, sheep, and horses in three counties in central Utah. Comments from the animal owners indicated the problem had existed for a number of months and was getting progressively worse. The postulated causes included: poisonous plants, pesticides, insecticides, malnutrition, infectious diseases, contaminated water, and industrial pollutants. An epidemiological study was conducted and it was found that the animals were eating vegetation with high levels of fluoride. Based on vegetative analyses, clinical signs, and lesions in the animals, fluoride toxicosis was diagnosed. Extensive controlled experiments were conducted to elucidate the disease and allow correlation of controlled findings with those from annual field surveys.

Installation of anti-pollution equipment greatly reduced the fluoride problems, although clinical cases still occur adjacent to the emitting source. In the peripheral and outlying areas, cases requiring a differential diagnosis constantly occur. Some have been due to various types of poisoning such as poisonous plants, pesticides, insecticides, and heavy metals from batteries, paint buckets, and some industrial operations.

B. Case Study 2

In another range area where poisonous plants and lead poisoning had been a problem, fluoride toxicosis was also diagnosed. Fluoride levels in the range vegetation are shown in Table 2.

TABLE 2

Fluoride in Vegetation from Rangeland near an Industrial Operation where Livestock Health Problems Occurred

Common name	Scientific name	F ppm
Western wheatgrass	*Agropyron spicatum*	60.2
Crested wheatgrass	*Agropyron cristatum*	58.6
Sunflower	*Helianthus anuus*	127, 50, 76.7
Salt grass	*Distichlis stricta*	82.1
Cheatgrass	*Bromus tectorum*	69.2
Mean of all vegetation over two-year period		55.5
(Control - low fluoride area) Cache Valley vegetation		8.0

Fluoride toxicosis in livestock and wildlife continues to be a serious problem in some agricultural and rangeland areas. Cases too often have been misdiagnosed and improperly evaluated.

VII. MOLYBDENUM TOXICOSIS

Molybdenum metabolism is intertwined with that of copper and inorganic sulfate. The relationship is very complex. Elements such as manganese, zinc, and iron affect this interaction (12).

Molybdenum and copper appear to be essential elements for plants and animals. Under natural conditions, however, uncomplicated molybdenum deficiency has not been substantiated.

Conditions classed as molybdenum poisoning (molybdenosis) occur primarily in cattle. The problem has also been diagnosed in sheep and horses. Young animals are more susceptible than adults. In England the condition is known as "Teart" scours and in New Zealand as "Peat" scours. It has also been seen in the Netherlands, Ireland, Canada, and the United States.

Normal vegetation usually contains 1 to 3 ppm of molybdenum and 8 to 11 ppm of copper. If animals also consume plants containing 10 ppm or more of molybdenum there is a good possibility of molybdenum toxicosis developing (13).

A. Case Study

In an area where chronic toxicosis in cattle had been diagnosed as due to industrial pollutants, poisonous plants, pesticides, and insecticides, some cattle started evidencing unthriftiness, emaciation, apathy, anemia, persistent water diarrhea, some evidence of impaired locomotion, and bleaching of hair. Grass samples in the area contained 2-5 ppm of molybdenum and clover samples contained 25-28 ppm of molybdenum. A diagnosis of molybdenum toxicosis was made.

VIII. COMBINED CAUSES

One complicated case history studied involved severe cattle death losses in an area where industrial pollutants, poisonous plants and infectious diseases had been troublesome. Ranges of elemental concentrations and known poisonous plants in the area of livestock losses are shown in Table 3.

TABLE 3

Range[1] of Elemental Concentrations (ppm) where Livestock Losses Occurred and Poisonous Plants Coexisted[2]

Sample	Mo	Cu	Fe	AL	NO_3	F
Stock water	.18-.36	2-42	8-35	6.9-371	5.6-7	<.14
Vegetation	3-15.6	10-178	83-1640	--	168-370	5-137
Soils	1.2-93	70-1522	800-40332	--	--	285-1380

[1]The range is for different locations and different sampling dates.

[2]African rue, Bitterweed, Desert baileya, Dock, Loco, Lupine, Milkweed, Nightshade, Red stem pea vine, Russian thistle, and Senecio.

After the surviving animals were given a fresh water supply and supplemental feed they gradually recovered. Based on the information available, the owner was informed that flood water containing excessive amounts of heavy metals was associated with the major portion of the death losses, but that the deaths of the younger, recently purchased animals that died acutely were caused by an infectious respiratory disease.

IX. GEOTHERMAL WATERS

Current impetus to locate and develop new energy sources such as geothermal water will undoubtedly continue. Water-associated environmental hazards that previously existed only with certain springs and geysers will, therefore, also likely increase.

Geothermal waters are usually contaminated with diverse chemical impurities of underground origin. Of particular concern are: heavy metals, fluoride, arsenic, molybdenum, nickel, selenium, lithium, silica, and some common salts. The concentrations of these elements vary from one location to another and from time to time within a given location (14). Fluoride content of geothermal waters used for livestock watering in an area where poisonous plants are also common is in Table 4.

TABLE 4

Fluoride Content of Stock Water

Water source	F mg/l
Range well - hot	6.9
Dairy well - warm	14.2
Ranch well - warm	11.5
Power wells - hot (not yet released)	5.4 - 10.4

Livestock from the area were examined and they had dental and bone lesions characteristic of chronic fluoride toxicosis.

X. DISCUSSION

Livestock and wildlife are exposed to a multitude of both naturally occurring and introduced toxic agents. The major sources of these toxic agents for livestock and wildlife are poisonous vegetation (15,16,17), industrial wastes (9), heavy metals (1), rodenticides, insecticides, fungicides, herbicides (13), feed additives, fertilizers, and biotoxins.

The toxic agents vary in their degree of toxicity due to the influences of many factors. Livestock are rarely exposed to some hazardous agents. Acute toxicosis is usually more easily recognized and spectacular than is chronic toxicosis. Standards for chronic toxicoses are difficult to establish. Chronic effects are often more significant than acute effects.

The toxicity of a toxic agent will vary with the route of exposure (air, soil, water, or vegetation). The usual route is oral, but may be dermal or by inhalation.

Much is known about how many substances individually induce toxicosis; however, the data in Table 5 illustrates the complexity in properly establishing tolerance levels when one substance is evaluated alone. This complexity is multiplied in the presence of more than one toxicant.

TABLE 5

Fluoride Tolerance[1] Levels in Feed and Water of Domestic Animals[2]

Species	Feed[3] ppm	Water[4] Mg/liter
Heifers, dairy and beef cattle	30	2.5 - 5
Dairy cattle, mature	40	4 - 8
Beef cattle, mature	50	6 - 10
Finishing cattle	100	12 - 15
Breeding ewes	60	6 - 9
Horses	60	4 - 10
Feeder lambs	150	12 - 15

[1]Biological availability depends on chemical composition. Dissolved F in water appears to be more readily assimilated than other forms.

[2]The values must be reduced proportionally when both water and feed contain appreciable amounts of fluorides.

[3]This is a suggested guide when F in the feed is essentially the sole source of fluoride.

[4]The average ambient air temperature and the physical and biological activity of the animals influence the amount of water consumed and hence the wide range of tolerance levels suggested. For active animals in a warm climate the lower values should be used as critical level indicators.

Much more needs to be known about critical levels of each toxicant and especially when two or more toxicants are involved. The alleviating, additive, or synergistic responses associated with the influence of two or more toxic agents in combination adds to the difficulty of properly diagnosing and evaluating some cases.

Possible interactions between poisonous plants and inorganic toxicants should not be overlooked. In times of stress such as occur with drought and inadequate nutrition, these problems are multiplied.

It is imperative that diseases be correctly diagnosed so that specific intelligent treatment can be prescribed and preventive measures recommended. In order to do this, the diagnostician must be an astute observer, thorough, alert to details, and learn to see what is looked at and hear what is said. After accumulating all the essential, factual information available, the diagnosis and recommendations must be based on that plus proven practical experience. One should not go beyond factual information or successful experience. It is important to determine whether the degree of toxic exposure was sufficient to induce the observed symptoms or lesions.

Safety and hazards are usually relative. We should consider and evaluate cost/benefit ratios and not routinely abandon a product nor condemn industry because it might prove hazardous under certain conditions.

XI. CONCLUSIONS

Poisonous vegetation and inorganic toxicants have caused death losses in animals throughout history. With increasing industrialization there is an increase in the number and complexity of toxicologic problems in livestock and wildlife. These problems are seldom induced by one toxic substance alone, but are usually the result of a combination of toxicants from multiple sources. The potential additive or synergistic influence of such combinations is of major concern. Overgrazing by animals is usually conducive to increased adverse effects of poisonous plants, inorganic toxicants or combinations thereof. These facts are important in both the diagnosis of toxicologic problems and in the management of land, water, and animals in prevention and treatment.

We have emphasized the nature and complexity of the problems and possible interactions caused by inorganic toxicants and poisonous plants and suggested that the competence of professionals from several disciplines are required to identify and solve the problems. This interdisciplinary approach should be utilized in research as well as in the diagnosis and evaluation of field toxicologic problems.

XII. REFERENCES

1. Buck, William B., Osweiler, Gary D., and Van Gelder, Gary A., "Clinical and Diagnostic Veterinary Toxicology," 2nd Ed. Kendall/Hunt Publishing Company, Dubuque, Iowa, 1976.
2. NRC (National Research Council), Committee on Biologic Effects of Atmospheric Pollutants, "Lead," National Academy of Sciences, Washington, D.C., 1972.
3. Schmidt, N., Brown, G., Devlin, E. L., Larsen, A. A., McCausland, E. D., and Saville, J. M., *Arch. Environ. Health* 23, 185-195 (1971).
4. Willoughby, R. A., MacDonald, E., McSherry, B. J., and Brown, G., *Vet. Rec.* 91, 382 (1972a).
5. Willoughby, R. A., Thirapatsokin, T., and McSherry, B. J., *Am. J. Vet. Res.* 33, 1165 (1972b).
6. Smith, H. A., Jones, T. C., and Hunt, R. D., *in* "Veterinary Pathology," 4th Ed., p. 965. Lea & Febiger Publishing Co., Philadelphia, Pennsylvania, 1972.
7. American Medical Association, "Efficacy and Safety of Fluoridation." Prepared in support of the Statement of the American Medical Association House of Delegates and

Council on Foods and Nutrition, Chicago, Illinois, 1975.
8. National Research Council, Committee on Animal Nutrition, Board on Agriculture and Renewable Resources. "Effects of Fluorides in Animals," National Academy of Sciences, Washington, D.C., 1974.
9. Shupe, J. L., *Am. Ind. Hyg. Assoc. J.* 31 (1970).
10. Shupe, J. L., *in* "Publikation der IV. Internationalen Tagung der Weltgesellschaft fur Buiatrik," 4, Zurich, Switzerland 1966.
11. Shupe, J. L., "Clinical and Pathological Effects of Fluoride Toxicity in Animals, ASP" (Elsevier · Excerpta Medica, Amsterdam, Holland, 1971.
12. Underwood, E. J., "Trace Elements in Human and Animal Nutrition," 3rd Ed. Academic Press, New York, 1971.
13. Radeleff, R. D., "Veterinary Toxicology," 2nd Ed. Lea and Febiger, Philadelphia, Pennsylvania, 1970.
14. Peterson, H. B., and Shupe, J. L., *in* "Proceedings of the International Salinity Conference," Texas Tech University, Lubbock, Texas, 1976.
15. Keeler, R. F., *Lloydia* Vol. 38, No. 1 (1975).
16. Kingsbury, J. M., "Poisonous Plants of the United States and Canada," Prentice-Hall, Englewood Cliffs, New Jersey, 1964.
17. Marsh, C. D., *U.S. Dep. Agric. Dep. Bull.* 1245 (1929).

EFFECT OF LAND USE ON PLANT POISONING OF LIVESTOCK IN AUSTRALIA

Selwyn L. Everist
Bribie Island, Queensland

I. ABSTRACT

Except in southern Australia and the humid east coastal belt, most of the beef and much of the wool in Australia is produced on native pastures or mixed pastures that are neither cultivated nor fertilized.

Management of native pastures and establishment, maintenance, and management of sown pastures produce profound changes in pattern, incidence, and severity of plant poisoning and species of plants involved. These changes are always accompanied by reduction in botanical complexity with a tendency towards monoculture, thus reducing the incidence of poisoning by native species and increasing poisoning by adventive weeds and the sown species themselves.

Productivity of sown fertilized pastures is so much greater that it is usually economically feasible to live with the problems rather than revert to less toxic but less productive species or cultivars.

Changes in management practices such as transporting livestock by road or rail rather than on the hoof shift the incidence of plant poisoning away from species that grow in the paddock or along stock routes to those that are abundant at the point of unloading.

Whatever the situation, recognition of toxic plants and knowledge of conditions under which they may become dangerous are essential for intelligent management.

In Australia there are virtually no regular seasonal movements of herds between 'summer' range and 'winter' range. Animals mostly remain on the same properties, often in the same paddocks, for 12 months each year. The only mass movements of livestock are those chosen by management or imposed by natural disasters such as droughts or floods.

II. GRAZING PRACTICES

The grazing of domestic livestock in Australia has been in progress less than 200 years. Most regions, except in the immediate vicinity of the very early settlements, have been occupied by Europeans for less than 150 years.

During that time there have been profound changes in patterns of agricultural and pastoral production. These have been reflected in changes in the nature, incidence and severity of plant poisining of livestock.

Today we can distinguish five major patterns of land utilization by livestock in Australia.

(a) Extensive grazing of native pastures on open range or in large paddocks, fenced and provided with watering points. In some of these areas the native trees and shrubs have been destroyed to stimulate growth of native grasses and forbs.

(b) Extensive grazing, usually in somewhat smaller paddocks, of sown pastures established without cultivation, e.g. on cleared and burnt scrub or forest land, not fertilized regularly.

(c) Intensive grazing of sown pastures, often rich in legumes, after complete destruction of the original plant cover. Fertilizer, usually phosphate, is applied regularly.

(d) Grazing of crops grown specifically for the purpose or of stubbles remaining after harvesting of grain or fodder crops. This practice is often supplementary to grazing of sown pastures.

(e) Feeding of crops without grazing, i.e. supplementary or lot feeding.

In the more humid areas, particularly in temperate and cool subtropical regions there has been progression from extensive grazing of native grasslands to intensive use of sown pastures but most of Australia's beef and much of its wool are still produced from native pastures (1).

We shall consider some of the poisonous plant problems encountered in each situation and trace the way in which changes in land use influence the incidence of plant poisoning and alter the importance of particular poisonous plants.

A. Native Pastures

In the first situation, animals depend entirely on native plants, except sometimes for a few adventive species (weeds). The nature, magnitude, and incidence of plant poisoning depends on the species and palatability of the toxic plants present and on factors that influence their toxicity or consumption by animals.

These factors include seasonal conditions, availability of other forage, animal species, and the condition and management of the animals. They have been discussed in detail elsewhere (2).

There are some native plants so palatable and poisonous that losses of livestock are virtually unavoidable. Country that carries these plants is not utilized for grazing at all, except in desperate circumstances such as severe drought.

This applies to most of the toxic species of *Gastrolobium* and *Oxylobium* in southwest Western Australia (3,4) and to the one species of *Gastrolobium* that extends from the northern part of Western Australia, across the Northern Territory to central and northern inland Queensland. These plants all contain substantial amounts of monofluoroacetic acid and wherever they occur in quantity it is necessary to destroy them before the land can be used safely for grazing by sheep or cattle.

Acacia georginae, the other Australian species that contains monofluoroacetic acid, poses serious problems in parts of the Northern Territory and northwest Queensland but its presence does not absolutely preclude the use of the land by livestock. Except for the seeds, this plant usually contains less fluoroacetic acid than most species of *Gastrolobium*. It is possible to run cattle or sheep on country where it grows, provided they are removed during dry spring and early summer months when grass is dry and unpalatable and seed pods from *Acacia* are produced in abundance (2).

Erythrophleum chlorostachys, a tree that is widespread in inland areas of northern Australia, presents somewhat different problems. On areas where the tree grows there is always a risk of poisoning, particularly on stock routes used by large numbers of cattle.

In an attempt to minimize the danger, trees on some properties and on stock routes have been cut down. However, in many places this exacerbated the problem instead of solving it. The cut stumps suckered freely, thus making available to grazing animals a plentiful supply of young, palatable, and highly toxic leaf material (2).

Uncontrolled grazing of native pasture can lead to changes in botanical composition that sometimes increase the risks of plant poisoning. If grazing pressure is heavy there is a tendency for more palatable species to be reduced in amount and for less palatable ones to increase. Sometimes the increasing species are potentially toxic but do not cause trouble in well managed pasture because they are not eaten in sufficient amounts or because the animals are too well nourished to be at risk.

Examples of such plants are *Swainsona spp.*, *Sarcostemma australe*, *Myoporum deserti*, and *Terminalia oblongata*.

In a region of erratic rainfall such as arid and semi-arid parts of Australia, drought can seriously reduce the perennial plant cover, leaving large areas of bare ground. When rain comes again, forbs and annual grasses many of which contain nitrate, oxalate, or cyanogenetic glycosides often grow in great abundance in these areas. Whether or not plant poisoning occurs in these situations depends on the intensity of grazing and the condition and management of animals. Sometimes losses can be disastrous.

Changes in the species of animal pastured can also bring new hazards. A good example is the widespread incidence of St. George disease in some semi-arid parts of southwestern Queensland and northwestern New South Wales. Some years ago, following a dramatic slump in wool prices and an almost simultaneous steep rise in the price of beef, whole properties formerly grazed exclusively by merino sheep were converted to beef cattle raising.

Small, inconspicuous annual species of *Pimelea* that were neglected by sheep were present on these properties and, since the sheep had eaten out the palatable grasses and forbs, these plants remained in great abundance, almost unnoticed because they were dead and dried up. When cattle were introduced into these paddocks, they either ate or inadvertently inhaled this dry material while grazing. As a result many of the cattle developed St. George disease, the cause of which was at that time unknown (5). It will be noted from the more detailed discussion of this syndrome at a later session of the Symposium that sheep are not susceptible to this disease.

B. Extensively Grazed Sown Pastures

Destruction of native vegetation and establishment of sown pasture always involves a reduction in botanical complexity and the range of forage species available to the grazing animal. This can influence poisonous plants problems in two ways. Firstly, it can reduce the risk of poisoning by eliminating many potentially toxic native species. Secondly, it can increase the danger if, as has sometimes happened, the pasture plants themselves or the weeds that come with them are potentially toxic.

On sown pastures used for extensive grazing there are two main danger periods, first during the establishment stage when regrowth of toxic native species may be plentiful and second some years after full establishment when one or two sown species have become dominant, livestock numbers have increased greatly and the animals have little or no choice of forage.

Examples of both situations are afforded by some areas in subcoastal central Queensland where *Acacia* scrubs were cleared, burned, and sown to mixtures of rhodes grass (*Chloris gayana*), buffel grass (*Cenchrus ciliaris*), and green panic (*Panicum maximum* var. *trichoglume*) about 15 years ago. During the first few years large amounts of *Trema aspera* came up on the cleared areas. When cattle from other districts were introduced to the new pastures, mortalities were often very heavy.

About 10 years later, on some of these same pastures and others developed in the same way, there was serious intoxication from buffel grass and green panic (6). Horses grazing on these pastures on more than 30 properties developed lesions of *osteodystrophia fibrosa*. Morbidity rates on different properties ranged from 1% to 100%.

Both the pasture plants involved contained soluble oxalate in concentrations ranging from 0.33% for green panic to 1.3% for buffel grass.

C. Intensively Grazed Sown Pasture

In the temperate regions of Australia and in humid subtropical and tropical areas along the east coast, sown pastures mostly fertilized regularly are grazed intensively in small units, mainly by dairy cattle, wool sheep, mutton sheep, or fat lambs. Many of these pastures present special plant poisoning problems.

There may be sporadic deaths due to toxic weeds that take

advantage of the increased soil fertility (1), e.g. variegated thistles (*Silybum*) and other thistles or plants that invade run-down and degraded old pasture, such as bracken (*Pteridium*), St. John's wort (*Hypericum*), ragwort (*Senecio jacobaea*), or heliotrope (*Heliotropium europaeum*).

The major problems arise from potential toxicity of the pasture plants themselves or of fungi or bacteria associated with them. There are about 5 major problems of this kind: (a) clover disease or estrogenic disease, (b) acute nitrite poisoning, (c) oxalate poisoning, (d) phalaris staggers, and (e) microbial intoxications associated with particular grass species. Kikuyu grass poisoning, first noted in New Zealand (7) has also been reported recently from Australia. There is a possibility that this too may be due to mycotoxins (8,9).

1. *Clover Disease*

This disease is widespread in southern Australia. It is most commonly associated with intensive grazing by sheep of particular cultivars of subterranean clover (*Trifolium subterraneum*) but a few other closely related leguminous pasture plants have also been involved. In the pastures concerned, animal numbers are high, there is rarely much alternative forage available and high breeding performance is crucial to the economics of the operation. The toxins involved are isoflavones, mainly *formononetin*. The syndrome is discussed in detail elsewhere (2).

Recent studies of estrogenic and non-estrogenic pastures in Western Australia (10,11) showed that when grazed exclusively on estrogenic clover pasture, only 65% of ewes were served during the first 16 days of joining compared with 75% on non-estrogenic pasture. Ovulation rates were low in both groups. On estrogenic pastures fertilization rates were low (73%) compared with those in ewes on non-estrogenic pasture (93%).

Abnormalities such as prolapse of the uterus and dystocia are frequently seen in ewes on these pastures.

It is unfortunate that the highly estrogenic strains of clover are usually those best suited to the districts where clover disease is most common. At present, no other pasture plants are available that can replace the toxic cultivars without seriously reducing carrying capacity and productivity.

2. *Acute Nitrite Poisoning*

This condition can occur in ruminants following ingestion of plants containing large amounts of nitrate. It is a common cause of sickness and death in livestock exposed to many native and introduced forbs and some grasses. In some pasture species nitrate can reach potentially toxic levels under the special conditions of season and weather described elsewhere (2). The pasture grass most commonly implicated in Australia is kikuyu grass (*Pennisetum clandestinum*), particularly when it is growing in nitrogen-enriched soil such as around stockyards or in heavily fertilized paddocks.

3. *Oxalate Poisoning*

Again there are many native plants and introduced weeds that contain potentially toxic amounts of soluble oxalates. In the present context we are concerned with pasture plants that are themselves potentially toxic for this reason.

Cenchrus and *Panicum* have already been mentioned under the heading of extensively grazed sown pastures. In the more intensively used pastures, the most important oxalate-containing plants are cultivars of the *Setaria anceps* - *S. sphacelata* group. They have been implicated in acute oxalate poisoning of cattle and chronic oxalate poisoning of horses (6,12,13,14,15,16).

In the field acute oxalate intoxication due to setaria has occurred only in hungry cattle shortly after transfer to new paddocks containing abundant young growth of these grasses.

4. *Phalaris Staggers*

Australian phalaris (*Phalaris aquatica* formerly *P. tuberosa)* is an important pasture plant on tablelands and western slopes of New South Wales and in northern Victoria and parts of South Australia. It is also grown in southwest Western Australia. It is a perennial species of high palatability and high productive capacity but capable of producing sudden death, convulsive spasms, and chronic 'staggers' in sheep.

Animals that have acute neuro-muscular symptoms frequently recover quickly and apparently completely after removal from toxic pasture. The toxic principles are reported to be dimethyltryptamine alkaloids.

The chronic syndrome known as 'phalaris staggers' is the most common form of phalaris poisoning. In animals affected by this syndrome, nervous symptoms persist after removal from the toxic pasture.

5. *Mycotoxicoses Associated with Particular Grass Species*

Perennial ryegrass (*Lolium perenne*) is associated with certain intoxications. Facial eczema is due to the presence on the ryegrass of *Pithomyces chartarum*, a parasitic fungus. Ryegrass staggers may be due to a toxin in the grass itself or to mycotoxin from a fungus associated with it (17).

Annual ryegrass or Wimmera ryegrass (*Lolium rigidum*) is also associated with a 'staggers' syndrome. That toxicity is due to the presence of a bacterium.

Several species of *Lupinus* are grown for pasture in temperate areas, mainly in southwest Western Australia and parts of South Australia. They are associated with two syndromes in sheep and cattle, lupine poisoning or transient intoxication and lupinosis.

The first condition is apparently due to the presence in the seeds of quinolizidine alkaloids or N-oxides of these bases. Intoxication usually follows consumption by livestock of large amounts of seeds. Driving and other disturbances can bring on symptoms but the alkaloids are excreted rapidly and their effects appear not to be cumulative. Lupinosis, the more serious disorder in Australia, is a chronic condition that occurs when sheep or cattle are feeding on dried-up lupins during periods of rainfall and high humidity in summer. The condition is apparently due to a mycotoxin produced by fungal growth that develops on the dry stemmy material under these conditions.

Intoxication from the ergot of paspalum (*Claviceps paspali*) occurs frequently on paspalum pasture during warm weather, mainly in northeastern New South Wales and coastal Queensland. It has also been reported from New Zealand. The symptoms are entirely neuromuscular. Gangrene, a feature of poisoning by ergot of rye (*Claviceps purpurea*) in Europe and North America, has not been recorded in cases of *C. paspali* poisoning.

D. Grazing of Crops and Stubbles

Risk of plant poisoning in grazing crops and stubble can arise from two sources, the crop plants themselves or the weeds that grow with them or after they are harvested.

Many of our most productive fodder crops are potentially toxic. Most cultivated species and cultivars of *Sorghum* are cyanogenetic and some of them can accumulate nitrate. Maize, oats, rape, lucerne or alfalfa, and other crop plants may also contain potentially toxic amounts of nitrate or other inorganic compounds of nitrogen. Goitrogenic compounds are usually present in cruciferous crops.

These potentially toxic crops are well known and appropriate management techniques have been developed so that they can be used without serious risk of animal intoxication.

During the last 25 years or so, other potentially toxic fodder crops have been introduced or tested on a large scale. These include the tropical legumes *Leucaena leucocephala* and *Indigofera spicata*, both of which contain toxic amino-acids.

Forage crop plants such as elephant grass or napier grass (*Pennisetum purpureum*) and pearl millet or bulrush millet (*P. typhoideum*) can accumulate oxalate in potentially toxic amounts and need to be handled carefully under some circumstances.

Lucerne or alfalfa (*Medicago sativa*), the 'king of fodders,' is also not without potential toxicity. Not only is it capable of producing bloat in ruminants but it and some related species of *Medicago* can produce photosensitization, may contain estrogenic isoflavones, or may accumulate potentially toxic amounts of nitrate.

It is obvious that high nutritive value is often associated with potential toxicity. As with highly productive pastures, it is necessary to accept these risks if we are to take advantage of the productive capacity of these plants. If conditions that lead to intoxication are understood it is possible to use the plants to advantage without serious risk.

Potentially poisonous weeds that commonly occur in crops, stubbles, or fallow fields in Australia include the oxalate accumulators *Oxalis pes-caprae*, *Emex australis*, and various species of *Rumex*, the nitrate accumulators *Silybum marianum*, *Carduus spp.*, and *Salvia reflexa*, and the alkaloid-containing plants *Argemone spp.*, *Datura spp.*, *Fumaria spp.*, and *Papaver spp.* In some situations *Malva parviflora* and *Stachys arvensis* have also been responsible for intoxication of livestock, mainly sheep.

E. Supplementary Feeding and Lot Feeding

The hand feeding of cut green material and/or grain to animals in confined areas is not without risk of plant poisoning. Cut green material and seeds of many of the sown species already mentioned can be toxic if fed in sufficient quantities.

Recently seeds of *Crotalaria retusa*, a native species, were responsible for poisoning pigs and poultry in the Northern Territory. The seeds were harvested with grain sorghum. They contain a very poisonous pyrrolizidine alkaloid and the plant itself is one of the major causes of pyrrolizidine alkaloidosis in horses in the Northern Territory. Change of land use has extended the hazard to include hand fed stock being offered contaminated grain.

The risks of aflatoxicosis when feeding peanut meal or sorghum meal contaminated with the fungus *Aspergillus flavus* are well known.

III. MANAGEMENT PRACTICES

Changes in management practices have brought profound changes in patterns of plant poisoning and in the importance of particular toxic plants.

For more than 100 years after European settlement, livestock were moved by walking them from place to place. Under these conditions the most frequent causes of plant poisoning were the plants that grew in the paddocks or along the stock routes. These were mainly native species such as *Gastrolobium spp.*, *Oxylobium spp.*, *Eremophila maculata*, *Brachyachne convergens*, *Sarcostemma australe*, *Nicotiana spp.*, *Myoporum deserti*, *Erythrophleum chlorostachys*, *Macrozamia spp.*, and *Trema aspera*.

For many years railways carried most of the long-distance traffic in livestock and the risks of acute plant poisoning at unloading points have always been recognized. Recent improvements in roads and motor vehicles, combined with increases in farm incomes due to higher productivity and higher prices, have resulted in the increased movement of livestock by road instead of by walking. Similarly, in remote regions there has been a tendency to replace horses by trail bikes or 4-wheel drive motor vehicles and to use helicopters for mustering rough country. Current low prices for beef have halted and reversed this trend in some regions but the new practices are still fairly widespread.

The effect of these changed management practices on the incidence of plant poisoning has been dramatic. Poisoning of travelling stock by native shrubs, forbs, and grasses along stock routes has become less common but there has been a marked rise in the number of cases of oxalate, nitrite, and cyanide intoxications at unloading points. Animals that have been starved and subjected to the stresses of mechanical transport for many hours arrive at their destination in a condition that makes them very susceptible to poisoning by these substances. Exposure to large amounts of native or naturalized plants that are cyanogenetic or are rich in oxalate or nitrate can have fatal results and some spectacular 'smashes' have been reported.

IV. CONCLUSION

Whatever the situation, it is apparent that recognition of the toxic plants present is a prerequisite for coping with the problems. If the potentially toxic plants are known, it is possible to find out the conditions under which they are likely to be dangerous and the steps that should be taken to avoid or counteract the dangers.

These steps may be removal or avoidance of the toxic plants themselves. More often they involve skillful management of the flocks or herds at risk.

Whatever the technique, without precise knowledge of the toxic plants concerned and their properties, the manager will be shooting in the dark.

V. REFERENCES

1. Moore, R. M., *in* "Australian Grasslands" (R. M. Moore, Ed.), Chap. 6, p. 87. Australian National University Press, Canberra, 1970.
2. Everist, S. L., "Poisonous Plants of Australia," Angus & Robertson, Sydney, 1974.
3. Cameron, J. M. R., *J. R. Soc. West Aust.* 59, 71-7 (1977).
4. Gardner, C. A., and Bennetts, H. W., "The Toxic Plants of Western Australia," West Australia Newspapers Ltd, Perth 1956.
5. Clark, I. A., *Aust. Vet. J.* 47, 123 (1971).
6. Walthall, J. C., and McKenzie, R. A., *Aust. Vet. J.* 52, 11-16 (1976).

7. Cordes, D. O., Coup, M. R., Harris, G. H., Davenport, P. G., and Busch, J., *N. Z. Vet. J.* 17, 77-81 (1969).
8. Martinovich, D., Mortimer, P. H., and di Menna, Margaret E., *N. Z. Vet. J.* 20, 57-8 (1972).
9. Smith, B., and Martinovich, D., *N. Z. Vet. J.* 21, 85-9 (1973).
10. Wroth, R. H., and Lightfoot, R. J., *Aust. Soc. Anim. Prod. Proc.* 11, 225-28 (1976).
11. Marshall, T., Beetson, B. R., and Lightfoot, R. J., *Aust. Soc. Anim. Prod. Proc.* 11, 229-32 (1976).
12. Seawright, A. A., Groenendyk, S., and Silva, K. I. N. G., *Aust. Vet. J.* 46, 293-6 (1970).
13. Jones, R. J., Seawright, A. A., and Little, D. A., *J. Aust. Inst. Agric. Sci.* 36, 41-3 (1975).
14. Groenendyk, S., and Seawright, A. A., *Aust. Vet. J.* 50, 131 (1974).
15. Jones, R. J., and Ford, C. W., *Tropical Grasslands* 6, 201-4 (1972).
16. Jones, R. J., and Ford, C. W., *Aust. J. Exp. Agric. and Anim. Husb.* 12, 400-6 (1972).
17. Letch, G. C. M., Falloon, R. E., and Christensen, M. J., *N. Z. J. Agric. Res.* 19, 233-42 (1975).

PERSPECTIVES IN PHYTOTOXIC RESEARCH

J. H. Whittem
Embassy of Australia, Washington, D.C.

I. ABSTRACT

Research into the phenomena associated with plant poisoning is justified by the need to improve supplies of animal protein and fiber for human welfare, the primary importance of the grazing animal in this enterprise, and the known occurrence, often in catastrophic proportions of sudden death or ill-thrift upon the ingestion of poison plants. The justification for this first meeting and publication of its proceedings is the preeminence of research in the U.S.A. and Australia in the field of phytotoxicology and the expectation of increased research results from the interaction at the meeting. This paper deals with institutional settings, choice of research topics and the role of workshops in cross fertilizing research programs. Two areas for intensified research programs are proffered, dealing with important but toxic native and improved species of grazing and browse plants. Modern aids to research are discussed, including machine readable data bases, remote sensing, and plant breeding. Some speculations are presented on the role of the rumen in detoxication and possible methods to improve it, and the potential importance of supplementary feeding of livestock at risk.

II. INTRODUCTION

In preparing an address for this first workshop of practicing poison plant research workers from Australia and the United States, I recall that one of the first tasks allotted to me by Professor H. R. Carne when I joined the Department of Veterinary Pathology at Sydney at the conclusion of the second world war was to see whether I could reproduce photosensitization by feeding guinea pigs on a diet of *Panicum effusum*. Although I was unsuccessful with the materials available, the task led me directly into the photosensitization literature, especially the South African geeldikkop papers, e.g., (1).

As the years went by I came to distrust increasingly the proposition that, under Australian conditions at least, *Tribulus terrestris* was toxic to sheep and now, of course, I wonder whether the real culprit is not a fungal agent, e.g., (2).

Subsequent participation in field and laboratory studies with *Indigofera linnaei* (3), *Acacia georginae* (4), and many plants containing pyrrolizidine alkaloids, e.g., (5), has maintained my interest in the field, caused me to stimulate you to meet here, and perhaps made it appropriate that I should presume to address you on your own business - phytotoxic research.

In preparing the paper, however, I found myself in some difficulties due to the length of time since I worked actively as a veterinary pathologist. In more recent years I have had responsibilities in the area of encouragement and administration of research, and some of my efforts here have been in the phytotoxic field. More recently my scientific base has been broadened by the experience of working in Washington with the opportunity to see much of modern science including disciplines quite new to me or not encountered (in their simpler form) since university days. I hope that these peculiarities of career and experience will prove to be useful here and that I may sow one or two seeds of new technical ideas to be transplanted across the Pacific and cross-fertilized by the disciplines represented here, which will serve as the basis for new experiments and more rewarding investigation of residual poison plant problems.

III. THE IMPORTANCE OF PHYTOTOXIC RESEARCH

The primary and sufficient justification for this meeting is to bring together for a workshop, discussion, and interaction, selected scientists from a number of disciplines in our two countries along with colleagues from elsewhere, in the expectation that science, the biosphere, and mankind will benefit thereby.

A more pragmatic justification for the meeting and its timing is the current growing concern in intellectual, academic, scientific, philanthropic, and governmental circles throughout the world in the global improvement of agriculture and increased food production.

If one believes, as I do, that human nutrition requires improvement over large areas of the globe, then the grazing ruminant animal represents the major key to aspirations for increased production of animal protein.

The ruminant animal can be raised comparatively cheaply in areas where it does not compete for use of arable land better dedicated to growth of crops for direct human consumption, and it does not need to compete directly for human foodstuffs. Ruminant animals then are destined to increase in numbers and to graze increasing areas of either native or "improved" sown pasture, since they provide high quality protein to feed and clothe the growing human population.

In either native pasture or sown pasture in areas traditionally devoted to livestock production, flocks can encounter sudden death, often in catastrophic proportions, or alternatively, slow debilitation and eventual death or disability, from ingestion of poisonous plants.

In important areas of the world such as East Africa, the success of unrelated research programs such as those on East Coast Fever and Trypanosomiasis being carried out at ILRAD will enable cattle to be grazed over larger tracts of presently unused country, and anyone even superficially knowledgeable about poisonous plants in that continent will agree that there will be many new phytotoxic problems to recognize and solve before the full benefit of increased animal production can be felt.

In addition, in important parts of the world, production and management of ruminant animals can be severely affected by poisoning of stock horses needed for seasonal work in the herds, e.g. (3,6).

It is important to reiterate that the grazing animal is at risk both from native plants and introduced pasture species; Australian experience and research has encompassed both types of occurrence.

Increased interest in intensive rearing of animals indoors or in feed lots on prepared concentrate rations has introduced another element into overall consideration of feed-borne toxicity, namely, mycotoxins, and there has been a commensurate growth of expertise and literature in this area. Apart from noting the increasing discovery of toxic fungal contamination of standing pasture grasses typified by ergot, and more recently sporadesmin, I do not propose to consider this topic. Culvenor (7) has produced a review of this area and we have excluded the subject from this conference since it has been frequently and recently discussed in depth.

IV. THE INSTITUTIONS OF PHYTOTOXIC RESEARCH

In the expectation that this will not be the last meeting of its kind, and in the hope that from it will arise an increment of interest in the study of poison plants, I would like to devote a few paragraphs to a brief review of the institutional anatomy of your discipline. Perhaps there are lessons here for research leaders and administrators alike. In my earlier paper I mentioned briefly that poison plant research had commenced in both Australia and the United States primarily at Agricultural Experiment Stations or their equivalent. From these diffuse beginnings, some obvious centers of excellence have developed. What are these centers of excellence, how do they grow, should they be encouraged, and if so, how?

Obviously, we are meeting in Logan, Utah, because this plesant city possesses a center of excellence in phytotoxicology - the USDA Poisonous Plant Research Laboratory. Kingsbury (8) has briefly alluded to it in his history of poisonous plant research on this side of the world.

The CSIRO Animal Health Research Laboratory at Parkville, Victoria, is clearly another and, in my view, is a practical consequence of the successful research program on toxemic jaundice and, later, pyrrolizidine alkaloidosis. It now possesses the additional advantage for a primarily veterinary institution of having Dr. Culvenor with his analytical facilities as well as a number of related disciplines.

It is interesting that such major centers have not always commanded all the relevant disciplines within their staffs. Neither Logan nor Parkville currently has a botanist on staff, though their botanical mentors are here today, while Logan lacks a histopathologist and Parkville lacks a blood and guts pharmacologist-physiologist. Apparently a center of excellence can readily obtain the services of enthusiastic and competent collaborators to fill such deficiencies.

Among other reasons for development of good phytotoxic research are the very old ones of sheer curiosity, combined with the more modern use of satisfactory postgraduate and postdoctoral experience and training so that an individual develops a reputation in the field, and problems, funds, and graduate students tend to be attracted to his institution. There are several prime examples at this meeting. In addition to teaching and research, some of these individuals become motivated to write, and produce comprehensive reviews of their subject, often of continent-wide scope and global relevance.

Finally, we should not overlook the fact that occasionally, research in some related area, for reasons quite irrelevant to death of livestock from poison plants, leads directly to competence and capacity in our area of interest. Dr. Culvenor would, no doubt, agree with me that he is here today partly because the Australian Government, during the second world war, decided to take a look at potential native Australian sources of medicinal alkaloids to guard against supplies from overseas being cut off by blockade or loss by enemy action of the regions where they were usually grown.

V. CHOOSING RESEARCH TOPICS

In both Australia and the United States the research dollar is becoming relatively scarcer and more difficult to corral, while the sophistication and therefore the cost of research (not to say the salaries of research workers) are increasing significantly. Consequently, research administrators demand increasingly compelling justification for research grants or the allocation of additional resources. Therefore, I thought that it might be useful to consider where we should be going and how best to start to get there. More precisely, I propose briefly to review what I have been able to find out about the content of recent research programs in both our countries, and attempt to generalize therefrom.

A quick look at American Journal of Veterinary Research for 1976 revealed papers on only *Halogeton* (9), *Astragalus* (10), and *Helenium* (11), which might be compared with the recent Australian Veterinary Journal output on *Pimelea*, *Macrozamia*, *Solanum*, and *Pennisetum* species.

However, searching using data bases yielded a much wider list of publications from both countries, including in the United States, *Astragalus, Crotalaria, Solanum, Jojoba, Florensia,* and *Phalaris spp.*, plus some references to experimental pyrrolizidine alkaloid studies. From European authors were papers on toxins in *Daphne, Medicago, Vicia,* and *Trichodesma spp.* In Australia, *Setaria* was added.

One might summarize by saying that recent publications suggest a worldwide interest in the pyrrolizidine alkaloids, an Australian preoccupation with *Pimelea spp.* and toxic fodder plants, while in America there is continued emphasis on *Astragalus*, the oxalate-producing species, and a few Texan species. The content of the papers, however, showed little discernible pattern - perhaps this does not matter.

American colleagues may have wondered at the recent spate of papers on the relatively obscure "St. George Disease" of cattle in Queensland and elsewhere, incriminating an equally unfamiliar genus - *Pimelea*. While I will leave it to my colleagues to present the result of their investigations, I should like to relate how the work got underway.

A number of us had been aware of an enzootic disease of cattle in the St. George district of Queensland characterized by chronic facial, intermandibular, and ventral edema. Some of us had seen cases of such a syndrome in Central Australia. As long ago as 1960 I had looked at a few sections of edematous tissue without picking up any clues.

In the late 1960s graziers in the affected area of Queensland began to ask for some work to be done and although it was perceived to be a local problem of the kind that CSIRO is usually reluctant to take up, the Chief of the CSIRO Division of Animal Health found himself under some pressure to react to the requests.

It was decided to call a meeting in Brisbane of the dozen or so scientists who had seen the disease in field or laboratory, along with representatives of the state government agencies most closely concerned, the University of Queensland, CSIRO, and the Australian Meat Research Committee (which provides funds for selected research programs).

We sat down for two days, 17 field veterinarians, botanists, chemists, pathologists, microbiologists, and research administrators, and pooled our experience and knowledge. The (unpublished) report of the meeting recorded that there had been discussion of the following alternative etiological possibilities, but remarked that there was no convincing evidence to support any of them: specific and general malnutrition, plant poisoning, intoxication from surface waters, water deprivation, hematozoan infection, and other infections including viruses!

Of course the report concluded with recommendations for further research, including pathological, physiological, biochemical, ecological, toxicological, botanical, and experimental studies. But interest had been kindled, cross-fertilization occurred, money was found, programs were commenced or accelerated, and in a surprisingly short time a number of experiments had incriminated *Pimelea spp.* as the cause of this disease.

It is to be hoped that a similar and even wider increment to knowledge of poison plant syndromes may follow this meeting if we sit down to the task of defining global and regional priorities and discuss them from the comparative point of view in this international and interdisciplinary gathering.

VI. MAJOR RESEARCH OBJECTIVES

Having regard to what I have already said on the importance of the grazing ruminant animal for increased production of animal protein in previously ungrazed tropical regions, and the possibility of the development of improved water economies (12) leading to development of "improved pastures" in more temperate but dry to semiarid areas, I would like to state, quite simply, two major, worthwhile goals for phytotoxic research work during the next decade.

First, multidisciplinary investigation of the toxicologic problems of *Leucaena leucocephala* should be expanded and internationalized, in addition to work on the toxicology of mimosine, e.g., Hegarty *et al.* (13), because of the potential importance of the species as a high-protein browse plant throughout the tropics where marked seasonal nutritional deficiencies occur.

Second, there is a need to develop and use a standard methodology for screening new and improved pasture species for phytotoxins before their dissemination over large acreages of grazing land. In Australia, at least, the list of poison problems from such sewn pasture species is now a long one, including high estrogen subterranean clovers, *Phalaris spp.* containing high levels of tryptamine alkaloids, *Lolium* (rye grass), *Cenchrus*, *Pannicum*, and a number of other species. Plant breeders and agronomists traditionally have not considered the potential toxicity of their products, and there is need for a whole new look at this area (14).

VII. SOME MODERN AIDS TO RESEARCH

A. Machine Readable Data Bases

1. *Bibliographic Services*

Involvement in the information revolution in the United States and specifically in setting up a retrospective literature search service at the Australian Embassy in Washington for Australian research scientists has prompted me to devote part of this paper to this topic. Experience suggests that as yet not all Australian research scientists or administrators are aware of the wide range of such services on line in the United States. Among the bases I used for bibliographic purposes for this general paper on phytotoxicological perspectives were Biosis Previews, Cain, and Medlars

II, where we searched both "Medline" and "Toxline" files. The latter is of specific interest and value to toxicologists, but unfortunately the file is not yet available in Australia. Thus the majority of searching must be done through the National Library of Medicine at Bethesda, Maryland, but this presents no problem.

I concluded that these data bases provide useful, cheap, and efficient biographical tools but that no base seems all-inclusive. Vocabularies vary somewhat and some listings depend on keywords appearing in title or abstract. Probably each research scientist should work to the base of his choice depending on topic and experience.

2. *Current Research Topics*

The SSIE (Smithsonian Science Information Exchange) base provides a different kind of service, covering on-going and recently completed research projects from over 1300 funding institutions, principally in the United States.

Searching the SSIE file for poisonous plants produced 37 citations of current projects, attributed to the USDA Poisonous Plant Research Laboratory, Logan, Utah, and state experiment stations and universities in seven Western and Southern states. It provides for each current project a statement of its objectives, the approaches envisaged, and a report, as well as offering information about staff, funds, sponsoring, and responsible institutions. The subscriber can thereby gain an overview of current activity in any field or research that he may be contemplating entering or funding.

3. *Numerical Data Bases*

Of special interest to our chemist colleagues perhaps, these bases provide numerical data in respect of compounds likely to be encountered, as an aid to their identification. Data on mass spectra, infrared and ultraviolet spectra, NMR, RAMAN, and fluorescent spectra, as well as crystallographic data are held in various data bases (15).

B. Remote Sensing

Modern trends in monitoring environmental parameters, meteorological trends and phenomena, and perhaps of special relevance, spectral irradiation from the earth's surface using sophisticated instrumentation such as NASA's multispectral scanner from ground, aircraft, or satellites can obviously be used to assist in dealing with some of the problems of poisonous plants.

Applications that readily come to mind include monitoring of rainfall situation favoring emergence of annuals such as *Heliotropium europeum* or *I. linnaei*, delineating affected areas in time to permit stock to be removed to safety, and development of regional range condition monitoring to enable strategic placement of stock to avoid favoring emergence of undesirable dominant weed species.

Those of us concerned in any way with the health and welfare of range animals should not overlook the potential contribution of remote sensing in remote underpopulated areas.

C. Plant Breeding

The success of the green revolution in developing varieties and wide crosses of conventional graminaceous species with improved growth characteristics, seasonal and day length adaptability, and even with improved amino-acid composition for human food should be a challenge to pasture agronomists to perform similar small miracles in ridding important pasture species of many of their more important toxic characteristics. We should be looking for strains of *Phalaris* without tryptamine alkaloids, or *Leucaena* without mimosine and so on.

Such work might be accompanied by work designed to examine the comparative situations so familiar to us all: why *A. georginae* is the only one of several hundred *Acacia* species that produces fluoroacetate, and then only at certain times; the influence of climate and season on toxicity of *Phalaris tuberosa*, and so on.

VIII. FURTHER WORK ON OLD IDEAS

Before I conclude this presentation I want to take the opportunity to discuss two or three conceptual approaches to the control of phytotoxic problems in Australia, which may have an application in this hemisphere. As usual, ideas arise from one's own circumstances and experiences, and you will have to bear with me if I illustrate the concepts with Australian examples. If you can apply them successfully to other circumstances in your own country, or region, you will gain merit thereby!

We have all pondered the mechanisms of intoxication and Everist (16) has expanded on the subject in his thought-provoking introductory chapters. I refer to "factors affecting toxicity" and to all the regional, seasonal, species, and other variations that occur. It seems to be that we should give more consideration to the role of the rumen than perhaps we have done in the past. The conventional attitude is that the liver is the principal site of detoxication mechanisms, and it well may be for those molecules which reach the circulation.

However, consider two phenomena. First, *I. linnaei* is toxic for Equidae but not for ruminants. I wonder what happens to the toxic principle if it is incubated in an artificial rumen? Second, sheep grazing *H. europeum* ingest pyrrolizidine alkaloids at levels an order of magnitude or so greater than the acute LD_{50} but still take two seasons of grazing to die of megalocytosis or chronic pyrrolizidine alkaloidosis.

The proposition then is straightforward, though elucidation of the technical answer may be some way off. How can we arrange to stimulate the ruminal microbes to degrade certain phytotoxins just a little more efficiently? Can we do it, for instance, by providing a small daily supplement of lucerne (alfalfa)? Perhaps we need a slogan "when in drought, feed your ruminal microbes!"

Turning to a related situation, can we nullify the toxic effects of some fodder plants by providing dietary supplements to the animals themselves? Hooper's interesting work on protection of horses from Birdsville disease by supplements of peanuts or arginine (17) arose from experimental observations (unpublished) in our early work that while we could kill horses by feeding them *I. linnaei* with a supplement of cereal hay, its replacement by lucerne hay proved disastrous to the experiment though, of course, eminently satisfactory to the horses.

I might be beginning to sound like an alfalfa seed salesman, but you know it has a reputation as the "king of fodders" in Australia and, to the best of my knowledge, does not contain poisonous alkaloids, phytoestrogens, or other phytotoxic principles.

IX. CONCLUSION

The elation experienced by research scientists when a critical experiment supports an important hypothesis has to be experienced to be believed. I still remember one night in Alice Springs during investigation of Georgina River Poisoning. We had performed the critical experiment - dosing our guinea pigs with watery extract of *A. georginae* and the experimental animals and the controls were caged on the front veranda of my residence.

There was a dinner party going on, in honor of Sir Rudolph Peters, F.R.S., who had interrupted a visit to the Australian National University to come and advise us on fluoroacetate poisoning and its associated phenomena and who was leaving the following day. Every few minutes one of the experimenters would tip-toe outside to monitor the guinea pigs. Finally, and fortunately after dinner was finished, the pigs commenced to die and the livers and kidneys were taken into trichloracetic acid and the next morning flown to Darwin and London, then to Peter's laboratory at Tennis Court Road, whence a day or two later came back the answer we were awaiting.

But we are not here to reminisce, rather to get on with the task and the challenge of exchanging knowledge of results and techniques that will be mutually useful.

Perhaps the greatest good that will come out of this meeting comprises new ideas generated in discussion within groups of us who are familiar only with our own problems - much light may be thrown upon hitherto obscure phenomena by consideration of comparative or contrasting phenomena. Therefore, let us proceed with the more substantial papers of this symposium, pausing to recollect the Pasteurian adage that chance favors the prepared mind and not forgetting Claude Bernard's admonition that the study of things caused should precede the study of the causes of things.

X. REFERENCES

1. Steyn, D. G., "Toxicology of Plants in South Africa," Central News Agency, Capetown, 1934.
2. Hore, D., *Aust. Vet. J.* 37, 312 (1961).
3. Rose, A. L., Banks, A. W., and McConnell, J. D., *Aust. Vet. J.* 27, 189 (1951).
4. Whittem, J. H., and Murray, L. R., *Aust. Vet. J.* 39, 168 (1963).
5. Jago, M. V., Lanigan, G. W., Bingley, J. B., Piercy, D. W. T., Whittem, J. H., and Titchen, D. A., *J. Pathol.* 98, 115 (1969).
6. Rose, A. L., Gardner, C. A., McConnell, J. D., and Bull, L. B., *Aust. Vet. J.* 33, 25 (1957).
7. Culvenor, C. C. J., *Aust. Vet. J.* 50, 69 (1974).
8. Kingsbury, J. M., "Poisonous Plants of the United States and Canada," Prentice-Hall, Englewood Cliffs, New Jersey, 1964.
9. Littledike, E. T., James, L., and Cook, H., *Am. J. Vet. Res.* 37, 661 (1976).
10. James, L. F., and Van Kampen, K. R., *Am. J. Vet. Res.* 37, 845 (1976).
11. Witzel, D. A., Ivie, G. W., and Dollahite, J. W., *Am. J. Vet. Res.* 37, 859 (1976).
12. Ambroggi, R. P., *Sci. Am.* 236, 21 (1977).
13. Hegarty, M. P., Court, R. D., Christie, G. S., and Lee, C. P., *Aust. Vet. J.* 52, 490 (1976).
14. Norris, D. O., *Trop. Grassl.* 96, 159 (1972).
15. Heller, S. R., Milne, G. W. A., and Feldmanor, R. T., *Science* 195, 253 (1977).
16. Everist, S. L., "Poisonous Plants of Australia," Angus and Robertson, Sydney, 1974.
17. Hooper, P. T., Hart, B., and Smith, G. W., *Aust. Vet. J.* 47, 326 (1971).

THE HAZARD OF PLANT TOXICITIES TO THE HUMAN POPULATION

Frederick W. Oehme
Comparative Toxicology Laboratory, Kansas State University

I. ABSTRACT

*The magnitude of human hazard from plant ingestion is suggested by the fact that plants are the second most frequent hazardous material ingested by children under 5 years of age and the fifth most frequent hazardous material ingested by humans of all ages. Common household and garden plants are among those most commonly ingested. A variety of potential clinical entities can be produced by most parts of these plants, including digestive tract disorders, cardiac irregularities, hallucinogenic effects, convulsions, and liver damage. To study some of these potential hazards rats were dosed with the flower or fruit, leaf, stem, or root of Chrysanthemum (*Chrysanthemum morifolium* Ramat.), Jerusalem cherry (*Solanum pseudocapsicum*), Dieffenbachia (*Dieffenbachia picta* Schott), Geranium (*Pelargonium clonesticum* Bailey), or Philodendron (*Philodendron cordatum* Kunth), and did not exhibit overt toxicity. Organ weight/whole body weight ratios were altered for liver, spleen, and heart, but daily weight gain was not affected. There is much to be learned about the relationship between experimentally induced plant ingestion in animals and actual human exposure.*

II. INTRODUCTION

The ingestion of plants by humans is a common occurrence in all age people. According to the 1975 records of the National Clearinghouse for Poison Control Centers (1), plants were the second most frequent substance ingested by children under 5 years of age, and plants were the fifth most common substance ingested by persons of all ages. While some of these patients did not show any effects, others had symptoms that required treatment or hospitalization, and some were fatally poisoned.

Only very small amounts of some plant parts (flowers, fruits or berries, leaves, stems, bark, or roots) may be necessary to cause dramatic effects. Some plants are poisonous if they are chewed or swallowed. Others poison by causing allergies, dermatitis, or mechanical injury. Some plants are harmful only if eaten or chewed at certain stages of their growth; others are toxic at all stages. Both the species of the plant and its stage of growth or the season of the year are important in determining the potential hazard. Table 1 provides a listing of garden and household plants that have been suspected of producing human toxicity together with the toxic portion(s) of the plant, the active principle(s), and a general description of the toxicity produced.

TABLE 1

Poisonous Plants, Active Principles, and General Symptomatology of Plants Commonly Considered Hazardous to Humans

Plant name	Poisonous parts and active principles	Signs and symptoms
Arnica	Flowers and roots	GI symptoms, drowsiness, coma
Arum family: *Caladium*, calla lily, dumbcane, *Dieffenbachia*, elephant's ear, *Colocasia*, *Alocasia*, *Philodendron*, *Dracunculus*, *Amorphophallus*	All parts (calcium oxalate, unidentified principles)	Severe burning of mucous membranes with swelling of tongue and throat, nausea, vomiting, diarrhea, salivation, rare direct systemic effects
Black locust (*Robinia pseudoacacia* L.)	Bark, foliage, and seed (phytotoxin)	Nausea, vomiting, weakness, depression
Bleedingheart or Dutchman's breeches (*Dicentra cucullaria*)	All parts (isoquinoline-type alkaloids such as apomorphine, protoberberine, and protopine)	Trembling, ataxia, respiratory distress, convulsions
Castor bean (*Ricinus communis* L.)	Seed (ricin, if chewed; if swallowed whole, the hard seed coat prevents absorption and poisoning)	Severe GI symptoms, convulsions, uremia
Crowfoot family: buttercup (*Ranunculus spp.*), cowslip or marsh marigold (*Caltha palustris*), larkspur (*Delphinium*), monkshood (*Aconitum spp.*)	All parts; for monkshood, especially roots and seeds	Paresthesia, burning sensation of mouth and skin, nausea, vomiting, hypotension, weak pulse, convulsions
Daphne (*Daphne mezereum*)	All parts (daphnin)	Abdominal pain, vomiting, bloody diarrhea, weakness, convulsions

TABLE 1 (Continued)

Plant name	Poisonous parts and active principles	Signs and symptoms
Deadly nightshade (*Atropa belladonna* L.)	Berries, leaves, and roots (atropine and related alkaloids)	Fever, rapid heartbeat, dilation of pupils, skin hot, flushed, dry
Elderberry, black and scarlet elder (*Sambucus spp.*)	Leaves, shoots, and bark (sambunigrin, a cyanogenic glycoside)	Nausea, vomiting, diarrhea
Foxglove (*Digitalis purpurea*)	Leaves (digitalis glycosides)	Nausea, diarrhea, stomach pain, severe headache, irregular heartbeat and pulse, tremors, convulsions
Poison hemlock (*Conium maculatum* L.)	All parts (alkaloid coniine)	GI symptoms, necrosis, muscular weakness, respiratory paralysis, convulsions
Hyacinth (*Hyacinthus orientalis* L.)	Bulb	Severe GI symptoms
Indian tobacco (*Lobelia spp.*)	All parts (α-lobeline)	Progressive vomiting weakness, stupor, tremors, contraction of pupils, coma
Rosary pea, jequirity bean, precatory bean, prayer bean, love bean, lucky bean (*Abrus precatorius* L.)	Poisoning unlikely unless bean (abrin) is chewed; causes agglutination and hemolysis even in weak dilution	After 1 to 3 days, severe GI symptoms; drowsiness, coma, circulatory collapse hemolytic anemia, oliguria, fatal uremia
Jessamine or yellow jessamine (*Gelsemium sempervirens*)	All parts (gelsemine and gelseminine)	Profuse sweating, muscular weakness, convulsions, respiratory depression
Thornapple, jimsonweed, stinkweed (*Datura spp.*)	All parts (atropine and related alkaloids)	Thirst, dilation of pupils, dry mouth, red skin, headache, hallucinations, rapid pulse, high blood pressure, delirium, convulsions, coma

TABLE 1 (Continued)

Plant name	Poisonous parts and active principles	Signs and symptoms
Lantana (*Lantana camara*), red sage, wild sage	All parts (lantanin), especially the green berries	Photosensitization with increase in severity from sunlight, acute symptoms resemble belladonna alkaloid (atropine) poisoning, salivation, lacrimation
Laurel: mountain (*Kalmia latifolia*), black (*Leucothoe davisiae*), sheep (*K. angustifolia* L.)	All parts (andromedotoxin)	Salivation, lacrimation, rhinorrhea, vomiting, convulsions, slowing of pulse, hypotension, paralysis
Lily-of-the-valley (*Convallaria majalis* L.)	Leaves and flowers (convallatoxin and other glycosides)	Irregular heartbeat, stomach upset
Mushrooms (*Amanita muscaria* and *Amanita phalloides*)	All parts (muscarine and phalloidine)	Muscarine produces sudden stomach cramps, thirst, watering of eyes and mouth, sweating, breathing difficulty, diarrhea, vomiting, mental disturbances, coma, convulsions. Phalloidine, after a delay of 6 to 24 hours, produces vomiting, diarrhea, liver damage and failure, followed in 2 to 10 days by circulatory failure and coma
Mistletoe (*Phoradendron serotinum*)	Berries (β-phenylethylamine and tyramine)	GI symptoms and bradycardia similar to digitalis
Narcissus family: daffodil, jonquil (*Narcissus spp.*)	Bulb	GI symptoms
Nutmeg (*Myristica fragrans*)	Seeds (myristicin)	Hallucinations and elation, stomach pain, red skin, dry mouth, drowsiness, stupor, double vision,

TABLE 1 (Continued)

Plant name	Poisonous parts and active principles	Signs and symptoms
		delirium. (Two nutmegs can be fatal.)
Oleander (*Nerium oleander*)	Leaves (oleandrin and nerioside)	Nausea, severe vomiting, stomach pain, dizziness, slowed pulse, irregular heartbeat, marked dilation of pupils, bloody diarrhea, drowsiness, unconsciousness, paralysis of lungs. (One leaf can kill an adult.)
Pokeweed, pokeberry, scoke, inkberry (*Phytolacca americana* L.)	All parts, especially root (saponin and glycoproteins in African species produce lymphocytes that resemble those in Burkitt's lymphoma.	Burning bitter taste in mouth, persistent vomiting, amblyopia, slowed respiration, dyspnea, weakness, tremors, and convulsions, peripheral blood plasmacytosis. (May be fatal.)
Rhododendron	All parts	Salivation, lacrimation, rhinorrhea, vomiting, convulsions, slowing of pulse, hypotension, paralysis
Rhubarb (*Rheum rhaponticum*)	Leaves only (oxalic acid)	Nausea, vomiting, abdominal pain, anuria, hemorrhages
Sweet pea (*Lathyrus spp.*)	All parts, but especially seeds (β-aminopropionitrile, α-γ-aminobutyric acid)	Paralysis, slow and weak pulse, respiratory depression, convulsions
Water hemlock or cowbane, beaver poison (*Cicuta spp.*)	Roots (resin cicutoxin)	GI symptoms, convulsions, respiratory depression
Wisteria (*Wisteria sinensis*)	Pods (resin and glycoside, wisterin)	Severe GI symptoms, collapse

TABLE 1 (Continued)

Plant name	Poisonous parts and active principles	Signs and symptoms
Yew (*Taxus spp.*)	All parts (alkaloid taxine)	GI symptoms, dilation of pupils, muscular weakness, coma, convulsions, cardiac and respiratory depression

III. GENERAL ETIOLOGICAL SYNDROMES

It is very difficult to prepare meaningful statistics on serious or fatal poisonings by plants because of incomplete reporting and limited means for physicians to obtain plant identifications. However, many published reference works and review articles are available on the potential hazard to humans of plant contact and ingestion (2-6). The general toxic syndromes and causative plant-chemical agents associated with the most frequent poisoning situations (7) may be reviewed with some advantage.

A. Gastroenteritis-Inducing Plants

The majority of plant intoxications in the United States occur from the ingestion of plants containing gastroenteric irritants. Symptoms range from burning in the mouth and throat when toddlers chew the leaves of such common household plants as from the vine growing on the window sill (*Philodendron* species) or of the dumbcane (*Dieffenbachia* species) in the big pot by the front door to severe vomiting, intestinal cramping, and purging diarrhea from the fresh roots and stems of the pokeweed (*Phytolacca americana*), *Wisteria* seeds, the berries of the spurge laurel (*Daphne* species), or the leaves of buttercups (*Ranunculus* species). The onset of the irritant response is variable depending upon the chemical nature of the toxin, the necessity for biological activation of the irritant, and to the various mechanisms which may be evoked for the elicitation of emesis or gastroenteritis. Many plants, which may cause only minor abdominal discomfort in an adult, may provoke profound emesis and diarrhea in a small child. Dehydration and electrolyte imbalance can develop rapidly and it may be necessary to institute replacement therapy to prevent shock.

Serious intoxications are produced by plants containing toxalbumins, e.g., the rosary pea (*Abrus precatorius*) and castor bean (*Ricinus communis*). Following ingestion of the chewed seeds of either of these plants there may be a considerable delay prior to the onset of symptoms. This is related to the quantity of material but typically the latent period is about two hours but may be a day or more. The clinical picture is one of severe hemorrhagic gastroenteritis with persistent nausea, emesis, colic, and profuse diarrhea. The severe dehydration may result in oliguria, and cardiovascular collapse. In non-fatal cases the period of intoxication is about three to ten days.

B. Digitalis-Containing Plants

Humans have been fatally poisoned by eating the berries, chewing on the leaves or flowers, or drinking water from vases containing the flowers of digitalis-containing plants such as lily-of-the-valley (*Convallaria majalis*), foxglove (*Digitalis purpurea),* and oleander (*Nerium oleander*). Initially there is a local irritation to the mouth and emesis. In contrast to the pure cardiac glycosides, poisoning by these plants will be associated with diarrhea and abdominal pain due to the presence of saponins and other irritants. Otherwise the intoxication is similar to that which is seen with digitalis overdosage.

C. Nicotine, Cytisine, and Coniine-Containing Plants

These alkaloids all exert similar actions from a toxicological viewpoint. A number of fatal poisonings have occurred in the Western states because parents have prepared "salads" from wild flora which include wild tobacco leaves (*Nicotiana* species). Cytisine poisoning is most commonly encountered in the persons who sell shell and eat the seeds from the pea-like pods of the golden chain tree (*Laburnum anagyroides*). Coniine intoxications follow nibbling of the parsley-like leaves or from eating the seeds from poison hemlock (*Conium maculatum*). Usually there is a spontaneous emesis within one hour and most commonly within 15 minutes of ingestion. This is accompanied by profuse salivation. Abdominal cramping is usually minimal and diarrhea is quite rare. One may anticipate headache, confusion, incoordination, hyperpyrexia, and sometimes mydriasis and tachycardia. Fatalities result from respiratory failure.

D. Atropine-Containing Plants

Although a number of plants in the United States contain atropine and its related alkaloids by far the most important in human poisoning is jimsonweed (*Datura stramonium*). Toxicity may be produced by eating the seeds or sucking the flowers. The early symptoms are mydriasis with blurring of vision due to loss of accommmodation and dryness of the mouth which presents as thirst followed by dysphagia and speech difficulties. The skin becomes hot, dry, and flushed, with a rash occasionally appearing about the face, ears, and neck. In more severe intoxications there is pronounced hyperpyrexia, delirium and hallucinations. Convulsions may appear in young children. Ultimately coma can develop.

Atropine poisoning mimics a variety of pathologic states such as encephalitis, meningitis, uremia, concussion, and overt psychosis. Exclusion can be made in that atropine poisoning consistently produces equal, bilateral pupillary dilation; hot, dry skin; and tachycardia. Young children are more sensitive to atropine poisoning because of their lower tolerance to elevated body temperature. Fatalities due to atropine-containing plant intoxications are uncommon and recovery, other than to the persistent mydriasis, is usually complete within 24 hours.

E. Convulsion-Producing Plants

In this country the principal plants responsible for producing convulsions as their primary toxic manifestation are the water hemlocks (*Cicuta* species). Since these plants are found only in wet, swampy areas they are more likely to be ingested by older children who mistake them for wild parsnips. Being encountered on hikes and camping trips, many persons may be involved in a single incident. Within 15 minutes to one hour after ingestion the patient experiences nausea, salivation, emesis, and tremors. This prodroma is followed quickly by multiple grand mal seizures. Death occurs secondary to prolonged anoxia encountered during the tonic contractions.

F. Mushrooms

If the rapid and reasonably accurate identification of poisonous plants is difficult for physicians, the identification of mushrooms is virtually impossible. The mushroom so frequently pictured in story books with the red cap covered in polka dot fashion with white spots is the *Amanita muscaria*. Mushrooms of this group produce manic excitement and hallucinations about two to three hours after ingestion, usually after an initial period of drowsiness. The central excitement usually does not exceed 3 to 4 hours.

There is a specific group of muscarine-containing mushrooms with which symptoms begin within 15 minutes of ingestion with sweating, salivation, and colic. Moist rales may be present. This toxin cannot cross the blood-brain barrier in sufficient quantity to produce central nervous system effects.

The remaining subgroup of toxic mushrooms with a rapid onset of action are those which produce primarily a severe gastroenteritis. Whereas wild mushrooms eaten by adults will almost invariably have been cooked, a process that markedly reduces or inactivates a number of irritants and even some major toxins, this is not the case with childhood experimentation which may well account for some of the pediatric fatalities following the ingestion of normally "non-toxic" species.

The most serious mushroom poisoning is that in which there has been a latent period of about 12 hours prior to the onset of symptoms. These mushrooms belong to the *Amanita phalloides* group. Such intoxications have a very grave prognosis. These mushrooms contain two classes of thermostable, cyclic polypeptides, the phallotoxins and the amatoxins, which have distinct pharmacological properties. The phallotoxins act initially, signaling the end of the latent period with nausea, emesis, painful colic, and a watery, sometimes bloody diarrhea. Following a symptom-free period of three to five days, during which the patient seems to be making a rapid recovery, the hepatorenal toxicity of the amatoxins becomes evident. If only a small quantity has been ingested only renal tubular necrosis is seen, whereas large doses may produce fatal hepatic damage before renal necrosis has had time to develop. Although both of these are seen clinically, more commonly a hepatorenal syndrome terminating in hepatic failure produced by intermediate dosage is encountered.

A high mortality is associated with mushroom intoxication in children.

IV. PLANTS MOST COMMONLY INGESTED

Of all the varieties of plants in gardens, households, and fields, certain types are more often encountered in potential human poisoning situations than others. These tend to be those that are commonly grown in or around the home and those plants that are most conspicuous and attractive to the passing individual. Table 2 lists in order of frequency the twelve plants reported most often ingested by children during 1975 (8).

TABLE 2

Plants (Excluding Mushrooms and Toadstools) Involved in Ingestion by Children Under 5 Years of Age in 1975 (8)

Name	Cases	% Total category
1. Philodendron *(Philodendron sp.)*	645	11.3
2. Pokeweed *(Phytolacca americana)*	402	7.0
3. Holly Berries *(Ilex sp.)*	333	5.8
4. Pyracantha *(Pyracantha sp.)*	306	5.3
5. Poinsettia *(Euphorbia pulcherrima)*	278	4.9
6. Dieffenbachia *(Dieffenbachia sp.)*	257	4.5
7. Woody Nightshade *(Solanum sp.)*	232	4.1
8. Black Elder *(Sambucus sp.)*	174	3.0
9. Jerusalem Cherry *(Solanum pseudo-capsicum)*	138	2.4
10. African Violets *(Saintpaulia spp.)*	125	2.2
11. Elephant Ear Plant *(Colocasia sp.)*	116	2.0
12. Begonia *(Begonia sp.)*	102	1.8
Total plants	5727	

V. EXPERIMENTAL STUDIES OF SELECTED FLORAL PLANTS

Since allegations of human hazard from floral plants occur periodically, most recently in relation to the increasing emphasis on safety in all areas of human environment, studies of such possibilities were reviewed. Experimental data to support or refute such allegations was sparse. Dosage trials were undertaken at Kansas State University to investigate what effects, if any, a group of selected ornamental plants may produce when administered in large doses to experimental animals.

A. Materials and Methods

Chrysanthemum (*Chrysanthemum morifolium*), Jerusalem cherry (*Solanum pseudocapsicum*), Dieffenbachia (*Dieffenbachia picta* Schott), Geranium (*Pelargonium clonesticum*), and Philodendron (*Philodendron cordatum*) were selected by the Society of American Florists as economically important plants. Twenty growing specimens of each of the plants for study in saleable condition were provided by cooperating florists. All plants were botanically identified and representative specimens preserved for later reference. Plants were maintained in the Kansas State University greenhouses under careful supervision to avoid chemical exposure and to maintain standardized growing conditions. After 60 days of cultivation, representative portions of roots, stems, leaves, flowers, or fruits were randomly collected for animal dosing. Twenty-three groups of albino male rats consisting of seven rats per group with each rat weighing 200-300 grams were randomly selected. Each rat was dosed via stomach tube with five grams (wet weight) per kilogram of body weight of the respective homogenized portion of the particular plant under study, as stipulated by the Federal Hazardous Substances Act Regulations of the Consumer Products Safety Commission (9). Homogenates of flower, leaf, stem, and root were administered from Chrysanthemum (*Chrysanthemum morifolium*); fruit, leaf, stem, and root were given from Jerusalem cherry (*Solanum pseudocapsicum*); leaf, stem, and root were utilized from Dieffenbachia (*Dieffenbachia picta* Schott); flower, leaf, stem, and root were administered from Geranium (*Pelargonium clonesticum*); and leaf, stem, and root were utilized from Philodendron (*Philodendron cordatum*).

All rats were housed in individual cages and were examined carefully for fifteen days following dosing. General health, food and water consumption, and body weight were carefully observed, and any indication of ill effects was noted and daily weight gains were calculated. All animals were humanely sacrificed on the sixteenth day following dosing. A gross post mortem examination was performed and all tissues visually examined. All major organs were weighed and the percent organ weight/total body weight was calculated.

Biological values for weight gain and organ weight/body weight ratios were summed and mean values determined for each experimental and control group. Statistical analyses were performed on the mean values from each group versus the respective control group for organ weight/body weight ratios and the slope of the daily weight gain. Student's "t" test was employed with significant differences established at P = 95% and highly significant differences at P = 99%.

B. Results

Clinical signs of disease or adverse health effects from administering the respective portions of the floral plants were not observed in any of the experimental animals. Feed consumption, weight gain, and general health were not significantly depressed in any of the experimental groups. The slope of the daily weight gain was significantly less (P = 95%) in the group receiving Dieffenbachia (*Dieffenbachia picta*) root when compared with the control group (See Table 3).

The results of the statistical evaluation of the organ weight/total body weight percentages are given in Table 3. The differences when compared with the control (P = 95%) were observed in the liver ratios of those groups receiving the Chrysanthemum (*Chrysanthemum morifolium*) leaf, Jerusalem cherry (*Solanum pseudocapsicum*) fruit, Dieffenbachia (*Dieffenbachia picta*) root, or Geranium (*Pelargonium clonesticum*) leaf or stem; in the spleen weights of those groups receiving Jerusalem cherry (*Solanum pseudocapsicum*) stem or root, or Geranium (*Pelargonium clonesticum*) flower or stem; and in the heart weights from animals receiving Chrysanthemum (*Chrysanthemum morifolium*) stem, Jerusalem cherry (*Solanum pseudocapsicum*) stem, or Dieffenbachia (*Dieffenbachia picta*) stem. Highly significant differences (P = 99%) were observed in liver weights from those rats receiving Jerusalem cherry (*Solanum pseudocapsicum*) leaf or Dieffenbachia (*Dieffenbachia picta*) stem; in kidney weights from rats receiving Jerusalem cherry (*Solanum pseudocapsicum*) leaf; in spleen weights from animals receiving Geranium (*Pelargonium clonesticum*) leaf or root, or Philodendron (*Philodendron cordatum*) leaf or root; and in heart weights of rats dosed with Chrysanthemum (*Chrysanthemum morifolium*) flower or leaf, or Geranium (*Pelargonium clonesticum*) root.

C. Discussion and Conclusions

The absence of clinical signs of toxicity or death in animals receiving the homogenized portions of the respective plants suggests that overt poisoning did not occur in rats under this experimental procedure. Lack of interference with general health and maintenance of body condition further supports this lack of toxicity.

The significant reduction in daily weight gain in the group

TABLE 3

Results of Student's "t" Test Evaluation of Organ/Body Weight Ratios from Rats Fed Various Parts of Selected Floral Plants

Plant and part	Organ weight represented as percent body weight: Liver	Kidneys	Spleen	Lungs	Heart	Brain	Daily weight gain
Chrysanthemum *(Chrysanthemum morifolium)*							
Flower	NS	NS	NS	NS	HS↑	NS	NS
Leaf	S↓	NS	NS	NS	HS↑	NS	NS
Stem	NS	NS	NS	NS	S↑	NS	NS
Root	NS	NS	NS	NS	NS	NS	NS
Jerusalem Cherry *(Solanum pseudocapsicum)*							
Leaf	HS↑	HS↑	NS	NS	NS	NS	NS
Fruit	S↑	NS	NS	NS	NS	NS	NS
Stem	NS	NS	S↓	NS	S↓	NS	NS
Root	NS	NS	S↓	NS	NS	NS	NS
Dieffenbachia *(Dieffenbachia picta)*							
Leaf	NS	NS	NS	NS	NS	NS	NS
Stem	HS↑	NS	NS	NS	S↓	NS	NS
Root	S↑	NS	NS	NS	NS	NS	S↓
Geranium *(Pelargonium clonesticum)*							
Flower	NS	NS	S↑	NS	NS	NS	NS
Leaf	S↑	NS	HS↑	NS	NS	NS	NS
Stem	S↑	NS	S↑	NS	NS	NS	NS
Root	NS	NS	HS↑	NS	HS↑	NS	NS
Philodendron *(Philodendron cordatum)*							
Leaf	NS	NS	HS↑	NS	NS	NS	NS
Stem	NS	NS	NS	NS	NS	NS	NS
Root	NS	NS	HS↑	NS	NS	NS	NS

NS = no significant difference
S = significant difference (95%)
HS = highly significant difference (90%)
↑ = increase in percent body weight
↓ = decrease in percent body weight

receiving Dieffenbachia (*Dieffenbachia picta*) root suggests some potential chronic internal (perhaps microscopic pathologic or biochemical) effect due to the administered plant portion. The variable significant and highly significant alterations in liver, kidney, spleen, and heart weights further suggests that the respective portions of the plant may have induced subclinical tissue alterations on a microscopic or biochemical level. The presence of effects in the liver, spleen, and heart, with little if any effects on kidney, lung, and brain weights, supports the concept that the alterations are related to circulating plant compounds that would insult the liver first and effect, via the circulating blood, spleen, and heart. The recognized stability of the lungs and brain to plant materials and the primary role of the kidneys as excretory organs are further supported by these observations.

These studies indicate that rats receiving large oral doses of flower or fruit, leaf, stem, or root of Chrysanthemum (*Chrysanthemum morifolium*), Jerusalem cherry (*Solanum pseudocapsicum*), Dieffenbachia (*Dieffenbachia picta*), Geranium (*Pelargonium clonesticum*), or Philodendron (*Philodendron cordatum*) do not develop clinical toxicity. Doses in excess of those administered in this study would likely be required to be consumed by other animals or humans to produce any toxicity. It is unlikely that the average child or adult would voluntarily consume such amounts. To exceed the dose used in this study, a forty-pound child would be required to chew and swallow in excess of 100 grams (3 1/3 ounces or 7 tablespoonfuls) of fresh plant material. Since Dieffenbachia (*Dieffenbachia picta*) root is an impractical material for human consumption, it is unlikely that any hazard is present for human consumption of this material.

The changes in organ weight/total body weight ratios cause concern for subtle alterations associated with consumption of the various plant parts. Although gross examination of the tissues revealed no visable evidence of damage, histopathological studies would be required to determine the type and degree of any organ pathology. While the observations of this study are valid for the experimental conditions and are as stipulated by the Federal Hazardous Substances Act Regulations, it is difficult to extrapolate them to potential exposure in humans. Such confirmatory data can only be secured by actual trials or clinical experience in that ultimate consumer; however, additional confidence in the applicability of these results to people could be obtained by further studies utilizing other animal species.

VI. NEEDS FOR BETTER EVALUATION OF HUMAN HAZARD FROM PLANTS

The problem of predicting human toxicity from potential ingestion or contact with plants is not easily solved. The usual source of well-documented case reports in humans has been diminished in recent years. For the physician, the problem is complicated by the difficulty in obtaining a history from a very young patient, by not knowing whether one is dealing with a solitary or multiple plant ingestion, and by the uncertainty of whether the toxicity is due to the plant *per se* or whether one is dealing with an insecticide, herbicide, or liquid fertilizer. In recent years, financial support for the chemical identification and pharmacological evaluation of plant toxins and for the investigation of the hazards of and new treatment procedures for plant poisonings has been minimal.

However, there is a sense of urgency and a realistic need to have better and more accurate information for use in emergency situations of human plant ingestions. Since human experimentation is impossible, studies are needed on the effects of various plants when ingested by more human-relevant species than rats. In particular, more specific and greater in-depth evaluations should be performed as part of such studies to detect possible subtle effects produced by the suspect plants. For even more definitive data, better reporting is needed of the effects of actual plant ingestions and whether or not poisoning (i.e., signs of toxicity) occurred as a result. Ingestion is not poisoning. Finally, the health profession must make a conscientious effort to document all cases of clinical poisonings in humans due to plants, so that the observed signs, clinical duration, and effect of treatment can be applied to benefit the next instance of human exposure to possibly toxic plants.

VII. REFERENCES

1. Bulletin, National Clearinghouse for Poison Control Centers, U. S. Department HEW, Food and Drug Administration, Bethesda, Maryland, February 1977.
2. Hardin, J. W., and Arena, J. M., "Human Poisoning from Native and Cultivated Plants," 2nd Ed. Duke University, Durham, North Carolina, 1973.
3. Kingsbury, J. M., "Poisonous Plants of the United States and Canada," Prentice-Hall, Englewood Cliffs, New Jersey, 1964.
4. Kingsbury, J. M., *Clin. Pharmacol. Ther.* 10, 163 (1969).
5. Kingsbury, J. M., *Clin. Toxicol.* 2, 143 (1969).
6. Lampe, K. F., and Fagerstrom, R., "Plant Toxicity and Dermatitis: A Manual for Physicians," Williams & Wilkins Co., Baltimore, 1968.
7. Lampe, K. F., *Pediatrics* 54, 347 (1974).
8. Bulletin, National Clearinghouse for Poison Control Centers, U. S. Department HEW, Food and Drug Administration, Bethesda, Maryland, April 1977.
9. Federal Hazardous Substances Act, Sec. 2(h)(1) as amended (15 USC 1261).

ECOLOGY OF POISONING

John M. Kingsbury
New York State College of Veterinary Medicine, Cornell University

I. ABSTRACT

Poisoning of vertebrates represents a toxic equation between specific actions of compounds that have arisen in one evolved part of the biota (plants) and specific systems in another (vertebrates). Pressure on plants to evolve defensive mechanisms is greater and more pervasive from herbivorous insects than from the larger herbivorous vertebrates. Secondary compounds of plants form a major defense against insects and may provide other direct benefits for the plant as well. The unusual molecular diversity of secondary compounds and the range of toxic effects they produce in the larger vertebrates have probably not evolved (in most cases) from advantages resulting from those effects, but are instead accidental characteristics of compounds evolved for other positive selective reasons.

II. INTRODUCTION

Why are some higher vascular plants poisonous to the larger domestic and wild vertebrates? Few authors have addressed this question in the past twenty years (1). Muenscher, in the standard American text on poisonous plants of a generation ago (2) summarized contemporary thinking in the following words: "Many hypotheses have been advanced to explain the significance of toxic substances produced in plants, as, that they are developed to protect the plants against herbivorous animals, are waste products, are stages in the processes of metabolism. Of these suggestions the first appears the least acceptable, and the last the most plausible."

Plants and animals have evolved from the same basic biological origins. The structure of the unspecialized plant or animal cell, the ultrastructure of the organelles within it, and the functions they perform are remarkably similar, and their basic biochemistry even more so. Even at the level of the whole organism, simple algae and protozoa possess intergrading characteristics, and the line separating plants from animals is not clear. The study of toxicity of vascular plants in relation to larger vertebrate animals can be approached, then, as the study of compounds evolved in one advanced part of the biota that promote a seriously deleterious reaction when they come in contact with systems evolved in another major part of the biota. In this sense, the study of plant poisons is an examination of an essence of the differences between plants and animals. It should always be possible (though sometimes difficult) to identify the specific reactants on either side of the toxic equation. Why each should be present (of what benefit to the plant or animal) is also worthy of consideration when the toxic equation is known in detail, and when it is understood, deepens insight into the nature of poisoning.

Poisonings emphasize evolutionary differences. The similarity between plant and animal cells is, however, the greater generalization. In consequence, a typical plant cell meets all or almost all of the fundamental nutritional needs of an animal, and animals from insects to vertebrates differ little if at all in their basic nutritional needs (3,4,5). All respiring systems nevertheless produce some end products which would eventually be poisonous to the producer or unspecialized consumer if allowed to accumulate or become concentrated in living cells (6). Cycles of production and consumption are seldom exactly complete or completely balanced. Early organisms, living and evolving in an aquatic milieu, could expel water soluble or lipid soluble metabolic wastes directly into the ambient aqueous environment. In the landward migration plants developed mechanisms by which such wastes were isolated or detoxified. Animals evolved specialized enzymes that detoxify certain wastes and excretory routes for others. The metamorphosis from tadpole to toad (7), or even the transition from neonatal to independent mammal (8), is accompanied by the appearance of detoxifying enzyme systems. Living on land brought increased diversity into the chemistry of organisms.

A tremendous advance in knowledge of the chemistry of organisms has taken place in the past two decades. The ability of the chemist to isolate, identify, and investigate the interesting reactions of the lesser or more complex compounds has been greatly enhanced by powerful new techniques and increasingly sensitive instrumentation. The systematic biologist has discovered in these compounds new potential for ordering plant and animal kingdoms and for resolving problems of taxonomy raised by older methods (9). Increasingly the ecologist has appreciated their significance in controlling biological interrelationships. Most important of all, the agricultural scientist finds these compounds central in the relationship of herbivore or pathogen to crop plant and sees possibilities for new methods of biological control of agricultural pests (5). Hundreds of research papers have appeared from these research stimuli in the past twenty years, and enough data are now on record that substantial patterns of relationship can be expected to emerge (10). Toxicity is one of these patterns. References cited in the following review are not intended to be complete, but only to provide access to the pertinent literature.

III. SECONDARY COMPOUNDS

The chemistry of plants has long been divided into primary compounds (those involved in the basic metabolism of the plant) and secondary compounds (those not so involved) (4). This is not a very rigorous definition. Most authors skirt the issue when dealing with secondary compounds by listing them rather than defining them. Lists include such things as glycosides, tannins, saponins, essential oils, organic acids, phenolics, terpenoids, steroids, flavonoids, cyanogenic glycosides, rotenoids, polyacetylenes, mustard oils, betaines, free amino acids, etc. (e.g. 11,12, 13,14). As is usual with such lists, the terms are not mutually exclusive because they are not organized in a single non-redundant conceptual scheme. Lists of secondary compounds in plants read like lists of poisons in poisonous plants texts (15).

Since most plants can meet the fundamental nutritional needs of a herbivore, success of feeding is related to the positive or negative characteristics of the secondary compounds in the plant (3). All vascular plants contain numerous secondary compounds and often some that are unique to the species. Whittaker (16) has proposed replacing the term "secondary compounds" with "allelochemics," defining the latter as non-nutritional chemicals produced by organisms of one species which affect the growth, health, behavior, or population biology of another. Toxicity is only a part (but an important part) of these relationships.

A conception of secondary compounds as toxic metabolic wastes goes back to the early 1800's (17). In the late 1800's, Stahl believed that plants used secondary compounds primarily for protection and that such compounds had evolved for that purpose as thorns had for mechanical protection (4). While most secondary compounds are potentially toxic to vertebrates given adequate exposure, it does not necessarily follow that these secondary compounds have evolved because of the benefits such potential toxicity confers on the possessor. The common idea that poisonous plants benefit in competition with harmless species when the herbivorous vertebrates that might feed on them are killed or injured is simplistic and unsatisfactory on closer scrutiny. The historical generalizations are no longer tenable without modification (18).

IV. ROLES OF SECONDARY COMPOUNDS

Work with insects dominates recent literature on effects of secondary compounds so much so that "herbivorous insect" has been abbreviated simply to "herbivore" in some reports (19). Insects are major predators of plants. Ehrlich and Raven have suggested (20) that the rapid diversification of angiosperms took place behind a screen of toxic secondary compounds found in terrestrial gymnosperms. The coevolution of angiosperms and insects has had since mid-Cretaceous (more than 100 million years) to operate. Some spectacularly refined interactions have resulted. Secondary compounds are all-important in the food-finding, feeding, and breeding (successful completion of life cycle) success of herbivorous insects. Responses to secondary compounds may be behavioral (attraction, stimulation, repulsion) or physiological (nutritional, inhibitional, toxic) (21,22). The behavioral responses depend on reactions that are commonly classified as taste, smell, touch, or sight. Taste and smell, particularly, may not represent the same kind of function that these terms describe for man's reactions to secondary compounds. Some insect species have developed specific mechanisms to isolate or detoxify certain otherwise dangerous secondary compounds and have profited from the resulting non-competitive access to plants containing them. These compounds may now function as attractants for these insects. In complex specializations for pollination, plants and insects have coevolved relationships beneficial to both based on specific flavonoid compounds in plants (23). Certain butterflies accumulate poisons from plants and thus defend themselves against ingestion by birds. Other innocuous butterflies mimic the appearance of poisonous ones thus acquiring protection from predation (24,25). Some herbivorous insects employ the seasonally changing concentration of secondary compounds in plants to control their own breeding season (26). Plants may in turn produce compounds (ecdysones) that act as hormones in insects and so interfere with normal metamorphosis (27). Insects can modify the growth responses of plants through the mediation of enzymes that act on secondary compounds to effect the reactivation of the plant's growth hormones, and a gall results (28).

These kinds of relationships are occasionally the result of a specific response by a herbivore to a specific compound in a plant. More often, however, the insect responds only after integrating specific reactions to many secondary compounds, some positive, some negative (18). Negative effects may not be immediately obvious (19). Similarly, the full ecological effect of allelochemic relationships among organisms cannot be appreciated by examining only the relationship between one predator and one host. The net effect of relationships mediated by secondary compounds is more complex. Each allelochemic event sets in motion a chain of actions throughout the interrelating populations inhabiting the area in question. Individual plants may specialize their capabilities for defense so that the total defensive effort of the plant population is greater for the individual members than each could have mustered on its own. Such mutually reinforcing communities have been called "defense guilds" (29). These webs of action, reaction, and interaction require a second order level of understanding of the toxic equation.

The impression arising from relationships like those outlined above is of a constant mutual pressure between herbivorous insects and plants over evolutionary time. Insects are genetically programmed to respond in predictable ways to secondary compounds genetically fixed in plants. Small genetic breakthroughs of advantage to one side, amplified rapidly by the selective characteristics of the advantage, are met by counter breakthroughs of defense or counteradvantage on the other side. The totality is a continuing, fine-tuned equilibrium between plants and herbivorous insects with occasional perturbations that may or may not self-correct in time.

Patterns may be emerging from these data concerning the nature of strategies used by herbivorous insects (and perhaps other herbivors) in relating attack and defense most efficiently to the available resources of the organism (30,31,32,33,34,35). Herbs, with brief life spans, usually in large populations, with massive means of dispersal, employ selective toxicity against specific herbivorous insects. By their numbers and fecundity, many escape attack or are vulnerable at most to a limited number of insects, so an elaborate generalized defense against all insects does not make a particularly good investment of resources for them. Long-lived woody plants on the other hand may produce few seeds per growing season, are inescapably found by herbivorous insects of various kinds over their life spans, and can benefit from a generalized defense against a spectrum of attack (often by tannin-mediated undigestibility).

Secondary compounds also mediate reactions between species of plants by which one species prevents another from living close to it (36). Inhibiting secondary compounds may be volatile (terpenes), diffusing through the air, they may pass directly from the plant into the soil surrounding it, or they may cycle into the soil through dead leaves and other plant litter (37,38).

The amounts, reactive pathways, and distribution in the plant give insight into possible additional functions of secondary compounds. Some exhibit high turnover rates (18), and important metabolic functions have been identified for a few, as, for example, the relationship of certain phenolics to dormancy and the breaking of dormancy in plants (28). The pool of phenolics is often secondary only to that of carbohydrates (39). As a rule, these compounds are readily degraded or respired. Much of the pool of phenolics is, however, metabolically inactive and may represent plant wastes rendered harmless by glycosylation. Tanin-complexed proteins cannot be digested (40). Isoflavonoids mimic steroids in structure and some may be steroid antimetabolites (23). Examination of the reactions of cyanogenic glycosides (12) shows clearly that the roles of just this one category of secondary compounds are multiple. In general plants are not profligate with nitrogen, especially if additional work is required to reach a stable end product. Yet cyanogenic glycosides are often concentrated in the older parts of stems or in bark where they are isolated from the reactive parts of the plants and can be considered excreted waste. They are also often concentrated in seeds where they are probably not wastes. Cyanogenic glycosides are known to participate importantly in the synthesis of asparagine from aspartic acid. On the other hand, their concentration in the plant is often far greater than can be explained by all possible metabolic roles known for them. Thus, cyanogenic glycosides are sometimes the inert end products of nitrogen metabolism removed from the reactions of the plant at the expense of energy and nitrogen, yet at other times they are functionally important in metabolism or concentrated in metabolically active locations. In either role, they benefit the plant as a defense mechanism against herbivorous insects (most but not all of which are susceptible to cyanide poisoning) or vertebrates.

The ease with which plants form new secondary compounds varies. Some compounds appear to be evolutionary relics, presisting tenaciously. Others, previously unknown, arise when two closely related species are hybridized (10). The genetics of alkaloid formation, well-examined, has proved to be unexpectedly complex.

In summary, secondary compounds or allelochemics are ubiquitous in plants, often abundant in amount, numerous, chemically heterogeneous, and taxonomically scattered or gathered among plant families (16). Some appear to be waste products, detoxified by the plant in various energy-expensive ways, or sequestered into cell walls, vacuoles, or heart wood, shedding bark, or senescent leaves. A few many be involved in important metabolic processes of the plant.

V. POISONOUS PLANTS AND LARGER VERTEBRATES

Most of the work to date on the toxicity of secondary compounds has been related to herbivorous insects. Vertebrates differ from insects in many behavioral and structural ways. One, simply, is size. Since vertebrates differ among themselves enormously in size, this discussion is limited to the larger domestic and wild mammals. When an insect goes foraging, it usually makes a meal (or even a lifetime consumption) from a single species of plant, a single plant, a single leaf on a plant, or even a single leaf in a single stage of development. Larger herbivorous vertebrates must necessarily move from plant to plant and usually from species to species to satisfy a single meal (continuous feeding) and may take several hours in the process, covering linear distances of a kilometer or more. It is evolutionarily easier for insects to evolve specific detoxification mechanisms to match the toxic characteristics of a limited diet than it is for the vertebrates. The heterogeneity of the diet of larger vertebrates, their smaller populations, lesser fecundity, and longer generation times compared with those of typical insects, make the evolution of specific detoxification mechanisms against the secondary compounds in plants slower and less certain. Instead, mammals appear to be generalists in detoxification. Mammalian livers possess a rich store of immediate and inducible mixed-function oxidases capable of detoxifying many classes of secondary compounds in various oxidative ways. Some invertebrates possess mixed-function oxidases as well (41), but not as richly.

Another important way in which vertebrates differ from insects is in the sensory reactions we imprecisely term taste and smell, and behavioral responses embodied in such words as curiosity, preference (volitional), and learning. Populations of insects exert a continuing pressure on a species of forage plant, a pressure that can adapt rapidly to defensive changes in the plant. The larger vertebrates, in contrast, display a more idiosyncratic element in their foraging. All husbandmen are familiar with the situation in which animals will explore (by eating) the foliage of trees or brush cut down in a pasture which they have totally ignored until then, though easily accessible. Animals that have been ranged in a limited area as the seasons change often are not poisoned by dangerous vegetation developing in it, yet animals newly introduced into the same range may immediately suffer considerable mortality. Young livestock are more adventurous in what they will eat than are older animals. These situations represent a summation of responses which may be called curiosity and learning. Certainly, individual large vertebrates can in a brief time and through limited encounters learn to recognize individual species of plants, associate unpleasantness with some of them, and avoid them. Individuals in a herd may have had differing exposures and learned different things. In consequence, they may react individually in different ways to a given plant species. Hunger plays a definite role, too. Barriers of taste and smell may be lowered at one time and raised at another (42). Situations have been discovered (43) in which insects are said to display learning and memory, but the element of individuality is less important and the situations are not exactly equivalent.

The fact that it takes the larger vertebrates a relatively long time to fill their gut is also important in poisoning. Many toxic compounds in plants are irritants. The first reaction to a stomach ache is to stop eating. A lethal dose, therefore, need not be consumed. Most mammals vomit, - a very effective way of ridding the system of dangerous ingesta whether of plant or animal origin. As a mammal, man has evolved a number of unique adaptations to protect himself against plant poisons. Apart from such modern inventions as the Food and Drug Administration, some of man's adaptations to secondary compounds may have had evolutionary significance for the species. It has been suggested (44) that the invention of cooking served in a major way to detoxify many otherwise dangerous foodstuffs and made it possible for man to move into new areas of the world.

The most advanced large vertebrates are mammals, and the most advanced angiosperms are monocots. Of the latter, the grasses are remarkably free of secondary compounds compared with plant groups generally. Grasses grow from the base of the plant in such a way that their growth is not stopped by having the top cut off. Moderate grazing, in fact, may improve a stand of certain grasses and reduce competition from other species (1). The effect is perhaps similar to the effect of repeated fire on prairie vegetation and could represent a mutually beneficial relationship between large herbivorous vertebrate and forage species based on (non)toxicity.

In summary, compared with insects the relation of herbivorous vertebrates to vegetational toxicity is less all-or-none.

What makes herbivorous vertebrates consume lethal quantities of a particular plant species is often the complex summation of a number of influences. When at the New York State College of Veterinary Medicine we try to duplicate or confirm a natural poisoning, the experimental animal often refuses to ingest any or more than a toxicologically insignificant amount of the material that was apparently eaten readily by another animal of that species at pasture or in the barn. Even more frustrating are the experiments with large animals in which plants known to be toxic have no apparent effect when placed directly in the animal's gut in large amount. We have had this kind of experience with *Cicuta maculata* (water hemlock) in cattle and *Taxus cuspidata* (yew) in deer. One of the major difficulties in experiments with large animals is the cost of the specimens needed for any kind of statistical analysis of results if mortality is the result needed. The kind of toxicity study easily done with small vertebrates or insects is usually not practical with the larger domestic species.

I have summarized elsewhere (45) examples showing that a species of plant can vary markedly (often from innocuous to lethal) with growing conditions, age, part of plant, genetics (variety), and even with sex of plant or with the individual specimen. Domestic animals likewise can vary in toxic reaction to a given exposure by breed, age, sex, nutritional history, and individual idiosyncrasy. Some (perhaps all) domestic animals will select against a species of plant on the basis of its bitterness alone as opposed to its toxicity (21). Sheep show no selectivity against cyanogenic strains of *Trifolium repens* when compared with cyanide-free strains of the same species (12).

Microsomal mixed-function oxidases found in the mammalian liver catalyse a large variety of detoxifications. Exact pathways and consequences of detoxification vary with species (8). In many cases enzyme induction takes place rapidly after challenge by a new toxicant or a suddenly increased level of one experienced only in small amounts before. The phenomenon of selective toxicity among species of animals may often relate to the presence or rapid enhancement of specific microsomal oxidases.

The larger wild herbivores appear not to be poisoned as frequently as our domesticated animals. An exact comparison is not possible because the wild fauna is not as closely monitored. But if this observation is correct, differences between wild and domestic animals can shed light on the phenomenon of poisoning itself. Some of the pertinent differences include the following. Wild animals are able to choose their diet from a greater diversity of botanical materials. Even when under situations of nutritional stress, they are still able normally to utilize several species of plants. The domesticated animal on the other hand may be afforded access in a sown pasture or in the barn to a very limited number of crop species. Unusual stresses of appetite may develop in domesticated species under special circumstances. For example, cattle in a lush pasture sought out bracken fern (*Pteridium aquilinum*), normally eaten only as a last resort, in an uncultivated corner of the pasture apparently to supplement a diet that was lacking in roughage (46). Chopped forage effectively eliminates the animal's normal ability to be selective. Thus pokeweed (*Phytolacca americana*) chopped with corn forage provoked purging diarrhea in a herd of cattle that would not have touched the plant in the pasture (47). Examples could be added almost endlessly. As soon as man takes over from the innate normal feed-selectivity of domesticated animals, their experiences become limited, their capacity to learn from individual experience seems to lessen, and the predictability of their responses seems to decrease the more unnatural the situation becomes (42).

Wild animals may possess a greater reservoir of detoxifying abilities than do domesticated species. While we could not kill a deer experimentally with yew, horses are easily killed (48) and natural cases in cattle have been confirmed at the New York State College of Veterinary Medicine.

VI. CONCLUSIONS

Secondary compounds have been abundantly elaborated in plants. Few systems in herbivorous vertebrates, including man, are immune to damage from one or more of them (49). Whatever the reason for their initial appearance, they now serve many advantageous functions in plants, the principal among which is defense. In the spectrum of defense capabilities the phenomenon of toxicity looms large. The war plants fight with such compounds appears primarily the war against herbivorous insects. Herbivorous vertebrates, in contrast, elicit from plants only a rear guard action.

This conclusion comes in part from observations cited earlier and in part from the nature of the toxic equation between plants and large herbivorous vertebrates. Feeny (32) points out that the defenses of plants against insect attack may be grouped into two broad categories based on the life style of the plant. Long-lived plants are certain to be found sometime (probably repeatedly) and suffer attack from one or more (probably many) herbivorous insects. They need and can afford to elaborate a generalized defense. Others by means of brief life cycles, high transient populations, and great reproductive or disseminating power, escape potential devastation from most insects. For them, a generalized defense is not worth the effort, but specific toxins may be worthwhile to meet specific recurrent insect attacks.

Just as the plant defense can be characterized broadly as generalized or specific, so in a sense can the animal attack. Insects mount specific attack against either generalized or specific defenses of plants. Such attacks are characterized by whatever qualities are necessary for continuous effective pressure on the host and an ability to change rapidly to match any changes in the host's defenses. Large herbivorous vertebrates on the other hand represent a generalized attack. Each animal grazes or browses over considerable distances and has access to a variety of plant species. To be successful in such a strategy, herbivorous vertebrates require and possess many ways of dealing effectively with most toxic secondary compounds.

Plants are poisonous for a variety of reasons. Among those reasons is the positive value of toxicity as a defense against herbivorous vertebrates. However, among the full spectrum of reasons, this one appears minor. Most poisonings of larger herbivorous vertebrates are probably the incidental consequence of ingestion of toxic secondary compounds present in plants for other reasons against which the animal's detoxification or protection mechanisms are inadequate.

VII. REFERENCES

1. Culvenor, C. C. J., *Search* 1, 103 (1970).
2. Muenscher, W. C., "Poisonous Plants of the United States," Macmillan, New York, 1939.
3. Beck, S. D. and Reese, J. C., *Recent Adv. Phytochem.* 10, 41 (1976).
4. Fraenkel, G. S., *Science* 129, 1466 (1959).
5. Fraenkel, G. S., *Entomol. Exp. Appl.* 12, 473 (1969).
6. Muller, C. H., *Science* 164, 197 (1969).
7. Brodie, B. B., and Maickel, R. P., *Proc. 1st Int. Pharm. Meeting* 6, 299 (1961).
8. Oehme, F. W., *Can. Vet. J.* 11, 69 (1970).
9. Swain, T., Ed., "Chemical Plant Taxonomy," Academic Press, New York, 1963.
10. Mabry, T. J., *Recent Adv. Phytochem.* 4, 273 (1972).
11. Harbourne, J. B., Ed., "Phytochemical Ecology," p. vii. Academic Press, New York, 1972.
12. Jones, D. A., *in* "Phytochemical Ecology" (J. B. Harbourne, Ed.), Academic Press, New York, 1972.
13. Levin, D. A., *Annu. Rev. Ecol. Syst.* 7, 121 (1976).
14. Southwood, T. R. E., *Symp. R. Entomol. Soc. London* 6, 3 (1973).
15. Kingsbury, J. M., "Poisonous Plants of the United States and Canada," Prentice-Hall, Englewood Cliffs, N. J., 1964.
16. Whittaker, R. H., *in* "Chemical Ecology," (E. Sondheimer and J. B. Simeone, Eds.), p. 43. Academic Press, New York, 1970.
17. Muller, C. H., *Recent Adv. Phytochem.* 3, 105 (1970).
18. Schoonhoven, L. M., *Recent Adv. Phytochem.* 5, 197 (1972).
19. Breedlove, D. E., and Ehrlich, P. R., *Science* 162, 671 (1968).
20. Ehrlich, P. R., and Raven, P. H., *Evolution* 18, 586 (1964).
21. Bate-Smith, E. C., *in* "Phytochemical Ecology," (J. B. Harbourne, Ed.), p. 45. Academic Press, New York, 1972.
22. Hsiao, T. H., *Entomol. Exp. Appl.* 12, 777 (1969).
23. Harbourne, J. B., *Recent Adv. Phytochem.* 4, 107 (1972).
24. Brower, L. P., *in* "Biochemical Coevolution," (K. L. Chambers, Ed.), p. 69. Oregon State University Press, Corvallis, 1970.
25. Rothschild, M., *Symp. R. Entomol. Soc. London* 6, 59 (1973).

26. DeWilde, J., Bongers, W., and Schooneveld, H., *Entomol. Exp. Appl.* 12, 714 (1969).
27. Williams, C. M., *in* "Chemical Ecology," (E. Sondheimer and J. B. Simeone, Eds.), p. 103. Academic Press, New York 1970.
28. Miles, P. W., *Entomol. Exp. Appl.* 12, 736 (1969).
29. Atsatt, P. R., and O'Dowd, D. J., *Science* 193, 24 (1976).
30. Ehrlich, P. R., *in* "Biochemical Coevolution," (K. L. Chambers Ed.), p. 1. Oregon State University Press, Corvallis, 1970.
31. Feeny, P., *in* "Coevolution of Plants and Animals," (L. E. Gilbert and P. H. Raven, Eds.), p. 3. University of Texas Press, Austin, 1975.
32. Feeny, P., *Recent Adv. Phytochem.* 10, 1 (1976).
33. McKey, D., *in* "Coevolution of Plants and Animals," (L. E. Gilbert and P. H. Raven, Eds.), p. 159. University of Texas Press, Austin, 1975.
34. Rhoades, D. F., and Cates, R. G., *Recent Adv. Phytochem.* 10, 168 (1976).
35. Whittaker, R. H., and Feeny, P. P., *Science* 171, 757 (1971).
36. Rice, E. L., "Allelopathy," Academic Press, New York, 1974.
37. Muller, C. H., *Bull, Torrey Bot. Club* 93, 332 (1966).
38. Muller, C. H., and del Moral, R., *Bull. Torrey Bot. Club* 93, 130 (1966).
39. Levin, D. A., *Am. Nat.* 105, 157 (1971).
40. Feeny, P., *Ecology* 51, 565 (1970).
41. Krieger, R. I., Feeny, P. P., and Wilkinson, C. F., *Science* 172, 579 (1971).
42. Arnold, G. W., and Hill, J. L., *in* "Phytochemical Ecology," (J. B. Harbourne, Ed.), p. 71. Academic Press, New York, 1972.
43. Gilbert, L. E., *in* "Coevolution of Plants and Animals," (L. E. Gilbert and P. H. Raven, Eds.), p. 210. University of Texas Press, Austin, 1975.
44. Leopold, A. C., and Ardrey, R., *Science* 176, 512 (1972).
45. Kingsbury, J. M., *Proc. Cornell Nutr. Conf. Feed Manuf.* p. 14 (1960).
46. Wells, H. E., *Agriculture* (Britain) 56, 204 (1949).
47. Kingsbury, J. M., and Hillman, R. B., *Cornell Vet.* 55, 534 (1965).
48. Lowe, J. E., Hintz, H. F., Schryver, H. F., and Kingsbury, J. M., *Cornell Vet.* 60, 36 (1970).
49. Kingsbury, J. M., *in* "Toxicology, The Basic Science of Poisons," (L. J. Casarett and J. Doull, Eds.), p. 591. Macmillan, New York, 1975.

BOTANICAL AFFINITIES OF AUSTRALIAN POISONOUS PLANTS

Selwyn L. Everist
Bribie Island, Queensland

I. ABSTRACT

Native toxic species of Angiosperms and Gymnosperms in Australia total about 430, distributed through 72 families. Only 9 families contain more than 10 native species. Families with the greatest numbers are Leguminosae (81), Solanaceae (54), Euphorbiaceae (20), and Gramineae (19). Except for a few families there is little positive correlation between toxicity and phylogeny at the family level. Some genera are generally toxic but a number of important poisonous species have none or few toxic relatives. Examples are given of families with a general distribution of similar toxins, of families in which many species contain toxins of different types and of families with an erratic distribution of toxic species. Examples are also given of similar toxins occurring in single genera in widely different families.

II. INTRODUCTION

Of 800 species of known poisonous plants recorded from Australia (1), 469 are native, 244 are naturalized, and 87 are commonly cultivated but not naturalized. The naturalized species include 65 that are widely grown for food, fodder, fibre, or ornament. The number of cultivated species does not include several known toxic plants that are grown only occasionally or in a few gardens.

Botanical affinities of native Australian species of poisonous plants will be the primary consideration in this discussion but in some cases it will be necessary to consider extra-Australian relatives of these plants.

Is there any consistent correlation between toxicity to animals on the one hand and the genetic make-up and presumed phylogeny of the plants on the other?

III. FAMILIES

Of the 469 native species listed, 16 are Pteridophytes, 22 are Fungi, and 2 are Algae. This leaves a total of 429 spermatophytes (Angiosperms and Gymnosperms) to be considered.

According to Burbidge (2) the native Angiosperms and Gymnosperms of Australia belong in 212 families. The known poisonous species fall into only 72 of these families. Table 1 lists these

TABLE 1

Distribution of Species by Families

Number of species					
Leguminosae	81	Rubiaceae	4	Boraginaceae	1
Solanaceae	54	Amaryllidaceae	3	Caryophyllaceae	1
Euphorbiaceae	20	Gyrostemonaceae	3	Combretaceae	1
Gramineae	19	Haloragidaceae	3	Cyperaceae	1
Proteaceae[1]	18	Meliaceae	3	Davidsoniaceae	1
Zamiaceae	18	Passifloraceae	3	Flagellariaceae	1
Chenopodiaceae	17	Rutaceae	3	Gentianaceae	1
Flindersiaceae[2]	16	Umbelliferae	3	Guttiferae	1
Thymelaeaceae	13	Zygophyllaceae	3	Icacinaceae	1
Ranunculaceae	10	Aizoaceae	2	Idiospermaceae	1
Myoporaceae	9	Amaranthaceae	2	Iridaceae	1
Xanthorrhoeaceae	9	Atherospermataceae	2	Juncaceae	1
Apocynaceae	7	Convolvulaceae	2	Lauraceae	1
Campanulaceae	7	Curcubitaceae	2	Linaceae	1
Compositae	7	Dysphaniaceae	2	Moraceae	1
Liliaceae	7	Goodeniaceae	2	Olacaceae	1
Winteraceae	6	Labiatae	2	Onagraceae	1
Barringtoniaceae	5	Loganiaceae	2	Oxalidaceae	1
Cycadaceae	5	Menispermaceae	2	Philydraceae	1
Urticaceae	5	Sapindaceae	2	Polygonaceae	1
Asclepiadaceae	4	Sterculiaceae	2	Rhamnaceae	1
Droseraceae	4	Verbenaceae	2	Scrophulariaceae	1
Myrtaceae	4	Anacardiaceae	1	Tetragoniaceae	1
Portulacaceae	4	Araceae	1	Ulmaceae	1

[1]Chemical evidence only: few field cases.
[2]Barks contain physiologically active compounds: no evidence of intoxications in livestock or man.

families in descending order of the number of native toxic species in each.

It will be noted that the families with the greatest numbers of toxic species include Leguminosae, Solanaceae, and Gramineae. Between them, these three families include almost all the major food and fodder plants of the world. Indeed, many of the naturalized and cultivated species grown as crop or pasture plants are potentially toxic to man and/or domestic animals.

In only a few families is the majority of plants consistently toxic. These families will be considered first.

The Cycadales, which earlier botanists regarded as one family (Cycadaceae) are probably the most primitive living seed-plants (3). About a quarter of the known species in this group are native to Australia, with 25 species in five genera, 5-7 species of *Cycas* (Cycadaceae), 2 species of *Bowenia*, 2 of *Lepidozamia*, and about 14 of *Macrozamia* (Zamiaceae) (4).

All species appear to be toxic. Consumption of seeds can cause severe gastro-intestinal disturbance, often accompanied by damage to the liver and development of neoplastic changes at various sites. Consumption of leaves over a long period of time leads to degeneration of proprioceptive pathways in the spinal cord and the development of irreversible posterior ataxia in cattle.

The carcinogenic and hepatotoxic agent in the seeds has been identified as methylazoxymethanol (MAM). It occurs combined with various sugars to form different glycosides in different species. The nature of the agent responsible for damage to the spinal cord is still not clear (1).

Most plants in the family Thymelaeaceae are unpalatable, but if leaves or fruits are eaten, they can produce severe, sometimes fatal gastro-intestinal disturbance. The toxic principle responsible for this effect is apparently a glycoside of dihydroxycoumarin. Repeated ingestion of smaller amounts of some plants, Notably several species of *Pimelea*, can produce vaso-constriction in the lungs of cattle, leading to cardiac dysfunction, hydrothorax, liver damage, and massive ventral edema. The toxic principle is *simplexin*, a diterpenoid ester (5).

Xanthorrhoeaceae is a family of 8 genera and about 60 species, all endemic in Australia except for a few species of *Lomandra* in New Guinea and New Caledonia. Different botanists have assigned these plants to different families, including Juncaceae and Liliaceae. There is still some doubt as to whether it is really a homogeneous family (6).

It seems likely that all species of *Xanthorrhoea* (about 15) can be toxic to cattle in the same way. The flower spikes of several species have been shown to produce loss of condition, dribbling of urine, and asymmetric posterior ataxia if eaten over a long period by animals in poor condition on mineral-deficient country.

In Australia, as in some other parts of the world, the family Euphorbiaceae has the reputation of being a "poisonous" family. Although about 300 species in this family are native to Australia, only 20 have been recorded as toxic. Many species, particularly in the genus *Euphorbia*, contain copious amounts of latex which is often corrosive to mucous surfaces and tender skin. Several species of *Euphorbia* and other genera in the family are cyanogenetic but are often eaten by livestock without ill effect. The presence of toxalbumins or phytotoxins is a feature of several naturalized species whose distribution is now almost cosmopolitan. These include *Ricinus* and *Jatropha*, the seeds of which are extremely poisonous. For many of the known toxic species in this family the nature of the toxic principle is unknown.

The family Gramineae is probably the most important plant family in the world. All the cereals, sugar cane, and thousands of pasture species belong to it. At the same time, the family also includes many toxic plants.

There appears to be no pattern in this toxicity. Many grasses are cyanogenetic or can accumulate potentially toxic amounts of nitrate. The presence of soluble oxalates in grasses is currently causing some concern in Australia. In tropical and subtropical areas several introduced species of *Cenchrus, Pennisetum,* and *Setaria* are being grown as pasture plants. There have been cases of acute oxalate poisoning in cattle and sheep but one of the main causes of concern is the development of osteodystrophia fibrosa in horses raised on these pastures.

Some grasses, most of them introduced pasture species, can accumulate dimethyltryptamine alkaloids, some act as hosts to fungi that are toxic to livestock.

Australian plants in the family Chenopodiaceae include 17 species that are potentially poisonous to livestock. Most of them accumulate oxalate and/or nitrate and a few are cyanogenetic. Despite this, many of the species are useful fodder plants under normal conditions. Intoxication occurs only when animals are under stress and have little or no alternative forage.

Dysphaniaceae, sometimes included in Chenopodiaceae, contains two species of *Dysphania* that are cyanogenetic. Both have been involved in field cases of livestock poisoning. In the context of this paper, it is noteworthy that these plants have many features in common with one small section in the genus *Chenopodium* and that those particular species are also cyanogenetic.

Another closely related family, Amaranthaceae, is generally regarded as quite wholesome and few field cases of poisoning by Australian species have been recorded. However, McBarron (7) has reported strong positive tests for nitrate for 12 species in this family, 5 of which are native, the remainder naturalized.

The two related families Apocynaceae and Asclepiadaceae are both commonly regarded as "poisonous families." Australian representatives do not support this generalization although some toxic native species do occur in each family.

In the family Apocynaceae, several species, both native and introduced, contain cardiac glycosides and some contain toxic alkaloids. The most important native species is *Alstonia constricta.* It contains several indole alkaloids.

The most toxic members of this family are the cultivated shrubs Oleander (*Nerium*) and the related *Thevetia*, both of which contain cardiac glycosides. Of particular chemical and pharmaceutical interest is *Catharanthus roseus*, a common tropical weed. More than 60 indole alkaloids have been isolated from this species (1).

Many of the plants in the family Asclepiadaceae contain latex that is corrosive in the same way as the latex from species of *Euphorbia*. Several also contain cardiac glycosides.

Two native species, *Hoya australis* and *Sarcostemma australe,* are definitely poisonous to livestock but produce no cardiac symptoms. They produce neuro-muscular symptoms identical with those caused by the ingestion of different species of *Asclepias*, both in Australia (where 3 are naturalized) and in other continents, including North America. No agreement has been reached concerning the nature of the toxic principle, but some authors believe it to be a resinoid (1,8).

Many species in the family Solanaceae contain physiologically active alkaloids or alkaloidal glycosides. These fall into three major groups:

1. Tropane alkaloids of the atropine type. These are found in 2 native species of *Duboisia* as well as introduced species of *Datura* and *Atropa*.
2. Pyridine alkaloids of the nicotine type. The endemic *Duboisia hopwoodii* and 19 endemic species of *Nicotiana* contain these, the first in very high concentration.
3. Steroidal alkaloidal glycosides of the solanine type. These are contained in many native and introduced species of *Solanum* and the closely related cultivated genus *Lycopersicon*.

IV. GENERA

More positive correlation between toxicity and botanical affinity may be noted at the generic level.

For example, although the family Leguminosae has more toxic native species than any other family, there is no general pattern of toxicity throughout the family. However, there are several genera of particular interest.

About 27 species of *Gastrolobium* and 7 out of the 35 known species of the closely related *Oxylobium* in Western Australia accumulate monofluoroacetic acid. Many of them are extremely toxic to livestock. It is remarkable that the same compound is found in only one species of the distantly related *Acacia* out of a total of more than 600 native Australian species in that genus. Fluoroacetic acid is also found in the unrelated *Dichapetalum* from southern Africa.

The genus *Erythrophleum* is represented in Australia by one endemic species in the monsoon tropical region. It is extremely toxic and usually contains alkaloidal esters of diterpenoid acids similar to those from the west African *E. guineense*. In one population from North Queensland only esters and amides of cinnamic acid were identified (1).

Swainsona is a genus of more than 50 species, all of them except one endemic in Australia. It is closely related to *Astragalus* of North America and species in both genera can produce similar lesions in the central nervous system and similar locomotory disturbance in livestock.

The genus *Crotalaria* contains more than 500 species and is widely distributed throughout the tropics. Many species in this genus contain pyrrolizidine alkaloids, most of which are hepatotoxic or otherwise injurious to animals, including man. In Australia there are several very toxic native species as well as naturalized ones and the plants are an important source of injury to horses in tropical areas. In Northern Territory, some of the native species have caused concern by appearing in weeds of grain sorghum crops and their seeds have contaminated the grain to such an extent that it has caused injury to poultry.

Pyrrolizidine alkaloids have not been found in other genera in the family Leguminosae but they occur commonly in plants of the unrelated family Boraginaceae and again in *Senecio*, one genus in the quite unrelated family Compositae (1,9).

An interesting native species is *Neptunia amplexicaulis*, known only from a restricted area in north-west Queensland. It accumulates large amounts of selenium. Although it is included in the broad definition of the family Leguminosae, it belongs to the subfamily Mimosoideae and is not at all closely related to *Astragalus*, several species of which are known selenium accumulators in North America.

The only other Australian species known to accumulate selenium is *Morinda reticulata*, a small shrub in the unrelated family Rubiaceae.

The very large and cosmopolitan family Compositae is quite well represented in Australia but it contains relatively few native toxic plants. Those it does contain mostly have little in common with each other.

Senecio has already been mentioned as a source of pyrrolizidine alkaloids. One native species of particular interest is *Wedelia asperrima* a small annual confined to tropical inland areas. If eaten in quantity by very hungry sheep or cattle it can cause pulmonary edema and sudden death. There is also congestion of the liver and degeneration of kidneys. Although the plant accumulates considerable quantities of nitrate, this does not appear to be the toxin responsible for the syndrome observed in the field. The toxin has been isolated and identified as *wedeliatoxin* (10), a glycoside containing nitrogen and of steroidal or pseudosteroidal nature.

A closely related American species, *Verbesina encelioides*, that is commonly naturalized in eastern Australia, can produce the same syndrome and it is likely that the active principle is similar.

In the family Myoporaceae which comprises about 150 species mostly from Australia and the South Pacific one genus, *Myoporum*, is notable for the presence of furanoid sesquiterpenes; many of which are hepatotoxic.

Eremophila maculata, one species in a large endemic Australian genus of the same family, is notable for the presence in the leaves of high concentrations of *prunasin*, a cyanogenetic glycoside, yielding HCN equivalents from 0.14% to 1.4%. Several other species of *Eremophila* contain furanoid sesquiterpenes (1).

In the family Convolulaceae there are 2, possibly 3, native species of *Ipomoea* that are toxic to cattle, sheep, and horses if the animals eat enough of them. The symptoms appear to be neuromuscular and somewhat resemble those produced by *Swainsona* and *Astragalus*. In the Western Australian *I. muelleri*, chromatographic tests suggested the presence of indole alkaloids of the

LSD type, but tests on the Queensland *I. calcbra* were inconclusive (1). It is interesting to note that several American species in this genus contain similar indole alkaloids.

The family Cyperaceae is very closely related to Gramineae. Unlike grasses, however, the family contains very few pasture plants. In Australia only one toxic native species, *Schoenus asperocarpus*, is known. The toxic principle is unknown (1).

Myrtaceae is one of the largest families in Australia but contains very few toxic species. A few species of *Eucalyptus* are cyanogenetic and most of them produce essential oils, some of which are mildly toxic. The most interesting toxic species in the family in Australia is *Rhodomyrtus macrocarpa*. Immature fruits of this species appear to be capable of causing irreversible degeneration of the optic nerves in man, leading to permanent blindness (1). There is still some uncertainty about the nature of the toxin. *Rhodomyrtoxin*, a complex benzofuran compound, was isolated from dried immature fruit but there is no experimental proof that this substance can injure the optic nerve in humans.

The family Rutaceae, although well represented in Australia, also contains relatively few native toxic species. Alkaloids of great chemical interest have been isolated from the bark of many species and essential oils are common in the leaves. There is no evidence that these are toxic. One interesting species is *Zieria arborescens* from Tasmania and southern Victoria. If eaten by livestock it causes respiratory embarrassment and pulmonary edema. Another species, *Z. laevigata* can be cyanogenetic.

Examples of isolated toxic species within otherwise innocuous families are afforded by *Melia* (Meliaceae), two species of *Trachymene* (Umbelliferae), and *Trema aspera* (Ulmaceae).

Melia azedarach var. *australasica* is the Australian representative of a widespread tropical species. The ripe fruits are poisonous to pigs, sheep, and children. They produce gastro-intestinal upset, accompanied by excitement and depression, weakened heart action and respiratory distress, usually followed by death within a few days. The exact nature of the toxic principle is not known but it is contained in the resinous portion of the alcoholic extract.

Trachymene ochracea and *T. cyanantha* can produce 'bent-leg' in lambs from ewes that have eaten the plants during late pregnancy and early lactation. The condition is characterized by bowing and effective shortening of the limbs, particularly the forelegs. There is rotation of the joints, lateral twisting of bones, and flaring at the metaphyses, sometimes accompanied by twisting of the distal shafts of metacarpal bones and thickening or shortening of the longbones (12). The nature of the toxic principle is unknown.

Trema aspera is a shrub or small tree, common in areas of high rainfall along the east coast of Australia. It is a frequent cause of poisoning in cattle and is also toxic to sheep and goats. Symptoms are depression or excitement, followed by muscular twitching, loss of tone in voluntary muscles, shallow jerky respiration, fast heartbeat, and uncontrolled leg movements, then coma, feeble heartbeat, and death. The toxic principle is *trematoxin*, a glycoside with a high molecular weight but whose composition has not yet been fully elucidated (1,13).

Toxic ferns and fern-allies (Pteridophyta) in Australia are mostly related to those from other parts of the world. Three species of *Pteridium* are native, one of them widespread in the Southern Hemisphere. These produce the same characteristic syndromes as related species in Europe and North America.

Of particular interest is the genus *Cheilanthes*, at least one species of which has been shown to produce the "bracken" syndrome in cattle. It can also produce ataxia, diarrhea, and respiratory distress in sheep under stress (1,11).

V. CONCLUSION

It is obvious that in large groups such as families there are few examples of positive correlation between phylogency and toxicity. In some genera and a few families there is sufficient correlation to allow fairly confident prediction whether a species is likely to be toxic. In the majority of families, however, this is not possible and it is necessary to look at each species (or sometimes a group of species) separately.

VI. REFERENCES

1. Everist, S. L., "Poisonous Plants of Australia," Angus & Robertson, Sydney, 1974.
2. Burbidge, N. T., "Dictionary of Australian Plant Genera," Angus & Robertson, Sydney, 1963.
3. Willis, J. C., "A Dictionary of the Flowering Plants and Ferns," (7th edition, revised by H. K. Airy Shaw), p. 315. Cambridge University Press, London, 1966.
4. Johnson, L. A. S., *Proc. Linn. Soc. N. S. W.* 84, 64-117 (1959)
5. Roberts, H. B., McClure, T. J., Ritchie, E., Taylor, W. C., and Freeman, P. W., *Aust. Vet. J.* 51, 325-326 (1975).
6. Lee, Alma T., *Contrib. N. S. W. Nat. Herb. Flora Ser.* 34, 1 (1966).
7. McBarron, E. J., *N. S. W. Dep. Agric. Sci. Bull.* 83, 6-7 (1966).
8. Kingsbury, John M., "Poisonous Plants of the United States and Canada," Prentice-Hall, Englewood Cliffs, New Jersey, 1964.
9. Bull, L. B., Culvenor, C. C. J., and Dick, A. T., "The Pyrrolizidine Alkaloids," North Holland Publ., Amsterdam, 1968.
10. Oelrichs, P. B., and Muller, W. A. *Toxicon* 10, 63-66 (1972).
11. Clark, I. A., and Dimmock, C. K., *Aust. Vet. J.* 47, 149-152 (1971)
12. Clark, L., Carlisle, C. H., and Beasley, P. S., *Aust. Vet. J.* 51, 4-10 (1975).
13. Oelrichs, P. B., *Phytochemistry* 7, 1691-1693 (1968).

THE ROLE OF RUMINAL MICROBES IN THE METABOLISM OF TOXIC CONSTITUENTS FROM PLANTS

Milton J. Allison
National Animal Disease Center, Agricultural Research Service, U.S. Department of Agriculture

I. ABSTRACT

Ruminal microbes interact with some of the toxic substances from plants and this interaction may be of great importance to the host. Examples are given for microbial degradation of toxic substances, production of toxic substances by the microbes, and toxicity due to induced changes in or inhibitions of the microbial population. Diets may induce a selection or change in the proportions of functional microbes so that rates of interaction with toxic substances are changed. In some cases this "adaptation" may be crucial to the well-being of the ruminant. For many toxic substances the interactions with ruminal microbes have not yet been adequately characterized.

II. INTRODUCTION

Most of the current information on the metabolic activities of ruminal microbes deals with degradation of the major constituents of plants with the concomitant production of volatile fatty acids, methane and microbial cells. Pregastric fermentation also plays an important but less studied role in the detoxification of various dietary substances such as oxalic acid, mimosine, and ochratoxin. In this respect, ruminal microbes may be considered as a "first line of active defense" (1).

The microbe-host relationship in the rumen, while basically a mutualistic one, may also have certain attributes of parasitism because the toxicity of some dietary substances may be induced or increased by the metabolic activities of the microbial population. Examples of this kind of interaction include reduction of nitrate to nitrite, production of equol from formonetin, and hydrolysis of cyanogentic glycosides. A given diet may also be considered toxic when it produces a marked change in the microbial population which leads to production of large quantities of a normal metabolite that is not toxic at usual concentrations but is toxic at higher concentrations. Examples of this include the production of the thiaminase I associated with polioencephalomalacia and the D(-) lactic acid associated with the acidosis of grain overload.

Because ruminal microbes perform essential functions, a substance can also be toxic due to its inhibitory effects on the microbial population. Examples of this include the effects of perloline, essential oils, and tannins (2).

Interactions between ruminal microbes and most toxic substances have not been extensively studied. Where information is available the activity studied has usually concerned the population as a whole. Information on rates of reactions or of interactions involving specific microbial species or their enzymes is rare. With some toxic substances, interactions with microbes may be inferred from differences in toxicity between ruminants and preruminants, antibiotic-treated ruminants or non-ruminants or between conventional animals and gnotobiotes.

The predominantly anaerobic microbial populations of the rumen are in many respects metabolically similar to the populations of the lower bowel of non-ruminants; thus information concerning metabolism of toxic substances in these environments is pertinent to the present topic. Some of the major transformations of anutrient compounds that are brought about by intestinal bacteria have been categorized (3,4,5). These include hydrolytic reactions, various kinds of reductive reactions, and degradation by decarboxylation, dealkylation, dehalogenation, deamination, and ring fission.

The breadth of the topic considered here is such that a review covering all aspects is difficult and certainly this attempt to synthesize available information is not complete. Other reviews that deal with certain aspects of this subject have been prepared (1,5,6).

III. NITROGEN COMPOUNDS

A. Proteins

In general, rates of protein degradation in the rumen are directly related to the solubility of a given protein in the rumen. It seems probable that the potent microbial proteolytic activity is of significant survival value with regard to toxic proteins. For example, purified toxin from *Clostridium botulinum*, type C. was rapidly detoxified by the mixed population of ruminal microbes from either cattle or sheep (7). Direct experimental evidence with toxic proteins from plants to support this position is limited, but the probable protective effects of ruminal proteolysis can be inferred from comparisons of toxicity between ruminants and non-ruminants.

Substances that inhibit proteolytic enzymes and growth of non-ruminants are distributed throughout the plant kingdom but are particularly abundant in seeds of legumes (8). The inhibitory substances are mostly heat-labile proteins that differ within and among species. The inhibitory factors from soybeans appear to act in the pig mainly by reducing the activities of intestinal trypsin and chymotrypsin (9). Some of the protease inhibitors cause pancreatic hypertrophy in certain species and thus their capacity to inhibit growth of non-ruminants is more complex than the mere inhibition of gastrointestinal protein digestion.

Toxic plant proteins that cause agglutination of red blood cells are called lectins or phytohemagglutinins and are widely distributed in various plants. The most potent of these is ricin, from the seed of the castor plant, *Ricinus communis* (10). Ricin is resistant to digestion by pancreatic juice (11), but there appears to be no direct experimental evidence concerning the fate of ricin in the rumen. When castor meal, containing 11.6 ppm ricin, was fed at 10-20% of the diet to dairy cattle, milk production was satisfactory, and the milk was apparently not injurious when fed to calves or rats (12).

Soluble proteins, especially Fraction 1 protein, have been implicated as one of many factors involved in pasture or legume bloat (13). The rate of degradation of this class of proteins may be important if the event sequence is as suggested by McArthur, *et al.* (14). Soluble Fraction 1 protein enters the microbial environment as an almost spherical particle. If the protein reaches the surface before it is attacked by microbial proteases it uncoils there, becomes insoluble and stabilizes the foam. On the other hand, increased rates of microbial degradation of salivary mucoproteins with antifoaming activity would tend to increase the stability of the foam. Reports of poisoning of ruminants by mushroom toxins are rare and it is generally assumed that the toxic peptides are degraded in the intestinal tract. Again, experimental evidence concerning this activity is lacking.

B. Amino Acids

Ruminal microbes clearly play an essential role in the pulmonary edema and emphysema induced by oral doses of L-tryptophan or indoleacetic acid. Microbial production of the apparent toxic agent, 3-methyl indole, can occur (15).

The non-protein, pharmacologically active amino acids from plants are discussed in several reviews (16,17,18). Relatively little is known about either the action of these amino acids on ruminal microbes or the extent of their degradation in the rumen. From knowledge of the degradation of other amino acids in the rumen it is reasonable to expect that degradation of these also is significant. In the case of mimosine, degradation to 3,4-dihydroxypyridine is known to occur in the rumen and evidence was obtained that selection of a mimosine-degrading population occurred in response to dietary mimosine (19).

L-3,4-Dihydroxyphenylalanine (L-Dopa) occurs in free form or as a *B*-glycoside in various legumes, and undergoes para-dehydroxylation to produce meta-hydroxy phenylacetic acid in conventional but not in germ-free rats (20). It seems reasonable to predict that this transformation (detoxication) also occurs in the rumen.

Canavanine, a close analog of arginine found in the seeds of many leguminous species (17), inhibits growth of fungi and some bacteria (16). Data on its interactions with ruminal microbes apparently are lacking, except for one experiment indicating that canavanine inhibited growth of *Bacteroides ruminicola* (21).

The neurotoxic acid, beta-n-oxalyl, alpha, beta-diaminopropionic acid, found in *Lathyrus sp.* (16) inhibited growth of *Saccharomyces cerevisiae* and *Neurospora crassa* but not that of *Escherichia coli* or *lactobacilli* in one study (22). In another study toxin from *Lathyrus sativa* inhibited growth of *E. coli*, *Staphylococcus aureus* and *Candida albicans* (23) but its effect on ruminal microbes is not known.

C. Organic Nitro Compounds

There is good evidence for the importance of the interaction between ruminal microbes and organic nitro compounds from plants. Miserotoxin from timber milkvetch (*Astragalus miser* var. *serotinus*) is hydrolyzed to produce glucose plus 3-nitropropionic acid in the acidic stomach of rodents, but in the rumen the nitro compound produced is 3-nitropropanol (24,25,26). Ruminants may be poisoned by either nitro compound but the alcohol is more potent, apparently because it is more rapidly absorbed (27,28).

The toxicity of crownvetch (*Coronilla varia*) for young growing non-ruminant animals was related to the concentration of 3-nitropropionic acid in the plant material (29). Toxicity was not observed for ruminants (30), and Gustine *et al.* (31) found that 3-nitropropionic acid supplied either free or as the di- or triester was degraded and detoxified during incubation *in vitro* with ruminal fluid. Studies using centrifuged rumen fluid showed that this activity was associated with the microbial cells. The products of metabolism were not identified but reduction of the nitro group seems probable. Factors that influence the rate of the detoxification are not known but if reduction of the nitro group is involved, the availability of metabolic hydrogen may be critical. Low rates of ruminal metabolism of 3-nitropropionic acid and/or dosage at rates too high to be compensated by degradation could cause the toxic symptoms that are sometimes seen in ruminants (27,32).

D. Nitrate and Nitrite

Ruminal microbes are able to reduce nitrate to nitrite and nitrite to ammonia. When excess nitrate is ingested, the toxic nitrite may accumulate and be absorbed from the rumen because the activity of nitrate reductase exceeds that of nitrite reductase (33,34). The rates of nitrate and nitrite reduction by a given population of ruminal microbes appears to depend upon the supply of fermentable energy sources which supply hydrogen for the reductions (35,36,37). Dietary factors may influence the selection of ruminal populations with different capacities for nitrate or nitrite reduction (38,39). Nakamura *et al.* (40) reported that ruminal microbes from sheep fed high-nitrate forages reduced nitrate to nitrite more rapidly than did microbes from sheep fed low-nitrate forages.

Nitrite has long been used in various foods as an inhibitor of microbial growth but its mode of action is poorly understood (41). It may be that when nitrite accumulates sufficiently in the rumen it causes a general inhibition of energy metabolism and thus reduces the rate of further reductive reactions.

Several nitrate-reducing species from the rumen utilize cytochrome-linked electron transport systems and Vries *et al.* (42) showed that anaerobic electron transport to nitrate in *Selenomonas ruminantium* and *Veillonella alcalescens* was linked to cytochrome b. A nitrate reductase from *Clostridium perfringens*, however, was linked to ferredoxin (43). Ferredoxin also participates in nitrite reduction by *Clostridium pasteurianum* (44), and it would not be surprising if ferredoxin, flavodoxin or another low potential electron-carrying protein were involved in nitrate and/or nitrite reduction by ruminal bacteria.

Several studies illustrate that profound changes in metabolism may occur due to the competition for electrons between nitrate or nitrite reduction and other hydrogen-utilizing reactions. With *V. alcalescens* cells grown on lactate, acetate production increased and the succinate pathway to propionate was greatly repressed by potassium nitrate (100 nM). A strain of *S. ruminantium* grew with glycerol as substrate when nitrate was available as a terminal electron acceptor but not when nitrate was absent (42). Methane production by a mixed ruminal population was markedly inhibited when nitrate was present (35).

Much information on microbial nitrate reductase has been obtained in studies with facultatively anaerobic bacteria (45,46, 47). Purified nitrate reductases from different species contain varying amounts of molybdenum and iron, and both of these appear to have functional roles. Factors that regulate the synthesis and activation of both the assimilatory and dissimilatory reductases have been studied, but such information is not yet available for nitrate reducers from the rumen.

E. Cyanide

Cyanogenic glucosides are readily hydrolyzed in the rumen. The rate of the reaction apparently depends upon the quantity and physiologic state of the microbes because the reaction is more rapid in fed than in starved animals. Glucosides in plant tissue are hydrolyzed more slowly than free glucosides (48,49). Little is known of interactions between cyanide and ruminal microbes (6). Growth of *Bacteroides ruminicola* was inhibited by KCN at 2×10^{-3} M and was prevented by 10^{-2} M KCN (21). Since hydrogen cyanide is rapidly absorbed, metabolism, if any, by rumen microbes after administration of acutely toxic doses is probably too slow to be of significance.

IV. ACIDS

A. Unsaturated Fatty Acids

Hydrogenation of unsaturated fatty acids by ruminal microbes is well known, and this activity may protect the animal when diets containing high quantities of certain acids are fed. Diets high in erucic acid (cis-13-docosenoic acid), which is found especially in rape seed, produce myocarditis and an accumulation of triglycerides in the rat heart. This did not occur when hydrogenated rape seed oil was fed (50). Erucic acid was transferred to the milk of rats but Mattson (50) states it is unlikely that this would occur in ruminants because of microbial hydrogenation in the rumen. Evidence for hydrogenation of ricinoleic acid from castor meal or oil by ruminal microbes has been obtained (12).

Cyclopropene fatty acids are found in seed lipids from many plants of the order Malvales. Several biological effects have been observed during feeding studies with cyclopropene acids (50) but probably the most important action is that as a cocarcinogen with aflatoxin (51,52,53). The work of Cook *et al.* (54) strongly suggests that cyclopropene fatty acids are hydrogenated by ruminal microbes.

B. Oxalic Acid

Toxicities due to high concentrations of oxalic acid in certain plants are common (55). There is good evidence that ruminants fed gradually increasing quantities of high-oxalate plants acquire the ability to tolerate large quantities of dietary oxalic acid and further that this tolerance depends upon the increased degradation of oxalic acid by ruminal microbes (56,57,58,59,60).

Oxalate-degrading aerobic bacteria have been isolated from rumen contents (61,62). Our evidence indicates that anaerobic rather than aerobic bacteria are responsible, but initial attempts to isolate these from sheep adapted to halogeton (*Halogeton glomeratus*) were not successful (63).

Increased rates of oxalate degradation by the microbes and thus tolerance for oxalate were acquired by gradually increasing the quantity of oxalate-containing plant material fed to either cattle or sheep. Increased degradation rates were also induced by intraruminal infusion of sodium oxalate (63). The most logical explanation for these results is that the proportion of microbes able to degrade oxalate increases by selection in response to the increased oxalate, a phenomenon also observed *in vitro* when a continuous fermenter was fed gradually increasing amounts of sodium oxalate (Allison, M. J. and Cook, H. M., unpublished observations).

The basis for the selection is not yet known, but our current hypothesis is that selection is related to use of oxalate as an energy source.

Oxalate is apparently split to carbon dioxide and formate, and the hydrogen from formate is used to synthesize methane. Oxalate degradation by mixed enrichment cultures is inhibited by a number of substances which are relatively specific inhibitors of methanogenesis. The oxalate degraders do not appear to be methanogens, however, since the cultures lost the capacity to degrade oxalate but not the capacity to produce methane after they were transferred to a medium containing formate rather than oxalate (64).

Hydrogen is toxic to the oxalate degrading system and thus an intimate relationship appears to exist between oxalate degrading organisms and hydrogen utilizing methanogenic organisms. This concept is supported by the finding that addition of fumarate and the hydrogen utilizing species, *Vibrio succinogenes*, to the enrichment culture stimulates oxalate degradation. If the organism that degrades oxalate is indeed not a methanogen, it must use some unknown mechanism to obtain energy for growth. Wolin (65) has discussed the theoretical basis for increased energetic efficiency when the partial pressure of hydrogen is maintained at a low concentration by hydrogen-using bacteria. The metabolic interactions in oxalate degradation appear to be similar to others in anaerobic ecosystems that have been described especially by Wolin, Bryant, and coworkers (65).

V. HETEROCYCLIC COMPOUNDS

A. Essential Oils

There is good evidence that a variety of essential oils inhibit ruminal microbes (6,66,67,68). Fortunately these oils are often produced by plants that are relatively unpalatable to ruminants. The importance of diversity in the diet in relation to detoxification of plants that contain such oils has been discussed (69). Some evidence is available for an adaptation which perhaps involves the selection of ruminal microbes able to tolerate or degrade certain essential oils (70).

B. Saponins

The possible involvement of saponins in various animal health problems is discussed by Reid (1). According to Clarke and Reid (13) saponins probably have no more than a minor role (if any) in legume pasture bloat. Saponin degradation in the rumen may explain the absence of certain toxic effects of saponins in ruminants (71). Saponin-fermenting *Butyrivibrio* have been isolated from the rumen (72), but relatively little is known about the rate or extent of saponin degradation in the rumen.

C. Estrogens

Interesting interactions occur between ruminal microbes and the phyto-estrogenic isoflavones that are especially abundant in *Trifolium sp.* (i.e., red clover, subterranean clover). Biochanin A and genistein are often inactive as estrogens when administered intraruminally to sheep but are highly active following parenteral administration to either sheep or rodents. This is explained by their degradation in the rumen to p-ethyl phenol, which is non-estrogenic (73,74). The apparent development of this degradative capacity after a few days on a genistein-rich pasture suggests the diet-induced selection of microbes capable of this degradation.

On the other hand formononetin is inactive in mice but active in sheep when it is administered intraruminally. This is due to the demethylation which can occur in the rumen to produce daidzein and subsequent conversion to the estrogenic substance, equol (75,76).

D. Gossypol

The polyphenolic pigment from cottonseed, gossypol, is toxic to non-ruminants but ruminants tolerate relatively large amounts of this substance well (77). Reiser and Fu (78) concluded from their experiments that free gossypol was rapidly bound by soluble proteins in the rumen, and that the bound gossypol was not released by proteolytic enzymes. No evidence for direct microbial involvement in detoxication was found. Gossypol inhibited growth of a variety of bacteria and yeasts (79), but I have not found a record of toxicity tests with ruminal microbes. Such tests as well as experiments to verify the nature of gossypol binding or detoxification should be conducted.

E. Alkaloids

An extensive review of the alkaloids found in herbage has been prepared by Culvenor (80), and these are also discussed in other papers of this symposium. Apart from information on the pyrrolizidine alkaloids or perloline, relatively little is known concerning interactions of these with ruminal microbes.

1. *Pyrrolizidine Alkaloids*

The detoxification of the pyrrolizidine alkaloids, heliotrine and lasiocarpine, by ruminal microbes has been described by Culvenor, *et al.* (81) and by Lanigan (82,83). The alkaloids are detoxified by reductive fission reactions and then converted to the common end product 7,α-hydroxy-1α-methyl-8α-pyrrolizidine. Anaerobic bacteria, a gram-negative coccus (84) and a gram-positive coccus, *Peptococcus heliotrinreducans* (85), capable of this reductive cleavage have been isolated. Both organisms use hydrogen gas or formate as hydrogen donors for the reductive reaction. In addition to the pyrrolizidines, *P. heliotrinreducans* could also use fumarate or nitrate as hydrogen acceptors.

Alkaloid-degrading bacteria are selected in the rumen in response to the addition of *Heliotropium europaeum* to the diet (86). In the rumen, these bacteria apparently must compete with methanogens for metabolic hydrogen, and thus, when methanogenesis was selectively inhibited with various chemicals, heliotrine reduction was accelerated (86,87). Since *P. heliotrinreducans* grew better when nitrate was present as an electron acceptor it would not be surprising if the rate of alkaloid degradation in the rumen was reduced by addition of nitrate.

The toxicity for rats of pyrrolizidine alkaloids from tansy ragwort (*Senecio jacobaea*) was reduced by incubation with rumen fluid from a steer but not by incubation with rumen fluid from a sheep (88). The reasons for this are unknown. Pretest differences in the selection of the active organisms may have been involved, although both of the donor animals were apparently fed the same roughage diet.

The foregoing studies of Lanigan are an excellent example of the degradation of toxic substances in the rumen particularly in that they illustrate the complex ecologic relationships that exist between the microbes.

2. *Perloline*

Bush *et al.* (89) observed poor performance of cattle grazing tall fescue (*Festuca arundinacea*) in the summer. They later found that cellulose digestion and volatile fatty acid production were inhibited when the alkaloid from tall fescue, perloline, was added (at $\leq$ 9.4 x 10^5M) to mixed populations of ruminal microbes (90). Growth of pure cultures of four different species of cellulolytic rumen bacteria was completely inhibited by 10^{-3}M perloline and was significantly inhibited by 5 x 10^{-4}M perloline. Ruminal protozoa were killed when incubated with 1.13 x 10^{-3}M perloline. The concentrations of perloline used could reasonably be expected in the rumen, and these workers suggest that the poor performance of cattle may be explained by the influence of perloline on the microbes. Inhibitory activity *in vitro* was due to the perlolidine moiety, and an intact β ring with no substitution at the 5-position was essential for maximal activity (91).

F. Phylloerythrin

Ruminal microbes are involved in bighead (geeldikkop) in sheep in that they produce phaeophytins from cholorophyll which are subsequently degraded to produce the photodynamic agent, phylloerythrin (92,93,94). Phylloerythrin usually causes no harm to the animal, but photosensitization occurs when other toxic agents impair the normal biliary excretion of phylloerythrin and the animals are subsequently exposed to sunlight.

VI. TOXIC SULFUR COMPOUNDS

Kale (*Brassica oleracea* var. *acephala*), if fed exclusively, produces a severe hemolytic anemia in cattle. The first sign of the disease is the appearance of refractile, stainable granules (Heinz-Erlich bodies) within the red blood cells. Smith (95) reported the results of a series of experiments which indicate that S-methylcysteine sulfoxide (SMCO) from kale is converted by ruminal microbes (probably via SMCO lyase and a subsequent reduction) to dimethyl disulfide. The latter compound produced a response characteristic of kale or SMCO poisoning in a goat. Pure cultures that had significant SMCO lyase activity were *Lactobacillus*, *Veillonella alcalescens*, *Megasphera elsdenii* and *Anaerovibrio lipolytica*. Smith (95) also proposed that methanethiol, produced by further reduction of dimethyl disulfide or from S-methylcysteine or methionine (96) has hemolytic potential.

Seed from *Crambe abyssinica* and from several *Brassica* species (e.g., *napus* and *campestris*) contain thioglucosides, which are progoitrins; when they are split by a thioglucosidase (Myrosinase), they form oxazolidine thiones (R and S goitrin) which are toxic to non-ruminants due to their antithyroid and, therefore, goitrogenic action. Ruminants are apparently less sensitive to these compounds (97). Virtanen *et al.* (98) reported that the goitrogens were not transferred in significant quantities to milk since they were apparently destroyed in the rumen. When progoitrin was incubated *in vitro* with ruminal fluid from a sheep, it was completely metabolized in 24 hr. Products of metabolism were 5-vinyl-1,3-thiazolidine-α-thione, 5-vinyl-1,3-thiazolidine-α-one, and other unidentified substances (99).

VII. SELENIUM

Dietary selenium can be converted in the reticulo-rumen to a form that is less available to the animal (100). Much of the ^{75}Se excreted in the feces of sheep that were fed clover grown on ^{75}selenite was insoluble and was probably present as elemental selenium or as metal selenides (101). Ruminal microbes apparently are responsible for the reactions producing these compounds and may also convert significant quantities of either inorganic or organic selenium into organic selenium compounds in microbial cells (102,103,104). The low net absorption of selenium (supplied as Na_2SeO_3) by sheep as compared with swine (105) and the mainly fecal rather than urinary excretion of selenium by ruminants may be related to metabolism of selenium in the rumen. If microbial conversion to a less easily absorbed form is significant on diets that contain high levels of selenium this would be another example of detoxication by ruminal microbes.

VIII. THIAMINASE

The thiamine-degrading enzyme, thiaminase I (EC 2.5.1.2), is present in bracken fern (*Pteridium aquilinum*) and in horsetail (*Equisetum arvense*). According to Evans (106) ruminants are less sensitive than non-ruminants to the effects of this enzyme, and this can be demonstrated when both are fed complete diets supplemented with low-temperature dried green bracken frond powder. Thiamine deficiency, however, was produced in sheep by supplementing their diet with bracken rhizome powder, which is a richer source of the enzyme (107). The rhizome powder destroyed about 80 ug of thiamine/min/g, and disease was produced when it constituted 15 to 25% of the diet. Increased tolerance to thiaminase I in ruminants, as compared to non-ruminants, could be due to degradation of the enzyme in the rumen, and/or to microbial production of the vitamin in excess of that destroyed.

There is increasing evidence that polioencephalomalacia (PEM) (108) or cerebrocortical necrosis (CCN) (109) is a thiamine deficiency disease associated with production of high levels of thiaminase I by ruminal microbes (110). The thiamine deficiency could be due to inadequate supply of the vitamin due to destruction of the enzyme and/or to production of antithiamine compounds depending upon the co-substrates available (5). Edwin *et al.* (111) found that the major co-substrate for the reaction in the rumen is Δ'-pyrroline, and that a product of the reaction with it plus thiamine was 1-(4-amino-α-methylpyrimidin-5-ylmethyl)-1-pyrrolinium chloride. This product was present in the brains of calves suffering from PEM and could be an important factor in the disease.

The disease is apparently induced by dietary manipulations, usually those in which roughage is replaced with grain or other readily fermented carbohydrates (112, 113). The proportion of ruminal butyrate increases and that of acetate decreases (112) and ethanol may accumulate (114). The ruminal environment is apparently changed so that a selection of greatly increased numbers of microbes which produce thiaminase I occurs.

Cultures of *Clostridium sporogenes* (115) and of aerobic thiaminase I-producing *Bacillus* species (116) have been isolated from rumens of animals affected with PEM. The concentrations of these thiaminase I-producing bacteria in the rumen have not been determined and further work is needed to clarify which microbes are involved and the factors that regulate selection of the organisms and/or their production of thiaminase I.

IX. MYCOTOXINS

The diversity of toxic substances produced by fungi suggests that various kinds of interactions with ruminal microbes may be found with these materials. Probably the best evidence for mycotoxin degradation in the rumen is that which showed that ochratoxin A is hydrolyzed at the peptide bond by ruminal microbes from cattle to produce nontoxic ochratoxin α. As with other ruminal peptidases, activity is associated with microbial cells rather than cell-free rumen liquor obtained by centrifugation (117). An ochratoxin A degradation rate of 0.67 nMols/hr/g was calculated for bovine rumen contents obtained from a slaughter house (118). The ochratoxin A degradation rate probably depends upon the nutritional environment (or physiologic state) of the microbes; Galtier and Alvinerie (117) found that samples of rumen contents obtained from a slaughter house were much less active than samples obtained by stomach tube from cows fed a concentrate-hay ration. Since in both of the above studies precautions were not taken to maintain anaerobic conditions during the *in vitro* incubations, further work to describe and quantitate degradation of ochratoxin A seems indicated.

The antimicrobial activity of fungal products are well known and this activity may be significant in the rumen. Brewer and coworkers (119,120,121) presented evidence which suggests that reduced growth rates of sheep, "Ovine Ill Thrift," in Nova Scotia is related to inhibition of ruminal microbes by antibiotics produced by fungi from soil or herbage. Aflatoxin B_1 incubated with ruminal contents *in vitro* at concentrations greater than 0.1 ug/ml, inhibited cellulose digestion, and production of total volatile fatty acids and ammonia (122). When aflatoxin B_1 (50 ug/ml) was incubated for 24 hours with rumen contents, no degradation of the toxin could be detected (123). Similar results were obtained in both *in vitro* and *in vivo* studies with aflatoxin B_1 at about 1/1000 the above concentrations (Richards, J., Fritz, K., and Allison, M. J., unpublished observations). Growth of pure cultures of *Streptococcus bovis* was inhibited by 75 ug/ml of aflatoxin B_1 (123).

When sporidesmin, a mycotoxin produced by *Pithomyces chartarum*, was incubated with cilliated ruminal protozoa there was no evidence of toxicity but rather an increase in the rate of gas production was seen (124).

Long-term (96 hr) *in vitro* digestibility of hay by microbes from the rumen of sheep was unaffected by ochratoxin A, aflatoxin B_1 or sterigmatocystin at 0.2 ug/ml. Some reduction in digestibility was observed with these substances at 1.4 ug/ml (125). Considering the differences between the *in vitro* conditions used and conditions in the rumen the data obtained seem inadequate to justify the conclusion by Pettersson and Kiessling (125) that these mycotoxins do not inhibit digestion by sheep ruminal microbes *in vivo*.

X. CONCLUSIONS

A principle underlying many interactions between ruminal microbes and toxic substances is that most reactions probably involve a dynamic interdependency between several microbial species. For example, detoxication by reductive processes (nitrite, unsaturated fatty acids, pyrrolizidine alkaloids) may involve interspecies hydrogen-transfer reactions and thus depend upon availability of fermentable substrates as well as competition that may exist between various pathways of terminal electron transfer.

Studies with several toxic substances (e.g., oxalic acid, mimosine, and pyrrolizidine alkaloids) indicate that rumen microbial population can be manipulated so that microbes are selected to increase the rates of specific detoxication reactions (69). Conversely, without an adequate understanding of the system, unfavorable manipulations of populations may inadvertently be made. It is proposed that application of knowledge concerning interactions between ruminal microbes and toxic substances may contribute significantly to control of various toxicity diseases. If this is true, the current bank of knowledge is not adequate.

XI. REFERENCES

1. Reid, C. S. W., *in* "Chemistry and Biochemistry of Herbage" (G. W. Butler and R. W. Bailey, Eds.), Vol. 3, p. 215. Academic Press, London, 1973.
2. Tagari, H., Henis, Y., Tamir, M., and Volcani, R., *Appl. Microbiol.* 13, 437 (1965).
3. Sheline, R. R., *Pharmacol. Rev.* 25, 451 (1973).
4. Walker, R., *Proc. Nutr. Soc.* 32, 73 (1973).
5. Prins, R., *in* "Nutrition and Drug Interrelations" (J. N. Hathcock and J. M. Coon, Eds.), Academic Press, New York, 1977.
6. James, L. F., Allison, M. J., and Littledike, E. T., *in* "Digestion and Metabolism in the Ruminant" (I. W. McDonald and A. C. I. Warner, Eds.), p. 576. University of New England Publishing Unit, Armidale, Australia, 1975.
7. Allison, M. J., Maloy, S. E., and Matson, R. R., *Appl. Environ. Microbiol.* 32, 685 (1976).
8. Liener, I. E., and Kakade, M. L., *in* "Toxic Constituents of Plant Foodstuffs" (I. E. Liener, Ed.), p. 7. Academic Press, New York, 1969.
9. Yen, J. T., Jensen, A. H., and Simon, J., *J. Nutr.* 107, 156 (1977).
10. Balint, G. A., *Toxicology* 2, 77 (1974).
11. Jaffe, W. G., *in* "Toxic Constituents of Plant Foodstuffs" (I. E. Liener, Ed.), p. 69. Academic Press, New York, 1969.
12. Robb, J. G., Laben, R. C., Walker, H. G., Jr., and Herring, V., *J. Dairy Sci.* 57, 443 (1974).

13. Clarke, R. T. J., and Reid, C. S. W., *J. Dairy Sci.* 57, 753 (1974).
14. McArthur, J. M., Miltimore, J. E., and Pratt, M. J., *Can. J. Anim. Sci.* 49, 69 (1964).
15. Carlson, J. R., and Dickinson, E. O., These Proceedings.
16. Bell, E. A., *in* "Toxicants Occurring Naturally in Foods," p. 153. National Academy of Sciences, Washington, D.C., 1973.
17. Hegerty, M. P., and Peterson, P. J., *in* "Chemistry and Biochemistry of Herbage" (G. W. Butler and R. W. Bailey, Eds.), Vol. 1, p. 1. Academic Press, London, 1973.
18. Hegerty, M. P., These Proceedings.
19. Hegerty, M. P., Court, R. D., and Thorne, P. M., *Aust. J. Agric. Res.* 15, 168 (1964).
20. Goldman, P., Peppercorn, M. A., and Goldin, B. R., *Am. J. Clin. Nutr.* 27, 1348 (1974).
21. Pittman, K. A., and Bryant, M. P., *J. Bacteriol.* 88, 401 (1964).
22. Mehta, T., Hsu, An-Fei, and Haskell, B. E., *Biochemistry* 11, 4053 (1972).
23. Rao, S. L. N., Adiga, P. R., and Sarma, P. S., *Biochemistry* 3, 432 (1964).
24. Williams, M. C., Van Kampen, K. R., and Norris, F. A., *Am. J. Vet. Res.* 30, 2185 (1969).
25. Williams, M. C., Norris, F. A., and Van Kampen, K. R., *Am. J. Vet. Res.* 31, 259 (1970).
26. Mosher, G. A., Krishnamurti, C. R., and Kitts, W. D., *Can. J. Anim. Sci.* 51, 475 (1971).
27. Williams, M. C., and James, L. F., *J. Range Manage.* 28, 260 (1975).
28. Williams, M. C., and James, L. F., These Proceedings.
29. Shenk, J. S., Wangsness, P. J., Leach, R. M., Gustine, D. L., Gabble, J. L., and Barnes, R. F., *J. Anim. Sci.* 42, 616 (1976).
30. Peterson, A. D., Baumgardt, B. R., and Long, T. A., *J. Anim. Sci.* 38, 172 (1974).
31. Gustine, D. L., Moyer, B. G., Wangsness, P. J., and Shenk, J. S., *J. Anim. Sci.* 44, 1107 (1977).
32. Morris, M. P., Pagan, C., and Warmke, H. E., *Science* 119, 322 (1954).
33. Fassett, D. W., *in* "Toxicants Occurring Naturally in Foods," p. 7. National Academy of Sciences, Washington, D.C., 1973.
34. O'Hara, P. J., and Fraser, A. J., *N. Z. Vet. J.* 23, 45 (1975).
35. Jones, G. A., *Can. J. Microbiol.* 18, 1783 (1972).
36. Lewis, D., *Biochem. J.* 49, 149 (1951).
37. Sinclair, K. B., and Jones, D. I. H., *Res. Vet. Sci.* 8, 65 (1967).
38. Sapiro, M. L., Hoflund, S., Clark, R., and Quin, J. L., *Onderstepoort J. Vet. Sci. Anim. Ind.* 22, 357 (1949).
39. Holtenius, P., *Acta Agric. Scand.* 7, 113 (1957).
40. Nakamura, Y., Yoshida, J., Nakamura, R., and Horie, H.,

Jpn. J. Zootech. Sci. 47, 63 (1976).
41. Hansen, J. N., and Levin, R. A., *Appl. Microbiol.* 30, 862 (1975).
42. Vries, W. de., Wijck-Kapteyn, W. M. C. van, and Oosterhuis, S. K. H., *J. Gen. Microbiol.* 81, 69 (1974).
43. Chiba, S., and Ishimoto, M., *J. Biochem.* 73, 1315 (1973).
44. Mortenson, L. E., Valentine, R. C., and Carnahan, J. E., *Biochem. Biophys. Res. Commun.* 7, 448 (1962).
45. Stouthamer, A. H., *in* "Advances in Microbiol Physiology (A. H. Rose and D. W. Tempest, Eds.), Vol. 14, p. 315. Academic Press, London, 1976.
46. Payne, W. J., *Bacteriol. Rev.* 37, 409 (1973).
47. Pichinoty, F., *Bull. Inst. Pasteur Paris* 71, 317 (1973).
48. Coop, I. E., and Blakely, R. L., *N. Z. J. Sci. Technol.* 30A, 277 (1949).
49. Tapper, B. A., and Reay, P. F., *in* "Chemistry and Biochemistry of Herbage" (G. W. Butler and R. W. Bailey. Eds.), Vol. 1, p. 477. Academic Press, London, 1973.
50. Mattson, F. H., *in* "Toxicants Occurring Naturally in Foods," p. 189, National Academy of Sciences, Washington, D.C., 1973.
51. Sinnhuber, R. O., Lee, D. J., Wales, J. H., and Ayres, J. L., *J. Natl. Cancer Inst.* 41, 1293 (1968).
52. Lee, D. J., Wales, J. H., and Sinnhuber, R. O., *Cancer Res.* 28, 2312 (1968).
53. Lee, D. J., Wales, J. H., and Sinnhuber, R. O., *Cancer Res.* 31, 960 (1971).
54. Cook, L. J., Scott, T. W., Mills, S. C., Fogerty, A. C., and Johnson, A. R., *Lipids* 11, 705 (1976).
55. James, L. F., These Proceedings.
56. Morris, M. P., and Garcia-Rivera, J., *J. Dairy Sci.* 38, 1169 (1955).
57. James, L. F., Street, J. C., and Butcher, J. E., *J. Anim. Sci.* 26, 1438 (1967).
58. Dodson, M. E., *Aust. Vet. J.* 35, 225 (1959).
59. Maymone, B., Tiberio, M., Dattilo, M., and Giacomino, A., *Ann. Sper. Agrar.* 16, 167 (1962).
60. Watts, P. S., *Aust. J. Agric. Res.* 8, 226 (1957).
61. Muller, H., *Arch. Mikrobiol.* 15, 137 (1950).
62. O'Halloran, M. W., *Proc. Aust. Soc. Anim. Prod.* 4, 18 (1962).
63. Allison, M. J., Littledike, E. T., and James, L. F., *J. Anim. Sci.* 45, (1977).
64. Dawson, K. A., and Allison, M. J., *Abstr. 77th Annu. Meet. Am. Soc. Microbiol.*, p. 180 (1977).
65. Wolin, M. J., *Am. J. Clin. Nutr.* 27, 1320 (1974).
66. Crane, A., Nelson, W. O., and Brown, R. E., *J. Dairy Sci.* 40, 1317 (1957).
67. Oh, H. K., Jones, M. B., and Longhurst, W. M., *Appl. Microbiol.* 16, 39 (1968).
68. Nagy, J. G., Steenoff, H. W., and Ward, G. M., *J. Wildl. Manage.* 28, 785 (1964).

69. Freeland, W. J., and Janzen, D. H., *Am. Nat.* 108, 269 (1974).
70. Oh, H. K., Sakai, T., Jones, M. B., and Longhurst, W. M., *Appl. Microbiol.* 15, 777 (1967).
71. Bondi, A., Birk, Y., and Gestetner, B., *in* "Chemistry and Biochemistry of Herbage" (G. W. Butler and R. W. Bailey, Eds.), Vol. 1, p. 511. Academic Press, London, 1973.
72. Gutierrez, J., Davis, R. E., and Lindahl, I. L., *Appl. Microbiol.* 7, 304 (1959).
73. Braden, A. W. H., Hart, N. K., and Lamberton, J. A., *Aust. J. Agric. Res.* 18, 335 (1967).
74. Shutt, D. A., Braden, A. W. H., and Lindner, H. R., *Aust. J. Agric. Res.* 20, 65 (1969).
75. Batterham, T. J., Shutt, D. A., Hart, N. K., Braden, A. W. H., and Tweeddale, H. J., *Aust. J. Agric. Res.* 22, 131 (1971).
76. Nilsson, A., Hill, J. L., and Davies, H. L., *Biochem Biophys. Acta* 148, 92 (1967).
77. Berardi, L. C., and Goldblatt, L. A., *in* "Toxic Constituents of Plant Foodstuffs" (I. E. Liener, Ed.), p. 211. Academic Press, New York, 1969.
78. Reiser, R., and Fu, H. C., *J. Nutr.* 76, 215 (1962).
79. Margalith, P., *Appl. Microbiol.* 15, 952 (1967).
80. Culvenor, C. C., *in* "Chemistry and Biochemistry of Herbage" (G. W. Butler and R. W. Bailey, Eds.), Vol. 1, p. 375. Academic Press, London, 1973.
81. Culvenor, C. C. J., Dann, A. T., and Dick, A. T., *Nature* 195, 570 (1962).
82. Lanigan, G. W., and Smith, L. W., *Aust. J. Agric. Res.* 21, 493 (1970).
83. Lanigan, G. W., *Aust. J. Agric. Res.* 21, 633 (1970).
84. Russell, G. R., and Smith, R. M., *Aust. J. Biol. Sci.* 21, 1277 (1968).
85. Lanigan, G. W., *J. Gen. Microbiol.* 94, 1 (1976).
86. Lanigan, G. W., *Aust. J. Agric. Res.* 22, 123 (1971).
87. Lanigan, G. W., *Aust. J. Agric. Res.* 23, 1085 (1972).
88. Shull, L. R., Buckmaster, G. W., and Cheeke, P. R., *J. Anim. Sci.* 43, 1247 (1976).
89. Bush, L. P., Streeter, C., and Buckner, R. C., *Crop Sci.* 10, 108 (1970).
90. Bush, L. P., Boling, J. A., Allen, G., and Buckner, R. C., *Crop Sci.* 12, 277 (1972).
91. Bush, L. P., Burton, H., and Boling, J. A., *J. Agric. Food Chem.* 24, 869 (1976).
92. Quin, J. I., Rimington, C., and Roets, G. C., *Onderstepoort J. Vet. Sci. Anim. Ind.* 4, 463 (1935).
93. Dawson, R. M. C., and Hemington, N., *Br. J. Nutr.* 32, 327 (1974).
94. Scheel, L. D., *in* "Toxicants Occurring Naturally in Foods," p. 558. National Academy of Sciences, Washington, D.C., 1973.
95. Smith, R. H., *Rep. Rowett Inst.* 30, 112 (1974).

96. Merricks, D. L., and Salsbury, R. L., *Appl. Microbiol.* 28, 106 (1974).
97. Van Etten, C. H., *in* "Toxic Constituents of Plant Foodstuffs" (I. E. Liener, Ed.), p. 103. Academic Press, New York, 1969.
98. Virtanen, A. I., Kreula, M., and Kiesvaara, M., *Z. Ernaehrungswiss. Suppl.* 3, 23 (1963).
99. Lanzain, A., Piana, G., Piva, G., Cardillo, M., and Rastelli, A., *J. Am. Chem. Soc.* 51, 517 (1974).
100. Butler, G. W., and Peterson, P. J., *N. Z. J. Agric. Res.* 4, 484 (1961).
101. Peterson, P. J., and Spedding, D. J., *N. Z. J. Agric. Res.* 6, 13 (1963).
102. Whanger, P. D., Weswig, P. H., and Muth, O. H., *Fed. Proc.* 27, 418 (Abstr.) (1968).
103. Hidiroglou, M., Heaney, D. P., and Jenkins, K. J., *Can. J. Physiol. Pharmacol.* 46, 229 (1968).
104. Hidiroglou, M., Jenkins, K. J., and Knipfel, J. E., *Can. J. Anim. Sci.* 54. 325 (1974).
105. Wright, P. L., and Bell, M. C., *Am. J. Physiol.* 211, 6 (1966).
106. Evans, W. C., *Bot. J. Linn. Soc.* 73, 113 (1966).
107. Evans, W. C., Evans, I. A., Humphreys, D. J., Lewin, B., Davies, W. E. J., and Axford, R. F. E., *J. Comp. Pathol.* 85, 253 (1975).
108. Jensen, R., Griner, L. A., and Adams, O. R., *J. Am. Vet. Med. Assoc.* 129, 311 (1956).
109. Terlecki, S., and Markson, L. M., *Vet. Rec.* 71, 508 (1959).
110. Edwin, E. E., Spence, J. B., and Wood A. J., *Vet. Rec.* 83, 417 (1968).
111. Edwin, E. E., Jackman, R., Machin, A. F., and Quick, M. P., *Biochem. Biophys. Res. Commun.* 70, 1190 (1976).
112. Loew, F. M., *J. Am. Vet. Med. Assoc.* 166, 219 (1975).
113. Lusby, K. S., and Brent, B. E., *J. Anim. Sci.* 35, 270 (1972).
114. Losada, H., Dixon, F., and Preston, T. R., *Rev. Cubana Cienc. Agric.* (English Ed.) 5, 369 (1971).
115. Shreeve, J. E., and Edwin, E. E., *Vet. Rec.* 94, 330 (1974).
116. Morgan, K. T., and Lawson, G. H. K., *Vet. Rec.* 95, 361 (1974).
117. Galtier, P., and Alvinerie, M., *Ann. Rec. Vet.* 7, 91 (1976).
118. Hult, K., Teiling, A., and Gatenbeck, S., *Appl. Environ. Microbiol.* 32, 443 (1976).
119. Brewer, D., Calder, F. W., MacIntyre, T. M., and Taylor, A., *J. Agric. Sci. Cambridge* 78, 257 (1972).
120. Brewer, D., Taylor, A., and Hoehn, M. M., *J. Agric. Sci. Cambridge* 78, 257 (1972).
121. Brewer, D., Duncan, J. M., Jerram, W. A., Leach, C. K., Safe, S., Taylor, A., Vining, L. C., Archibald, R. McG, Stevenson, R. G., Mirocha, C. J., and Christiansen, C. M., *Can. J. Microbiol.* 18, 1129 (1972).

122. Fehr, P. M., and Delage, J., *C. R. Acad. Sci. Paris Ser. D* 270, 550 (1970).
123. Mathur, C. F., Smith R. C., and Hawkins, G. E., *J. Dairy Sci.* 59, 455 (1976).
124. Shaw, B. A., and Wright, D. E., *N. Z. J. Agric. Res.* 15, 512 (1972).
125. Pettersson, H., and Kiessling, K. H., *Swed. J. Agric. Res.* 6, 161 (1976).

III. SIMPLE PHYTOTOXINS

Chairman: James H. Whittem

SELENIUM IN PLANTS AS A CAUSE OF LIVESTOCK POISONING

O. E. Olson
South Dakota State University

I. ABSTRACT

Soils in some areas of the world contain such high concentrations of selenium that they produce plants toxic to livestock. Some plants grow only in these seleniferous soils, are referred to as primary selenium indicators, and concentrate high levels of the element in their tissues. Others, referred to as secondary selenium absorbers, can accumulate rather high concentrations of the element when growing on seleniferous soils. A third class of plants, grasses, and grains as well as many others, absorb less selenium, but still often contain enough to be toxic.

Three major types of selenium toxicosis have been described. "Blind staggers' is suggested as a chronic type toxicosis resulting from long-term ingestion by sheep and cattle of the primary indicators or secondary absorbers in less than acutely toxic amounts. There is some reason to question the role of selenium in causing this syndrome. "Alkali disease" occurs in poultry, swine, cattle, and horses that consume grains, forages, or pasture plants containing usually less than 50 but more than 5 parts per million of the element over a period of many weeks or months. Acute selenium toxicosis results when grazing animals consume the primary selenium indicators in amounts sufficient to cause a very rapid toxicosis. Control in all types of selenium toxicoses requires avoidance of seleniferous feeds.

II. INTRODUCTION

Reviews of the problem of selenium poisoning (selenosis) in animals are numerous. The first detailed review was by Moxon (1), and the most comprehensive was by Rosenfeld and Beath (2). The reader is referred to these for many of the details that space precludes recording here. Other more recent reviews on selenium (3,4,5,6) cover the chemistry, biochemistry, role in nutrition, and other similar topics. The following is a brief overview of the problem.

The history of the discovery of selenium as an important, naturally occurring livestock toxicant has been covered in the above reviews, but certain aspects of this history seem important to this discussion, and they will be included. It should be pointed out, for instance, that it was through a cooperative effort of scientists with the United States Department of Agriculture and the Wyoming and South Dakota Agricultural Experiment

Stations that several previously unexplained toxicoses or maladies in farm animals were found to be caused by the ingestion of plants containing high concentrations of selenium. This was in the early 1930's. A flurry of interest in research on the problem over about a decade was followed by a lull until the late 1950's, when the findings of Schwarz and Folz (7) stimulated a rapidly expanding interest in the element as an essential nutrient, and consequently some additional interest in its toxic effects. We are left, nevertheless, with much to learn about selenium poisoning as it occurs in the field under natural conditions.

Rosenfeld and Beath (2) have described various types of selenosis, as follows:

- Chronic selenosis
  - "Blind staggers" type
  - "Alkali disease" type
  - Experimental
- Acute selenosis
- Other types

These will be discussed in about the order shown, omitting any separate consideration of the experimental chronic type. Before doing so, however, it seems appropriate to summarize what is known of the occurrence of selenium in nature, the formation of seleniferous soils, and the accumulation of selenium by plants.

III. SELENIFEROUS SOILS

The earth's crust has been estimated to contain an average of about 0.1 part per million (ppm) of selenium (4). Some soils contain considerably more than this, enough more so that plants growing in them are toxic.

In the United States, such soils have usually weathered from sedimentary rocks of high selenium content. The principal source of the element in these rocks is thought by many to have been volcanic gases, the selenium in these gases having been deposited in and precipitated from the shallow seas during formation of the sedimentary rocks. High selenium contents of some ferruginous Hawaiian soils have also been suggested to result from volcanic action. On the other hand, highly seleniferous soils of Ireland seem to have been formed on redeposition of the element by reduction in a poorly drained basin containing much organic matter, after its first having been leached and transported from sedimentary rocks at a higher level (8). Canadian workers (9) have reported some concentration of selenium in soils formed from lacustrine deposits, probably through a similar process. An alluvial seleniferous sand in Israel apparently derived the element from a higher lying limestone (10).

Selenium occurs in soils in various forms. In unweathered rock and in soils of the more arid areas, it may occur as an iron selenide or as the free element (4). In either form, its availability to plants would be very low (11). The reason certain Hawaiian soils of high selenium content grow plants of low selenium content has been suggested to be the fixation of the element as a basic iron selenide (7), and at least some of the insoluble selenium in soils may exist as selenite in this form or tightly adsorbed on iron colloids (12). No doubt, some organic forms of the element derived from plant residues are also present, and these may be soluble and available to plants (13). Perhaps the most soluble and the most significant form of the element in terms of its availability to plants is selenate (14).

The distribution of available forms of selenium in the soil profile can have an important effect on its uptake by plants. Particularly in the somewhat arid areas, the soluble and thus the more readily available forms may in large part leach from the surface and redeposit at lower depths. Thus, more will be available to deep rooted plants than to shallow rooted ones (15). Nevertheless, soluble selenium in the second and third foot of the soil profile can contribute significantly to the selenium content of such crops as grasses, and must be taken into account in assessing the potential of a soil to produce seleniferous crops.

In the United States, Wyoming, and South Dakota are most well-known for their soils of excessive selenium contents, but such soils are also found to some extent in other states of lower rainfall. A number of other countries have reported seleniferous areas, but none to date appear as extensive as those in the United States (2).

IV. SELENIUM IN PLANTS

Plants contain selenium in widely varying amounts. The most significant causes for this variation are discussed below.

The kind of plant is important in determining its selenium content, as reviewed by Rosenfeld and Beath (2). According to these authors, certain plants are restricted to seleniferous soils and often have very high selenium content, some as much as 10,000 ppm on a dry basis. These they call primary selenium indicators, and included are various species of *Astragalus*, *Xylorrhiza (Machaeranthera)*, *Oonopsis (Haplopappus)*, and *Stanleya*. Some of these have very offensive odors.

Rosenfeld and Beath also refer to secondary selenium absorbers which they describe as accumulating moderate amounts of selenium (probably several hundred ppm) when growing in soils of high available selenium content. These include some species of *Aster*, *Atriplex*, *Grindelia*, and certain other genera.

Finally, crop plants, grasses, and a number of weeds absorb lesser quantities, usually not more than 50 ppm on soils of high available selenium content. The crop plants are involved in selenosis in poultry and swine, while it is the grasses and other non-accumulators that are largely responsible for the "alkali disease" syndrome in grazing animals. This is probably because the animals avoid the primary and secondary indicators if other forage is available.

In addition to the kind of plant, the part of the plant is also important in determining selenium content. Seeds usually contain more than leaves, which contain more than stems. The selenium content decreases with advancing maturity in most cases. The chemical form of the selenium in the soil affects plant uptake of the element, selenate appearing to be very available. While sulfate reduces selenate uptake by plants in greenhouse studies, sulfur additions to soils in the field have been found to have no effect on selenium uptake. Some plants contain volatile selenium compounds that are lost on drying, especially on drying at high temperature.

Shrift (16) listed the following selenium compounds as having been reported in plants: Se-methylselenocysteine, selenohomocystine, selenocysteineseleninic acid, Se-propenylselenocysteine selenoxide, γ-L-glutamyl-Se-methylseleno-L-cysteine, selenocysteine, selenocystathionine, selenomethionine, selenomethionine selenoxide, Se-methylselenomethionine, dimethyldiselenide, selenopeptides, and a selenowax. For some of these compounds, the data for their existence are not convincing. Hamilton (17,18) has reported the presence of Se-methylselenocysteine selenoxide in onions and cabbage, and Lewis *et al.* (19) have reported the presence of dimethylselenide in cabbage. Dimethylselenide and, especially, dimethyldiselenide are no doubt almost entirely responsible for the loss of selenium on the drying of some plants and for the odor associated with plants of high selenium concentrations. In addition to the above organic compounds, selenate and selenite have also been reported to occur in plants (20). The toxicities of some of these compounds have not been studied, and, since many of them may occur in any one plant, evaluation of the toxicity of the plant based on its total selenium content is hardly possible.

Shrift (16) also suggested that within the genus, *Astragalus*, the indicator species synthesize largely the Se-methylselenocysteine from the selenium they absorb, while the non-indicators synthesize largely the Se-methylselenomethionine. He has also suggested that the formation of non-protein amino acids containing selenium by the accumulator plants is a mechanism by which the plants protect themselves against the toxicity of the element.

V. CHRONIC SELENOSIS

As pointed out previously, two types of chronic selenosis have been described. These are the "blind staggers" and the alkali disease" types.

A. "Blind Staggers"

Work with the "blind staggers" type of selenium poisoning has been almost entirely confined to the Wyoming Agricultural Experiment Station. Rosenfeld and Beath (2) thoroughly summarized this work, and unless otherwise indicated the following discussion is taken from their summary.

According to the Wyoming workers, the "blind staggers" syndrome appears in cattle and sheep that consume primary selenium indicator and/or secondary selenium absorber plants of moderate selenium content over a considerable period of time. They have produced the syndrome by feeding seleniferous weeds of the above types to both cattle and sheep. However, they have not reported having produced it by feeding selenium compounds, and the reports of Maag *et al.* (21) and Glenn *et al.* (22,23) have raised some doubt that selenium is the cause. It is possible that selenium may act in conjunction with other compounds in the weeds, of course, but it is also possible that alkaloids or some other nonseleniferous biologically active compound(s) are the cause of the observed signs of toxicosis. Additional research seems necessary to clarify this matter.

The "blind staggers" syndrome expresses itself in three stages. In the first stage, inappetence and some impairment of vision have been noted. Affected animals may wander in circles and disregard objects in their paths. In the second stage, the severity of the above signs increases. The front legs become weak and cannot support the animal. In the third stage, the tongue and swallowing mechanisms become paralyzed, respiration is labored and quickened, there is obvious evidence of abdominal pain, the animal grates its teeth, and there is excessive salivation. The body temperature is subnormal, the cornea becomes cloudy, the eyelids are swollen, and the mucous membranes of the mouth are pale. The third stage usually appears suddenly, and death often follows within a few hours, apparently as the result of respiratory failure. Gradual loss of weight is common.

Recovery from the disease is often incomplete because mature animals lack vigor and young animals are stunted. A delayed action of the poison has been noted; clinical signs appeared up to several months after animals were removed from seleniferous feeds. The disease is not as easily diagnosed in sheep as it is in cattle, since the three stages are not as clearly differentiated.

The gross and microscopic pathology of the syndrome have been described in detail by Rosenfeld and Beath. They indicate that "there is superimposed upon a chronic process an acute reaction which may be due to ingestion of extremely toxic plants or to sudden liberation of selenium stored in various organs because of some stress or secondary damage to the organs."

Treatment consists of drenching with copious quantities of warm water and injection of strychnine sulfate. After a day or two, there seems to be some advantage in drenching with a solution of iron, quinine sulfate, and nux vomica. Laxatives should be avoided. Prostigmine has also been used in treatment.

B. "Alkali Disease"

In 1934, Franke and his associates (24) described the "alkali disease" syndrome, basing their report on a field survey made before selenium was discovered as its cause. Some examples of what they found are shown in Figure 1. A few years later, Draize

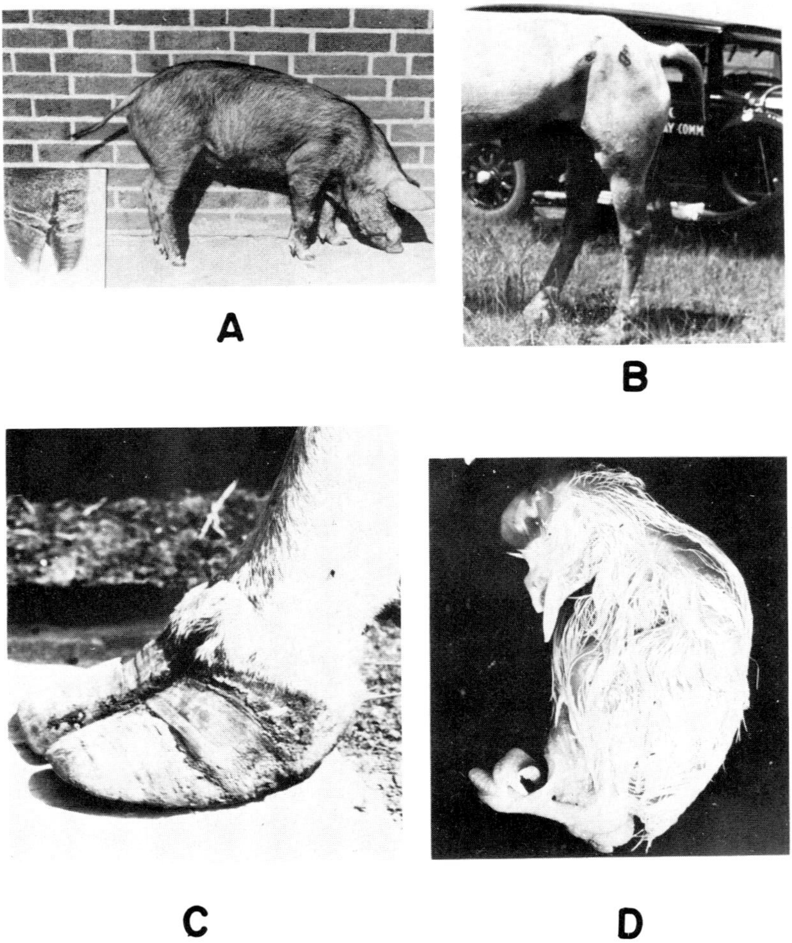

Fig. 1. *Some examples of the "alkali disease" syndrome photographed by early workers in the field: (A) thin hair coat and cracked hoof (inset) in swine; (B) emaciation and loss of hair from tail in horse; (C) cracked hoof in cow; and (D) malformed chick embryo. All these signs have been reproduced in these animals by feeding selenium compounds.*

and Beath (25), and Moxon (1) expanded on the description of the malady. The following pathological signs were usually observed: loss of long hair from the mane and tail of horses and from the switch of cattle; loss of body hair from swine; sore feet with inflammation at the coronary band in horses, cattle, and swine, followed by lateral cracking and other deformities of the hoof; lack of vitality and emaciation in horses, cattle, and swine, on occasion to the point of death; lesions at the base of the horns in cattle similar to those of the hoof, but less pronounced; decreased hatchability of chicken eggs due to malformation of the developing embryo. Chicks that did hatch often had a "greased" appearance and were weak.

Anemia, liver atrophy and cirrhosis, atrophy of the heart, erosion of the joints of the long bones, deterioration of the bone marrow, some kidney lesions, and histological changes representative of a chronic intoxication were also found to be quite prevalent in horses and cattle. Sheep were not mentioned in any of the early reports as suffering from the "alkali disease" syndrome, and the author has not observed any chronic effects of the element on sheep other than a severely reduced rate of reproduction when the animals grazed pastures that produced the typical syndrome in cattle.

Except for chickens, no effects on reproduction were described by the early workers. However, such effects have been noted in rats fed grains from toxic areas (26), in swine on diets containing added inorganic selenium (27), and in cattle on seleniferous range (28,29,30).

1. *Selenium as the Causative Agent*

It seems proper at this point to review the research that confirms selenium as the cause of "alkali disease," since some fairly recent reports have suggested otherwise. Maag and his associates (21) have, for instance, reported experiments in which cattle were administered oral doses of sodium selenate over a period of many months. They observed few typical signs of "alkali disease." In addition, Glenn *et al.* (22,23,31) report in much detail on the toxicosis produced by daily oral administration of sodium selenate to sheep at toxic and subtoxic levels over extended periods. They observed no chronic toxicity and no effect on reproduction, although a large portion of the animals consumed lethal amounts of the element. The results with sheep are not entirely unexpected, since the "alkali disease" syndrome had not been observed in these animals by the early workers. Concerning the observations on cattle made by Maag and his associates, it has been suggested (1,2, see Discussion on p. 138 of Ref. 32) that only the organic forms of selenium produce the "alkali disease" syndrome, but the following indicates otherwise.

The establishment of selenium as the cause of "alkali disease" began with the discovery of the element in wheat and soils from affected areas (Robinson 33). Franke and Potter (34) then fed rats diets containing different grains from farms with histories of the malady and recorded the pathologic effects. Later (35) they found sodium selenite added to similar diets containing normal grains "virtually identical with the natural plant toxicant" as far as the clinical signs it produced. They also found the toxicant to be mostly concentrated in the protein fraction of grains (36), that the same was true for selenium (37), the hydrolysates of isolated toxic proteins were toxic and contained selenium but that when the element was removed from them they were not (38).

At about this same time, Munsell *et al.* (39) reported that rats fed diets containing various levels of selenium added as seleniferous wheat produced increasing toxicosis with increasing selenium content. Further, feeding selenite produced toxicosis identical to that produced by toxic grain. Finally, wheat grown in a sand culture containing selenate produced the same signs and lesions as did that grown in a toxic area while that from a culture without added selenium did not. Later, Rhian and Moxon (40) found that diets containing added inorganic selenium salts produced effects in dogs very similar to those produced by diets containing toxic wheat.

Franke and his coworkers next found that inorganic selenium reduced yeast fermentation (41) as had proteins from toxic grains (42). By feeding grains from affected areas, they also reproduced the low hatchability of eggs and deformities in chick embryos that had been reported from the field (43), correlated the effects of the toxic grains on chickens on farms in affected areas with those produced experimentally (44) and with the selenium contents of the diets containing naturally toxic grains (45), and reproduced monstrosities in egg embryos by the injection of inorganic selenium salts into eggs (46). In addition, Moxon (1) reported that feeding inorganic selenium to laying hens caused decreased hatchability of eggs and malformed embryos.

Schoening (47) produced loss of hair and hoof lesions typical of "alkali disease" in swine by feeding corn from an affected area and containing 10 ppm of the element. Corn from the same area but containing 5 ppm of selenium and corn from an area with no history of the syndrome caused none of the signs. Later, Miller and Schoening (48) produced "alkali disease" in swine by feeding sodium selenite. Moxon (49) also reproduced the syndrome in swine by feeding a diet containing seleniferous corn, and Wahlstrom and associates (27,50) did the same by feeding diets containing added sodium selenite.

Miller and Williams (51) fed sodium selenite in the feed to three horses and a mule. The principal signs of toxicity noted were emaciation, listlessness, looseness of the hair of the mane and tail, and some softness and scaling of the horny wall of the hoof, none of these signs being as outstanding as those described for field cases. Lesions of the heart, liver, spleen, and kidneys resembled those for field cases of the syndrome.

Olson and Embry (52) fed selenite added to the diet at 18 ppm of selenium to five heifers over a period of 231 days, observing typical signs of "alkali disease" in one of the animals. This is consistent with field observations at a seleniferous ranch (53,54) where only a small percentage of the animals in a herd showed visual signs of the poisoning.

Since the "alkali disease" syndrome was observed in cattle, horses, swine, and poultry within the same area of land and most often on the same farm or ranch, there seems little doubt of a common cause. Further, in view of what has been presented above, there seems no doubt that the cause is selenium. Finally, since the syndrome has been so often produced experimentally by feeding either toxic grains or inorganic selenium, it seems that both organic and inorganic forms of the element can cause "alkali disease," although it is well known that not all forms are equally toxic. Available data indicate that feeds containing over 5 but usually less than 50 ppm of the element are involved.

2. *Control Measures*

The prevention of "alkali disease" at present requires limitation of selenium intake. The use of bromobenzene to stimulate urinary excretion of the element has been suggested as a means of reversing the effects of the element (55), but has not proved efficacious (53). Arsenic, known for its prevention of chronic selenosis under closely controlled conditions (56,57) has not been found effective in range animals, where control of intake of both arsenic and selenium is difficult (53). Linseed oil meal contains something that prevents chronic selenosis in rats (58) and in poultry (59), but under practical feeding conditions for swine and range cattle it has not been found useful (53,57). To date, the only practical control measures have been based on management. These have included the avoidance or limitation of seleniferous feeds. With range animals, this demands a mapping program based on knowledge of the geology of the area and on plant analysis. Emphasis has also been placed on proper protein nutrition to somewhat reduce the effects of excessive selenium intake, as suggested by some experimental work (1,60).

3. *Diagnosis*

Diagnosis of the "alkali disease" type of selenosis is usually based on usual clinical signs as already described. Draize and Beath (25) have described the gross and microscopic pathology of the toxicosis in detail, and their observations may be somewhat helpful in diagnosis. Blood analyses indicate what the present level of selenium intake is. Hair analyses indicate what the long term ingestion has been. Based on its experimental findings (53, 61) and field observations, the South Dakota Agricultural Experiment Station uses the following guidelines for diagnosis (62):

Selenium (ppm) in Blood	Hair	
Under 1.0	Under 5.0	Chronic selenosis should not be expected.
1.0--2.0	5.0--10.0	Suggests a borderline problem.
Over 2.0	Over 10.0	Selenium intake excessive and selenosis can be expected. However, animals with these levels will not necessarily exhibit signs of the toxicosis.

VI. ACUTE SELENOSIS

In the field, acute selenosis results from the ingestion of a sufficient amount of primary indicator or other plants containing high levels (several hundred ppm or more) of selenium, usually at a single feeding. Cattle and sheep are most commonly involved, but apparently horses and swine can be also. As many as 340 sheep have been reported to have died within 24 hours after consuming *Astragalus bisulcatus* plants. The plants involved are rather unpalatable, and animals will avoid them unless pastures are sparse (2).

The clinical signs of the poisoning have been described as follows (63). The affected animal's posture and movement are abnormal at first and these signs soon become more pronounced. Watery diarrhea, increased excretion of urine, and dilated pupils are observed. Prostration and apparent unconsciousness precede death due to respiratory failure. Duration of the illness is from a few hours to several days. The poisoning has been reproduced by the forced feeding of highly seleniferous plants and by the administration of selenium compounds.

The pathology of the toxicosis has been detailed by Beath and his associates (25,64). The most obvious pathological changes were found to be hemorrhages due to capillary damage and necrosis.

Death usually occurs before the disease can be diagnosed, and there is no known treatment for counteracting the poison. Normally it occurs under conditions where there would be no time to use remedies were any available (2).

Diagnosis is usually based on the observation that the animals have consumed highly seleniferous weeds. Analysis of rumen contents for selenium might be helpful in confirming the element as the cause of deaths, but there are few data to help in interpreting the results of such an analysis.

VII. OTHER TYPES OF SELENOSIS

Brown (65) has suggested that selenium might have a predisposing role in Geeldikkop and enzootic icterus of sheep in South Africa. To date, this has not been clearly established. Lathyrism was at one time suggested as being caused by selenium (66), but now this is known not to be the case. The widely varying conditions (kind of animal, chemical form of the element, route, rate, and level of dosage, etc.) under which selenium toxicity has been studied have given rise to a wide variety of reactions of the element on the animal body. Thus, there may be found sets of clinical signs that suggest other types of the toxicoses than those listed by Rosenfeld and Beath. Indeed, variations from the classical signs can be expected in the field as well (67).

VIII. REFERENCES

1. Moxon, A. L., *S. D. Agric. Exp. Stn. Bull.* 311 (1937).
2. Rosenfeld, I., and Beath, O. A., "Selenium," Academic Press, New York, 1964.
3. "Selenium in Nutrition," National Academy of Sciences, National Research Council, 1973.
4. "Medical and Biological Effects of Pollutants. Selenium," National Academy of Sciences, National Research Council, 1976.
5. Klayman, D. L., and Günther, H. H., "Organic Selenium Compounds: Their Chemistry and Biology," John Wiley & Sons, New York, 1973.
6. Zingaro, R. A., and Cooper, W. C., "Selenium," Van Nostrand Reinhold, New York, 1974.
7. Schwarz, K., and Folz, *J. Am. Chem. Soc.* 79, 3292 (1957).
8. Fleming, G. A., and Walsh, T., *Proc. R. Ir. Acad.* 58, (Sec. B, No. 7), 151 (1957).
9. Thorvaldson, R., and Johnson, L. R., *Can. J. Res.* 18, 138 (1940).
10. Ravikovitch, S., and Margolin, M., *KTAVIM* 7, 41 (1957).
11. Moxon, A. L., Olson, O. E., and Searight, W. V., *S. D. Agric. Exp. Stn. Tech. Bull.* 2 (1950).
12. Byers, H. G., Miller, J. T., Williams, K. T., and Lakin, H. W., *U. S. Dep. Agric. Tech. Bull.* 601 (1938).
13. Beath, O. A., Eppson, H. F., and Gilbert, C. S., *J. Am. Pharm. Assoc.* 26, 394 (1937).
14. Byers, H. G., *U. S. Dep. Agric. Tech. Bull.* 530 (1936).
15. Olson, O. E., Whitehead, E. I., and Moxon, A. L., *Soil Sci.* 54, 47 (1942).
16. Shrift, A., *in* "Organic Selenium Compounds: Their Chemistry and Biology" (D. L. Klayman and W. H. H. Günther, Eds.), p. 763. Interscience, London and New York, 1973.
17. Hamilton, J. W., *Adv. Front. Plant Sci.* 30, 189 (1975).
18. Hamilton, J. W., *J. Agric. Food Chem.* 23, 1150 (1975).
19. Lewis, B. G., Johnson, D. M., and Broyer, T. C., *Plant Soil* 40, 107 (1974).
20. Beath, O. A., and Eppson, H. F., *Wyo. Agric. Exp. Stn. Bull.* 278 (1947).
21. Maag, D. D., Orsborn, J. S., and Clopton, J. R., *Am. J. Vet. Res.* 21, 1049 (1960).

22. Glenn, M. W., Jensen, R., and Griner, L. A., *Am. J. Vet. Res.* 25, 1479 (1964).
23. Glenn, M. W., Jensen, R., and Griner, L. A., *Am. J. Vet. Res.* 25, 1486 (1964).
24. Franke, K. W., Rice, T. D., Johnson, A. G., and Schoening, H. W., *U. S. Dep. Agric. Circ.* 320 (1934).
25. Draize, J. H., and Beath, O. A., *J. Am. Vet. Med. Assoc.* 86, 753 (1935).
26. Franke, K. W., and Potter, V. R., *J. Nutr.* 12, 205 (1936).
27. Wahlstrom, R. C., and Olson, O. E., *J. Anim. Sci.* 18, 141 (1959).
28. Dinkel, C. A., Minyard, J. A., and Ray, D. E., *J. Anim. Sci.* 22, 1043 (1963).
29. Minyard, J. A., *S. D. Farm Home Res.* 12 (No. 1), 1 (1961).
30. Dinkel, C. A., Minyard, J. A., and Ray, D. E., *S. D. Farm Home Res.* 15 (No. 1), 13 (1964).
31. Glenn, M. W., Martin, J. L., and Cummins, L. M., *Am. J. Vet. Res.* 25, 1495 (1964).
32. Maag, D. D., and Glenn, M. W., *in* "Selenium in Biomedicine" (O. H. Muth, J. E. Oldfield, and P. H. Weswig, Eds.), AVI Publishing Co., Inc., Westport, Connecticut, 1967.
33. Robinson, W. O., *J. Assoc. Off. Agric. Chem.* 16, 423 (1933).
34. Franke, K. W., and Potter, V. R., *J. Nutr.* 8, 615 (1934).
35. Franke, K. W., and Potter, V. R., *J. Nutr.* 10, 213 (1935).
36. Franke, K. W., *J. Nutr.* 8, 609 (1934).
37. Franke, K. W., and Painter, E. P., *Cereal Chem.* 13, 67 (1936).
38. Franke, K. W., and Painter, E. P., *J. Nutr.* 10, 599 (1935).
39. Munsell, H. E., Devaney G. M., and Kennedy, M. H., *U. S. Dep. Agric. Tech. Bull.* 534 (1936).
40. Rhian, M., and Moxon, A. L., *J. Pharmacol. Exp. Ther.* 78, 249 (1943).
41. Moxon, A. L., and Franke, K. W., *Ind. Eng. Chem.* 27, 77 (1935).
42. Franke, K. W., and Moxon, A. L., *J. Nutr.* 8, 625 (1934).
43. Franke, K. W., and Tully, W. C., *Poult. Sci.* 14, 273 (1935).
44. Franke, K. W., and Tully, W. C., *Poult. Sci.* 15, 316 (1936).
45. Poley, W. E., and Moxon, A. L., *Poult. Sci.* 17, 72 (1938).
46. Franke, K. W., Moxon, A. L., Poley, W. E., and Tully, W. C., *Anat. Rec.* 65, 15 (1936).
47. Schoening, H. W., *North Am. Vet.* 17, 22 (1936).
48. Miller, W. T., and Schoening, H. W., *J. Agric. Res.* 56, 831 (1938).
49. Moxon, A. L., *Proc. S. D. Acad. Sci.* 21, 34 (1941).
50. Wahlstrom, R. C., Kamstra, L. D., and Olson, O. E., *J. Anim. Sci.* 14, 105 (1955).
51. Miller, W. T., and Williams, K. T., *J. Agric. Res.* 61, 353 (1940).
52. Olson, O. E., and Embry, L. B., *Proc. S. D. Acad. Sci.* 52, 50 (1973).
53. Dinkel, C. A., Minyard, J. A., Whitehead, E. I., and Olson, O. E., *S. D. Agric. Exp. Stn. Circ.* 135 (1957).

54. Moxon, A. L., Rhian, M. A., Anderson, H. E., and Olson, O. E., *J. Anim. Sci.* 3, 299 (1944).
55. Moxon, A. L., Schaefer, A. E., Lardy, H. A., Dubois, K. P., and Olson, O. E., *J. Biol. Chem.* 132, 785 (1940).
56. Moxon, A. L., *Science* 88, 81 (1938).
57. Wahlstrom, R. C., Kamstra, L. D., and Olson, O. E., *S. D. Agric. Exp. Stn. Bull.* 456 (1956).
58. Halverson, A. W., Hendrick, C. M., and Olson, O. E., *J. Nutr.* 56, 51 (1955).
59. Jensen, L. S., and Chang, C. H., *Poult. Sci.* 55, 592 (1976).
60. Rosenfeld, I., and Beath, O. A., *Am. J. Vet. Res.* 7, 52 (1946).
61. Olson, O. E., Dinkel, C. A., and Kamstra, L. D., *S. D. Farm Home Res.* 6 (No. 1), 12 (1954).
62. Olson, O. E., and Fox, D. G., *S. D. Beef Cattle Handb.*, File 312.
63. Beath, O. A., Gilbert, C. S., Eppson, H. F., and Rosenfeld, I., *Wyo. Agric. Exp. Stn. Bull.* 324 (1953).
64. Rosenfeld, I., and Beath, O. A., *Wyo. Agric. Exp. Stn. Bull.* 275 (1946).
65. Brown, J. M. M., *Ann. N. Y. Acad. Sci.* 104, 504 (1963).
66. Rudra, M. N., *Nature* 170, 124 (1952).
67. Approved for publication by the Director of the Agricultural Experiment Station of South Dakota State University.

MANIFESTATIONS OF INTOXICATION BY SELENIUM-ACCUMULATING PLANTS

Kent R. Van Kampen and Lynn F. James
Utah State University and Poisonous Plant Research Laboratory, Agricultural Research Service, U.S. Department of Agriculture

I. ABSTRACT

A selenium-accumulating indicator plant, Astragalus bisulcatus, *previously recognized as toxic and thought to be a cause of chronic selenium toxicity described as Blind Staggers, was fed experimentally to sheep. Clinical signs of emaciation, depression, neurological disturbances, and pathologic changes of neurovisceral cytoplasmic vacuolation were observed microscopically in the experimental sheep. These changes are similar to those observed in locoweed poisoning. It is suggested that the principle toxic agent(s) in* Astragalus bisulcatus *is similar to that of the true locoweeds rather than being selenium related. Further studies feeding other seleniferous indicator plants are being conducted.*

II. INTRODUCTION

In a paper published in 1946, Irene Rosenfeld and O. A. Beath described the pathology attributed to selenium poisoning (1). They classified selenium poisoning into three categories. First, acute; second, sub-acute; and third, chronic poisoning. The characteristic lesions ascribed to acute and sub-acute poisonings were multiple hemorrhages and fibrosis of many body organs. They sub-classified the chronic form into two diseases. "Alkali Disease" was characterized by hair loss, weight loss, hoof deformities, and swollen joints. "Blind Staggers" was characterized by incoordination, impaired vision, and paralysis. Although they mentioned examining many body tissues, no reference was made of examination of the central nervous system. Both of the chronic diseases were attributed to the continuous ingestion of sub-lethal levels of selenium contained in plants.

These descriptions have been propogated in most Veterinary Pathology textbooks (2,3). The acute form and one of the chronic forms ("Alkali Disease") of selenium toxicity have been confirmed by experimental feeding of selenium to ungulates (1). The second chronic form, "Blind Staggers," has not been experimentally reproduced by feeding selenium, but has been associated with ingestion of selenium-containing plants.

III. SELENIUM-CONTAINING PLANTS

Seleniferous plants have been subdivided into non-indicator and indicator plants (4,5). Non-indicator plants contain selenium bound to protein and the selenium is relatively insoluble in water. The indicator plants requiring selenium for growth are found only where significant levels of selenium are present. Selenium in the indicator plants is water soluble. It has been suggested that the indicator plants are deep rooted and transport selenium from the deeper areas in the soil profile to the surface where it becomes available to the more shallow rooted grasses and cereal crops (5). Alkali Disease has been attributed to the ingestion of non-indicator plants (6) while Blind Staggers has been associated with ingestion of indicator plants.

IV. EXPERIMENTAL DESIGN

Astragalus bisulcatus is a selenium-accumulating indicator plant which has not been classified as a locoweed, but placed with other types of plants causing chronic selenium poisoning (4,7). Since clinical signs of Blind Staggers and locoweed poisoning are similar, an experiment was designed to compare lesions in sheep fed *Astragalus bisulcatus* with those fed selenium-containing alfalfa hay and those fed sodium selenite.

V. RESULTS

Ewes fed *Astragalus bisulcatus* (180 ppm Se) for 30 days at the rates of 110 or 230 grams per day, did not have clinical or pathologic signs of poisoning. Ewes fed for a similar period, but at a rate of 340 grams of *Astragalus bisulcatus* per day, had typical neural-visceral cytoplasm vacuolation of the Purkinje cells of the cerebellum, hepatocytes of the liver, tubular cells of the kidney, ascinar cells of the pancreas and follicular cells of the thyroid gland (Fig. 1). Mild vacuolation was also observed in the neurons of the plexus of Auerback in the intestine. These lesions were similar to those in locoweed poisoning (8). Serum levels of alkaline phosphatase and SGOT increased in peripheral circulation.

No lesions were found in ewes fed selenium-containing alfalfa hay (12.9 ppm Se). Sheep could not be enticed to eat diets containing sodium selenite.

In subsequent trial, pregnant ewes were fed a mixture of alfalfa hay, *Astragalus bisulcatus*, barley, and molasses from the 30th day of gestation until the lambs were born. The ewes and lambs were then killed and examined for lesions. Prior to being killed, the ewes became depressed, emaciated, and had neurological disturbances typical of locoweed poisoning. All of the ewes had typical vacuolar lesions in the liver and pancreas. Two of the lambs had degenerative vacuolar lesions of the thyroid and kidney.

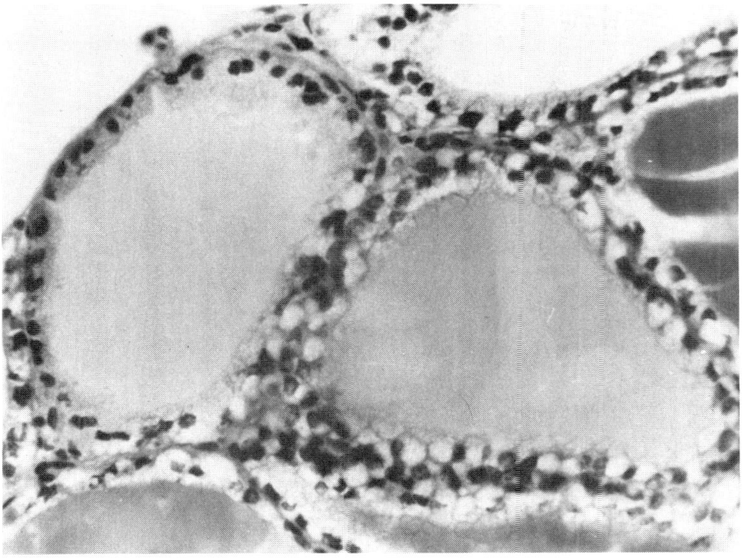

Fig. 1. *Cytoplasmic vacuolation of follicular cells of the thyroid gland from a ewe fed* Astragalus bisulcatus *at 340 g/day.*

Four lambs were dead or died at birth. These results are similar to those found by James *et al.* in locoweed poisoning (9).

VI. DISCUSSION

Rosenfeld and Beath stated that there is little toxic material in *Astragalus bisulcatus* other than selenium (5). Our research would indicate that in addition to a high level of selenium, *Astragalus bisulcatus* contains agents similar to those found in the true locoweeds. Lesions of selenium toxicity described by Rosenfeld and Beath were not observed. Perhaps the condition described as Blind Staggers is actually chronic locoweed poisoning. *Astragalus* species, reported as causing true locoweed poisoning, do not contain significant amounts of selenium, so we find it difficult to attribute the lesions in our experimental sheep to the selenium content of *Astragalus bisulcatus*. The proported chronic selenium intoxication, as it relates to Blind Staggers, must be further investigated by feeding *Astragalus bisulcatus*, other seleniferous plants, and varying types of seleniferous compounds to ungulates.

VII. SUMMARY

A selenium-accumulating indicator plant, *Astragalus bisulcatus*, previously recognized as toxic and thought to be a cause of chronic selenium toxicity described as Blind Staggers, was fed experimentally to sheep. Clinical signs of emaciation, depression, neurological disturbances, and pathologic changes of neurovisceral cytoplasmic vacuolation were observed microscopically in the experimental sheep. These changes are similar to those observed in locoweed poisoning. It is suggested that the principle toxic agent(s) in *Astragalus bisulcatus* is similar to that of the true locoweeds rather than being selenium. Further studies feeding other seleniferous indicator plants are being conducted.

VIII. REFERENCES

1. Rosenfeld, Irene, and Beath, O. A., *Wyo. Agric. Exp. Stn. Bull.* 275 (1946).
2. Jubb, K. V., and Kennedy, P. C., "Pathology of Domestic Animals," 2nd Ed., Vols. 1 and 2. Academic Press, New York, 1970.
3. Smith, H., Jones, T. C., and Hunt, R. D., "Veterinary Pathology." Lea and Febiger, Philadelphia, 1972.
4. Kingsbury, J. M., "Poisonous Plants of the United States and Canada." Prentice-Hall, Englewood Cliffs, New Jersey, 1964.
5. Rosenfeld, Irene, and Beath, O. A., "Selenium," pp. 61-226. Academic Press, New York, 1964.
6. Moxon, Alvin L., *S. D. Exp. Stn. Bull.* 311 (1937).
7. Beath, O. A., Draize, J. A., and Eppson, H. F., *Wyo. Agric. Exp. Stn. Bull.* 189 (1932).
8. Van Kampen, Kent R., and James, Lynn F., *Pathol. Vet.* 6, 413-423 (1969).
9. James, L. F., Shupe, J. L., Binns, W., and Keeler, R. F., *Am. J. Vet. Res.* 28, 1379-1388 (1967).

OXALATE POISONING IN LIVESTOCK

Lynn F. James
Poisonous Plant Research Laboratory, Agricultural Research Service
U.S. Department of Agriculture

I. ABSTRACT

Oxalate poisoning is of great importance throughout the world. Oxalate poisoning in livestock occurs primarily from the ingestion of oxalate containing plants. The oxalate in these plants occurs in association with a number of different cations. It now appears that the toxic effects these various oxalate compounds have on animals may be modified by the cation with which they are associated. Some of these effects are discussed in this paper.

II. INTRODUCTION

Oxalic acid (oxalate) poisoning of livestock, household pets, and people is of great importance throughout the world. Oxalic acid is an organic dicarboxylic acid that readily forms insoluble salts with calcium and magnesium. Its principal soluble salts are sodium, potassium, and ammonium oxalate. Oxalic acid and its soluble salts are both corrosive and systemic poisons (1).

Oxalate poisoning in livestock results principally from ingesting oxalate-producing plants. Because these plants are palatable, they may sometimes form a large part of a ruminant's diet. To be potentially dangerous, the plants must contain 10% or more oxalic acid on a plant dry-weight basis. The principal oxalate-producing shrubs and forbs, which occur throughout the world, belong to the genus *Rumex* or genera of the Chenopodiaceae and Oxalidaceae families. Recently, certain grasses have been shown to accumulate harmful amounts of oxalate.

Plants that produce substantial amounts of oxalate generally fit into one of two groups (2): (a) those with a sap pH of about 2, with the oxalate anion present chiefly as acid oxalate ($HC_2O_4^-$) (*Oxalis pes-caprae* and some species of *Rumex*); and (b) those with a sap pH of about 6, with the oxalic acid present chiefly as the oxalate ion ($C_2O_4^=$) (some Chenopodiaceae).

The oxalate of group 1 plants occurs primarily as acid potassium oxalate, that of group 2 plants as soluble sodium oxalate and the insoluble calcium and magnesium oxalates (2).

The grasses that produce oxalate do so at a level lower than that of the above-listed shrubs and forbs. *Setaria sphacelata*, a grass in Australia, is thought to contain oxalate as ammonium oxalate (3,4).

Two of the principal oxalate-producing plants of the world,

soursob (*Oxalis pes-caprae* of Australia) and halogeton (*Halogeton glomeratus* of western United States), have traveled beyond their native countries. Soursob was introduced into Australia from South Africa and halogeton into the U.S. from Asia (5).

Most oxalate-producing plants are palatable to livestock; therefore, the management of ruminants at risk due to these plants can be critical under certain conditions. For example, cattle and sheep readily graze halogeton. Under conditions where sheep have grazed it excessively, more than 1200 sheep have been poisoned at one time; and under many conditions, 100-800 deaths have been documented.

III. COMPARATIVE ANIMAL RESPONSE TO OXALATE POISONING

Animal response to halogeton intoxication varies with species of animal and species of plant (kind of oxalate) consumed. In halogeton poisoning (sap pH 6-sodium oxalate), only acute intoxication has been described (6,7); but with soursob poisoning (sap pH 2-acid potassium oxalate), chronic, subacute, and acute forms of intoxication have been described (8). Sheep poisoned on soursob will respond to treatment with calcium borogluconate (8), but those poisoned on halogeton will not (6). The signs of poisoning caused by the two species also differ.

Cattle fed on paddy straw in India (9) or on certain grasses (2% oxalate) in Peurto Rico developed a negative calcium balance (10,11), but sheep fed halogeton (6% oxalate) did not (12).

Cattle in Australia were poisoned when they ate *S. sphacelata* (6.9% oxalate). The oxalate was present in the plants as ammonium oxalate (3). This level of oxalate would be considered non-toxic in some of the Chenopodiaceae such as halogeton.

Horses in Australia grazing *S. sphacelata* developed osteodystrophy fibrosa, a degenerative condition of the bone (13). This condition in horses is associated with a calcium and phosphorus imbalance in the diet. Apparently, the oxalate interfered with the horses' calcium metabolism.

Rumen bacteria can degrade oxalate to a non-toxic form (14-16) if given time to become conditioned. A sheep must be fed low doses of oxalate for about 4 days before the bacteria are fully conditioned. Such conditioning results in a nearly 30% increase in the level of oxalate required to kill the sheep.

Recently, another oxalate-producing plant, bassia (*Bassia hyssopifolia*), was fed to sheep to test its toxicity (17). On the basis of oxalate fed, bassia was lethal at about one-half the dose rate of halogeton. The rumen bacteria failed to adapt to the oxalate in the bassia as they do to that in halogeton. Analysis of bassia plants showed that they were relatively high in potassium and low in sodium and suggests that the soluble oxalate in the bassia exists as acid potassium oxalate.

Michael suggested that the cationic constituent should be considered in correlating oxalate toxicity with clinical effects (2).

The bassia/halogeton comparison indicates that he is probably right. Also, cattle, sheep, and horses apparently differ in their responses to oxalate.

IV. SIGNS OF POISONING AND ASSOCIATED PATHOLOGICAL CHANGES

Halogeton poisoning in sheep is characterized by rapid and labored respiration, depression, weakness, coma, and death. A few animals may have convulsions, and some exhibit mild tetany. The hypocalcemia occurring in animals poisoned by halogeton should result in a greater frequency of tetany than is observed (18,19). The gross pathology of halogeton-poisoned animals includes hemorrhages and edema of the rumen wall; there may be ascites, and the kidneys may be swollen. Micropathology includes additional hemorrhages and crystals of calcium oxalate in the rumen wall, oxalate crystals in the tubules of the kidney, and microhemorrhages in the medulla oblongata (7). Some crystals have been observed in the wall of the arteries in the rumen. A marked hypocalcemia is accompanied by an increase in plasma phosphorus, magnesium, and sodium. The extent of the changes in blood electrolytes during halogeton poisoning is related to the time it takes the animal to die (18). Changes in plasma potassium were seen only occasionally. When death is somewhat delayed, plasma urea nitrogen increases markedly. Motility of the gastrointestinal tract becomes greatly depressed shortly after intoxication begins (19).

Acute soursob poisoning is characterized by hypocalcemia with accompanying tetany (8). Sheep with subacute soursob poisoning may move with a stiff gait or on their knees, and they may become recumbent. The appetite remains normal. The principal problem in chronic soursob poisoning is kidney damage, which is usually manifested at times of stress.

Bassia is another oxalate-producing plant of the Chenopodiaceae family (17). Signs of poisoning by bassia include weakness, incoordination, coma, and tetany. Serum calcium decreased markedly and serum glutamic oxaloacetic transaminase (SGOT) increased. The increase in SGOT levels, however, was less than that expected in acute halogeton poisoning. On an oxalate basis, the lethal dose of bassia for sheep is about one-half that of halogeton. Sheep fed slightly less than lethal amounts of bassia over a period of several days died. The signs of poisoning resembled those of acute halogeton intoxication except that the sheep poisoned on bassia had a greater tendency to develop tetany and incoordination than those poisoned on halogeton. As indicated, the bassia was much higher in potassium and lower in sodium than halogeton and this suggests a different form of oxalate.

In several feeding experiments, pure sodium or potassium oxalate have been tested rather than plant material. Small doses of the pure compounds are tolerated by sheep. The pure compounds had a strong tendency to produce hyperemia and edema of the rumen (20). Sheep fed small doses of sodium or potassium oxalate became anorectic. Thus, results obtained with pure compounds cannot be readily compared with those obtained with plant materials.

Cattle that grazed on halogeton and were then driven experienced difficulty in locomotion (21). After the animals were driven a short distance, some became stiff, first in the front and then in the hind legs. Some of the animals forced to move, after walking had become very labored, died.

V. OXALATE METABOLISM

Oxalate placed in the rumen (22) may: (a) be degraded by rumen bacteria; (b) combine with calcium to form insoluble calcium oxalate and thus become unavailable for absorption; or (c) be absorbed from the rumen into the blood stream where it can combine with calcium to produce hypocalcemia or interfere with other body processes.

The insoluble calcium oxalate may crystallize in various tissues, especially the kidneys and rumen wall.

In vitro and *in vivo* methods have proved that oxalate can be degraded to a non-toxic form by certain rumen bacteria (14,15). The rate of degradation varies with several factors (14). These factors include: (a) the time when the animal is fed relative to the time when ingesta is collected; (b) solid or liquid parts of ingesta analyzed; and (c) levels of oxalate fed. High levels of oxalate in an *in vitro* system inhibit cellulose fermentation and oxalate degradation. This inhibition was particularly noticeable when the ingesta was collected from sheep not pre-fed oxalate (halogeton) and suggests that the rumen microorganisms may be overwhelmed by a high oxalate concentration. Field observations and feeding trials indicate that the animal becomes intoxicated only when it eats excessive halogeton in a relatively short period of time. If preconditioned by 4 days of low-level consumption, a sheep can then consume larger amounts of halogeton per day with no harmful effects. The preconditioning increases the lethal dose about 30% (22).

When the rumen microflora are not able to degrade incoming oxalate, it may be absorbed into the blood stream. If this amount exceeds 20 to 30 mg percent oxalate, calcium oxalate may be crystallized in the kidney.

A sheep loses its normal tolerance to oxalate when the oxalate is placed directly into the abomasum (23). Calcium oxalate will form in the rumen at pH 5-7; however, it evidently becomes soluble and is absorbed on reaching the abomasum (at pH 1.5-3). Calcium oxalate infused into the abomasum at a calculated lethal dose, however, does not kill sheep. Balance trials with sheep and cattle suggest that all calcium oxalate consumed is excreted in the feces (9,10).

Intravenous oxalate infusion studies indicate a considerable difference between lethal oral dosages and how much oxalate had been absorbed by animals dying of oxalate poisoning (24). Because gastrointestinal motility nearly stops shortly after the feeding of a lethal dose of halogeton, absorption of oxalate may cease early in the process of intoxication and thus limit the total amount of oxalate absorbed. The difference between the oral dose and that absorbed indicates that it takes little of the compound to exert its effect on the rumen bacteria and rumen motility.

VI. OXALATE INTOXICATION

If a cow or sheep consumed too much halogeton in a relatively short time, it dies (12). We assume that under these conditions, the ability of the rumen microorganisms to degrade oxalate is exceeded and oxalate is absorbed. In contrast, small amounts of halogeton do not harm cattle or sheep. Harmful effects have been observed, however, in animals grazing sublethal amounts of bassia.

Death has generally been attributed to hypocalcemia in acute cases of oxalate poisoning and to uremia resulting from kidney damage in chronic cases (25). We question whether hypocalcemia is the sole cause because sheep made hypocalcemic by dialysis or EDTA infusion do not die. Also, blood calcium levels can be maintained in sheep or cattle poisoned on halogeton, and they will still die. A sheep can survive 3-4 days after a bilateral nephrectomy, which is much longer than most sheep live after being poisoned by halogeton. Also, the occlusion of renal tubules is not an essential feature of oxalate nephritis.

Further, a number of other factors have been implicated in deaths associated with oxalate consumption. For example, in halogeton and bassia poisoning, hemorrhagic rumenitis and shock may contribute to death. Oxalate also competitively inhibits enzymatic reduction of oxalate and non-competitively interferes with the reduction of lactate. In addition, oxalate interferes with succinic dehydrogenase and possibly with enzymes activated by calcium and magnesium metabolism. Taken together this suggests that an interference with energy metabolism contributes to death in oxalate poisoning (18). Oxalate-induced stasis of the gastrointestinal tract changes the pH in both the abomasum and rumen, and hemorrhage and edema of the rumen could both be factors in ultimate deaths.

Sheep given a normally lethal dose of halogeton and then force-fed water do not die (24), if bloat is controlled. The excess water apparently flushes the oxalate from the system.

Because oxalate-producing plants are high in soluble salts, their ingestion tends to increase an animal's water intake and urine excretion. Additionally, as oxalate in the diet increases, consumption of other feed decreases. This can obviously have an adverse effect on weight gains. As indicated, certain oxalate-producing plants also interfere with calcium metabolism in cattle and horses.

Preliminary feeding trials with sheep fed low levels of bassia (6% oxalate) resulted in an increase in serum glutamic oxaloacetic transaminase (SGOT) levels and a varied response in serum calcium and magnesium levels. Sheep fed at less than one-half the calculated lethal dose of oxalate in bassia died after being fed more than 7 days. Microscopic changes were similar to those observed in halogeton poisoning.

Calves on full feed of kochia (*Kochia scoparia*) (3.5% oxalate) had a gradual increase in SGOT, an increased blood clotting time, and a mild decrease in serum calcium at about the 6th week of feeding. No effects were noted in sheep fed kochia (26).

Certainly, various effects do indicate that oxalate poisoning is a complex phenomenon.

VII. CONCLUSIONS

Oxalate poisoning remains a complex and poorly understood phenomenon. Signs of poisoning vary with the animal species and the chemical form of the oxalate. There are apparently as many dissimilarities as similarities among the effects of the different types of oxalate on the different species of animals.

VIII. REFERENCES

1. Brown, A., and Gettler, O., *Proc. Exp. Biol. Med.* 19, 204-208 (1922).
2. Michael, P. W., *Aust. Vet. J.* 35, 431-432 (1959).
3. James, M. P., Seawright, A. A., and Steele, D. P., *Aust. Vet. J.* 47, 9-17 (1971).
4. Seawright, A. A., Groenedyk, S., and Silva, K. I. N. G., *Aust. Vet. J.* 46, 293-296 (1970).
5. Kingsbury, J. M., "Poisonous Plants of the United States and Canada," Prentice-Hall, Englewood Cliffs, New Jersey, 1964.
6. Cook, C. W., and Stoddart, L. A., *Utah Agric. Exp. Stn. Bull.* 364 (1953).
7. Van Kampen, K. R., and James, L. F., *Am. J. Vet. Res.* 30, 1779-1783 (1969).
8. Smith W., *J. Agric. South Aust.* 54, 377-378 (1951).
9. Talapata, S. K., Ray, S. C., and Sen, K. C., *J. Agric. Sci.* 38, 163-173 (1948).
10. Morris, M. P., and Garcia-Revira, J., *J. Dairy Sci.* 38, 1169 (1955).
11. Garcia-Revira, J., and Morris, M. P., *Science* 120, 1089 (1955).
12. James, L. F., and Butcher, J. E., *J. Anim. Sci.* 36, 1233-1238 (1972).
13. Walthall, J. C., and McKenzie R. A., *Aust. Vet. J.* 52, 11-16 (1976).
14. James, L. F., Stout, J. C., and Butcher, J. E., *J. Anim. Sci.* 26, 1438-1444 (1967).
15. Allison, M. J., Littledike, E. T., and James, L. F., *J. Anim.*

Sci., In press.
16. Watts, P. S., *Aust. Agric. Res.* 8, 266-270 (1957).
17. James, L. F., Williams, M. C., and Bleak, A. T., *J. Range Manage.* 29, 284-285 (1976).
18. James, L. F., *Can. J. Comp. Med.* 32, 539-543 (1968).
19. Littledike, E. T., James, L., and Cook, H., *Am. J. Vet. Res.* 37, 661-666 (1976).
20. James, L. F., Stout, J. C., Butcher, J. E., and Binns, W., *J. Anim. Sci.* 27, 718-723 (1968).
21. James, L. F., *J. Am. Vet. Med. Assoc.* 156, 1310-1312 (1970).
22. James, L. F., Butcher, J. E., and Van Kampen, K. R., *J. Range Manage.* 23, 123-127 (1970).
23. Dodson, M. E., *Aust. Vet. J.* 35, 225-233 (1959).
24. James, L. F., and Johnson, A. E., *J. Am. Vet. Med. Assoc.* 157, 437-442 (1970).
25. James, L. F., *Clin. Toxicol.* 5, 231-243 (1972).
26. James, L. F., Unpublished data (1977).

ORGANO-FLUORINE COMPOUNDS IN PLANTS

T. McEwan
Animal Research Institute, Yeerongpilly, Queensland

I. ABSTRACT

A brief review is presented of the occurrence of organo-fluorine compounds in plants and of the effects of feeding plants with fluoride. The influence of fluorine location in a molecule on toxicity is discussed and the toxicities of a range of organo-fluorine compounds, both naturally occurring and synthetic, are summarized.

Distribution of fluoroacetate in Acacia georginae *is considered and the various findings are related to the incidence of poisoning of sheep and cattle in the field. Difficulties in detection of organo-fluorine compounds are emphasized and possible areas of further investigation are indicated.*

II. INTRODUCTION

General interest in the carbon-fluorine compounds began to expand in the early 1940's when Marais reported the occurrence of monofluoroacetic acid as the toxic principle in the South African plant *Dichapetalum cymosum* (1). Although the possibilities of such compounds as chemical warfare agents generated some enthusiasm during the war years, it was not until the late 1960's that general interest in the field began to expand. However, during the interval the biological significance of many forms of organically bound fluorine became evident. For example, it was found that the introduction of fluorine into the steroid hormones could greatly enhance their biological action. Furthermore changes could be qualitative as well as quantitative, that is, the type of biological action could be changed as well as the amount.

As interest in organo-fluorine compounds increased, Sir Rudolph Peters and Dr. P. W. Kent thought that a meeting with an interdisciplinary approach might clarify problems and stimulate further work. The result was the "Symposium on Carbon-Fluorine Compounds: Chemistry, Biochemistry, and Biological Activities" held at the Ciba Foundation, London, 13th-15th September 1971. There were twenty-five contributors from almost as many research groups. The papers presented and the discussion sessions were edited and were published in 1972 (2), providing a broad view of the whole field. Continuing interest is illustrated by the list of approximately 650 entries under "fluoro-" in the cumulative index of Biological Abstracts, July-December 1976. It seems relevant, therefore, to review the present knowledge of organo-fluorine compounds, especially in relation to their occurrence in plants.

III. OCCURRENCE

Of the known natural occurrences of organo-fluorine compounds the incidence of fluoroacetate is by far the most extensive. Following the initial identification in *Dichapetalum cymosum* (1) it was also detected in *Acacia georginae* in Australia (3) in the Brazilian plant *Palicourea marcgravii* (4) and in a large number of Australian plants, varieties of *Gastrolobium* and *Oxylobium*, of the family Leguminosae (5,6). All of these plants are toxic to animals, but the most toxic appear to be *Gastrolobium bilobum* and *Oxylobium parviflorum* from West Australia. The dry leaf of these plants has contained up to 1.25% fluoroacetate so that about 30 g fresh leaf would be sufficient to kill a sheep.

The toxicity of another South African plant *Dichapetalum toxicarium* is concentrated mainly in the seed and is predominantly caused by ω-fluorooleic acid. Also present is ω-fluoropalmitic acid and possibly also ω-fluoromyristic and ω-fluorocapric acids (7,8). Further examination of the organo-fluorine compounds extracted from these seeds has resulted in the detection of three other compounds, one of which has been purified (2a). This compound has a molecular weight of 472 and an empirical formula (from high resolution mass spectrometry) of $C_{27}H_{49}O_5F$ although it normally exists as a hydrate in association with $1\frac{1}{2}H_2O$. It probably contains a carbonyl group, four hydroxyls, a $-CH_2-CH_2F$ group, at least sixteen methylene groups and two rings. An interesting feature is the isolation from the same source of a non-fluorinated analogue which shows very similar properties and spectra. The only difference in structure appears to be $-CH_2-CH_3$ in place of $-CH_2-CH_2F$. A further interesting point was that the concentration ratio of fluoro-compound to non-fluoro was approximately 1:10, very similar to the ratio of ω-fluorooleic acid to oleic acid reported in seed from the same plant.

An unusual naturally occurring organo-fluorine compound is the antitrypanosomal antibiotic, nucleocidin, which was first isolated from a Streptomyces and reported in 1957 (9). It was twelve years later before the presence of fluorine in the molecule was demonstrated (10). This compound has been assigned the structure of a nucleoside 1 in which the fluorine is attached to the carbohydrate moiety.

IV. EFFECTS OF FEEDING PLANTS WITH FLUORIDE

The most likely source of the fluorine bound in organic compounds was fluoride from the soil. Many experiments have supported this idea, at least in the cases of those plants which are known to produce organo-fluorine compounds. For example,

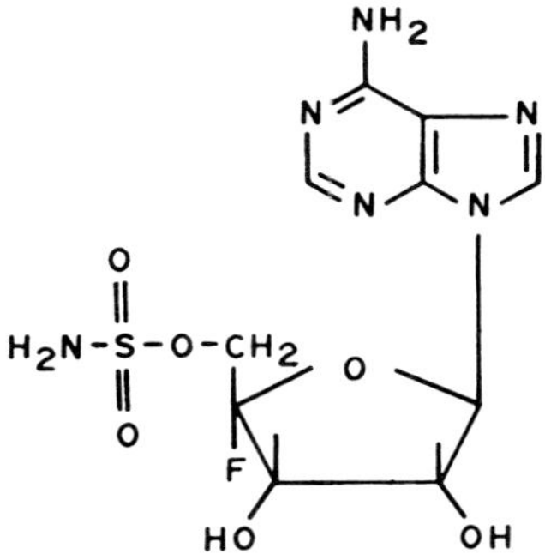

1

Weinstein (11) found that *Acacia georginae* seedlings varied in susceptibility to sodium fluoride damage so that he could select those which were most resistant. These fluoride-resistant seedlings produced high concentrations of fluoroacetic acid when incubated with sodium fluoride. Under similar conditions no fluoro-acids were detected in hay, soybean, crested wheat grass, corn, alfalfa or tomato. Peters (12,13) also investigated *Acacia georginae* seedlings and found that more fluorine was absorbed and more "organic" fluorine synthesized when the nutrient was more acid - pH 4.0 compared with pH 6.5.

Homogenates of *Acacia georginae* have also been treated with fluoride by Peters (14). The volatile products of this treatment were difficult to trap and it was suspected that vinyl fluoride might have been liberated. Further investigations showed other volatile fluorine compounds one of which has been tentatively identified as fluoroacetone. Addition of sodium fluoride to the homogenate increased the liberation of volatile fluorine by a factor of ten. Preuss (15) has reported that a tissue culture from a stem section of *Acacia georginae* will also produce fluoroacetate when fed with sodium fluoride.

Dichapetalum spp. are also capable of converting fluoride into fluoroacetate. For example, isolated leaves of *Dichapetalum toxicarium* produced 200 mg fluoroacetate/kg after ten days with their petioles in 10^{-3} M sodium fluoride (16). It is believed (17) that the fluoroacetate is synthesized in the young leaves of this plant, stored in the small leaves adjacent to the flowers and withdrawn by the embryo seeds to be converted to the long-chain fluoro-acids.

Numerous attempts have been made to detect organo-fluorine

compounds in plants exposed to relatively large amounts of fluoride, either atmospheric or in solution. Results have generally been negative but some indications of the presence of fluoroacetate and fluorocitrate have been found. Lovelace (18) has reported the presence of quite high levels (179 mg fluoroacetate/kg; 896 mg fluorocitrate/kg) in forage crops from a pasture mix which contained *Medicago sativa* and *Agropyron cristatum* collected within two miles of a phosphate plant. However, fluoride levels on the pasture were high and major clinical symptoms were those of fluoride intoxication although blood citrate levels were elevated.

Fluorocitrate, in very small amounts, has also been detected in lettuce plants fed with fluoroacetate (19,2b). Peters (2c) reports trace amounts of fluorocitrate in an extract of commercial tea. Tea, of course, can have very high concentrations of fluoride but previous examinations have failed to detect organofluorine compounds. Peters suggests that the presence of trace amounts of fluorocitrate may be rather general in plants and has also identified it in fluorosed bones from cattle (20). It is uncertain whether this fluorocitrate was produced within the animal or stored following ingestion in the forage.

Other fluoro-acids, fluorobutyric and fluorohexanoic acids, have been tentatively identified as metabolic products obtained when brewer's yeast was treated with fluoroacetate (21). No indication of the position of the fluorine atoms in the molecules was given.

V. DISTRIBUTION IN PLANTS

Distribution of organo-fluorine in some fifteen plants has been discussed in detail by Hall (22) who studied plant specimens which were collected in the appropriate parts of the world, air dried, packed in polythene bags and dispatched to England. On arrival the plants were separated into leaf, bark, roots, thick and thin stem, and in some samples seeds. These samples were analyzed for fluoride obtained after a selection of treatments: ashing for total fluoride; acid-labile fluoride; "organic" fluoride; water soluble fluoro-compounds; and fluoro-compounds soluble in alkaline propanol. Hall's major findings were that there were wide variations both within and between plants in both organic and inorganic fluorine and in the ratios between them. The Brazilian plant *Palicourea marcgravii* had far more fluorine in the leaves than any other species and 61% of this was organic. All of the samples of *Acacia georginae* leaf analyzed had rather low organo-fluorine content but this is not unusual since the leaf of this plant is usually of low toxicity. It is used as a drought feed for sheep in the area. The only leaf material of *Acacia georginae* which frequently contains high levels of fluoroacetate is young leaf, particularly leaf of suckers growing from the root stock of grubbed out plants. A surprising finding, however, was the very low organo-fluorine content found in the seed of *Acacia georginae*. While fluctuations occur in the field most analytical examinations have shown concentrations of fluoroacetate around 10-40 mg/kg with occasional samples, especially of young immature seed reaching 400 mg/kg (23). Perhaps of relevance in this context is a more recent finding by Vickery and Vickery (16) related to loss of fluoroacetate from leaf and from extracts of *Dichapetalum toxicarium*. When a sample of leaf was air-dried and kept for two months in humid air the concentration dropped from 600 mg fluoroacetate/kg to 60 mg/kg whereas a replicate sample, oven dried at 100° C and kept for two months in a sealed plastic bag retained the whole 600 mg/kg. Similarly, aliquots of a sterilized aqueous extract were stored either open to the atomosphere or sealed. Fluoroacetate disappeared from the open container but was retained in the sealed aliquot. This loss of fluoroacetate was attributed in both cases to the action of an unidentified micro-organism. Hall's samples could have been similarly attacked.

In many studies problems may arise through the actual compound containing the fluoroacetate moiety within the specific plant. In the seed of *Acacia georginae* the ease of extraction with organic solvents suggests that free monofluoroacetic acid is present (23). Similar solvent extraction data suggest that in the leaf of *Dichapetalum cymosum* the fluoroacetate is present as the potassium salt (1). Recently, Vickery and Vickery (16) have shown that fluoroacetate present in *Dichapetalum toxicarium* leaf is water-extractable but will not partition from the acidified aqueous extract into ether. When the neutralized extract is boiled for 30 minutes and reacidified, fluoroacetic acid could then be extracted with ether. The nature of the initial complex was not determined.

VI. SYNTHETIC FLUORO-COMPOUNDS

Goldman (2d) briefly summarizes some biosynthetic possibilities for the formation of organo-fluorine compounds. Some products of microbial transformations are very difficult to prepare by other means. For example, D(+)-fluorosuccinate is one of the products of metabolism of p-fluorophenylacetate in the protein of *E. coli* when the organism is grown in the presence of the fluoro-compound. Although such transformations are limited by the ability of micro-organisms to grow on substrates containing fluorine, the vast number of micro-organisms available and their adaptability make this approach a promising means of preparation of many kinds of fluorine-containing compounds.

Saunders (2e) has discussed the chemical synthesis of a range of compounds in which the carbon-fluorine bond is present. He states that some 300 compounds were synthesized. Among these were the methyl, ethyl, n-propyl and isopropyl fluoracetates, methyl α-fluoropropionate, methyl α-fluoroisobutyrate, fluoroethanol, 2-fluoroethyl-fluoroacetate, fluoroacetyl chloride, chloroacetyl fluoride, and fluoroacetyl fluoride, as well as a range of ω-fluoro acids and several cyclic compounds. Kent (2f) has reviewed the preparation of fluorocarbohydrates and has tabulated the properties of numerous fluoro- trioses, tetroses, pentoses, and hexoses and their derivatives. Fluorine can be inserted in place of most hydroxyl groups in the carbohydrate molecule. Fluorine can also be introduced into steroids and Wettstein (2g) has provided a brief review of the methods involved. Once again, one or more fluorine atoms may be introduced into a range of positions within the molecule. Many fluorinated amino acids have also been prepared and 5-fluorouracil and its derivatives have been extensively studied.

VII. TOXICITY

Quantitative toxicity data about the organo-fluorine compounds is not very plentiful. Fluoroacetic acid toxicity has been examined rather thoroughly and the variation in response of different species is illustrated in Table I taken in part from Garner's Veterinary Toxicology (24).

TABLE I

Oral Lethal Doses of Monofluoroacetic Acid

Species	Dose (mg/kg)	Species	Dose (mg/kg)
horse	0.5 - 1.75	cat	0.3 - 0.5
sheep	0.25 - 0.5	fowl	10 - 30
goat	0.3 - 0.7	quail	about 400
pig	0.3 - 0.4	man	4 - 7

Poisoning by fluoro-acetate, in short-term dosing, is essentially cumulative. Six days of dosing at one sixth of a lethal dose per day is usually fatal.

Toxicity of other fluoro-acids has been determined by Saunders (25,2e) and related to the toxicity of fluoroacetic acid. Compounds in the remaining discussion have been classified simply as "toxic," meaning of the same order of toxicity as fluoroacetate, or as "non-toxic," meaning the compound is of a low order of toxicity and does not cause fluoroacetate type intoxication. Methyl, ethyl, propyl, and isopropyl esters of fluoroacetic acid (2) are toxic. On the other hand methyl α-fluoropropionate (3) and methyl α-fluoroisobutyrate (4) are non-toxic.

$F\text{-}CH_2COOR$

2

toxic

$CH_3CH(F)\text{-}COOCH_3$

3

non-toxic

$CH_3\text{-}C(CH_3)(F)\text{-}COOCH_3$

4

non-toxic

There is a striking alternation in the toxicities of the ω-fluorocarboxylic esters:

FCH_2COOR	toxic
$F(CH_2)_2COOR$	non-toxic
$F(CH_2)_3COOR$	toxic
$F(CH_2)_4COOR$	non-toxic
$F(CH_2)_5COOR$	toxic
$F(CH_2)_7COOR$	toxic
$F(CH_2)_{10}COOR$	non-toxic

These toxicities are consistent with the β-oxidation of fatty acids in the living body:

$$RCH_2CH_2COOH \longrightarrow RCOOH + CH_3COOH$$

In the series $F(CH_2)_nCOOH$ when n is odd the end product is FCH_2COOH but when n is even the compound is oxidized to the non-toxic FCH_2CH_2COOH. The toxicity is dependent on the production of FCH_2CO^- grouping. This finding is supported by data on the acyl halides and ethyl fluoroformate.

FCH_2COCl fluoroacetyl chloride	toxic
$ClCH_2COF$ chloroacetyl fluoride	non-toxic
FCH_2COF fluoroacetyl fluoride	toxic
$FCOOC_2H_5$ ethyl fluoroformate	non-toxic

Compounds in which the β-position is blocked so that β-oxidation cannot occur are also non-toxic. Structures 5-8 are illustrations.

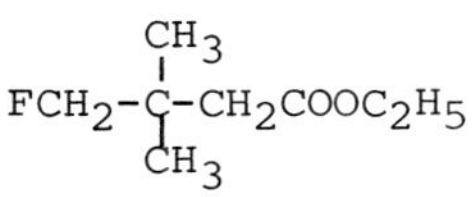

5

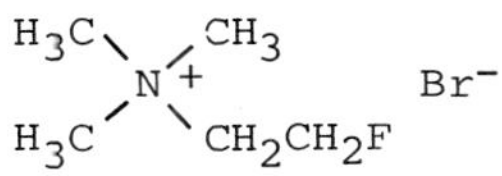

6

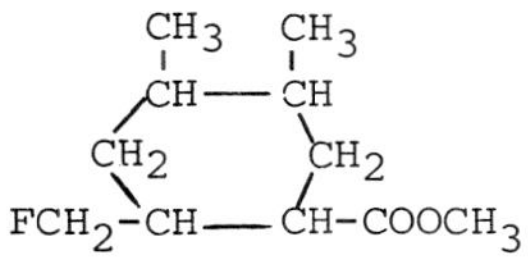

7

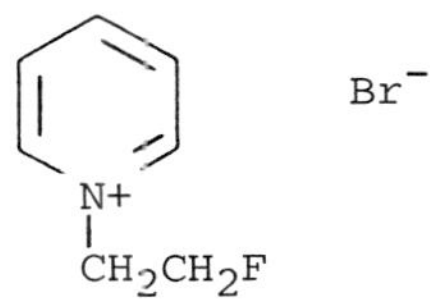

8

On the other hand 2-fluoroethanol is readily oxidized to $F\text{-}CH_2COOH$ and is toxic. The ester 2-fluoroethyl fluoroacetate has greatly enhanced toxic properties - about twice that of methyl fluoroacetate, weight for weight. Fluoroacetamide and several substituted amides are also toxic:

FCH_2CONH_2 fluoroacetamide	toxic
$FCH_2CONHCH_3$ N-methyl fluoroacetamide	toxic
$FCH_2CONHCH_2CH_2Cl$ N-chloroethyl fluoroacetamide	toxic
$FCH_2CON(CH_2CH_2Cl)_2$ N,N—di—(chloroethyl) fluoroacetamide	toxic

The LD_{50} values for intraperitoneal injection of a range of α-fluoromalonates and α-fluoroalkanoic acids have been reported by Pattison and co-workers (27). Fluoro-steroids have a wide range of biological effects. Wettstein (2h) has provided a review of their hormonal activities.

VIII. FIELD TOXICITY OF PLANTS

In field situations, the actual concentration of organo-fluorine compounds in a plant varies and consequently so does the toxicity. The actual hazard to livestock is related to both the toxicity and the likelihood that the animals will consume sufficient to harm them. Assessment of possible consumption is a management problem but toxicity can be related to analytical determinations. However, if the analysis is specific for fluoroacetate then other toxic fluorine compounds may be missed or the extraction process may not be adequate to remove all the biologically available fluoroacetate. On the other hand determination of total organic fluorine could include compounds which are relatively harmless.

Acacia georginae is rather unusual for a toxic plant in that it is often freely eaten by animals without harmful effect. Local graziers believe that some areas in which *Acacia georginae* is predominant are "poison" while others are "safe." Analytical investigation has so far found no significant differences between selections of plants from the two classifications. However, such distinctions may have a factual basis, since marked variations in fluoroacetate content have been observed between plants even though there seems to be a similar range of values present in groups of plants from the different areas.

In my opinion, *Acacia georginae* produces symptoms of toxicity in animals only when at least one of the following applies:

(a) Animals have no other feed.

(b) Animals are severely stressed by heat, exercise, or fright.

(c) Pods are available in sufficient quantity so that animals consume large amounts.

(d) Suckers of high fluoroacetate content are available.

(e) Fluoroacetate levels in leaf or pod are unusually high.

Sheep, on a good diet, seem to be able to handle an intake of about 2 mg fluoroacetate per day and perhaps more although animals on poorer rations seem to be more susceptible. Jarret and Packham in 1956 reported that lucerne or gluten seemed to protect animals against continued dosing with sublethal amounts of fluoroacetate (2 mg daily). Recent work at the Animal Research Institute (28) indicates that any protection by gluten or urea against continued ingestion of fluoroacetate is minimal and would be essentially useless as a safeguard against field intoxication.

Dichapetalum cymosum is very poisonous in spring (mid-August to the end of November) and autumn (March to May) because at these times the plant produces highly toxic new leaves (29). At no time is the plant non-toxic. Similarly, *Dichapetalum toxicarium* is always toxic but the toxicity is lowest during the initial stages of seed production in May and June, when production of young leaves is halted. Low fluoroacetate content of leaf in September has been attributed to the leaching action of heavy rain (17).

IX. DETECTION OF FLUORINE

Fluorine is ubiquitous in the environment. In fact, fluorine-free situations exist only in systems from which the fluorine has been rigorously excluded. Consequently if fluorine is not detected in a given system, the methods of detection should be checked for sensitivity and the procedures used examined for processes during which fluorine could be lost. Fluorine can form bonds with carbon which vary from extremely strong to very weak and the compounds formed cover the whole range of organic chemistry. Thus the detection technique must be designed specifically for the compounds involved or be sufficiently general to handle all possible compounds. Fortunately, high resolution mass spectrometry and some of the newer techniques of nuclear magnetic resonance spectroscopy are capable of providing the necessary generality. Sensitivity in the NMR techniques has been vastly increased by the use of Fourier transform techniques which have improved the signal to noise ratio by 10^3. Location of the fluorine has also been facilitated by the development of heteronuclear spin decoupling so that the proton spectrum can be recorded while the resonance frequency of the fluorine is being irradiated. Any protons coupled to the fluorine are then detected. The major remaining limitations are in the processing of materials before insertion into the instruments. Fluorine compounds may be readily lost, either by volatility, by difficulties in extraction, by absorption on to other components of the system or even, in low concentrations, by adsorption on to the walls of the containers. If biological activity is not lost along with the fluorine there is no problem, but if organo-fluorine compounds are present it is likely that their loss is also a loss of activity.

X. CONCLUSION

The range of information presented in this paper has illustrated that the presence of organo-fluorine compounds is not restricted to the higher plants. The data show that many systems are capable of synthesizing the carbon-fluorine bond or converting the compounds formed into others. It seems unlikely that this capacity has not been utilized extensively in natural processes especially since incorporation of fluorine can greatly enhance biological activity. One area in which this possibility could be investigated is the field of mold intoxications - a rapidly expanding area of knowledge. Toxic isolates of many molds have been reported and their biological actions described. It is apparent that many of the toxins involved are present in very small amounts and are extremely active. Naturally, isolation and purification of the active materials have proven difficult. It is possible that some of the difficulties could be caused by the presence of fluoro- and non-fluoro- analogues of ranges of closely related biologically active compounds. Small changes in location of a fluorine atom might cause little change in chemical or physical property but could alter biological activity both qualitatively and quantitatively.

It seems possible also that the range of biological activity available through adjustments of fluorine atom location could be a factor in the resistance of some plants to attack by micro-organisms. Even if nature has neglected this area of activity research workers now are actively synthesizing and testing fluorine compounds to try to develop more effective means of combating the destructive effects of micro-organisms. Only one fluorine-containing antibiotic, nucleocidin, has been mentioned. Others must follow.

The similarity in size between the fluorine and hydrogen atoms has been used in explanation of the way in which compounds such as fluoroacetate pass through metabolic pathways until their modifications cause a lethal blockage [the "lethal synthesis" described by Peters (30)]. Many attempts are being made to use this approach in the treatment of cancer. One idea is to try to set up a "lethal synthesis" specific for the cancer cell. In other words, compounds are being made which, it is hoped, will be rejected by normal cells but accepted into the metabolism of cancer cells and then kill by blocking essential pathways.

Workers involved with the chemistry of biologically active materials should therefore be aware of the possible presence of fluorine and be aware of the difficulties in detection of fluorine compounds. In short, remember to look for organo-fluorine in biologically active systems.

XI. REFERENCES

1. Marais, J. S. C., *Onderstepoort J. Vet. Sci. Anim. Ind.* 20, 67 (1944).
2. Elliott, K., and Birch, J. (Eds.), "Carbon-Fluorine Compounds, Chemistry, Biochemistry, and Biological Activity," A Ciba Foundation Symposium, (a) p. 163; (b) p. 119; (c) p. 64; (d) p. 345; (e) pp. 9-27; (f) pp. 169-208; (g) pp. 282-286; (h) pp. 286-298. Associated Scientific Publishers, Amsterdam, 1972.
3. Oelrichs, P. B., and McEwan, T., *Nature (London)* 190, 808 (1961).
4. de Oliveira, M. M. *Experientia* 19, 586 (1963).
5. McEwan, T., *Nature (London)* 201, 827 (1964).
6. Cannon, J. R., Unpublished results (1964).
   Aplin, T. E. H., *J. Agric. West. Aust.* 8, 42 (1967); 8, 200 (1967); 10, 248 (1969); 10, 327 (1969); 10, 517 (1969); 12, 12 (1971); 12, 154 (1971).
7. Peters, R. A., Hall, R. J., Ward, P. F. V., and Sheppard, N., *Biochem. J.* 77, 17 (1960).
8. Ward, P. F. V., Hall, R. J., and Peters, R. A., *Nature (London)* 201, 611 (1964).
9. Thomas, S. O., *et al.*, *Antibiot. Ann.* 716 (1956-57); Hewitt, R. I., *et al.*, *Antibiot. Ann.* 722 (1956-57).
10. Morton, G. O., *et al.*, *J. Am. Chem. Soc.* 91, 1535 (1969).
11. Weinstein, L. H., *et al.*, *Environ. Res.* 5, 393 (1972).
12. Peters, R. A., *Rev. Roum. Biochim.* 4, 79 (1967).
13. Peters, R. A., Murray, L. R., and Shorthouse, M., *Biochem. J.* 95, 724 (1965).
14. Peters, R. A., and Shorthouse, M., *Nature* 231, 123 (1971).
15. Preuss, P. W., Colairto, L., and Weinstein, L. H., *Experientia* 26, 1059 (1970).
16. Vickery, B., and Vickery, M. L., *Phytochemistry* 14, 423 (1975).
17. Vickery, B., and Vickery, M. L., *Phytochemistry* 11, 1905 (1972).
18. Lovelace, J., Miller, G. W., and Welkie, G. W., *Atmos. Environ.* 2, 187 (1968).
19. Ward, P. F. V., and Huskisson, N. S., *Biochem. J.* 113, 9P (1969).
20. Peters, R. A., and Shorthouse, M., *Biochem. J.* 113, 9P (1969).
21. Aldous, J. G., *Biochem. Pharmacol.* 12, 627 (1963).
22. Hall, R. J., *New Phytol.* 71, 855 (1972).
23. Oelrichs, P. B., and McEwan, T., *Queensl. J. Agric. Sci.* 19, 1 (1962).
24. "Garner's Veterinary Toxicology," 3rd Ed. (E. G. C. Clarke

and M. L. Clarke, Eds.), pp. 266-268. Robert Maclehose and Co., Glasgow, 1967.
25. Saunders, B. C., *Endeavour* 36 (1960).
26. Jarrett, I. G., and Packham, A., *Nature (London)* 171, 580 (1956).
27. Pattison, F. L. M., Buchanan, R. L., and Dean, F. H., *Can. J. Chem.* 43, 1700 (1965).
28. Laws, L., *et al.*, In preparation (1977).
29. Vickery, B., and Vickery, M. L., *Vet. Bull.* 43, 537 (1973).
30. Peters, R. A., Buffa, R., Wakelin, R. W., and Thomas, L. C., *Proc. R. Soc. B* 140, 497 (1953).

IV. PLANT HEPATOTOXINS

Chairman: Selwyn Everist

PYRROLIZIDINE ALKALOID POISONING - PATHOLOGY WITH PARTICULAR REFERENCE TO DIFFERENCES IN ANIMAL AND PLANT SPECIES

P. T. Hooper
Arid Zone Research Institute

I. ABSTRACT

Of the plant genera containing pyrrolizidine alkaloids studied, Crotalaria spp. *and* Trichodesma incanum *cause the broadest spectrum of organ pathology, notably hepatic and respiratory disease, renal megalocytosis, and sometimes severe renal nephrosis in pigs.* Senecio spp. *can cause respiratory disease in some pigs, rats, and mice but not in horses, cattle, and sheep. Few diseases other than hepatoses has been reported in animals poisoned by* Heliotropium spp., Amsinckia spp. *and* Echium spp.

Pigs were quantitatively the most sensitive of the animals studied, then chickens, cattle, horses, rats, and mice; sheep and goats were the most resistant. Although sheep were resistant to the chronic effects, they were quite sensitive to acute poisonings.

Pyrrolizidine alkaloids cause 3 main effects, necrosis, edema followed by fibrosis, and chronic megalocytosis of cells by inhibition of mitosis. The varied effects in the liver are probably related to the severity and duration of poisonings. In the lungs, the occurrence of intestitial pneumonia depends on the vascular activity of the plant's alkaloids as well as the sensitivity of the species. Megalocytosis in an extra hepatic organ not only depends on the passage of the alkaloid's active metabolites past the liver to the organ but also upon active cell division in that organ.

II. INTRODUCTION

Plants containing pyrrolizidine alkaloids cause overt diseases most commonly in the liver, occasionally in the lungs, and rarely in the kidneys (1,2,3). Occasionally, other organs can be affected by coincidental or secondary changes.

This paper summarizes the varied effects of plants containing the alkaloids on the organs of domestic and laboratory animals. Emphasis will be made on the light microscopic pathology.

III. PATTERNS OF DISEASE CAUSED BY DIFFERENT ALKALOIDS AND PLANT GENERA

The most important genera of pyrrolizidine alkaloid-containing toxic plants are *Crotalaria, Senecio, Heliotropium, Trichodesma,*

Amsinckia, and *Echium* (4). All are hepatotoxic. Other genera are known to contain pyrrolizidine alkaloids but await further clarification as causes of loss in domestic animals (5) (Culvenor, personal communication). *Crotalaria spp.* cause disease in the broadest range of tissues in most domestic species. It is often pneumotoxic in horses (6,7,8,9,10), cattle (11,12), sheep (13,14), goats (15), and pigs (3,16) as well as hepatotoxic. In pigs it is severely nephrotoxic (3,16,17). *Trichodesma incanum* has similar effects to *Crotalaria spp.* in horses and cattle (18,19,20).

Although most *Crotalaria spp.* have been shown to be pneumotoxic to horses (6,10), there is a striking exception in *C. retusa,* an important cause of disease in horses in northern Australia. This plant in the same area has been shown to be pneumotoxic in pigs (16), and horses can develop pulmonary disease by poisoning with another *Crotalaria sp., C. crispata* (10). Yet, horses have developed only hepatic disease when poisoned by *C. retusa* (21,22) (Hooper, unpublished observations).

Senecio spp. are primarily hepatotoxic. *Senecio jacobaea* has produced pulmonary disease in pigs (23) but this could be an inconsistent change (24). Rats and mice develop pulmonary disease when poisoned with *S. jacobaea* (25,26) and *S. magnificus* (Hooper, unpublished observation). However, there have been no reports of significant pulmonary disease in cattle, sheep, horses, or chickens in spite of many field observations and feeding experiments (4). Renal megalocytosis and occasional mild nephroses occur in most species poisoned with *S. jacobaea* (23,24) (Hooper, unpublished observations.

Heliotropium spp., Amsinckia spp., and *Echium spp.* are hepatotoxic. Pigs and rarely sheep and cattle also develop renal megalocytosis (R. G. Russell, C. J. Walker, personal communications, and Hooper, unpublished observations). Pulmonary disease has been recorded in laboratory animals acutely poisoned experimentally by some purified alkaloids extracted from these genera (27).

IV. QUANTITATIVE SUSCEPTIBILITY OF DIFFERENT ANIMAL SPECIES

There is a wide range in the susceptibility of different animal species to poisoning by plants containing pyrrolizidine alkaloids. Sheep have often been used in many parts of the world to graze on pastures regarded as dangerous to cattle. In fact, Dollahite (28) showed that it took over 20 times as much *Senecio spp.* to poison sheep and goats as that which killed cattle. Similar results have been obtained by poisoning sheep, cattle, rats, mice, and chickens with *Senecio jacobaea* (Hooper, unpublished observations). Sheep required more than 2.0 kg of dried plant/kg body weight (BW) to poison them compared with a mean of 1.5 kg/kg BW mice, 0.5 kg/kg BW rats, 0.14 kg/kg BW cattle, and 0.05 kg/kg BW chickens. When poisonings by *C. retusa* were compared, pigs were about 5 to 10 times as susceptible as chickens (16). Indirect evidence from many papers published (summarized in 4,29) suggests that horses seem to be about as sensitive as cattle. Overall, the approximate ratios of quantities of plant material required to poison the various species listed are about 200 for sheep (nearly = goats); 150 for mice; 50 for rats; 14 for cattle (nearly = horses); 5 for chickens; and 1 for pigs. Extreme ranges in susceptibility to acute poisoning have also been noted (30).

It has been suggested that the broad range in sensitivities is due to varying rates of conversion of pyrrolizidine alkaloids to active metabolites, the pyrroles (31,32). Shull, Buckmaster, and Cheeke (32) provided evidence that it was not ruminal metabolism which accounts for the differences between sheep and cattle. However, Lanigan (33) has shown that ruminal microflora detoxification of the alkaloids in sheep could be important and can be accelerated. One reason for susceptibility of pigs could be the sensitivity of a vital organ, the lungs. However, most of the rats in the above comparison died from pulmonary disease while the more sensitive cattle and chickens died from hepatic disease. The severe pulmonary disease in the rat could have accounted for its greater sensitivity to *S. jacobaea* than mice.

Resistance to chronic disease does not necessarily infer resistance to acute disease. Sheep died soon after single intraperitoneal injections of senecionine at 60 mg/kg BW, lasiocarpine at 30 mg/kg, and fulvine at 45 mg/kg (Hooper, unpublished observations). The *S. jacobaea* used in the above experiments contained approximately 0.27% toxic alkaloids (C. C. J. Culvenor, personal communication) which means they were poisoned by a minimum of 5,400 mg/kg BW. The toxicities of the alkaloids in *S. jacobaea*, jacobine, jaconine, and seneciphylline, seem to be only slightly less than that of senecionine, lasiocarpine, and fulvine (34). Thus the chronic toxic dose of *S. jacobaea* was of the order of 100 times the acute toxic dose. This compares with a chronic:acute ratio of some alkaloids in rats of about 4:1 or 5:1 (35). Sheep are thus quite susceptible to acute poisoning and field cases of acute poisonings by plants have been reported (7,14,36,37,38).

The quantitative susceptibility has been shown in laboratory animals to vary with sex and age (39,40), and can be altered by a variety of physical and chemical factors which influence hepatic metabolism (30,39,40,41). In domestic animals, cobalt bullets in the rumen did not protect sheep against *H. europaeum* poisoning (42). Dietary protein and the sulphur-containing amino acid, cysteine, afforded some protection against *S. jacobaea* in poisoning of rats (43,44). Cysteine did not protect rats against chronic heliotrine hepatosis (Hooper, unpublished observation), but this may have been a dose effect. Another sulphur containing amino acid, methionine, showed some promise as a treatment for horses poisoned by *Senecio spp.* (45) but was ineffective against hepatoses in horses poisoned by *C. retusa* (Hooper and Pitt, unpublished observations).

V. COMPARATIVE PATHOLOGY OF PYRROLIZIDINE ALKALOID POISONING

Pyrrolizidine alkaloids exert their effects on tissues by either causing necrosis, inhibiting mitosis and thereby causing megalocytosis, or acting directly on blood vessels and causing edema and vascular disease.

A. Liver

The principle hepatic lesions are acute necrosis (2), chronic parenchymal megalocytosis (1), and veno-occlusive disease (2). Other changes which can also occur include cytoplasmic invaginations, cytoplasmic inclusion globules, portal fibrosis, bile duct proliferation, regeneration nodules, and/or tumors (1,2).

The author has seen all of the above changes in horses, sheep, cattle, pigs, mice, rats, guinea pigs, rabbits, and chickens. Pathology of disease in any animal's liver probably reflects more on its quantitative sensitivity to plant (or alkaloid) toxicity and rate of intake, rather than a tendency of an individual species to develop disease in a particular way. Except for pneumotoxic effects in rats, the more resistant species (sheep, mice, and rats) respond to experimental feeding of Australian plants containing pyrrolizidine alkaloids by slowly developing megalocytosis over many months. The same doses expressed as percentages of feedstuffs offered, cause single cell necrosis, portal fibrosis, and veno-occlusive disease in cattle, and necrosis and bile duct proliferation in chickens. If, however, levels are increased substantially or more highly toxic plants or purified alkaloids are used, then necrosis, fibrosis, and bile duct proliferation develop in sheep, mice, and rats. Conversely, slowly developing megalocytosis can occur in sensitive species at low dosages.

Necrosis of periacinar distribution occurs similarly in most domestic and laboratory animals. Single cell necrosis is common in chronic disease. Irregular patterns of necrosis can occur in some species, for example chickens (2) (Hooper, unpublished observation) and any animal in which there is acute toxic insult superimposed on previous chronic disease. Hepatic necrosis has been seen in field cases in sensitive species such as cattle and horses (21,22,36) and even in resistant species, sheep, after eating comparatively large quantities of toxic plant (7,36,37,38).

A general description of megalocytosis has been provided by Bull (46) and Schoental and Magee (47). Megalocytosis is a residual, progressive disease (47,48,49) following an interaction between the antimitotic effect of the alkaloids (50) and a stimulus for regeneration (51,52). There are minor differences between species in megalocyte morphology. The megalocytes are larger in horses and smaller in chickens compared with other species (Hooper, unpublished observation). Cytoplasmic invaginations are pink (hematoxylin and eosin) staining globules inside the large nuclei (47) in all species, and are pockets of cytoplasm enveloped by the large nuclei (53,54). They are probably non-specific sequelae of nuclear swellings, and are present in other intoxications, for example, copper, cycad, or carbon tetrachloride poisonings in sheep (Hooper, unpublished observation) and some neoplastic and preneoplastic conditions (55).

If there is intermittent intoxication in any species, a more likely event in natural disease, regeneration nodules with small hepatocytes arise from cells escaping the antimitotic effects. Cattle and horses show a more mottled nodulation due to greater bile retention than in sheep (Hooper, unpublished observation).

The appearance and development of hepatic venous occlusion was discussed by McLean (2). The occlusion can be recognized as edema then fibrosis in and around hepatic veins in animals with repeatedly severe but sublethal hepatic insults. The toxic injury must be sustained for at least six days for venous occlusion to occur (56,57). Animals affected with a single exposure are more likely to regenerate with megalocytosis without fibrosis. In Australia, in sheep, the resistant species, veno-occlusive disease is rare because the plant species most likely to cause poisonings, *Heliotropium europaeum* and *Senecio jacobaea*, are insufficiently toxic. On the other hand, fibrosis is a common finding in the more sensitive animal species, particularly cattle (58,59). Sheep are still capable of developing the disease, for example, by 4 to 8 repeated injections of lasiocarpine at about 0.5 LD_{50} at 2 daily intervals (Hooper, unpublished observation). Studies with rats can be confusing because of congestion due to right side heart failure associated with severe pulmonary vascular disease.

Intensely eosinophilic cytoplasmic inclusion globules were described and discussed by Bull (46) and occur in all species. They are probably non-specific enlarged lysosomes or cytosegrosomes (60,61) or some even may be compacted, phagocytozed red cells (62). Portal fibrosis and bile duct proliferation are common, non-specific features of hepatic disease. A rarely reported change is that of osseous metaplasia of hepatic parenchymal tissue (63,64). Cavities in hepatic parenchyma have been reported in mice (62,65).

B. Lungs

Edema, fibrosis, epithelialization, and/or emphysema occur in the lungs of horses, cattle, sheep, and pigs in response to poisonings by some plants. The changes are characteristic of interstitial pneumonia (66) and probably not pathognomonic for pyrrolizidine alkaloid poisoning. The edema seems to start as a swelling of alveolar walls followed by exudation of protein-rich fluid into the alveoli, desquamation of macrophages, and interstitial fibrosis. Epithelialization and emphysema follow later. The epithelialization can be either cuboidal or columnar.

Pulmonary vascular disease affecting larger vessels is not a major characteristic in domestic animals as it is in rats (2,67) and young *Macaca arctoides* monkeys (68,69). Large cells, pulmonary megalocytes with cytoplasmic invaginations, are also commonly seen in alveolar lining cells and alveolar macrophages in rats (70,71,72) and pigs (23), but not horses and pigs poisoned by *Crotalaria spp.* (Hooper, unpublished observation). They can occur without evidence of other disease in the alveoli and bronchi of mice poisoned by *S. jacobaea* (65).

C. Kidneys

The most frequent renal alteration is megalocytosis. These nuclear and cytoplasmic enlargements or hypertrophies, which rarely contain cytoplasmic invaginations, occur usually in the epithelial cells of the proximal tubules and thick loops of Henle. Rats with spectabiline poisoning are unusual in that glomeruli and thin loops of Henle are the areas affected. The glomeruli and proximal tubules are severely affected in pigs with severe *Crotalaria spp.* poisoning (3,16,17). Renal megalocytosis is a common feature in pigs poisoned by at least 4 different genera containing a variety of toxic alkaloids (3,23) (C. Walker and R. Russell, personal communications) and is a common finding in feral pigs in northern Australia grazing in areas in which there are plants containing pyrrolizidine alkaloids (Hooper, unpublished observation). Megalocytosis has been seen occasionally in *C. retusa* poisoning of horses; in sheep and mice poisoned by *S. jacobaea* but not in sheep poisoned by *H. europaeum*; in rats poisoned by spectabiline and fulvine but not heliotrine, lasiocarpine, and senecionine (Hooper, unpublished observation); in vervet monkeys with chronic retrorsine poisoning (73); and in free living baboons which had access to pyrrolizidine alkaloid-containing plants (74).

In pigs, uremic nephroses have been recorded caused by *Crotalaria spp.*, (3,16,17). The kidneys could be the worst affected organs, accompanied by severe pneumonias and occasional severe hepatoses. Megalocytosis affected both the glomeruli and renal tubules and nephrosis followed in both areas. The damage in the glomeruli occurred in endothelial as well as epithelial cells (3,17). Moderate renal nephrosis accompanying severe hepatosis occurred in 2 calves experimentally poisoned by *S. jacobaea*, in 8 of 25 lambs poisoned by monocrotaline and lasiocarpine (Hooper, unpublished observation), in sheep poisoned by *S. longilobus* (75) and in rats by fulvine (76).

Vascular disease accompanied the severe nephroses in pigs caused by *C. spectabilis* (3). A number of workers have reported glomerular changes in rats poisoned with monocrotaline or *C. spectabilis* (70,77,78). The author has not seen similar changes even after examining a large number of rats poisoned by monocrotaline, fulvine, and spectabiline (Hooper, unpublished observations). Metaplastic changes of Bowman's capsules have been reported in vervet monkeys poisoned by retrorsine (73) and chickens poisoned by *C. retusa* (16).

D. Gastrointestinal Tract

Incidental lesions have often been reported in the stomachs and intestines in field and experimental cases of poisonings by pyrrolizidine alkaloids but are difficult to identify as specific results of the alkaloids themselves. Severe ulceration and histological changes consistent with mitotic inhibition of enteroblasts, have been reported in rats and sheep following dosages with high levels of purified alkaloids (79,80). The severe disease in sheep was accompanied by edema and ulceration of the gall bladder. Gastric ulceration occurred in a high proportion of pigs poisoned by *C. spectabilis* (3), *H. lasiocarpum* (81), and *E. lycopsis* (C. Walker, personal communication), but not by *C. retusa* (16). No histological description of the lesion, presumably in the squamous mucosa, has been provided. Rectal prolapses have been reported in cattle (82,83), probably as physiological responses to edema in the intestines of cattle following fibrosis in the liver.

E. Megalocytosis and Vascular Disease in Other Organs

A number of changes in other organs have been reported which, because of their nature, are probable direct effects of pyrrolizidine alkaloids. Megalocytosis has been seen in the pancreas and adrenal glands of pigs poisoned by *C. retusa* (16) and the Harderian glands of rats poisoned by fulvine and spectabiline (Hooper, unpublished observation). Vascular degeneration has been seen in the arteries in the mesenteries (84), pancreas (85), and the heart (86).

F. Laminitis and Esophageal Disease

Crotalaria spp. have caused laminitis in cattle and sheep in southern Africa and India (7,87,88,89,90). The condition may not be due to the pyrrolizidine alkaloid content of the plants (Smit, personal communication).

In north Queensland, Australia, there is a condition in horses characterized by ulceration of the esophagus and squamous mucosa of the stomach, known as "esophageal disease" or "Chillagoe horse disease." Culvenor and Smith (91) cited the work of Newton and Skerman who reproduced the disease by feeding *C. aridicola* and *C. trifoliastrum*. The ulceration is associated only with moderate liver lesions (92).

G. Carcinogenic and Radiomimetic Effects

Hepatomas were seen in association with regeneration nodules and megalocytosis in 1 sheep and 1 ox turned off pastures containing *H. europaeum* (Hooper, unpublished observation). Some pyrrolizidine alkaloids have been assessed as potential natural carcinogens to man (93). The alkaloids can act synergistically with other carcinogens (94,95). They are potent carcinogens in their own right (96,97). They are present in some grains mixed into prepared feedstuffs (16), and can pass into cows' milk (98). The levels in milk may be extremely low and not cause immediate disease (99), especially to a comparatively resistant species such as the rat. Overt severe hepatic disease in man has been controlled in some areas where its cause has been identified (100), but it is still being recognized in various parts of the world (93,101,102, 103,104) and the very long-term effects of intermittent consumption of very low levels of alkaloids are not known. Long-term effects due to such consumption of very small quantities may not be easy to recognize because of the low intermittent levels and the histopathology which can resemble other diseases such as some mycotoxicoses (105,106,107). Histological signs of disease were seen in pigs fed *C. retusa* seeds at levels as low as 0.004% in sorghum grain for only about 4 months (16) and there was contamination in grain sorghum which would have been undetected if it had not been fed to pigs at the time.

Pyrrolizidine alkaloids can act as antitumor agents (108), be teratogenic and abortigenic (15,16,109,110,111,112,113), mutagenic (2), and cause chromosome damage (2,114). Chromosome damage has been observed in the blood of people with veno-occlusive disease caused by *C. fulva* (115). Other possible radiomimetic activities include gastrointestinal disease; leucopenia in laboratory animals (116,117,118) and in a calf (119); but leucocytosis in milking cows (98); repression on lymph follicles and thymuses in rats (85, 120,121,122,123), and horses (18,20); suppression of leucocyte cultures (124); anemia in pigs (125,3), chickens (126,127,128, 129), sheep (128), and laboratory animals (119,120,130); repression of hemopoiesis in rat fetuses (108); wool loss in sheep (131); black hair loss in pigs (125,132,133,3); delayed feather development in poultry (A. Ross, J. Tucker, personal communication); and testicular degeneration in mice (134), and *Drosophila melanogaster* flies (135, 136).

H. Central Nervous Disease, a Probable Secondary Effect

Neurological signs are common in horses, cattle, and sheep probably due to a non-specific effect of liver disease, hyperammonemia (22,137,138,139). Spongy degeneration of the central nervous system in cattle, sheep, and pigs (140,141,142) and Alzheimer type II cells (143) are probably mediated in the same way.

I. Other Probable Secondary Effects

Some of the changes reported are probably secondary effects. These could include hemolysis in sheep associated with advanced hepatic disease and concurrent high liver copper levels (138), some anemias associated with kidney disease (3,16), pancreatic edema and fibrosis (144,145,146), cerebral hemorrhage, edema and congestion in rat brains (77,134,147), endocardial and epicardial hemorrhages, terminal pulmonary edema, congestion and edema of the gastrointestinal tract often interpreted as "gastroenteritis," and other edemas associated with hepatic disease.

J. Effects of the Metabolic Products, the Pyrroles

The effects of pyrrolizidine alkaloids on the various organs appear to be directly mediated by pyrrolic metabolites or pyrroles produced in the liver by action of microsomal enzymes on the parent alkaloids (148,149). A summary of evidence supporting the activity of pyrroles has been prepared by Mattocks (150).

Pyrroles can cause alterations in livers, kidneys, and lungs similar to parent pyrrolizidine alkaloids (151,152) and there can be more widespread suppression of mitosis (153,154,155) as well as carcinogenesis (156,157). Pyrroles also exert vascular effects in lungs and directly on other vessels such as those in rat cremaster muscles (151,158,159) and have analagous effects to their parent alkaloids, on cell cultures (160,114). The antimitotic effects of alkaloids and pyrroles are exerted on DNA (161,162,163).

VI. DISCUSSION

Overall, the patterns of disease in various organs are consistent with "spillover" passage of pyrroles. A striking example is the severe damage caused by lasiocarpine to the gall bladder and intestines of sheep and the intestines of rats when injected at near fatal dose rates (80). Toxicity of an alkaloid reflects its rate of metabolism to a pyrrole (40) and therefore it seems reasonable that "pyrrole spillovers" will be more likely at higher dosages.

Experimental work with rats suggests that the chemical structures of toxic pyrrolizidine alkaloids which are hepatotoxic should also be pneumotoxic when applied at higher dosages (27). The hepatotoxic effect could outweigh the pneumotoxic effect to such a degree that the latter is not expressed. The problem becomes complicated in plant poisonings because there is no simple relationship between the acute effects of the alkaloids and their chronic effects (31), and further complicated when a third effect of pyrrolizidine alkaloids is considered, that on blood vessels. The latter effect is probably responsible for most of the severe interstitial pneumonias by initially causing edemas of alveolar walls, and may be a big factor in the severe nephroses of pigs (17). Some animals are more sensitive to vascular disease and therefore more likely to develop pneumonic disease.

If "pyrrole spillover" is to account for extra hepatic diseases, it must account for the varied presence and absence of the various components of those diseases. Variation in the expression of disease not only depends on the presence and quantity of pyrroles but also the reactions of the host tissues. These reactions will probably be either changes due to reactions from edema or else if there is active cell division, megalocytosis. The active cell division can even occur in alveolar macrophages following edema. It is reasonable to believe that necrosis is less important outside the liver. Interstitial pneumonia can occur without megalocytosis. This may be due to the absence of cell division at the time when there is passage of the pyrroles. The converse (80) could be due to insensitivity of the host's vascular system. Cell turnover could be higher in the kidneys than in the lungs which could account for renal megalocytosis in the absence of pulmonary disease. It certainly accounts for the severe enteric lesions in acute disease.

Comparing *Crotalaria spp.* with *Senecio spp.*, *Crotalaria spp.* has more potent pneumotoxic effects and this must be due to greater predilection of the *Crotalaria spp.* for vascular effects. In the genera in which there are less extra-hepatic effects, there may be less "spillover," possibly due to lower toxicity.

Although this paper has highlighted the development of extra hepatic disease, the diseases in the livers are the most important causes of losses recognized in domestic animals with all plant genera. Subtle diseases may exist, for example due to contamination of grains in prepared feedstuffs, so an understanding of the complex pathology of the diseases is desirable.

VII. ACKNOWLEDGMENTS

The author is grateful for his term as a postgraduate student at the University of Melbourne (Professor K. V. F. Jubb) where some of the unpublished work was accomplished. Thanks are due to Drs. C. Culvenor, J. Peterson, and M. Jago for advice, and to Mrs. P. Newman for the difficult task of typing.

VIII. REFERENCES

1. Bull, L. B., Culvenor, C. C. J., and Dick, A. T., *in* "The Pyrrolizidine Alkaloids," p. 157. North Holland Publishing Company, Amsterdam, 1968.
2. McLean, E. K., *Pharmacol. Rev.* 22, 429 (1970).
3. Peckham, J. C., Sangster, L. T., and Jones, O. H., *J. Am. Vet. Med. Assoc.* 165, 633 (1974).
4. Bull, L. B., Culvenor, C. C. J., and Dick, A. T., *in* "The

Pyrrolizidine Alkaloids," p. 1. North Holland Publishing Company, Amsterdam, 1968.
5. Bull, L. B., Culvenor, C. C. J., and Dick, A. T., *in* "The Pyrrolizidine Alkaloids," p. 21. North Holland Publishing Company, Amsterdam, 1968.
6. Theiler, A., *7th/8th Rep. S. Afr. Dep. Agric. Vet. Serv.*, p. 59 (1918).
7. Steyn, D. G., *in* "The Toxicology of Plants in South Africa," South African Central News Agency, 1934.
8. Marais, J. S. C., *Onderstepoort J. Vet. Sci. Anim. Ind.* 20, 61 (1944).
9. Watt, J. M., and Breyer-Brandwijk, M. G., *in* "The Medicinal and Poisonous Plants of Southern and Eastern Africa," p. 584. E. S. Livingstone, Edinburgh and London, 1962.
10. Gardiner, M. R., Royce, R., and Bokor, A., *J. Pathol. Bacteriol.* 89, 43 (1965).
11. Sanders, D. A., Shealy, A. L., and Emmel, M. W., *J. Am. Vet. Med. Assoc.* 89, 150 (1936).
12. Berry, D. M., and Bras, G., *North Am. Vet.* 38, 323 (1957).
13. Steyn, D. G., and de Kock, G., *18th Rep. Dir. Vet. Serv. Anim. Ind.*, p. 947 (1932).
14. Laws, L., *Aust. Vet. J.* 44, 453 (1968).
15. Lewis, J. C., *Rep. N. T. Vet. Stock Dep. 1912*, p. 133 (1912).
16. Hooper, P. T., and Scanlan, W. A., *Aust. Vet. J.* 53, 109 (1977).
17. McGrath, J. P. M., Duncan, J. R., and Munnell, J. F., *J. Comp. Pathol.* 85, 185 (1975).
18. Smirnov, F. E., Grosheva, C. A., and Stoljarova, A. G., *Uzb. Inst. Vet. Sborn. Nauch. Tr.* 13, 173 (1959).
19. Smirnov, F. E., Grosheva, C. A., and Stoljarova, A. G., *Uzb. Inst. Vet. Sborn. Nauch. Tr.* 13, 195 (1959).
20. Smirnov, F. E., and Stoljarova, A. G., *Uzb. Inst. Vet. Sborn. Nauch. Tr.* 13, 186 (1959).
21. Rose, A. L., Gardner, C. A., McConnell, J. D., and Bull, L. B., *Aust. Vet. J.* 33, 25 (1957).
22. Rose, A. L., Gardner, C. A., McConnell, J. D., and Bull, L. B., *Aust. Vet. J.* 33, 49 (1957).
23. Harding, J. D. J., Lewis, G., Done, J. T., and Allcroft, R., *Pathol. Vet.* 1, 204 (1964).
24. Bull, L. B., Culvenor, C. C. J., and Dick, A. T., *in* "The Pyrrolizidine Alkaloids," p. 137. North Holland Publishing Company, Amsterdam, 1968.
25. Burns, J., *J. Pathol.* 103 Piii (*Proc. Pathol. Soc. G. B. Ir.)* (1971).
26. Hooper, P. T., *J. Pathol.* 113, 227 (1974).
27. Culvenor, C. C. J., Edgar, J. A., Jago, M. V., Outteridge, A., Peterson, J. E., and Smith, L. W., *Chem. Biol. Interact.* 12, 299 (1976).
28. Dollahite, J. W., *Southwest. Vet.* Spring (1972); p. 223 (1972)
29. Bull, L. B. Culvenor, C. C. J., and Dick, A. T., *in* "The Pyrrolizidine Alkaloids," p. 133. North Holland

Publishing Company, Amsterdam, 1968.
30. Mattocks, A. R., *Chem. Biol. Interact.* 5, 227 (1972).
31. White, I. N. H., Mattocks, A. R., and Butler, W. H., *Chem. Biol. Interact.* 6, 207 (1973).
32. Shull, L. R., Buckmaster, G. W., and Cheeke, P. R., *J. Anim. Sci.* 43, 1247 (1976).
33. Lanigan, G. W., *Aust. J. Agric. Res.* 23, 1085 (1972).
34. Bull, L. B., Culvenor, C. C. J., and Dick, A. T., *in* "The Pyrrolizidine Alkaloids," p. 141. North Holland Publishing Company, Amsterdam, 1968.
35. Bull, L. B., Culvenor, C. C. J., and Dick, A. T., *in* "The Pyrrolizidine Alkaloids," p. 159. North Holland Publishing Company, Amsterdam, 1968.
36. Mugera, G. M., *Bull. Epizoot. Dis. Afr.* 18, 389 (1970).
37. Forsyth, A. A., *in* "British Poisonous Plants," M.A.F.F. Bulletin No. 161, 2nd Ed., p. 99, H.M.S.O., London, 1968.
38. Bull, L. B., Culvenor, C. C. J., and Dick, A. T., *in* "The Pyrrolozidine Alkaloids," p. 16. North Holland Publishing Company, Amsterdam, 1968.
39. Jago, M. V., *J. Pathol.* 105, 1 (1971).
40. Tuchwever, B., Kovacs, K., Jago, M. V., and Beaulieu, T., *Res. Comm. Chem. Pathol. Pharmacol.* 7, 459 (1974).
41. Newberne, P. M., Chan, W. C. M., and Rogers, A. E., *Toxicol. Appl. Pharmacol.* 28, 200 (1974).
42. Lanigan, G. W., and Whittem, J. H., *Aust. Vet. J.* 46, 17 (1970).
43. Cheeke, P. R., and Garman, G. R., *Nat. Rep. Inter.* 9, 197 (1974).
44. Buckmaster, G. W., Cheeke, P. R., and Shull, L. R., *J. Anim. Sci.* 43, 464 (1976).
45. Retief, G. P., *J. S. Afr. Vet. Med. Assoc.* 33, 405 (1962).
46. Bull, L. B., *Aust. Vet. J.* 31, 33 (1955).
47. Schoental, R., and Magee, P. N., *J. Pathol. Bacteriol.* 74, 305 (1957).
48. Bull, L. B., And Dick, A. T., *J. Pathol. Bacteriol.* 78, 483 (1959).
49. Bull, L. B., and Dick, A. T., *Aust. J. Exp. Biol. Med. Sci.* 38, 515 (1960).
50. Peterson, J. E., *J. Pathol. Bacteriol.* 89, 153 (1965).
51. Jago, M. V., *Am. J. Pathol.* 56, 403 (1969).
52. Jago, M. V., *Aust. J. Exp. Biol. Med. Sci.* 48, 93 (1970).
53. Svoboda, D., and Soga, J., *Am. J. Pathol.* 48, 347 (1966).
54. Allen, J. R., and Carstens, L. A., *Am. J. Vet. Res.* 31, 1059 (1970).
55. Sobel, H. J., Schwartz, R., and Marguet, E., *Arch. Pathol.* 87, 179 (1969).
56. Bras, G., and McLean, E. K., *Ann. N. Y. Acad. Sci.* 111, 392 (1963).
57. McLean, E. K., *J. Pathol.* 103, PvII (1971).
58. McLennan, M. W., Dodson, M. E., and Rac, R., *Aust. Vet. J.* 48, 480 (1972).

59. Bull, L. B., Culvenor, C. C. J., and Dick, A. T., *in* "The Pyrrolizidine Alkaloids," p. 181. North Holland Publishing Company, Amsterdam, 1968.
60. Kerr, J. F. R., *J. Pathol. Bacteriol.* 93, 167 (1967).
61. Kerr, J. F. R., *Pathology* 1, 83 (1969).
62. Ruebner, B. H., Watanabe, K., and Wand, J. S., *Am. J. Pathol.* 60, 247 (1970).
63. Schoental, R., and Benstead, J. P. M., *Br. J. Cancer* 17, 242 (1963).
64. Carlton, W. W., *J. Am. Vet. Med. Assoc.* 151, 345 (1967).
65. Hooper, P. T., *J. Pathol.* 113, 227 (1974).
66. Omar, A. R., *Vet. Bull.* 34, 371 (1964).
67. Kay, J. M., and Heath, D., *in* "Crotalaria Spectabilis - The Pulmonary Hypertension Plant," Charles C. Thomas, Springfield, U.S.A., 1969.
68. Allen, J. R., and Chesney, C. F., *Exp. Mol. Pathol.* 17, 220 (1972).
69. Chesney, C. F., and Allen, J. R., *Am. J. Vet. Res.* 34, 1577 (1973).
70. Hayashi Y., and Lalich, J. J., *Proc. Soc. Exp. Biol. Med.* 124, 392 (1967).
71. Valdivi, E., Sonnad, J., Hayashi, Y., and Lalich, J. J., *Angiology* 18, 378 (1967).
72. Kay, J. M., Smith, P., and Heath, D., *Thorax* 24, 511 (1969).
73. Van der Watt, J. J., Purchase I. F. H., and Tustin R. C., *J. Pathol.* 107 279 (1972).
74. McConnell, E. E., Basson, P. A., De Vos, V., Myers, B. J., and Kuntz, R. E., *Onderstepoort J. Vet. Res.* 41, 97 (1974).
75. Harris, P. N., Henderson, F. C., and Chen K. K., *Arch. Pathol.* 64, 297 (1957).
76. Persaud, T. V. N., Putzke, H. P., Tessman, D., and Bienengräber, A., *Acta Histochem.* 37, 369 (1970).
77. Masugi, Y., Oami, K., Aihara, K., Hashimoto, K., and Hakozaki, T., *Acta Pathol. Jpn.* 15, 407 (1965).
78. Carstens, L. A., and Allen, J. R., *Am. J. Pathol.* 60, 75 (1970).
79. Bull, L. B., Culvenor, C. C. J., and Dick, A. T., *in* "The Pyrrolizidine Alkaloids," p. 153. North Holland Publishing Company, Amsterdam, 1968.
80. Hooper, P. T., *J. Comp. Pathol.* 85, 341 (1975).
81. Bourkser, G. V., cited by McLean, E. K., *Pharmacol. Rev.* 22, 433 (1970).
82. Fowler, M. E., *J. Am. Vet. Med. Assoc.* 152, 113 (1968).
83. Wiltjer, J. C., and Walker, C. E. J., *Aust. Vet. J.* 50, 580 (1974).
84. Schoental, R., and Magee, P. M., *J. Pathol. Bacteriol.* 78, 471 (1959).
85. Allen, J. R., and Carstens, L. A., *Am. J. Vet. Res.* 31, 1059 (1970).
86. Blaustein, H. L., Blaustein, A., and Rosenblat, M., *Arch. Pathol.* 79, 335 (1965).

87. Theiler, A., *Union S. Afr. Agric. J.* 1, 10 (1911).
88. Steyn, D. G., *Onderstepoort J. Vet. Sci. Anim. Ind.* 7, 169 (1936).
89. Jackson, J. J., Needham, A. J. E., and Lawrence, J. A., *J. Rhodesian Sci. Assoc.* 53, 10 (1968).
90. Watt, J. M., and Breyer-Brandwijk, M. G., *in* "The Medicinal and Poisonous Plants of Southern and Eastern Africa," p. 578 E. & S. Livingstone, Edinburgh and London, 1962.
91. Culvenor, C. C. J., and Smith, L. W., *Aust. J. Chem.* 15, 121 (1962).
92. Anon, *1959/60 Annu. Rep. Queensl. Agric. Stock Dep.* p. 35 (1960).
93. W.H.O., I.A.R.C. Working Group *in* "I.A.R.C. Working Group on the Evaluation of the Carcinogenic Risk of Chemicals to Man: Some Naturally Occurring Substances," W.H.O. International Agency for Research on Cancer, p. 332, 1975.
94. Newberne, P. M., and Rogers, A. E., *Plant Foods Man.* 1, 23 (1973).
95. Reddy, J. K., Rao, M. S., and Jago, M. V., *Int. J. Cancer* 17, 621 (1976).
96. Harris, P. N., and Chen, K. K., *Cancer Res.* 30, 2881 (1970).
97. Svoboda, D. J., and Reddy, J. K., *Cancer Res.* 32, 908 (1972).
98. Dickinson, J. O., Cooke, M. P., King, R. R., and Mahomed, P. A., *J. Am. Vet. Med. Assoc.* 169, 1192 (1976).
99. Johnson, A. E., *Am. J. Vet. Res.* 37, 107 (1976).
100. Barnes, J. M., *M. B. Pharm. Bull.* 25, 2 (1976).
101. Rose, E. F., *S. Afr. Med. J.* 46, 1039 (1972).
102. Williams, A. O., and Schoental, R., *Trop. Geogr. Med.* 22, 201 (1970).
103. Tandon, B. N., Tandon, R. K., Tandon, H. D., Narndranathan, M., and Joshi, Y. K., *Lancet* 2, 271 (1976).
104. Mohabbat, O., Srivastava, R. N., Shafig Younos, M., Sedig, G. G., Merzad, A. A., and Aram, G. N., *Lancet* 2, 269 (1976).
105. Newberne, P. M., and Butler, W. A., *Cancer Res.* 29, 236 (1969).
106. Carlton, W. W., and Tuite, J., *Toxicol. Appl. Pharmacol.* 17, 289 (1970).
107. Friis, P., Hasselager, E., and Krogh, P., *Acta. Pathol. Microbiol. Scand.* 77, 559 (1969).
108. Culvenor, C. C. J., *J. Pharm. Sci.* 57, 1112 (1968).
109. Sundareson, A. E., *J. Pathol. Bacteriol.* 54, 289 (1942).
110. Bhattacharyya, K., *J. Pathol. Bacteriol.* 90, 151 (1965).
111. Newberne, P. M., *Cancer Res.* 28, 2327 (1968).
112. Green, C. R., and Christie, G. S., *Br. J. Exp. Pathol.* 42, 369 (1961).
113. Persaud, T. V. N., and Hoyte, D. A. N., *Exp. Pathol.* 9, 59 (1974).
114. Armstrong, S. J., Zucherman, A. J., and Bird, R. G., *Br. J. Exp. Pathol.* 53, 145 (1971).
115. Martin, P. A., Thorburn, M. J., Hutchinson, S., Bras, G., and

Miller, C. G., *Br. J. Exp. Pathol.* 53, 374 (1972).
116. Carlton, W. W., *J. Am. Vet. Med. Assoc.* 151, 845 (1967).
117. Levin, G. S., and Novachenko, S. I., *Farmakol. Toksikol.* 32, 170 (1969).
118. Shtenberg, I., and Orlova, N. V., *Vopr. Pitan.* 14, 27 (1955).
119. Coulson, C. B., Davies, P. J., and Evans, W. C., *J. Comp. Pathol.* 70, 199 (1960).
120. Harris, P. N., Rose, C. L., and Chen, K. K., *Arch. Pathol.* 64, 152 (1957).
121. Harris, P. N., Anderson, R. C., and Chen, K. K., *J. Pharmacol. Exp. Ther.* 78, 372 (1943).
122. Harris, P. N., Anderson, R. C., and Chen, K. K., *J. Pharmacol. Exp. Ther.* 79, 133 (1943).
123. Schoental, R., *Nature* 179, 361 (1957).
124. Bick, Y. A. E., and Jackson, W. D., *Aust. J. Biol. Sci.* 21, 469 (1968).
125. Emmel, M. W., Sanders, D. A., and Henley, W. O., *J. Am. Vet. Med. Assoc.* 37, 43 (1935).
126. Emmel, M. W., *J. Am. Vet. Med. Assoc.* 44, 205 (1937).
127. Emmel, M. W., and Sanders, D. A., *Univ. Fla. Agric. Exp. Bull.* p. 574 (1942).
128. Bourkser, G. V., *Gig. Sanit.* No. 6, 24 (1947).
129. Simpson, C. F., Waldroup, P. W., and Harms, R. H., *J. Am. Vet. Med. Assoc.* 142, 264 (1963).
130. Schoental, R., *Biochem. J.* 60, i-ii (1955).
131. Steyn, D. G., and Van der Walt, S. J., *Farming S. Afr.* 20, 445 (1945).
132. Gibbons, W. J., *Mod. Vet. Pract.* 47, 84 (1966).
133. Gibbons, W. J., *Mod. Vet. Pract.* 48, 52 (1967).
134. Rosenfeld, I., and Beath, O. A., *Am. J. Clin. Pathol.* 15, 407 (1945).
135. Clark, A. M., *Z. Vererbungsl.* 91, 74 (1960).
136. Clark, A. M., *Z. Vererbungsl.* 94, 115 (1963).
137. Gibbons, W. J., *Mod. Vet. Pract.* 50, 79 (1969).
138. Bull, L. B., Dick, A. T., Keast, J. C., and Edgar, S., *Aust. J. Agric. Res.* 7, 281 (1956).
139. Bull, L. B., Scott-Rodgers, E., Keast, J. C., and Dick, A. T., *Aust. Vet. J.* 37, 37 (1961).
140. Hooper, P. T., Best, S. M., and Murray, D. R., *Res. Vet. Sci.* 16, 216 (1974).
141. Hooper, P. T., *Acta Neuropathol.* 31, 325 (1975).
142. Hooper, P. T., *Acta Neuropathol.* 31, 343 (1975).
143. Finn, J. P., and Tennant, B., *Cornell Vet.* 64, 136 (1974).
144. Bras, G., and Hill, K. R., *Lancet* 271, 161 (1956).
145. Schoental, R., *Voeding* 16, 268 (1955).
146. Schoental, R., and Magee, P. N., *J. Pathol. Bacteriol.* 78, 471 (1959).
147. Davidson, J., *J. Pathol. Bacteriol.* 40, 285 (1935).
148. Mattocks, A. R., *Nature (London)* 217, 723 (1968).
149. Jago, M. V., Edgar, J. A., Smith L. W., and Culvenor, C. C. J., *Mol. Pharmacol.* 6, 402 (1970).

150. Mattocks, A. R., *Proc. 5th Int. Congr. Pharmacol.* 2, 114 (1973).
151. Butler, W. H., Mattocks, A. R., and Barnes, J. M., *J. Pathol.* 100, 169 (1970).
152. Butler, W. H., *J. Pathol.* 102, 15 (1970).
153. Peterson, J. E., Samuel, A., and Jago, M. V., *J. Pathol.* 107, 175 (1972).
154. Hsu, I. C., Allen, J. R., and Chesney, C. F., *Proc. Soc. Exp. Biol. Med.* 144, 834 (1973).
155. Allen, J. R., and Hsu, I. C., *Proc. Soc. Exp. Biol. Med.* 147, 546 (1974).
156. Allen, J. R., Hsu, I. C., and Carstens, L. A., *Cancer Res.* 35, 997 (1975).
157. Shumaker, R. C., Robertson, K. A., Hsu, I. C., and Allen, J. R., *J. Nat. Cancer Inst.* (1976).
158. Plestina, R., and Stoner, H. B., *J. Pathol.* 106, 235 (1972).
159. Hurley, J. V., and Jago, M. V., *Pathology* 8, 7 (1976).
160. Armstrong, S. J., and Zuckerman, A. J., *Br. J. Exp. Pathol.* 53, 138 (1971).
161. Curtain, C. C., *Chem. Biol. Interact.* 10, 133 (1975).
162. Hsu, I. C., Chesney, C. F., and Allen, J. R., *Proc. Soc. Exp. Biol. Med.* 142, 1133 (1973).
163. Samuel, A., and Jago, M. V., *Chem. Biol. Interact.* 10, 185 (1975).

RECENT STUDIES ON MECHANISMS OF CYTOTOXIC ACTION OF PYRROLIZIDINE ALKALOIDS

A. R. Mattocks
Medical Research Council (U.K.)

I. ABSTRACT

The use of synthetic and semisynthetic analogues has assisted our understanding of mechanism of various toxic actions of pyrrolizidine alkaloids. Hepatotoxicity is influenced by structural features which affect metabolism of the alkaloids to pyrrole derivatives, and also by the chemical reactivity of the pyrrolic metabolites. Antimitotic activity like that of the alkaloids is also found with simple bishydroxymethyl pyrroles; it is much less common with monofunctional than with bifunctional alkylating agents.

Bifunctional hydroxymethylpyrrole esters also produce delayed lung damage like that caused by some alkaloids, whereas acute lung damage is caused by many monofunctional hydroxymethylpyrrole esters. Tissue distribution and metabolic studies have been made using tritiated semisynthetic and synthetic esters with similar hepatotoxicity to natural pyrrolizidine alkaloids.

The results described are useful for planning more detailed future studies on pyrrolizidine toxicity.

II. INTRODUCTION

Many different pyrrolizidine alkaloids are toxic to animals and sometimes to humans. Availability of a range of compounds has enabled relationships between chemical structures and biological activity to be studied. We are interested in liver and lung damage caused by the alkaloids, and most of our experimental work has been done with rats. I want to describe some of our recent results and try to reach a few conclusions about some aspects of pyrrolizidine toxicity. However, much of this work is still incomplete and is liable to provide as many new questions as answers.

While the natural alkaloids provide a wide range of structures, chemically prepared or modified compounds are very useful in experimental work in the following ways. (a) The most toxic natural pyrrolizidine esters, like retrorsine, are difficult or impossible to synthesize, but semisynthetic esters of natural amino-alcohols such as retronecine can be used to study effects of different acid moieties on metabolism and toxicity (1,2) and can be used as radioactive compounds of high specific activity (3). (b) Variation of the basic moiety has helped define structural features necessary for toxicity. For example, the totally synthetic synthanecine A bis-N-ethylcarbamate has most of the toxic effects in rats of pyrrolizidine alkaloids such as monocrotaline (4). (c) The use of pyrrolic alcohols and esters has allowed the study of chemical properties and biological effects of potential reactive metabolites of the alkaloids and synthetic analogues. (d) Specifically tritium labelled semisynthetic and synthetic alkaloid analogues and their pyrrole derivatives have been prepared. Thus, retronecine can be oxidized to the aldehyde and this reduced to ^{3}H-retronecine with tritiated borohydride, then converted to a toxic ester (3,5).

III. METABOLISM AND HEPATOTOXICITY

Death of an animal with liver necrosis within a few days after being given an alkaloid is always associated with the presence of pyrrolic metabolites in the liver a short time after dosing (6). Primary pyrrolic metabolites are chemically reactive alkylating agents, probably responsible for the cytotoxic effects. Factors affecting toxicity are: (a) the proportion of the alkaloid which is converted to pyrroles; (b) the rate of conversion to pyrroles; and (c) the chemical reactivity of the initially formed pyrrolic metabolite. These factors affect the rate of deactivation to non- or less-toxic secondary metabolites and also the distribution of reactive metabolite to other target organs, such as lungs.

A. Factors Affecting Conversion of Alkaloids to Pyrroles.

The aminoalcohols (necines) are evidently not metabolized to pyrroles. The ester alkaloid must remain unhydrolyzed in order for conversion to pyrrole to take place. Ester hydrolysis is reduced and pyrrole production increased by increased steric hindrance around the ester groups. Table 1 shows pyrrole metabolite levels in rat livers 2 hr after i.p. injections of some natural and semisynthetic retronecine esters. First, about 15 x more pyrrole is formed from diesters than mono-esters; compare (i) with (ii) and (v) with (vi). This is partly due to increased lipophilicity in the diesters. But the tetrahydroxy diester (iii) gives more pyrrole than (i). However, the lower pyrrole formation from (iii) compared with (ii) does appear due to lower lipid solubility rather than sterochemical factors, since acetylation to the even bulkier (iv) restores pyrrole metabolism almost to the level of (ii). Second, the nature of the acid moiety greatly affects pyrrole formation. The N-ethylcarbamates give much more pyrrole than the tiglates; compare (i) with (v); (ii) with (vi) and (vii). This might be due to the greater resistance of carbamates to enzymic hydrolysis. Cyclic retronecine diesters are more efficiently converted to pyrroles than 'open' diesters [compare (viii) and (ix) with (ii)]; the exceptionally high value for retrorsine (ix) might be due to greater resistance to hydrolysis or to optimal

TABLE 1

Pyrrolic Metabolites in Livers of Male Rats 2 hr after Retronecine Esters were Administered Intraperitoneally

Compound

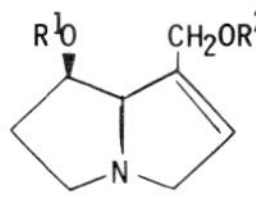

	R^1	R^2	Relative liver pyrrole level (Ehrlich colour) per 1 mmole dose
(i)	H	Me(H)C=C(Me)CO- (tigloyl)	0.047
(ii)	tigloyl	tigloyl	0.30
(iii)	both Me–CH(OH)–C(OH)(Me)–CO-		0.135
(iv)	both Me–CH(OAc)–C(OAc)(Me)–CO-		0.75
(v)	H	EtNHCO-	0.20
(vi)	EtNHCO-	EtNHCO-	2.91
(vii)	EtNHCO-	tigloyl	1.69
(viii)	Monocrotaline		2.08
(ix)	Retrorsine		6.6

binding to the dehydrogenating enzyme.

Data of this kind are useful for designing synthetic or semi-synthetic compounds for experiments on pyrrolizidine-type toxicity.

Further information is obtained using synthetic alkaloid analogues (Table 2). Many aliphatic esters, e.g. (i)-(v) give low yields of pyrrolic metabolites. Pyrrole levels are higher with the more hindered esters (vi) and (vii), and much higher with the carbamate (viii) and phosphate (ix). Both phosphates and carbamates can act as esterase inhibitors (7). It is likely that ester hydrolysis is a major detoxication mechanism. Thus in rats predosed with the esterase inhibitor tri-*o*-cresylphosphate (TOCP), the liver pyrroles from (i) and (ii) are greatly increased. When the tiglate (ii) was administered to male rats (300 mg/kg i.p.), metabolites found in a 24 hr urine sample were: pyrroles 3%, pyrrolines 91%; pyrroline N-oxides 13% (total recovery 107%). Of the pyrrolines, no diester and only a trace of monoester was found, i.e. nearly all the ester was hydrolyzed. In contrast, after giving the carbamate (viii) (40 mg/kg), the urine contained pyrroles 7.5%, N-oxides 1.8%, and solvent-extractable pyrrolines 23.8%, identified as mainly unhydrolyzed carbamate by n.m.r. spectroscopy.

Metabolism to pyrroles is also affected by the aminoalcohol

TABLE 2

Pyrrolic Metabolite Levels in Livers of Male Rats 2 hr after Intraperitoneal Administration of Various Esters of Synthanecine A

Compound	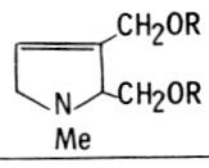	Relative Liver Pyrroles after dose of 1 mmole per kg Body Weight	
	R		
(i)	$COCH_3$	0.045	(0.34 after TOCP)
(ii)	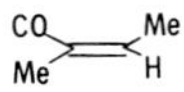	0.07	(0.77 after TOCP)
(iii)	COOEt	0.11	
(iv)	COOPh	practically nil	
(v)	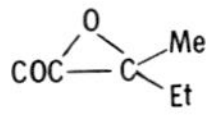	0.15	
(vi)	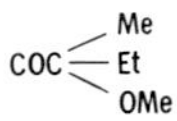	0.30	
(vii)	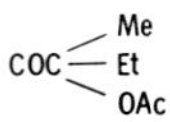	0.78	
(viii)	CONHEt	3.59	
(ix)	$PO(OEt)_2$	2.5	(TOCP = tri-o-cresylphosphate)

structure. Table 3 compares the N-ethylcarbamates of various synthetic aminoalcohols (synthanecines). The double bond is almost essential [compare (i) with (iv)]. Ring substituents increase pyrrole formation. Pyrrole is not formed from (ii) but is formed in good yield from the methyl homologue (iii) and even more from the diester (iv)-(vi).

B. Factors Affecting Toxicity of the Pyrrolic Metabolites

In most cases pyrrolizidine alkaloids and analogues cause liver damage in proportion to their conversion to pyrrolic metabolites. The latter are alkylating (electrophilic) agents and can react with thiols. Thus glutathione (GSH) in the liver can partially protect against subacute pyrrolizidine toxicity and there are several examples in the literature. My colleague Ian White has shown that the LD_{50} of retrorsine in male rats (42 mg/kg in controls) is increased to 83 mg/kg by pretreating them with cysteine and decreased to 23 mg/kg by pretreatment with 2-chlorethanol which depletes liver GSH to 25% of controls (8).

Another factor which might influence the toxicity of pyrrolic

TABLE 3

Pyrrolic Metabolites and Hepatotoxicity in Rats Administered Synthetic Carbamates Analogous to Pyrrolizidine Alkaloids

	Structure (R = CONHEt)	Relative Liver Pyrrole Level (2 h) per dose of 1 mmol/kg	Hepatotoxicity: Subacute LD_{50} mmol/kg	Relative liver pyrrole level per LD_{50} dose
(i)	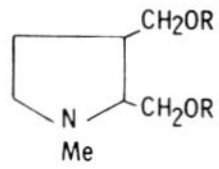	0.11	NT (R)	-
(ii)	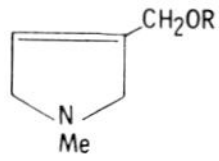	pract. nil	NT	-
(iii)	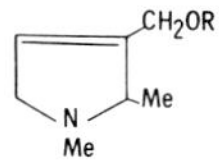	0.5	NT (R)	-
(iv)	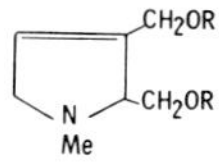	3.59	0.15	0.54
(v)	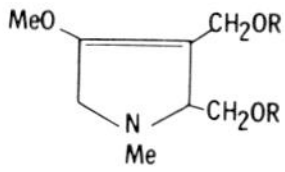	1.5	0.28	0.42
(vi)	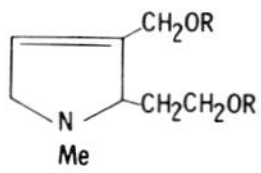	1.5	0.4	0.60

NT = hepatotoxicity not seen with single dose.

NT (R) = No hepatotoxicity after repeated large doses

metabolites is their chemical reactivity. They can act both as electrophiles, through their activated ester groups, and also as nucleophiles, like most pyrroles. Highly reactive metabolites could be deactivated, e.g. by hydrolysis or polymerization, before reaching sites of toxic action. Polymerization might be regarded as 'self-deactivation.' For instance amoebae treated in aqueous media with dehydromonocrotaline had a layer of polymer on the mucopolysaccharide coating of the cell membrane, and pockets of insoluble polymer were later found within the amoebae (M. Ord, unpublished results).

We measured the relative electrophilic and nucleophilic reactivities of hydroxymethyl pyrroles related to natural or synthetic alkaloids, using their reactions with 4-*p*-nitrobenzylpyridine and Ehrlich reagent respectively. Using excess reagents, pseudo first-order rate constants were obtained from which relative half-lives of the pyrroles were calculated (Table 4). Compounds with the highest reactivity to both reagents, such as (ii) and (v),

TABLE 4

Relative Chemical Reactivities of some Hydroxymethyl Pyrroles

	Hydroxymethylpyrrole		Half life (min) of reaction with Nitrobenzylpyridine (50°)	Ehrlich Reagent (30°)
(i)	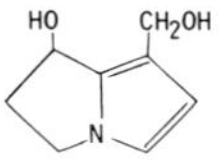	(Dehydroretronecine)	20.8	16.9
(ii)	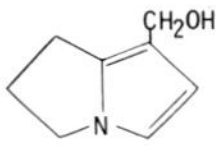	(Dehydrosupinidine)	0.82	0.6
(iii)	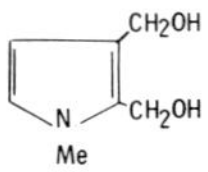		7.2	23.9
(iv)	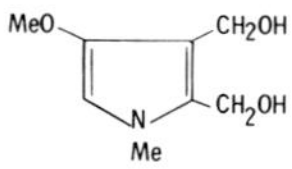		2.9	0.77
(v)	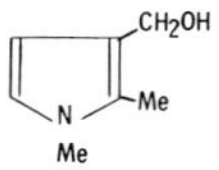		0.94	0.7
(vi)	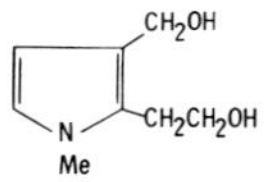		2.24	2.4

should polymerize most readily, while (i) and (iii) should be more stable. Table 5 compares the hepatotoxicity of some pyrrolizidine and analogues esters, and the tendency of pyrroles from them to polymerize; usually the most toxic compounds give the more stable pyrroles.

IV. ANTIMITOTIC ACTION IN THE LIVER

Antimitotic action, the most characteristic delayed effect of many pyrrolizidine alkaloids, may be manifested by the appearance of giant hepatocytes if the liver is stimulated to regenerate, by the necrogenic action of the alkaloid itself, or by some other form of liver injury (9). Antimitotic activity is seen not only with pyrrolizidines and their pyrrolic metabolites, but also in bishydroxymethylpyrroles and their esters and in pyrrolines which can be metabolized to them (Table 6). Giant hepatocytes are often seen after compounds are administered which are, or can be

TABLE 5

Comparison of Hepatotoxicities of some Pyrroline Esters

Compound (R = CONHEt)	approx. subacute LD_{50} mmol/kg	Relative tendency of pyrrolic metabolites to polymerize
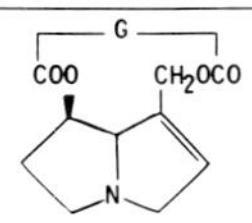 (Monocrotaline)	0.3	low
(Retrorsine)	0.1	low
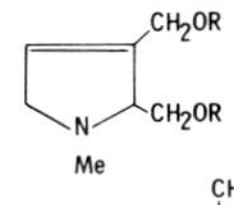	0.15	low
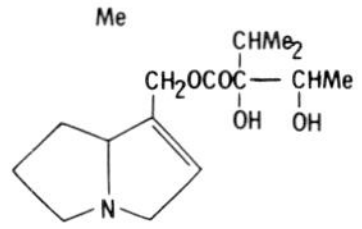 (Supinine)	Very high > 3.5	high
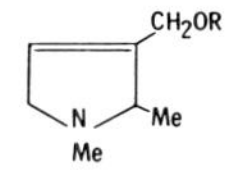	not toxic (?)	high
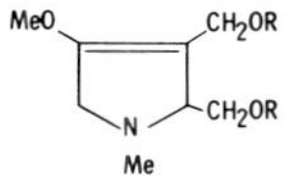	0.28	medium
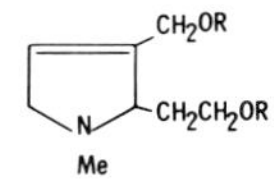	0.4	medium

metabolized to, bifunctional alkylating agents. Giant hepatocytes are uncommon after monofunctional agents are administered. Thus, tissue reactions leading to antimitotic effects are greatly enhanced by bifunctionality although this is not essential. The simplest compound to produce antimitotic effects in rat liver is 1-methyl-2,3-bishydroxymethylpyrrole. Giant hepatocytes are produced if administration of this compound (25-40 mg/kg) is followed several days later by administration of a liver damaging agent (dimethylnitrosamine, 30 mg/kg or, less effectively, multiple doses of thioacetamide, 50 mg/kg). The compound 2,3-bishydroxymethyl-5-methyl-1-phenylpyrrole, which itself causes some liver necrosis, gives very striking giant cells in rat liver when administered alone in doses above 70 mg/kg or at 25 mg/kg if followed by dimethylnitrosamine. However, some pyrroles known to have antimitotic activity, such as dehydroretronecine at 50 mg/kg, do not produce giant hepatocytes when administered even when followed by dimethylnitrosamine.

TABLE 6

Ability of some Pyrrolizidine and Pyrroline Esters to Produce Giant Hepatocytes in Rat Liver

Structure (R = various groups)	Compound	Giant hepatocytes
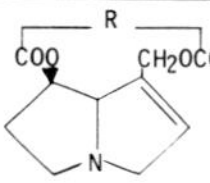	Retrorsine Monocrotaline etc	+ +
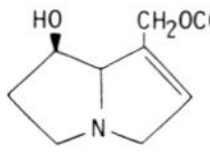	Indicine (M)	+
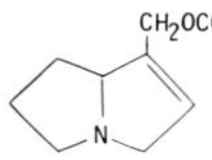	Supinine (M)	+
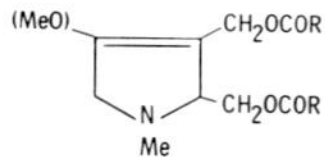	Synthanecine esters	+ +
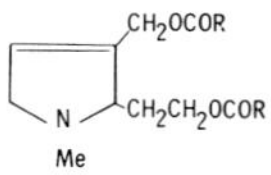	(M)	–
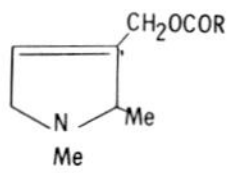	(M)	–

M = multiple doses

V. CARCINOGENIC ACTIVITY

Pyrrolizidine alkaloids are rather poor carcinogens; persistent dosing of alkaloids such as monocrotaline or lasiocarpine can cause liver tumors (10,11). We have not yet seen hepatomas in rats surviving single or multiple doses of synthetic analogues but very large liver nodules have been obtained with synthanecine A bis-N-ethylcarbamate (P. M. Newberne, unpublished). Possibly the antimitotic activity of pyrrolizidines might inhibit tumor development. Thus some alkaloids and dihydropyrrolizine derivatives have antitumor activity and some of our synthetic pyrroles, such as 2,3-bishydroxymethyl-1-methyl-pyrrole and its 4-methoxy-derivative have significant inhibitory activity against the Walker tumor in rats. However, the bis-N-ethylcarbamate of 2-hydroxyethyl-3-hydroxymethyl-1-methylpyrroline, which causes liver necrosis like pyrrolizidines and the hepatocarcinogen dimethylnitrosamine, is not antimitotic but has produced no tumors or other liver damage in rats surviving up to 2 years after repeated doses.

VI. LUNG TOXICITY

Toxic effects of some pyrrolizidine alkaloids to lungs can be reproduced with reactive pyrrolic esters like dehydromonocrotaline (Table 7, i) administered intravenously (12). A large single dose causes death after about 1 day with damage to lung capillaries and massive pleural effusion, which a sublethal dose might cause proliferation of alveolar tissue and death after 3-6 weeks. Other dehydroretronecine esters like the diacetate (ii) are similarly toxic (13) and this is general with reactive ester of hydroxymethyl pyrroles and indoles. Many cause acute damage, the indole

TABLE 7

Acute and Delayed Lung Toxicity of Pyrrolic Esters

	Compound (R = CONHEt)	Approx. LD_{50} mg/kg, iv, ♂ rats (1 - 2 days)	Delayed lung toxicity (3-5 weeks) approx. mg/kg
Bifunctional: (i)	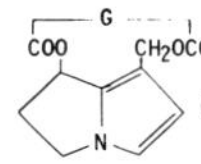 (Dehydromonocrotaline)	10	5 - 10
(ii)	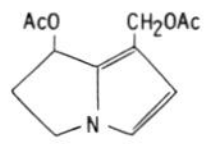	15	7 - 10
(iii)	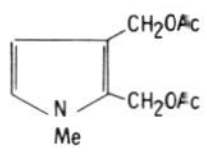	9	7 - 12
(iv)	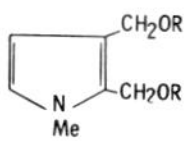	13	6 - 10
(v)	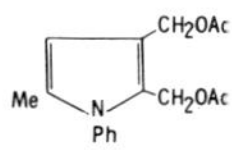	10.5	10 - 12
Monofunctional: (vi)	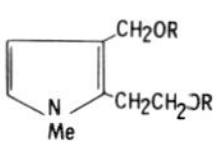	11	-
(vii)	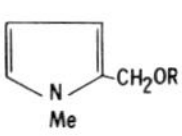	27	-
(viii)	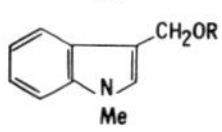	2	-

(viii) being especially potent, but we have only seen the delayed lung lesion with pyrroles which are bifunctional alkylating agents. Thus bifunctionality is important, and may be essential, for the development of delayed pneumotoxicity.

After intravenous administration to rats of the pneumotoxic ^{3}H-2,3-bisacetoxymethyl-1-methylpyrrole (Table 8, i), tissue distribution of radioactivity was measured. Compared with the pyrroline (ii), which requires liver metabolism for activation, the main difference was a 10 x higher level of ^{3}H in the tissues (blood, lungs) first exposed to the injected compound. Allowing for the quantities injected, rats administered (i) contain a quarter the metabolite in liver but twice the amount in lungs compared with rats administered (ii). When (i) was administered subcutaneously, most of the ^{3}H remained at the injection site (tail) and the lungs escaped damage. Injury to an organ is associated with the interaction of chemically reactive pyrrole with the susceptible tissue.

TABLE 8

Tissue Distribution of Radioactivity from Tritiated Pyrrole and Pyrroline Esters in Male Rats

Compound: (★ = position of ^{3}H)	(i) 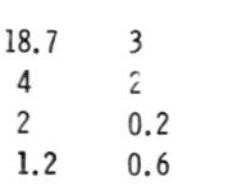		(ii) 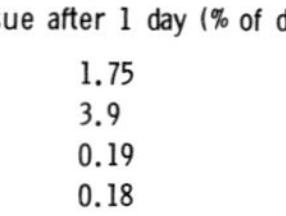	(iii) 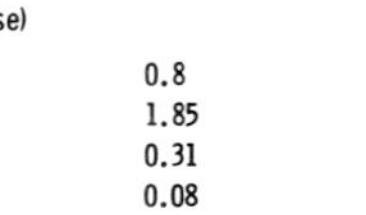
Dose (mg/kg, tail):	9	9	40	120
Route of injection:	i.v.	s.c.	i.v.	i.v.
Activation:	Already reactive		Requires metabolism	Requires metabolism
Tissue	^{3}H in tissue after 1 day (% of dose)			
Blood	18.7	3	1.75	0.8
Liver	4	2	3.9	1.85
Lungs	2	0.2	0.19	0.31
Kidneys	1.2	0.6	0.18	0.08
Spleen	1.1	0.3	0.27	0.06
Glandular stomach	1.6	0.2	0.04	0.02
Urine	51	-	40	81
Faeces	12	-	30	12.7
Injection site (tail)	~ 2	~ 90	-	-

VII. DISTRIBUTION AND TISSUE BINDING OF SEMISYNTHETIC ALKALOID ANALOGUES

Tritium from the retronecine carbamate (Table 8, iii) has a similar tissue distribution in rats to that from the analogue (ii) The most susceptible organ (liver) has the highest level (3,14). The ^{3}H in glandular stomach is very low. In contrast, the hydroxypyrrole corresponding to (iii), dehydroretronecine, gives a high level of binding to this organ (15) and hence is unlikely to be a major metabolite in the bloodstream of rats given (iii) (16). While we cannot synthesize a highly toxic natural alkaloid, synthetic and semisynthetic compounds are now available for radioactive tracer studies.

VIII. CONCLUSIONS

Experiments on the relationships between structure, metabolism and biological activity have given us a good idea of the main parameters necessary for a compound to have pyrrolizidine-like cytotoxicity. We need to know a lot more about the reactions of toxic metabolites with tissue constituents, or 'biochemical lesions' which lead to the pathological effects seen after poisoning by these alkaloids, and we now have a background of understanding and an armory of compounds to make possible investigations at this deeper level.

IX. REFERENCES

1. Schoental, R., and Mattocks, A. R., *Nature* 185, 842 (1960).
2. Mattocks, A. R., *J. Chem. Soc. (C)* 2698 (1969).
3. Mattocks, A. R., *Xenobiotica,* In press (1977).
4. Mattocks, A. R., *J. Chem. Soc.* (Perkin I), 707 (1974).
5. Mattocks, A. R., *J. Chem. Res. (S)* 40 (1977).
6. Mattocks, A. R., *Chem. Biol. Interact.* 5, 227 (1972).
7. Aldridge, W. N., and Reiner, E., "Enzyme Inhibitors as Substrates," North Holland Publishing Co., Amsterdam, 1972.
8. White, I. N. H., *Chem. Biol. Interact.* 13, 333 (1976).
9. Jago, M. V., *Am. J. Pathol.* 56, 405 (1969).
10. Newberne, P. M., and Rogers, A. E., *Plant Food Man* 1, 23 (1973).
11. Svoboda, D. J., and Reddy, J. K., *Cancer Res.* 32, 908 (1972).
12. Butler, W. H., Mattocks, A. R., and Barnes, J. M., *J. Pathol.* 100, 169 (1970).
13. Mattocks, A. R., *Nature* 228, 174 (1970).
14. Mattocks, A. R., and White, I. N. H., *Chem. Biol. Interact.* 15, 173 (1976).
15. Hsu, I. C., Shumaker, R. C., and Allen, J. R., *Chem. Biol. Interact.* 8, 163 (1974).
16. White, I. N. H., and Mattocks, A. R., *Chem. Biol. Interact.* 15, 185 (1976).

PREVENTION OF PYRROLIZIDINE ALKALOID POISONING—ANIMAL ADAPTATION OR PLANT CONTROL?

C. C. J. Culvenor
CSIRO Division of Animal Health

I. ABSTRACT

Investigations into the protection of sheep from poisoning by Heliotropium europaeum *are summarized. Inhibition of methanogenesis in the sheep rumen by means of iodoform, designed to increase conversion of alkaloids into 1-methylenepyrrolizidine derivatives, gives a small degree of protection. Manipulation of liver enzyme levels by induction and inhibition is unpromising because rats so treated respond in opposite ways to lasiocarpine and heliotrine, the main toxic alkaloids of* H. europaeum. *Immunization with N-carboxyalkyl-senecionine conjugates leads to decreased survival time in rats given continued, low doses of senecionine. The resulting antibodies form reversible complexes with senecionine and prolong the alkaloid clearance time. 6-Succinyloxysenecionine conjugates, designed to induce antibodies forming irreversible complexes, are under test.*

II. INTRODUCTION

The poisoning of livestock by pyrrolizidine alkaloids in Australia occurs in varied circumstances. In some areas recognized diseases follow regular and largely unavoidable exposure to pyrrolizidine-containing plants. The most important of these diseases is probably that in sheep due to the consumption of *Heliotropium europaeum*, a disease to which possibly 100 million sheep are exposed to some extent over 20,000 square miles in the south-eastern states. Generally the effects are chronic and the outcome can be substantial mortalities after two or three heavy exposures. In less severe circumstances, sheep may have their useful life reduced from about 8 to 5-6 years.

Other recognized hepatotoxic species are *Echium plantagineum*, *Crotalaria* species, and *Senecio jacobaea*. *Echium plantagineum*, commonly known as Paterson's Curse or Salvation Jane, is a weed of intermediate rainfall areas in all southern states overlapping to some extent with heliotrope. Its lower alkaloid content leads to less overt poisoning than that due to heliotrope but outbreaks occur in sheep, cattle, horses, and pigs. *Crotalaria retusa* and *C. crispata* were largely responsible for Kimberley Horse Disease which, in the past, caused considerable losses among station horses in northern Australia, especially in the Kimberley region. The current level of losses from these and other *Crotalaria* species is unknown. *Senecio jacobaea* is a hazard in the high rainfall areas of Victoria, Tasmania, and southern Western Australia.

There are many species in these and related genera which are accessible to stock to some degree and can be expected to contribute to a much wider, low-level intake of pyrrolizidine alkaloids. The hazard extends beyond the grazing of natural stands to the contamination of grains and prepared rations for pigs and poultry. Several poisoning episodes of the latter type have occurred in recent years, a major outbreak involving *Crotalaria retusa* seed in sorghum (1) and others of lesser extent due to *Heliotropium europaeum* seed in wheat screenings and pig rations (Russell and Pass, unpublished data). The need for careful surveillance of grains and rations is illustrated by Hooper's finding that 0.02% *C. retusa* seed in the diet (8 ppm monocrotaline) leads to high mortality in pigs and as little as 0.004% seed (1.6 ppm monocrotaline) causes a moderate degree of megalocytosis.

Under Australian conditions of large land holdings and high labor costs, it is largely impracticable to control weeds such as *Heliotropium europaeum* and *Echium plantagineum* adequately by herbicides or related measures, or to prevent access of stock to infested areas. It is not uncommon for *Heliotropium europaeum* and particularly *Echium plantagineum* and *Senecio jacobaea* to be controlled by grazing with sheep which, despite the poisoning which occurs, is regarded as the most advantageous course of action. Management procedures help to some degree; e.g. grazing infested pastures with animals destined for slaughter, giving supplementary feed to reduce the intake rate of alkaloid and grazing while the weeds are a seedling stage and of comparatively small bulk.

Possible prophylactic measures, which would enable grazing to take place without serious poisoning, have been under investigation in the CSIRO Division of Animal Health and have focused on protection of sheep from heliotrope poisoning. The three methods explored in depth have been enhanced destruction of alkaloid in the rumen, reducing the metabolic activation of the alkaloids, and protective immunization. Although none can be regarded as specially promising at the present time, work is continuing and the results obtained may be of value elsewhere.

III. ENHANCED DESTRUCTION OF ALKALOID IN THE RUMEN

Sheep are naturally equipped with the ability to detoxify a substantial proportion of ingested pyrrolizidine alkaloids in the rumen. Heliotrine and lasiocarpine and probably most other hepatotoxic alkaloids are reduced in sheep rumen liquor to the corresponding (non-toxic) 1-methylenepyrrolizidine derivatives (2,3). This form of detoxification is applicable also to ingested alkaloid N-oxides which are rapidly reduced by other rumen microorganisms to the tertiary base.

The organism responsible for the conversion of heliotrine to

7α-hydroxy-1-methylene-8α-pyrrolizidine is normally present at a low level in the rumen but is markedly stimulated by the addition of heliotrope to the diet (4). It has been isolated and characterized as a new species, *Peptococcus heliotrinreducans* (5). It was found to use molecular hydrogen as a hydrogen source and to compete poorly for this substrate with methanogenic bacteria. The rate of metabolism of heliotrine is markedly increased in the presence of inhibitors of methanogenesis such as carbon tetrachloride, chloroform, iodoform, and chloral hydrate (6).

On this basis, pen-feeding trials are now being conducted (Lanigan, unpublished results) to determine whether the administration of iodoform will protect sheep fed a ration containing 50% *H. europaeum*. Iodoform was chosen as an inhibitor on the grounds of convenience of administration. In one trial, a pellet of iodoform was placed in the sheep's rumen where it dissolved slowly. However, sheep so treated died at the same rate on a heliotrope diet as did the untreated controls, apparently because the hepatotoxicity of iodoform outweighed any protective effect. In a second trial, the iodoform is being given twice daily during periods of heliotrope-feeding which are of 3 months duration, alternating with 3 months of normal dry rations. The results to date (Table 1) indicate that the lowest dose rate of iodoform, 31 mg twice daily, delays the onset of liver damage but does not achieve long term protection. Another group, receiving a dose rate of 15.5 mg iodoform twice daily is now under investigation.

TABLE 1

Mortalities in Sheep Given Iodoform and a Heliotrope-Containing Diet, Alternating with a Normal Diet

Group[1]	Cumulative deaths at commencement of 2nd heliotrope period	3rd heliotrope period	4th heliotrope period
A. Heliotrope alone	2/7	5/7	5/7
B. Heliotrope with iodoform (62 mg twice daily)	2/7	5/7	7/7
C. Heliotrope with iodoform (31 mg twice daily	0/6	4/6	4/6

[1]Each group initially contained eight sheep. Non-specific deaths reduced the numbers to 7 in groups A and B and to 6 in group C.

The original observations indicated that the reduction of heliotrine was stimulated by supplementary vitamin B_{12} (2). This was not supported by the studies of Russell and Smith (7) or by field and pen trials of the protective effect of cobalt-containing pellets placed in the rumen (8,9). The field trial was inconclusive because of seasonal conditions and the pen trial failed to demonstrate a protective effect.

IV. MANIPULATION OF LIVER METABOLISM

The known metabolic changes undergone by pyrrolizidine alkaloids after absorption are illustrated for heliotrine in Fig. 1 (10, 11). The metabolites are formed very largely if not completely in liver cells. Hydrolysis and N-oxidation are detoxifying changes. Demethylation produces a product of lower toxicity. Oxidation gives the pyrrolic dehydroalkaloid and (after hydrolysis) dehydroaminoalcohol, which are fully responsible, so far as is known, for the acute and chronic toxicity of the alkaloids. The dehydroalkaloids are so reactive that they have their main effect in, and are destroyed in, the liver and the lung. The dehydroaminoalcohols are comparatively stable and circulate in the blood to reach other organs and tissues.

In general, the opportunities for decreasing the effect of the alkaloids in the animal are (a) enhancing the rates of hydrolysis

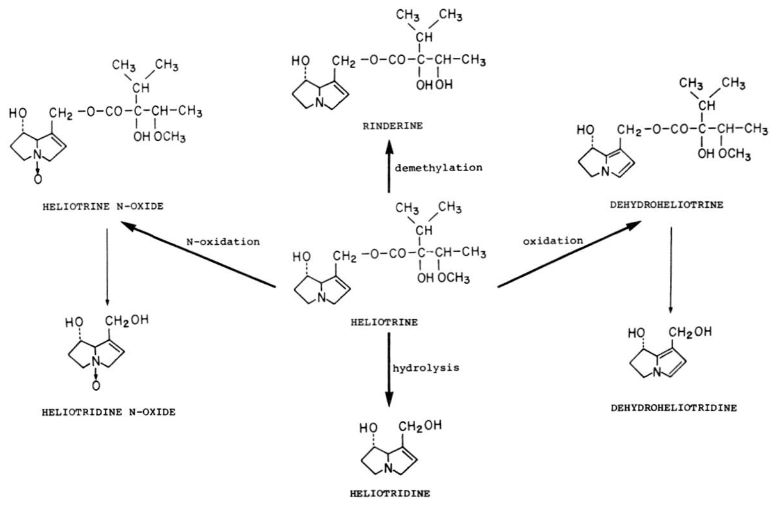

Fig. 1 *Metabolism of heliotrine in liver.*

and N-oxidation, (b) decreasing the extent of formation of the toxic metabolites, and (c) removing alkaloid from circulation by other means such as excretion or immunization. In the liver, esterases are found primarily in the microsomal fraction and they are found to be subject to induction and inhibition (12,13). The esterases are said to be only weakly active in hydrolyzing pyrrolizidine alkaloids *in vitro* but apparently they are effective against less sterically hindered pyrrolizidine esters since diacetylretronecine is hepatotoxic in rats only if an esterase inhibitor is given also (14,15). From the viewpoint of protection the esterases seem worthy of further attention. Conversion of the alkaloids into the N-oxides and toxic pyrrolic metabolites is effected by the mixed function oxidases of the microsomal fraction which also are subject to induction and inhibition (11,16,17). There are differences in responses to modifying factors which suggest that the two reactions are brought about by different oxidase systems (17,18,19,20).

Inhibition of the mixed function oxidase system would be expected to prevent formation of the toxic metabolites and so be effective in achieving protection of animals. However study of the effects of inhibition and induction by Jago and Mattocks reveals a more complicated picture. Only with certain alkaloids, e.g. heliotrine and monocrotaline, does inhibition of the liver enzymes lead to protection and induction to increased toxicity (16,19,21; Jago, unpublished results). With lasiocarpine in rats of both sexes the reverse is found; inhibition of the liver metabolizing enzymes with SKF 525 A (2-diethylaminoethyl 2,2-diphenylvalerate hydrochloride) or thioacetamide results in more rapid death; and induction with phenobarbitone or 3β-hydroxy-20-oxo-5-pregnen-16α-carbonitrile (PCN) has a protective effect (16, 22; Jago, unpublished results). Fulvine resembles lasiocarpine in that enzyme induction leads to protection (23), whereas retrorsine is peculiar in that both induction and inhibition have given a protective effect (21).

When examined *in vitro*, microsomes from induced rat liver showed an increased rate of formation of pyrrolic metabolites from all alkaloids tested. The reason for the unexpected outcome *in vivo* is not yet clear. Preliminary results with lasiocarpine (Jago, unpublished results) suggest that the rate of production of pyrrolic metabolites *in vivo*, as indicated by their levels in the blood, do not always parallel the microsomal production *in vitro*. Similarly Mattocks has shown a closer relationship between toxicity and the level of total pyrrolic metabolites found in the liver 2 hours after administration of alkaloid than with the rate of microsomal pyrrole production *in vitro* (21). The level of pyrrolic metabolites must be related both to the rate of *in vivo* production and to the availability of nucleophilic target sites. It is therefore possible that the overall clearance time of alkaloid from the blood influences toxicity. There is evidence to this effect from immunization experiments (below), which suggest that low levels of alkaloid for a long time are more lethal than an equivalent amount at high level for a short time. Lasiocarpine, in particular, is excreted very slowly if at all (10) and partial inhibition of the liver oxidase system may considerably extend its clearance time. Enzyme induction may possibly decrease toxicity through a differential increase in the rate of N-oxide formation over pyrrolic metabolites. However, in the case of retrorsine, the increase in N-oxide formation was the smaller (17).

The unfortunate aspect of these results is that enzyme induction and inhibition produce opposite results for heliotrine and lasiocarpine, the two main constituents of *Heliotropium europaeum.* Protection by these methods thus seems unlikely for heliotrope poisoning although they might be applicable in other instances of pyrrolizidine alkaloid poisoning. The issue is further complicated by the fact that liver enzyme levels in the grazing animal are already subject to influence by chemical constituents in food plants and by chemical treatments such as anthelmintics. Certain flavones and the anthelmintic, phenothiazine, are enzyme inducers (24,25) but there is no specific information on the more commonly used thiabendazole group of anthelmintics.

V. PROTECTIVE IMMUNIZATION

There has been little exploration of the potential of immunization for protection against alkaloids and other toxic plant constituents. In investigating its application to pyrrolizidine alkaloids, our experiments to date have been concerned mostly with senecionine.

Protein conjugates were first sought by quaternizing an alkaloid with a halogenated acid or ester and linking the product to bovine serum albumin (BSA) through the agency of 1-(3'-dimethylaminopropyl)-3-ethylcarbodiimide. Ethyl bromoacetate gave the expected quaternary derivatives but the acids obtained by selective hydrolysis did not link readily to protein, probably because of steric hindrance. Ethyl β-iodopropionate did not give quaternary derivatives, a failure which was ascribed to instability of the product with its potential for elimination of the original alkaloid. Methyl γ-iodobutyrate gave the required derivatives, that from senecionine being obtained crystalline. This product, N-(carboxypropyl)-senecionine (CPS), combined readily with BSA to give the conjugate, CPS-BSA. A conjugate, CMS-BSA, derived from N-(carboxymethyl)-senecionine, was also prepared.

The conjugates induced antibodies in rabbits which were directed very largely against the senecionine derivative. The protective effect of immunization was tested in rats given 0.1 LD_{50} senecionine (3.6 mg/kg in females), 3 times per week, the dosing schedule being chosen to avoid possible overloading of antibodies. Survival times were lower in the immunized animals than in the control groups including a group immunized with BSA alone (Table 2; Buttery, unpublished results). The BSA-immunized

TABLE 2

Survival Times of Immunized Rats given 3.6 mg/kg Senecionine (0.1 LD50), 3 Times per Week

Groups	Survival Times (days) Expt. 1	Expt. 2
Control	182	129
BSA immunized	154	77
CPS-BSA immunized	106	42
CMS-BSA immunized		60

group is believed to have suffered non-specific stress from injections of Freund's adjuvant and might be regarded as the true control group. The lowered survival time of rats immunized with the senecionine conjugates is thought to be due to the reversible nature of the complexing of antibody with senecionine. A dissociating complex will act as a storage site for alkaloid and extend the period for which senecionine circulates in the blood. This effect was confirmed by a series of blood assays for total senecionine in normal and CPS-BSA immunized rats dosed with senecionine (Fig. 2). The total senecionine levels were higher in the immunized rats and detectable for a much longer period. However an *in vitro* study of the binding of senecionine by CPS-BSA-induced antibodies (Buttery, unpublished results) indicates that the level of free senecionine should be only 1% of the total senecionine.

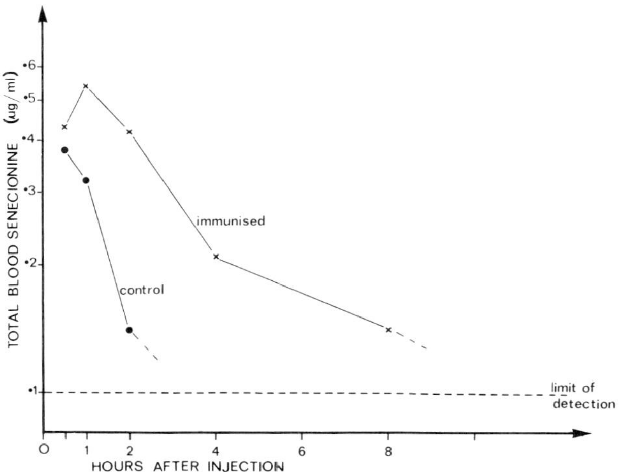

Fig. 2. *Total blood senecionine in normal and CPS-BSA-immunized rats after a dose of 3.6 mg/kg i.p.*

An attempt is now being made to produce an irreversible antibody-senecionine complex by directing antibodies against the allylic ester part of the molecule. This grouping has some reactivity against SH and NH_2 groups (26) and when held in close proximity with protein in the antibody cleft, it is possible that reaction will occur. To achieve this, we used anacrotine which can be regarded as senecionine with a convenient 6-OH attaching group on the opposite side of the molecule from the allylic ester grouping. Anacrotine was reacted with succinic anhydride to give a half-ester which was linked to thyroglobulin by means of the water soluble carbodiimide. The conjugate is now under test in rats.

It must be recognized, of course, that the rate of irreversible binding would be limited to the rate of production of antibodies. An estimate of the latter rate (Buttery, unpublished results) gives a maximum binding capacity of about 1.5 mg alkaloid/kg/day. For a sheep ingesting heliotrope as 50% of the diet, the alkaloid intake may be in the order of 50 mg/kg/day so that immunization will be able to cope only if the alkaloid entering the blood stream does not exceed 3% of the total ingested.

So far we appear only to have uncovered some of the problems in the immunization approach. However there are pointers to ways in which the technique might be used more successfully. For example, better results may be obtained with more hydrophilic alkaloids such as heliotrine and monocrotaline for which urinary excretion rates are higher and significant levels of free alkaloid will be maintained for a shorter period.

VI. PROTECTION WITH THIOLS OR OTHER NUCLEOPHILES

Because toxic metabolites are alkylating agents, the simplest rationale for protecting animals is to administer a high dose of a thiol compound or other reactive nucleophile which might react with and mop-up the toxic metabolites. This approach has been shown in several laboratories to increase the survival time of rats given an approximate LD_{50} of alkaloid. Hayashi and Lalich (27) found protection against monocrotaline in rats given 300 mg/kg cysteine or 150 mg/kg mercaptoethylamine 15 minutes before the alkaloid. An additional degree of protection was obtained with a second injection of cysteine 60 minutes after the alkaloid. Jago (unpublished results) found similar protection in rats given 300 mg/kg cysteine before and after heliotrine or lasiocarpine. The method depends on achieving high thiol levels inside the liver cell. White (28) has recently shown that this occurs, 200 mg/kg cysteine increasing liver glutathione or total non-protein thiol levels to a maximum which is double the level in normal rats. Such a dose reduced the level of bound pyrrolic metabolites in liver 2 hrs after dosing with retrorsine to 60% of the level in rats not given cysteine and increased the LD_{50} of retrorsine from 42 to 82 mg/kg.

Despite the measure of protection which is achieved, the method has never seemed a practical one to apply to livestock. Oral administration of cysteine to sheep would be the least costly route but protection by oral administration has not yet been demonstrated. In addition heavy losses of cysteine would be expected in the rumen. However, the development of encapsulated food supplements capable of passing through the rumen and investigated originally for use in boosting the intake of S-aminoacids for increased wool yield in sheep (29), may enable a practical double-benefit supplement to be applied to sheep or cattle in certain situations. Perhaps the most appropriate opportunity for trial of encapsulated cysteine supplements would be in dairy cattle exposed to *Echium plantagineum* or *Senecio jacobaea*, since the economics of the industry and access to animals for daily administration of the food supplement are more favorable. However the amount of cysteine administered would probably have to be kept high. Only one trial of cysteine against chronic pyrrolizidine alkaloid toxicity has been recorded (30) and in this instance no protection was observed against heliotrine, given in doses of 0.1 LD_{50} 3 times per week. The lack of protection may have been because the accompanying dose of cysteine, 30 mg/kg, was too low.

VII. BIOLOGICAL CONTROL OF PYRROLIZIDINE ALKALOID PLANTS

With no adequate method of prophylactic treatment of animals yet in sight, methods for biological control of pyrrolizidine alkaloid plants have come under consideration.

The main search for biological methods of controlling *Heliotropium europaeum* and *Echium plantagineum* has been taken up by the CSIRO Division of Entomology and an investigation into the predators and parasites of these plants in the Mediterranean region is being carried out at the CSIRO Biological Control Unit, Montpellier, France. The moth, *Callimorpha jacobaeae* or Cinnabar Moth, has been twice introduced into Victoria as a control agent for *Senecio jacobaea* but failed to become established because of extensive predation by insects and birds (31).

In the Division of Animal Health, an unusual approach based on our work on the role of pyrrolizidine alkaloids in the life cycle of certain insect species (e.g. 32), is also being tried. Numerous species of the butterfly families, Danainae and Ithomiinae, and the moth family, Arctiidae, are known to secrete derivatives of pyrrolizidine alkaloids. The butterflies obtain the alkaloid intermediates after emerging as adults, when the males seek out dead and withering pyrrolizidine plants and suck up alkaloid-containing juices. The Danainae convert the alkaloids, apparently via the toxic dehydroalkaloids, into 1-formyl-or 7-keto-pyrrolizines which are secreted on a "hair-pencil" at the end of the male body and used to facilitate mating (32). Several species of Ithomiinae convert the acid portion of alkaloids such as indicine into a lactone which is secreted on a "costal fringe" on the wings and acts as a repellent to other males (33). The role of the alkaloid derivatives appears to be vital to the butterflies and the alkaloids are sought out and inbibed by the males most avidly.

Many species of the Arctiidae, such as *Callimorpha jacobaeae*, and, in Australia, *Utetheisa pulchelloides*, use pyrrolizidine alkaloid plants as larval hosts and so have ready access to alkaloids. We have found that several species of Australian Arctiids, including *Utetheisa pulchelloides*, a predator of *Heliotropium europaeum* and *Echium plantagineum*, possess coremata at the end of the male body superficially resembling the hair-pencils of the male Danainae. Secreted on the coremata are the same 1-formyl- and 7-keto-pyrrolizines found on the hair-pencils of the Danainae (34; Edgar, unpublished results). It seems likely that the compounds have the same function, facilitation of mating, in the Arctiids as in the Danainae.

Uthetheisa pulchelloides has a strong feeding preference for pyrrolizidine alkaloid species and there is some evidence that the alkaloids are actually a necessary feeding stimulus for the larvae. We hope to use this requirement or preference for alkaloids to have the moth assist replacement of natural *Heliotropium europaeum* by a non-alkaloid strain. If a non-alkaloid strain can be developed and oversown with the natural strain, *Utetheisa* should selectively eat the natural strain. There are some obvious problems for such an approach but we are aiming at the first objective of a non- or very low-alkaloid strain of heliotrope. Since any other insect predators specific to *Heliotropium europaeum* and related species of Boraginaceae are also likely to have requirements for the alkaloids, insect predators introduced for control purposes should also encourage replacement by an alkaloid-free strain of *H. europaeum*.

VIII. ANIMAL ADAPTATION OR PLANT CONTROL

In relation to heliotrope poisoning of sheep, the question implied in the title can be answered only by time. The only prophylactic treatment of sheep with some promise at present is the release of an inhibitor of methanogenesis in the rumen. A considerable improvement in the results of this treatment could stem from the development of a non-hepatotoxic inhibitor. In the short term, the best hope of reducing the poisoning of sheep is probably the introduction of new predators of *Heliotropium europaeum* to reduce the amount of plant material available. However there is need also for close ecological study to improve management procedures and it might even be necessary to consider breeding sheep more resistant to pyrrolizidine alkaloids.

In other examples of pyrrolizidine poisoning, one or the other of the above methods may be effective and our experiences may prove a useful starting point.

IX. PREVENTION OF HUMAN POISONING

Pyrrolizidine alkaloids poison people as well as animals and documentation of human exposure and human poisoning is increasing. Recent examples are studies of carcinogenic plant drugs containing pyrrolizidine alkaloids in Japan (35-38) and substantial outbreaks of poisoning in India and Afghanistan due to consumption of grains containing seed of *Crotalaria* and *Heliotropium* species, respectively (39,40). Concern is increased by knowledge of the very low effective dose levels of some alkaloids (1,3,5), their confirmed carcinogenicity (41), their wide availability and a general lack of recognition of their occurrence and effects by most people even in advanced societies. Much of the fatal human poisoning occurs among poorly informed populations in isolated regions, frequently living in difficult circumstances. The key to prevention must be avoidance rather than prophylaxis but, in general, it seems that governments will take no action until after large scale outbreaks have occurred.

I suggest there is need for a world-wide survey, possibly under WHO auspices, of specific hazardous situations where pyrrolizidine alkaloid containing plants are associated with human populations through presence in agricultural or animal grazing areas or through known or suspected herbal usage. If it could combine full available botanical, chemical, epidemiological, and ethnic knowledge, and were presented both in a detailed report and in the form of pamphlets which governments could use for directly informing populations at risk, such a survey might contribute effectively to reducing this form of human poisoning.

X. REFERENCES

1. Hooper, P. T., *Aust. Vet. J.* 53, 109 (1976).
2. Dick, A. T., Dann, A. T., Bull, L. B., and Culvenor, C. C. J., *Nature (London)* 197, 207 (1963).
3. Bull, L. B., Culvenor, C. C. J., and Dick, A. T., "The Pyrrolizidine Alkaloids," p. 219. North Holland, Amsterdam, 1968.
4. Lanigan, G. W., *Aust. J. Agric. Res.* 21, 633 (1970).
5. Lanigan, G. W., *J. Gen. Microbiol.* 94, 1 (1976).
6. Lanigan, G. W., *Aust. J. Agric. Res.* 22, 123 (1970); 23, 1085 (1972).
7. Russell, G. R., and Smith, R. M., *Aust. J. Biol. Sci.* 21, 1277 (1968).
8. Whittem, J. H., *Aust. Vet. J.* 42, 395 (1966).
9. Lanigan, G. W., and Whittem, J. H., *Aust. Vet. J.* 46, 17 (1970).
10. Bull, L. B., Culvenor, C. C. J., and Dick, A. T. "The Pyrrolizidine Alkaloids," p. 215. North Holland, Amsterdam, 1968.
11. Jago, M. V., Edgar, J. A., Smith, L. W., and Culvenor, C. C. J.

Mol. Pharmacol. 6, 402 (1970).
12. Schwark, W. S., and Ecobichon, D. J., *Can. J. Physiol. Pharmacol.* 46, 207 (1968).
13. Ecobichon, D. J., *Comp. Biochem. Physiol.* 23, 925 (1967).
14. Mattocks, A. R., *Nature (London)* 228, 174 (1970).
15. Mattocks, A. R., *in* "Phytochemical Ecology" (J. B. Harbourne, Ed.), p. 179. Academic Press, London, 1972.
16. Tuchweber, B., Kovacs, K., Jago, M. V., and Beaulieu, T., *Res. Commun. Chem. Pathol. Pharmacol.* 7, 459 (1974).
17. Mattocks, A. R., and White, I. N. H., *Chem. Biol. Interact.* 3, 383 (1971).
18. White, I. N. H., Mattocks, A. R., and Butler, W. H., *Chem. Biol. Interact.* 6, 207 (1973).
19. Mattocks, A. R., and White, I. N. H., *Chem. Biol. Interact.* 6, 297 (1973).
20. Gillette, J. R., *Adv. Pharmacol.* 4, 219 (1966).
21. Mattocks, A. R., *Chem. Biol. Interact.* 5, 227 (1972).
22. Jago, M. V., *J. Pathol.* 105, 1 (1971).
23. Khaliq, S. U., *Cardiovasc. Res.* 7, 655 (1973).
24. Wattenberg, L. W., and Leong, J. L., *Cancer Res.* 25, 365 (1965).
25. Wattenberg, L. W., Page, M. A., and Leong, J. L., *Cancer Res.* 28, 934 (1968).
26. Culvenor, C. C. J., Dann, A. T., and Dick, A. T., *Nature (London)* 195, 570 (1962).
27. Hayashi, Y., and Lalich, J. J., *Toxicol. Appl. Pharmacol.* 12, 36 (1968).
28. White, I. N. H., *Chem. Biol. Interact.* 13, 333 (1976).
29. Solomon, D. H., *Nature (London)* 261, 258 (1976).
30. Hooper, P. T., Ph.D. Thesis, Univ. of Melbourne, p. 118, 1972.
31. Schmidl, L., *Weed Res.* 12, 37 and 46 (1972).
32. Edgar, J. A., *Philos. Trans. R. Soc. London Ser. B* 272, 467 (1975).
33. Edgar, J. A., Culvenor, C. C. J., and Pliske, T. E., *J. Chem. Ecol.* 2, 263 (1976).
34. Culvenor, C. C. J., and Edgar, J. A., *Experientia* 28, 627 (1972).
35. Hirono, I., Mori, H., and Culvenor, C. C. J., *Gann* 67, 125 (1976).
36. Hirono, I., Shimizu, M., Fushimi, K., Hori, H., and Kato, K., *Gann* 64, 527 (1973).
37. Furuya, T., Hikichi, M., and Itaka, Y., *Chem. Pharm. Bull.* 24, 1120 (1976).
38. Furuya, T., Murakami, K., and Hikichi, M., *Phytochemistry* 10, 3306 (1971).
39. Tandon, B. N., Tandon, R. K., Tandon, H. D., Narndranathan, M., and Joshi, Y. K., *Lancet* ii, 271 (1976).
40. Mohabbet, O., Srivastava, R. N., Younos, M. S., Sediq, G. G., Merzad, A. A., and Aram, G. N., *Lancet* ii, 269 (1976).
41. International Agency for Research on Cancer, Monographs on the Evaluation of Carcinogenic Risk of Chemicals to Man, Vol. 10, Lyon, 1976.

THE TRANSFER OF PYRROLIZIDINE ALKALOIDS FROM *Senecio jacobaea* INTO THE MILK OF LACTATING COWS AND GOATS

John O. Dickinson and Robert R. King
VCAPP, Washington State University

I. ABSTRACT

A study was conducted to determine if pyrrolizidine alkaloids from Senecio jacobaea *(tansy ragwort) are passed into milk of lactating milk goats. Four does were given dried tansy ragwort via rumen cannula at a dosage of 1% of body weight per day for 20 days. Chemical assay of pyrrolizidine alkaloid content in the dried plants averaged 0.15% by weight. Five separate alkaloids were isolated from plant materials. Specific alkaloids jacoline and jacobine were isolated from milk.*

Condition of does and kids was monitored via measurement of blood leukocyte count, and serum protein, albumin, and globulin content. Sorbitol dehydrogenase values were used to assess liver function. No significant changes in any of the parameters were observed in either does or kids. Mean pyrrolizidine alkaloid content of milk samples assayed was 233 μg/100 ml.

II. INTRODUCTION

There are more than 1,200 species of senecio in the world. Several of these species contain a varying number of pyrrolizidine alkaloids. Certain molecular configurations of these alkaloids are hepatotoxic and are considered carcinogenic by some pathologists (1,2,3,4). *Senecio jacobaea* (tansy ragwort), a plant that contains pyrrolizidine alkaloids, has been responsible for death losses of cattle and horses in California, Oregon, and Washington (5,6,7). It has been suggested that pyrrolizidine alkaloids might be transferred to the milk of cattle consuming contaminated pastures, hay, or silage (7,8,9). Because of the widespread prevalence of tansy ragwort in the western part of the state of Washington, a serious concern has been expressed for the human population in that area. The major importance, of course, is with reference to milk from cows because of the large quantity of milk consumed by the human population. However, the potential danger of these alkaloids in milk of dairy goats could conceivably present an isolated type of problem. Even though dairy goat milk is not consumed in as large a quantity by the human population, it is often consumed as the entire milk supply by a small number of people in a given area. Therefore, the chance of repeated exposure to the alkaloids through this milk will, in fact, be much greater than any other commercial dairy product. The susceptibility of cattle and goats to the damaging effect of the pyrrolizidine alkaloids is quite different (6,10). In general, cattle are quite susceptible and death losses are frequently reported. Goats seem to be more resistent to the alkaloids but little information is available in the literature concerning the lethality of the alkaloids in goats (11). Goats are, in fact, used for the control of tansy ragwort and other species of senecio because of their increased tolerance to the plant (10). This tolerance may or may not have any relationship to the amount of alkaloid that could conceivably be passed in the milk.

In newborn rats that suckled dams treated with pyrrolizidine alkaloids, liver lesions and death have been reported even though lactating rats were uneffected (9). Similar toxicologic studies involving bovine milk have been reported (8). Milk from cows receiving tansy ragwort was administered to young rats and mice; death rates among the treated and control groups were not significantly different (12). In a recent study lactating cows and nursing calves were utilized (8). Histopathologic changes were not detected in the calves even though the cows died and had lesions typical of pyrrolizidine alkaloid poisoning. In all these studies the pyrrolizidine alkaloid content of the plants or the milk was not determined. It, therefore, seemed advisable to conduct studies following a similar experimental method by analyzing both plants and milk for pyrrolizidine alkaloid content and, therefore, enable us to state positively whether the alkaloids can pass into milk of both dairy cows and of dairy goats. The work with cows was reported previously (13). We report here the work with goats.

III. MATERIALS AND METHODS

Four milk goats were freshly prepared with rumen canulas. These goats ranged in age from 2-5 years and were of the Toggenburg and Alpine breeding. The kids born to these does were separated from their dams and fed milk twice a day. The study was begun within two weeks after parturition.

Plant materials used in the feeding procedures were collected from fields near Puyallup, Washington. Both the first year rosette and second year plants were harvested and air dried after transporting to Pullman. The plants were chopped to a fine consistency and stored at 20° C. After this preparation and prior to feeding the materials to the goats, a spectrophotometric assay was performed on the plants to determine the pyrrolizidine alkaloid content.

The dried tansy ragwort was administered by the rumen canulas to each goat at a dosage rate of 1% of body wt/day. The quantity was given in one dose following the morning milking. The feeding trials were continued for a period of 3 weeks. During the feeding periods, each of the four kids was given milk from its dam. The amount approximated 150 ml of milk per kg per day. During the study, alfalfa-grass hay was fed *ad libidum* to the goats. In addition, each goat received 1.5 kg per day of the Washington State University dairy ration (65% barley, 15% corn, 10% beet pulp, 5% molasses, 0.5% trace mineralized salt, 2% sodium tripolyphosphate, 2.4% field peas, and 0.1% vitamin A). Body weights of does and kids were recorded on a weekly basis. The animals were observed daily for signs of illness. All animals were necropsied at the end of the trials and examined carefully for the presence of lesions.

Blood was collected prior to the study and at biweekly intervals during the study. Blood tests for sorbitol dehydrogenase (14) total protein,[1] globulin,[2] and albumin[3] content were performed. Leukocyte counts were recorded electronically.[4]

Milk samples were collected twice daily and assayed for pyrrolizidine alkaloid content by a modification of the method of Mattocks (15). The modification involved final detection of the alkaloids by the use of a gas chromatograph.[5] Pooling of samples was used to make these determinations. Chromatographic studies were used to separate and identify the individual alkaloids (16).

IV. RESULTS

Plant assays are given (Table 1). Specific alkaloids isolated from the plant and identified chromatographically were jacobine,

TABLE 1

Distribution of Pyrrolizidine Alkaloids in Tansy ragwort

Age of plant	Condition for analysis	Pyrrolizidine alkaloid content (% dry weight)[1] Root	Stem	Leaf	Flower	Whole plant[2]
First year (Rosette)	Air-dry	0.31	0.12	0.17	Not available[3]	0.17
	Fresh frozen, then air-dry	--	--	--	--	--
Second year	Air-dry	0.33	0.11	0.16	0.37	0.18
	Fresh frozen, then air-dry	--	--	--	0.09	0.03

[1]Values represent an average of more than 5 samples taken from various sites around the Olympia-Puyallup area.
[2]Does not include root.
[3]Plants flowers 2nd year.

[1]Dade Chemical Co., St. Louis, Missouri
[2]Sigma Chemical Co., St. Louis, Missouri.
[3]American Monitor Corporation, Indianapolis, Indiana
[4]Coulter Electronics, Inc., Hialeah, Florida
[5]Dr. M. P. Cooke, Department of Chemistry

jacodine, jacoline, jaconine, and jacozine. A record of the body weight of the does through the duration of this experiment is depicted graphically (Fig. 1). No appreciable weight loss by the does was recorded through the 20-day duration of the experiment. The milk flow remained approximately the same during this 20-day period of administration of the dry tansy ragwort (Fig. 2). The kids gained weight and appeared normal during the entire study. Blood serum albumin values were recorded (Fig. 3). Albumin-globulin ratios were not calculated because of the demonstration of the limited value of this in earlier work with cows. Total leukocyte count and serum sorbitol dehydrogenase values are presented (Fig. 4).

Necropsy findings were essentially negative as far as the does were concerned. No evidence of typical pyrrolizidine alkaloid toxicosis (megalocytosis, portal fibroplasia, centrilobular necrosis) (2) were detected. In addition, no gross or microscopic lesions of any type were observed in the kids.

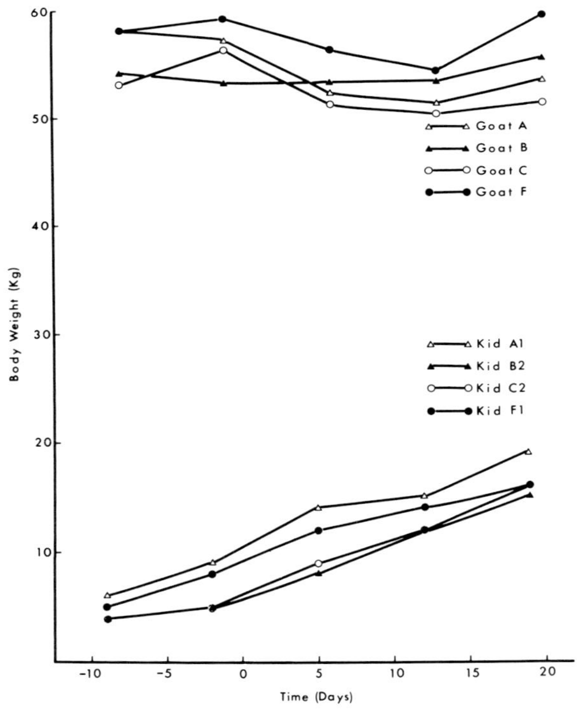

Fig. 1. *Body weight of 4 lactating goats fed tansy ragwort and of 4 kids consuming this milk.*

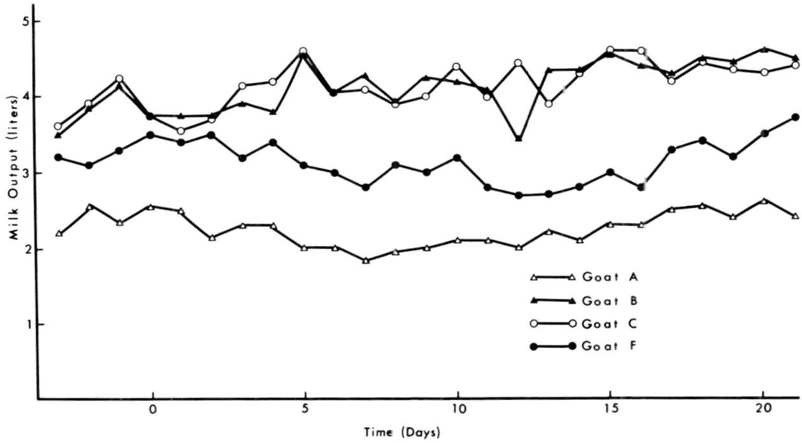

Fig 2. *Daily milk output by 4 goats fed tansy ragwort.*

The result of chemical analysis of milk samples for pyrrolizidine alkaloids are listed (Table 2). The percentage of recoveries by this modified method was much higher than the earlier 20% figure reported in the work with cows (17). For purposes of comparison, the recovery rate was considered to be 100% in this particular analysis. The percentage was based on values obtained from milk samples to which known amounts of jocaline had been added. Chromatographic examination identified jacoline as being present in the milk in the largest quantity. A significant amount of jacobine was also present and could be identified from the chromatographic peak. Milk samples were frozen prior to analysis. No attempts were made to relate the variation of pyrrolizidine alkaloid content to the time of the tansy ragwort administration.

TABLE 2

Concentration of Pyrrolizidine Alkaloids in Milk from Treated Does

Animal identification	PA content in milk (μg/100 ml) Mean concentration	Standard deviation
A	194	27.3
B	186	13.4
C	381	31.1
F	303	17.7

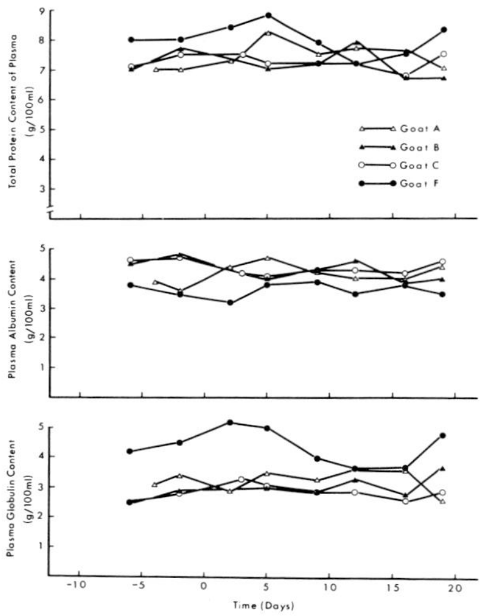

Fig. 3. *Protein content of blood plasma from 4 lactating goats fed tansy ragwort.*

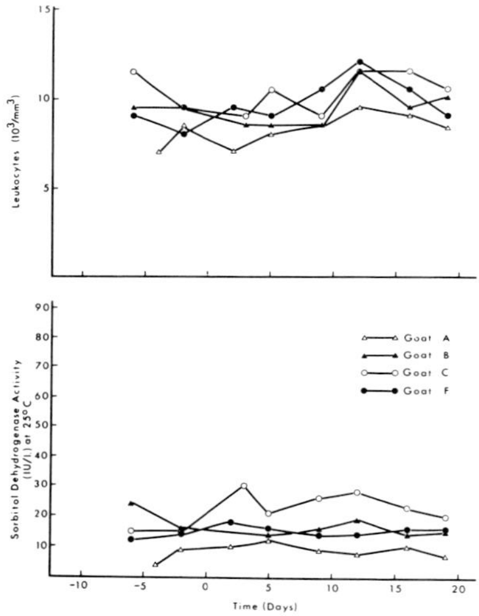

Fig. 4. *Leukocyte and sorbitol dehydrogenase changes in 4 lactating goats fed tansy ragwort.*

V. DISCUSSION

Pyrrolizidine alkaloid content of the entire tansy ragwort plant approximated that used in the study with cows (17). There was no apparent significant difference between first and second year plant growth. The portions of the plant with the highest concentrations were the blossom and the root. The root, of course, has no significance in this study although small portions were occasionally ground and utilized. The high content of the blossom does have significance from the standpoint of its incorporation of the alkaloids into honey produced by bees in areas of high tansy ragwort concentration. Assays were performed on a few honey samples. In all instances, they were found to contain a significant concentration of the pyrrolizidine alkaloid (2). The plant material fed to the goats in this experiment was a mixture of first and second year plants and no effort was made to distinguish between the two because of the similarity of the pyrrolizidine alkaloid content.

It was found, during the course of this study, that the finely ground plant material does not retain pyrrolizidine alkaloids well on storage. A rather large amount of material approximating something in excess of 800 pounds of dried tansy ragwort plant was finely ground and stored in burlap sacks for later use in feeding trials. The material remained in storage for approximately six months. At the end of this period, the new studies were begun and this material was to be fed to the animals involved. An assay of the plant material at that point revealed that the alkaloid content had dropped from .16% to .012%. This value was checked several times and, as a result, the prepared and dried material was not utilized for study. New, fresh plant material was harvested and dried for use in this study.

Body weight loss and reduced milk flow in goats comparable to cows were not demonstrated. This correlates very well with expected results as the tolerance of goats to the pyrrolizidine alkaloids has been well established (10).

The plasma levels of albumin, globulin, and total protein in does and kids remained essentially normal throughout the entire duration of the study. This, of course, was contrary to the results observed with the cows where the albumin levels dropped rather suddenly as the liver damage increased (13).

Blood Leukocyte count remained essentially normal in all animals throughout the duration of the study. In cattle, a rather sharp rise was recorded (13).

Blood sorbitol dehydrogenase activity remained essentially normal throughout the 20-day period. This correlates extremely well with the lack of liver lesions in the animals utilized. This enzyme assay is, of course, a specific liver function but not specific for pyrrolizidine toxicosis. In the study with cows, the increase in sorbitol dehydrogenase levels correlated quite closely with the development of the liver lesions (13).

Pyrrolizidine alkaloids were isolated and identified from the milk produced by the does. Evidence of the presence of jacoline and jacobine in the milk was confirmed by chromatographic examination. In the case of cow's milk, the alkaloid that was isolated was jacoline. However, the development of a more sensitive assay for the detection of the pyrrolizidine alkaloids may account for the presence of two alkaloids in the milk from the goats and only one in the milk from the cows. Additional studies are planned to assay samples of cow's milk which contain the pyrrolizidine alkaloids in an attempt to isolate alkaloids in addition to jacoline.

As was true in the case of the calves, the young kids demonstrated no lesions typical of pyrrolizidine alkaloid toxicity and, from all standpoints, appeared to remain quite healthy during the duration of this project. The potential danger to human beings drinking the milk from either goats or cows appears to be slight based on the evidence presented in these two experimental projects. However, a number of questions remain unanswered. Not the least of these is the question of the carcinogenecity of the pyrrolizidine alkaloids themselves. This is an area of scientific disagreement which is in need of additional study.

VI. REFERENCES

1. Allen, J. R., Hsu, I. C., and Carstens, L. A., *Cancer Res.* 35, 997-1002 (1975).
2. Bull, L. B., Culvenor, C. C. J., and Dick, A. T., "The Pyrrolizidine Alkaloids," John Wiley and Sons, New York, 1968.
3. Newberne, P. M., and Rogers, A. E., *Plant Foods Manage.* 1, 23-41 (1973).
4. Schoental, R., *Cancer Res.* 28, 2237-2246 (1968).
5. Anon, "Tansy Ragwort, an Increasing Problem in Western Oregon," Oregon State Extension Circular, p. 796, 1971.
6. Duby, G. D., *Mod. Vet. Pract.* 56, 185-188 (1975).
7. Muth, O. H., *J. Am. Vet. Med. Assoc.* 153, 310-312 (1968).
8. Johnson, A. E., *Am. J. Vet. Res.* 37, 107-110 (1976).
9. Schoental, R., *J. Bacteriol. Pathol.* 77, 485-495 (1959).
10. Dollahite, J. W., *Southwest. Vet.* (Spring) 223-226 (1972).
11. Gilruth, J. A., Twelfth Report of the Department of Agriculture, New Zealand, p. 206, 1904.
12. Dickinson, J. O., *West Vet.* 12, 26-27 (1974).
13. Dickinson, J. O., *West Vet.* 14, 11-13 (1976).
14. Wiesner, I. C., Raunsley, H. M., Brooks, F. P., and Senior, J. R., *Am. J. Dig. Dis.* 10, 147-151 (1965).
15. Mattocks, A. R., *Anal. Chem.* 39, 443-447 (1967).
16. Kery, A., *Acta Agron. Acad. Sci. Hung.* 24, 3-9 (1975).
17. Dickinson, J. O., Cooke, M. P., King, R. R., and Mohamed, P. A., *J. Am. Vet. Med. Assoc.* 169, 1192-1196 (1976).

TETRADYMIA TOXICITY - A NEW LOOK AT AN OLD PROBLEM

A. Earl Johnson
Poisonous Plant Research Laboratory, Agricultural Research Service
U.S. Department of Agriculture

I. ABSTRACT

We have previously shown that Artemisia nova *(black sagebrush) is a preconditioning plant that sheep must eat if photosensitization is to occur after they have ingested* Tetradymia spp. *Further study of the toxicity of these two plants to sheep revealed the plants to be highly synergistic in their action on sheep. Serum enzymes, glutamic oxaloacetic transaminase (SGOT) and lactic dehydrogenase (LDH), in sheep were elevated 30- to 90-fold for SGOT and 3- to 10-fold for LDH in sheep that had consumed both plants, but they were not elevated in sheep that had eaten one or the other of the two plants. Furthermore,* A. nova*, a nutritious and valuable range plant, was lethal to sheep under some conditions when even moderate amounts were consumed in a 2- to 3-day period. Several laboratory-based experiments attempting to experimentally produce photosensitization in sheep by first feeding* A. nova *and then* Tetradymia spp. *were largely unsuccessful. Similar field experiments on range sheep that had been eating* A. nova *were highly successful; this result indicated that additional unknown factors or conditions must be present to consummate this toxic syndrome.*

II. INTRODUCTION

Tetradymia poisoning in sheep in Utah and some adjacent states has plagued livestockmen for most of this century. The 2 species responsible for most poisonings are *Tetradymia glabrata* and *Tetradymia canescens*. *Tetradymia glabrata*, commonly called little leaf horsebrush or coal oil brush, is a bushy shrub that may grow up to a meter high and is found in semi-desert foothill areas. It becomes green early in the spring, quickly produces buds and flowers, sheds leaves, and becomes dormant from mid-summer until the next spring. *Tetradymia canescens*, called little gray horsebrush or spineless gray horsebrush, is found in mountain foothills and is green from early June until September.

Tetradymia glabrata is one of the first plants to become green in the spring and thus is available to sheep in western Utah and eastern Nevada at a crucial time when herds are being moved from winter range to summer range. Herds, each containing several thousand sheep, are often forced to move through extensive stands of *Tetradymia*; and in periods of spring storminess, drought, or other stress situations, sheep may consume more than normal amounts and thus may be affected by a variety of afflictions including general debilitation, abortion, photosensitization, loss of herding instinct, and death.

Tetradymia canescens, which greens later than *T. glabrata* is usually available when food selection on the range is good; thus, losses most often occur when sheep are confined and have consumed other forage first. *Tetradymia canescens* is less toxic than *T. glabrata*, and thus there may be fewer death losses. Other afflictions stated here for *T. glabrata* may occur, however, and debilitating losses can be serious.

Although many thousands of sheep have died from consuming these plants, relatively little work has been done on them. Fleming and coworkers in Nevada in 1922 (1) were some of the first to experimentally feed *T. glabrata* to livestock. They called it spring rabbit brush and conducted extensive feeding trials in which they described in detail signs of poisoning and gross pathology of both acute and chronic poisonings. They reported the toxin to be a resin and to be cumulative and established some levels of toxicity. Fleming was aware that the plant caused degeneration of the liver, but reported death to be due to cardiac failure. More recently, Jennings and coworkers (2) have isolated a furan compound from *T. glabrata* and determined that it is hepatotoxic.

Clawson and Huffman in the 1930's became interested in both *T. glabrata* and *T. canescens* and their relationship to a condition in sheep commonly called "bighead." This condition is a photosensitization caused by exposure to sunlight of uncovered or bare skin in the sheep. Affected areas become irritated and may itch or burn. Hyperemia develops and tissues swell greatly as a result of edema. In severe cases there may be loss of wool, skin ulceration, secondary infection, and permanent damage such as blindness.

When edema is severe, the head may be greatly enlarged; thus, the term "bighead." Clawson and Huffman, by experimental feeding of *T. glabrata* to sheep and subsequently exposing them to the sun, produced "bighead" with relative ease in 9 of 16 sheep and thus incriminated *Tetradymia* as the causative agents (3). They were aware of Rimington's work incriminating phylloerythrin, a breakdown product of chlorophyll, as the phototoxic agent in "geeldikkop" (4), and they assumed the photosensitization in "bighead" to be of a similar nature. Clare (5) later also made the same assumption and classed "bighead" as a secondary photosensitization involving phylloerythrin.

Clawson and Huffman in later feeding trials to sheep had much difficulty in causing photosensitization with *T. glabrata* and attempted to show that other range plants were related to the problem. They did not report their work because of the death of Clawson. After many feeding trials in a 4-year period, I also concluded that there must be predisposing factors (6). The experimental results of Clawson's last efforts were obtained, and the work that incriminated *Artemisia sp.* as preconditioning agents to

Tetradymia photosensitization was reported (7).

This paper reports further investigations into the toxic relationships of *Artemisia* and *Tetradymia* in sheep.

III. EXPERIMENT 1

Having recognized that *Artemisia nova* (black sage) could precondition sheep for *Tetradymia*-related photosensitization, we attempted to extract with water the substance responsible for the preconditioning. Thus, a measured amount of finely ground new growth from *A. nova* was extracted for 24 hours; the water was drained and expressed, and water extract and residue were retained for experimental feeding to sheep.

Three sheep were fed by stomach tube daily for 3 days freshly ground new growth from *A. nova* at the rate of 10 g of *A. nova*/kg of the sheep's body weight per day (1 sheep died on day 3 and did not receive the 3rd dose). Three sheep were fed water extract and 3 were fed residue daily for 4 days. Each feeding was from an amount of *A. nova* representing 10 g of *A. nova*/kg of the sheep's body weight. On the day after the last feeding each of the 9 sheep and a group of 3 previously untreated sheep was administered a single dose of 12.5 g of *T. canescens*/kg of body weight.

Three additional sheep were fed *A. nova* only for 3 days at 10 g of *A. nova*/kg of body weight. Another sheep was also fed *A. nova* water extract for 4 days and one other *A. nova* residue for 4 days as above. These last 2 animals were killed 2 days later and examined postmortem, and tissues were taken for histopathology.

Blood samples were taken from all sheep before the start of the experiment, and every few days during the experiment, and lactic dehydrogenase (LDH)[1] and serum glutamic oxaloacetic transaminase (SGOT)[1] were determined, primarily to monitor tissue damage. All animals were kept in full sunlight each day to observe possible signs of "bighead."

Two of 3 animals in the first group fed ground *A. nova* only for 2 and 3 days died on days 3 and 6. The survivor, after a few days listlessness, recovered. In general, the rest of the sheep that were fed either ground *A. nova*, *A. nova* extract, *A. nova* residue, or *T. canescens* alone, other than a brief period of depression in some instances, were affected very little. Blood chemical determinations (SGOT and LDH) also were not significantly changed. In sheep fed ground *A. nova*, *A. nova* water extract, and *A. nova* residue followed by *T. canescens*, however, SGOTs increased up to 20-fold and LDHs increased up to 10-fold; These increases indicate extensive tissue damage. After approximately 20

---

[1]Dade Chemical Company, Miami, Florida. (Mention of a trade name, proprietary product, or specific equipment does not constitute a guarantee or warranty by the U.S. Department of Agriculture and does not imply its approval to the exclusion of other products that may be suitable.)

days, all sheep appeared to be normal, and SGOTs and LDHs had returned to normal. Only two sheep became moderately photosensitized: one had been fed ground *A. nova* and then *T. canescens*, and one had been fed *A. nova* residue and then *T. canescens*.

The objective of this experiment was to extract with water the compound in *A. nova* responsible for the preconditioning effect in *Tetradymia* photosensitization. Because only 2 sheep were photosensitized, results are inconclusive. Perhaps of much greater significance was the finding of the synergistic effect of the 2 plants. This finding indicates to the livestockman that extra caution must be exercised in trailing sheep through *Tetradymia* when they have recently eaten *A. nova*. Also of significance was the finding that 2 of 3 sheep in one group died from being fed relatively small amounts of *A. nova* for 2 and 3 consecutive days; this finding indicates too the need for caution in moving sheep too rapidly into areas where no other feed except *A. nova* is available. This latter finding was not too surprising because *Artemisia tridentata* (big sage) has similar effects (8).

The fact that both water extract and residue acted synergistically with tetradymia indicates that extraction was probably incomplete but that the synergistic compound is likely water soluble.

IV. EXPERIMENT 2

In experiment 1, we determined that *A. nova* used to precondition sheep for *Tetradymia* studies may be lethal to sheep if given at the rate of 10 g/kg body weight per day for 3 days. In this experiment we preconditioned 10 sheep with *A. nova* at a much lower rate: 1.1 g of *A. nova*/kg of the sheep's body weight on day 1 followed by 2.2 g/kg on days 2 through 6, a total of 12.1 g/kg. On day 8, four of these sheep were fed growing tips of freshly collected *T. canescens* at the rate of 12.5 g/kg, and 4 others were similarly fed *T. glabrata* at 7.5 g/kg of plant. The 2 other sheep were held as controls. Four more sheep, not preconditioned, were also fed *T. canescens* at 12.5 g/kg and 4 others were fed *T. glabrata* at 7.5 g/kg. All sheep were kept in bright sunlight for the 2 days after *Tetradymia* feeding. Blood for chemical determinations was collected before the start of the experiment and frequently during the experiment to confirm findings in experiment 1.

As in experiment 1, only 1 sheep preconditioned with *A. nova* and fed *T. canescens* and 1 preconditioned with *A. nova* and fed *T. glabrata* developed "bighead." Serum enzymes, SGOT and LDH, were slightly elevated in sheep fed *T. canescens* and *T. glabrata* only and were essentially unchanged in sheep preconditioned with *A. nova*. Both SGOT and LDH were elevated maximally in sheep preconditioned with *A. nova* and fed *T. canescens* (as in experiment 1) and *T. glabrata*. Two sheep fed *A. nova* and then *T. canescens* died after 1 week, as did 1 sheep fed *A. nova* and then *T. glabrata*; the others returned to apparent normality in 2 to 3 weeks.

Results of this experiment indicate that single feedings of *T. canescens* at the rate of 12.5 g of *T. canescens*/kg of the sheep's body weight and *T. glabrata* at the rate of 7.5 g/kg are not harmful to sheep unless they have been fed small doses of *A. nova* for several days. Thus, there is indeed a synergistic relationship of the 2 plants as they relate to toxicity in sheep. Only preconditioned sheep developed "bighead," but the small number so affected (25%) was disappointing.

The extremely high SGOT values in preconditioned sheep fed *T. canescens* and *T. glabrata* are of interest in that increases this great (80- to 90-fold) are seldom encountered. Although SGOT and LDH increases are not specific for liver damage, we assumed that because histopathological study revealed liver injury, this liver injury was the main source of the high serum SGOT. Perhaps other tissues are involved.

V. EXPERIMENT 2 (SUPPLEMENTAL STUDY)

Two sheep were each fed *T. canescens* at the rate of 12.5 g of *T. canescens*/kg body weight for 3 consecutive days. Also, 2 sheep were each fed *A. nova* at 7.5 g/kg on 3 consecutive days and then fed *T. canescens* at 12.5 g/kg. All sheep were exposed to bright sun for 2 days after *Tetradymia* feedings.

No photosensitization occurred. Blood enzymes, SGOT and LDH, were normal on day 3 of *T. canescens* feeding, but one SGOT increased 3-fold 4 days after the last feeding. Sheep fed *A. nova* had normal values the last day of *A. nova* feeding but were elevated maximally after *T. canescens* feeding. Sheep not preconditioned can apparently tolerate 3 times the dose of *T. canescens* that may be lethal if they have been preconditioned with *A. nova*.

VI. EXPERIMENT 3

In experiments 1 and 2, we determined that sheep preconditioned with either large or small doses of *A. nova* and then fed *T. canescens* or *T. glabrata* were more severely damaged than sheep not preconditioned with *A. nova* and that sheep fed *T. cansecens* only at the rate of 12.5 g/kg body weight were not heavily insulted. Results also showed that animals in experiment 1 and 2 were not as easily photosensitized as expected. We assumed that this difficulty in experimentally producing photosensitization was due to improper preconditioning. Thus, in experiment 3, four sheep in 1 group were each fed *A. nova* at the rate of 2.5 g/kg body weight for 7 days; one-half of the daily dose was given in the morning and one-half in the evening. Four sheep in another group were similarly fed *T. glabrata* for 7 days at 1.25 g/kg per day. Four sheep in the third group served as controls and were not preconditioned. In an effort to insure that all animals received the intensity of sunlight that resulted in "bighead" in field toxicities the 3 groups were transported to the semi-desert area where "bighead" frequently occurs. There *T. glabrata* was collected and fed to all sheep at 7.5 g/kg in a single feeding. Animals were then exposed to the bright sunlight of the desert area for 2 days.

No animals became photosensitized. Serum enzymes, SGOT and LDH, as expected, were not abnormally elevated after preconditioning. However, an unexpected finding contrary to those in the previous 2 experiments was that LDH and SGOT were not significantly increased 3 days after *T. glabrata* was fed to the animals preconditioned with *A. nova*. The only apparent explanation is that the relatively small amount of *A. nova* given in a split dosage (1.25 g/kg morning and evening) was small enough for the toxin therein to be metabolized to non-toxic levels. Thus, no effect was elicited, and no preconditioning resulted. Preconditioning with small doses of *T. glabrata* was also ineffective. The rationale for attempting preconditioning with *T. glabrata* was that trailing sheep often forage small amounts of plants as they move along, and small amounts of *T. glabrata* over long periods of time might sensitize the animal to the plant.

VII. FIELD EXPERIMENTS

As a result of the difficulty experienced in producing photosensitization in the 3 experiments just reported and other experiments supplementary to them, we seriously suspected that even though *A. nova* exerted a definite synergistic effect on *Tetradymia* toxicity, other factors must be functioning to produce photosensitization in field toxicities that were not functioning in experimentally produced toxicities. To confirm this suspicion, we conducted in 4 separate years a series of experiments that had an underlying premise that range sheep are more susceptible to photosensitization than farm-reared sheep fed dry hay or grass. These experiments are summarized in Table 1. All have the same basic plan: farm-reared sheep fed alfalfa hay or grass were taken to range areas where "bighead" occurs. An equal number of sheep were taken from range herds in that area. Sheep in both groups were confined in shade-free pens and given equal amounts of *T. glabrata* by stomach tube, after which all sheep were exposed to bright sun for 2 days.

Twelve of 19 range sheep fed *T. glabrata* experimentally developed signs of "bighead" varying from mild to severe. Twenty-seven of 27 farm-reared sheep had no "bighead" symptoms.

The lack of uniformity of response in range sheep, as yearly results were compared, corresponded with the response that was seen in field outbreaks. *Tetradymia glabrata* is most often eaten when in the bud stage and when the buds are high in water content and plant growth is luxuriant. Some years, this stage of growth may last only a few days or 1 or 2 weeks; in extreme dry years (as in 1977), there are few buds and no growth. Thus, time for conducting experiments is short and must be correlated with the

TABLE 1

Summary of Field Feeding Trials of Tetradymia glabrata *to Farm-Reared and Range Sheep*

Number of sheep	Pretreatment	Daily dosage, *T. glabrata* g/kg	No. days	Results	Plant condition
1972 Experiment					
3(F)[1]	Dry hay	5.9	1	No changes	Young buds,
3(R)[2]	Range feed	7.1	1	2 bighead, 1 depression	but many plants with no buds
2(F)	Dry hay	3.9	2	No changes	
2(R)	Range feed	4.5	2	1 mild bighead, 1 depression	
1973 Experiment					
4(F)	Green grass	5.0	1	No changes	Slow growth,
4(F)	Dry hay	5.0	1	No changes	late in
4(R)	Range feed	5.0	1	No changes	season, dry
1974 Experiment					
2(F)	Green grass (*A. nova*)[3]	7.5	1	Both died	Young buds, fair growth,
2(R)	Range feed (*A. nova*)[3]	7.5	1	1 died,[4] 1 depressed	but somewhat dry
6(F)	Dry hay	7.5	1	No changes	
4(R)	Range feed	7.5	1	3 mild, 1 severe bighead	
1976 Experiment					
6(F)	Dry hay	7.0	1	No changes	Very young
6(R)	Range feed	7.0	1	1 died,[4] 5 bighead	buds, fair moisture

[1]Farm-reared sheep.
[2]Range sheep.
[3]*A. nova* dosage: 3.7 g/kg of the sheep's body weight for 2 days and 5.0 g/kg for 1 day.
[4]Death due to unrelated complications.

availability of range sheep. Plant growth varies with water and temperature, and extremes of both occur in *Tetradymia* areas. Growth was good in 1972 and 1976 and fair in 1974; and in these years range sheep could be obtained which had been eating *A. nova* in the previous 1 to 2 days. Table 1 results reflect these conditions; results were positive in these 3 years. In 1973, plant growth was slow and several weeks late, and the only range sheep that could be obtained had eaten no *A. nova* for approximately 5 days; thus, results were negative. *Tetradymia glabrata* dosages in range sheep and farm-reared sheep in 1972 did not have good correlation, and in 1973 were perhaps a little low. The experiments in years 1974 and 1976 were needed for confirmation of results. Because of remoteness of the field experimental area, blood chemical determinations were not made. These may have been enlightening.

Results of these field trials leave little doubt that other factors, in addition to the preconditioning effect of *A. nova* are important in the development of tetradymia-related photosensitization in sheep. They may be as simple as the time-dose relationship, or they may be more complicated and relate to the difference in rumen microorganism types or numbers in range and in farm-reared sheep; they may be nutritional and relate to a vitamin or other nutrient shortage; or we may not be dealing with a secondary photosensitization at all. We have assumed that because *T. glabrata* and *T. canescens* contain hepatotoxic compounds, damage to the liver is of the type that prevents excretion of phylloerythrin into the bile and that phylloerythrin is the phototoxic agent.

Phylloerythrin has not been shown to be in the peripheral circulation of sheep photosensitized in this syndrome; and the hepatic histopathological lesion does not give clues as to whether phylloerythrin is leaking into the arterial circulation. These phases of this very interesting toxicity problem are currently being investigated.

VIII. ACKNOWLEDGMENT

The author wishes to acknowledge the most able assistance of Robert Adamson and the sacrifice of his personal time especially in the conducting of the field experiments.

IX. REFERENCES

1. Fleming, C. E., Miller, M. R., and Vawter, L. R., *Univ. Nev. Agric. Exp. Stn. Bull.* 104 (1922).
2. Jennings. P. W., Reeder, S. K., Hurley, J. C., Caughlan, C. N., and Smith, G. D., *J. Org. Chem.* 39, 3392-3398 (1974).
3. Clawson, A. B., and Huffman, W. T., *Nat. Woolgrower* 27, 13-16 (1937).
4. Rimington, C., and Quin, J. I., *Onderstepoort J. Vet. Sci. Anim. Ind.* 3, 137-157 (1934).
5. Clare, N. T., *in* "Advances in Veterinary Science" (C. A. Brandly and E. L. Jungherr, Eds.), Vol. 2, p. 182-211. Academic Press, New York, 1955.
6. Johnson, A. E., *Can. J. Comp. Med.* 38, 406-410 (1974).
7. Johnson, A. E., *Am. J. Vet. Res.* 35, 1583-1585 (1974).
8. Johnson, A. E., James, L. F., and Spillet, J., *J. Range Manage.* 29, 278-280 (1976).

TOXIC CONSTITUENTS AND HEPATOTOXICITY OF THE PLANT *Tetradymia glabrata* (ASTEROCEAE)

P. W. Jennings, S. K. Reeder, J. C. Hurley, J. E. Robbins,
S. K. Holian, A. Holian, P. Lee, J. A. S. Pribanic, and M. Hull
Montana State University

I. ABSTRACT

In the early 1900's, Fleming, Clawson, and Huffman discovered that the plant Tetradymia glabrata *which grew in northwestern U.S. was responsible for fatalities of sheep. Numbers of fatalities as high as 1000 sheep were observed to occur at one time. From their investigations, it was concluded that the plant contained components causing hepatotoxicity and perhaps photosensitization.*

In 1967, we began to study the plant with hopes of identifying the toxic substances in the plant and their mode of action. As a result, three compounds have been isolated and chemically characterized as furanoeremophilanes. Subsequent studies showed that one of these substances, Tetradymol, is metabolized by the mixed function oxidase enzymes to a metabolite which is even more toxic. Finally, these furanoeremophilanes have been shown to express their toxicity by uncoupling oxidative phosphorylation from electron transport.

II. HISTORICAL INTRODUCTION

In the spring of 1967, Dr. Reeder and I began a study on the isolation and structure identification of the toxic components of the plant *Tetradymia glabrata* (Asteroceae), Senecioneae tr., having the common names, littleleaf horsebrush, spring rabbitbrush, and coal oil brush. Kingsbury's book on poisonous plants of the U.S. (1), containing a summary of all the previous investigations, related that the plant had been shown to be toxic to sheep with as many as 1,000 deaths at a single time. It also indicated that in addition to the plant components causing death, they might also be responsible for photosensitization. The exact chemical components responsible for these maladies were not known, according to Kingsbury.

At the Nevada experiment station, Fleming (2) and his coworkers worked from 1918 through 1922 establishing the conditions for toxicity through forced feeding experiments. They were successful in demonstrating that *T. glabrata* was fatal to sheep. They were unaware that the plant produced photosensitization. Attempts at isolating the toxins were not realized although they did show the toxin to be extractable from the plant by hexane and acetone. Fleming suggested that the acetone extract contained a cardiotoxin.

We have never been able to verify this conclusion.

In the years 1935-37, Clawson and Huffman (3) of the Utah experiment station reported in the *National Wool Grower* that their results of forced feedings and deaths of sheep were the same as those reported by Fleming. They were successful in developing the symptoms of photosensitization by forced feeding *Tetradymia glabrata* to animals on the range. In an additional series of feeding experiments, Huffman (4) co-fed over 40 plants with *T. glabrata*, finding that only *Artemisia tridentata* or *A. nova* produced the symptoms of photosensitization. All investigators had found the liver to have lesions after forced feeding experiments. No further work was published prior to our investigations in 1967.

We duplicated the previous workers' forced feeding experiments co-feeding 3 of the 40 plants, finding no activity with *T. canescens*, but death of sheep with *T. glabrata* (5). Using only the new growth and flower buds, death of sheep was attained by forced feeding approximately 2-3 lb of plant or 2-3% of the animal's body weight. Autopsy of the poisoned animals revealed the liver to be necrotic, friable, and tan in color. The gall bladder was extended and the lungs showed considerable congestion. The kidneys showed some yellow discoloration. There was a smell of ammonia upon initially opening the body cavity. At the microscopic level the liver showed centrolobular necrosis and some evidence of fatty degeneration. The lungs showed extreme congestion, alveolar emphysema, and intra-alveolar hemorrhage. Cardiac tissue showed a few sub-epicardial hemorrhages. Other tissues were normal.

While the poisoned animal was still alive, the bromosulfophthalein (BSP) clearance test and the concentration of ammonia in the blood were measured. The BSP clearance test (time necessary for the liver to remove 1/2 of the dye, BSP, from the blood) showed an increase from 3-7 minutes for normal sheep to as high as 70 minutes for drugged sheep. Likewise, the blood ammonia level went from 4 μg/ml in normal sheep to 13-24 μg/ml in drugged sheep. Thus it is apparent that hepatodysfunction of some sort may readily be assumed.

III. ISOLATION AND CHARACTERIZATION OF THE TOXIC CONSTITUENTS OF *Tetradymia glabrata*

Hexane and acetone extracts of the new growth and flower buds were administered orally to sheep, resulting in the same response as had been observed previously by forced feeding whole plant. Forced feeding of the plant material remaining after extraction gave no toxic response, indicating the toxin had been extracted. No adverse effects such as death were noted on feeding hexane or acetone in amounts similar to those which might have contaminated the extract.

Due to the small amount of compound obtained from various isolation steps beyond the crude extractions, a small animal was needed to assay for toxins. A variety of animals, including mice, rats, rabbits, gerbils, and guinea pigs were initially used to screen the extracts for toxins. All animals used showed similar symptoms of the poisoning, such as lethargy, hiding in corners, coma, and death. Except for the gerbils, all livers showed necrosis and, except for the rabbit's liver which exhibited periportal necrosis, the others showed centrolobular damage. Mice were used to assay for toxin and two compounds were isolated following the pathway which has been published (6a). A thin-layer chromatogram of the crude hexane extract of the plant, and corresponding mouse feeding experiments are shown in Figure 1.

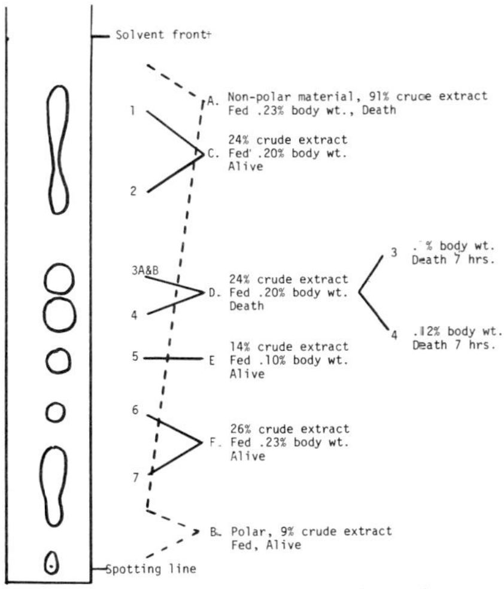

*Mice were used as test animals for the above feeding experiments.
+Anasil S tlc, developed in 40:60 n-hexane:diethyl ether.

Fig. 1. *Chromatogram of crude hexane extract.*

The thin-layer spot labeled 3 was later resolved into two components and will be referred to as henceforth as 3A and 3B. Compound 3A was shown to be toxic, but 3B was not. Thin-layer spots labeled 4 and 3A were subsequently shown to be Tetradymol and Tetradymadiol ester, having the structures I and II (6).

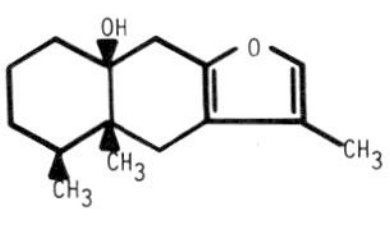

I

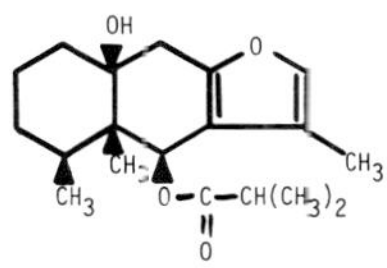

II

Both compounds are white crystalline solids with the following physical characteristics:

	Tetradymol	Tetradymadiol ester
Melting point:	92-92.5° C	100-100.5° C
M^+ m/e:	234	320
Base peak m/e:	109	124
λmax	222 nm (logε 3.83)	215 nm (logε 3.80)
$[\alpha]_D^{25}$	+56 (MeOH)	-56 (MeOH)

The key to the structure proof of these types of compounds is the mass and nuclear magnetic resonance spectra. The mass spectra are classical in that a low intensity parent ion is usually seen with the base peak resulting from the cleavage pattern diagrammed below where we see the mass spectral fragmentation for tetradymol m/e 234 M^+ (37%), m/e 109 (100%):

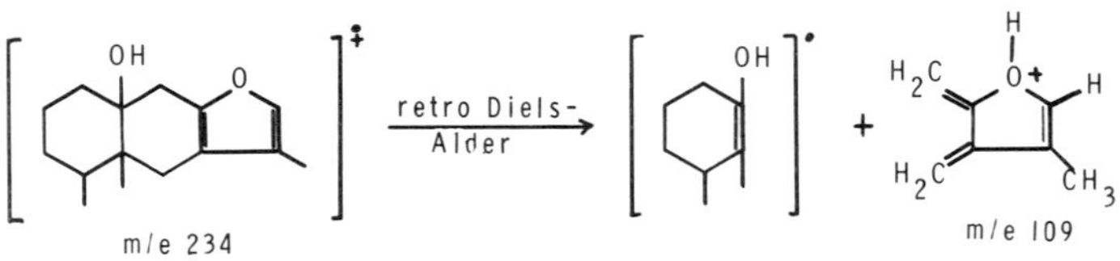

The nmr spectra of these furanoeremphilanic compounds exhibit easily-identifiable peaks for the furan hydrogen and the three methyl groups. Equally important, however, are the protons at carbon positions 6 and 9. We (6) have shown these to have a chemical shift between 2.1 and 3.5 ppm with each pair of hydrogens displayed as an AB or AX quartet. The protons having the β configuration at these two positions are upfield of the protons with the α configuration. The configuration of the methyl group at carbon position 4 is difficult to assess but had been assigned the β configuration in all known furanoeremophilanes. Two recent X-ray crystal structures in this series confirmed this assignment (6).

Several additional compounds have been synthesized from compound II as shown below in Figure 2.

Compounds I, II, and III have been shown to be toxic while compounds VII and VIII are not toxic. We have not had enough sample to test compounds IV, V, and VI. The LD_{50} of the toxic compounds are shown below:

Compound	LD50 (mg/kg)
I	275 orally
	94 IP
II	375 orally
	400 IP
III	113 IP

Recently, we have isolated a new compound which exhibits resonances in the nmr spectrum that are characteristic of furano-

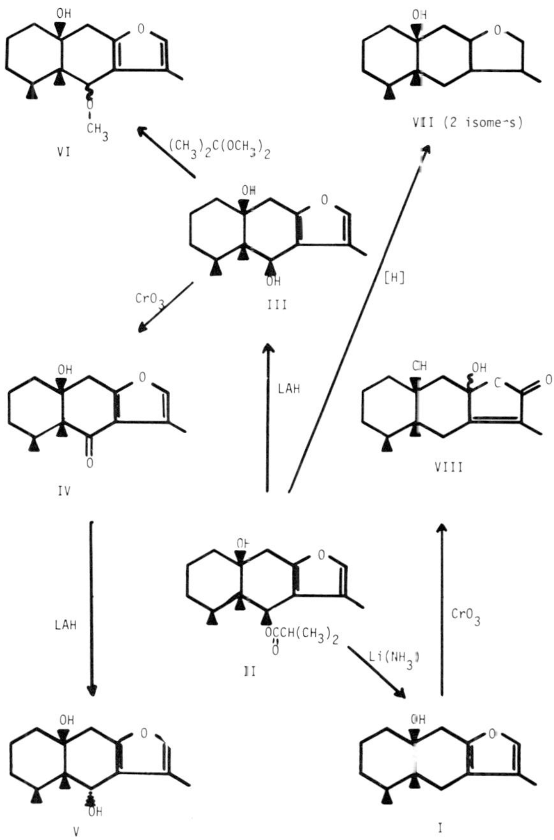

Fig. 2. *Chemical modifications of furanosesquiterpenes.*

eremophilanes with both C-6 and C-9 substituted. Also there is evidence for one isobutyl ester function. A major peak of the mass spectral fragmentation is at 140 m/e. The data would support the following structure which is accompanied by the postulated mass spectral fragments.

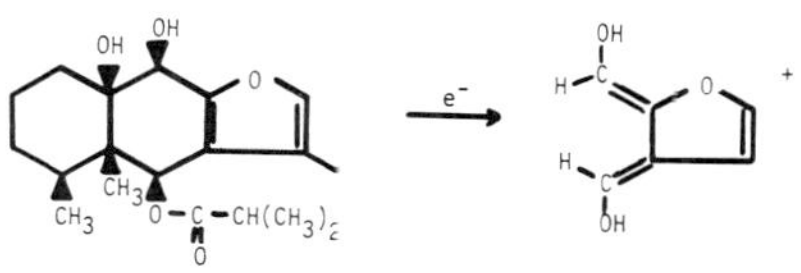

IV. TOXICITY CHARACTERIZATION

Since the most abundant toxin recovered from the plant was

tetradymol, most of our toxicity studies are with it (7). Ehrlich's reagent, which is normally used to visualize these toxins on thin-layer plates, was used in solution for analysis.[1]

Due to its lipid solubility, tetradymol was found fairly evenly distributed throughout the body tissues and organs from intraperitoneal administration. However, oral administration of toxin resulted in about half of it remaining in the stomach for over eight hours. The other body tissues still contained a fairly even distribution. The fact that a significant portion of tetradymol remains in the stomach probably explains why the oral LD_{50} is so much higher than the LD_{50} for IP injection. Experiments were conducted which showed tetradymol to be stable *in vitro* at pH values of 1 and in the stomach from *in vivo* studies.

Histological investigation of the following tissues: stomach, upper and lower intestine, liver, lung, heart, brain, pancreas, and kidney, revealed that the liver was the only affected organ. The damage to this organ was described as centrolobular necrosis which was subsequently shown to be time-dependent. Some swelling to the centrolobular cells was found two hours after oral administration with increased cellular degeneration continuing to a maximum at 8-10 hours when cell differentiation became difficult. The nuclei after 10 hours indicated karyorrhexis and blood-filled sinusoids were abundant. Periodic acid-Shiff stain of these liver slices also indicated glycogen depletion. This type of time-dependent liver degeneration was achieved with a 350 mg/kg oral dosage.

Further studies with microsomes isolated from the liver of mice, which were pretreated with phenobarbital, showed tetradymol to be a Type I binder (8) with the mixed function oxidase (MFO) system. At very high concentrations of tetradymol (1.5 mM), there was indication of slight Type II binding. These results suggested that the mixed function oxidase system is probably metabolizing tetradymol and that the metabolite should be investigated for toxicity. To this end, several experiments were run on mice which had been pretreated with various agents, dosed with 350 mg/kg of tetradymol and then allowed to succumb to the toxic action. The results are shown in Table 1.

A reduction in the death time of mice pretreated with phenobarbital and 3-methylcholanthrene strongly suggests that the MFO system metabolizes tetradymol to a new compound which is a more potent toxin. This hypothesis is further substantiated by experiments using a pretreatment of SKF 525A or piperonyl butoxide. These two agents block the MFO system, preventing metabolism of tetradymol and formation of the new, more potent toxin, and thus allow the animal to live longer. In pretreatment experiments 4 and 5, cysteine will enhance while diethylmaleate will block glutathione conjugation. The conclusion from the cysteine experiment

---

[1]This method is sensitive to 0.2 mg/ml of tetradymol with accuracy of ±0.5 μg. The standard curve used for this analysis is $y = 66x - 4.7$ where y = concentration and x = O.D. at 750 nm.

TABLE 1

Death Time Studies

Pretreatment	Death (Hrs)	T Test P Values
Control	7.48±1.67	
Phenobarbital	5.53±1.70	0.1165
3-Methylcholanthrene	5.17±1.08	0.0635
SKF 525A	13.55±1.86	0.0013
Piperonyl butoxide	17.90±2.90	0.0006
Cysteine	9.18±0.48	0.1014
Diethylmaleate	6.32±0.71	0.2513
Salicylamide	11.23±3.01	0.0561
Olive oil	7.05±3.01	0.7498
Ethanol	9.73±1.02	0.0529

is that conjugation ties up tetradymol or its metabolite or both resulting in a reduction of their toxic action. Blocking conjugation with diethylmaleate reduces the rate of removal of toxin. Salicylamide, which was supposed to block uridine diphosphate-glucuronic acid conjugation, should have decreased the death time as did diethylmaleate. Further work showed that salicylamide, in addition to its conjugation blocking properties, also binds to the MFO system as a Type I binder. Thus, it is competing with tetradymol for oxidation and preventing formation of the more potent metabolite.

Histological investigation of the mice livers from the pretreatment experiments were illuminating. In contrast to the typical centrolobular liver necrosis found with standard tetradymol administration, pretreatment with phenobarbital and then administration of tetradymol resulted in necrosis at the peripheral regions of the lobule. This is consistent with phenobarbital increasing the concentration of the MFO system in the lobule so that more toxic metabolite is formed earlier while tetradymol is diffusing toward the central vein (9). Pretreatment with 3-methylcholanthrene differed markedly from the phenobarbital experiment. While its administration as a pretreatment followed by tetradymol resulted in a slightly shortened death time compared to pretreatment with phenobarbital, the centrolobular cellular damage to the liver was mild after 5-6 hours. These results strongly suggest that there are at least two different metabolites generated from the MFO system with the substrate, tetradymol. The following model could explain these results:

Tetradymol + mouse → $necrosis_o$ + death
Phenobarbital + tetradymol + mouse → $metabolite_1$ + $necrosis_1$ + death.
$Metabolite_1$ + mouse → $necrosis_1$+ death.
3-Methylcholanthrene + tetradymol + mouse → $metabolite_2$ + $necrosis_o$ + death.
$Metabolite_2$ + mouse → death.

In other words, 3-methylcholanthrene produces a different metabolite than phenobarbital. Both metabolites are capable of killing the animal but the one from phenobarbital causes more severe liver necrosis. Since it is already known that phenobarbital and 3-methylcholanthrene enhance two different MFO or cytochrome P-450 (Cyt P-450) systems (10), it is possible to have two different metabolites. Extension of the above-mentioned model to include the other experiments in Table 1 leads to the conclusion that the death time of mice should be directly proportional to the concentration of Cyt P-450 and inversely proportional to Cyt P-450 blocking agents like SKF 525A. Thus experiments designed to maximize the Cyt P-450 concentration in the liver should result in a death time mostly attributable to the metabolite, while experiments designed to block metabolsim of tetradymol should result in death times attributable mostly to tetradymol.

Results of experiments to maximize the concentration of Cyt P-450 are shown in Figure 3 as a semi-reciprocal plot.

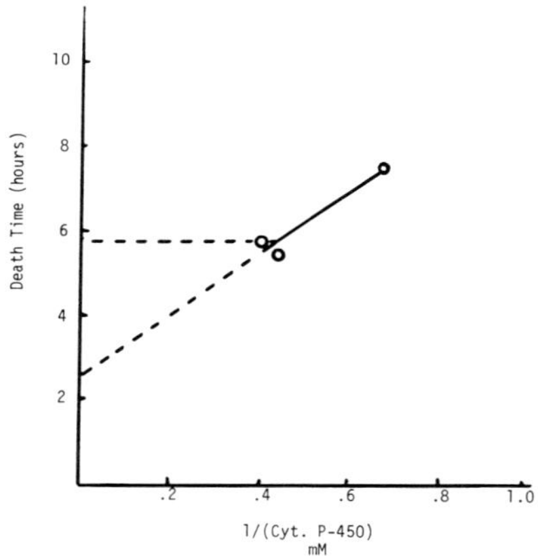

Fig. 3. *Death time vs mixed function oxidase enzyme concentration.*

Extrapolation, which is not necessarily justifiable due to the meager amount of data, suggests that a death time of 2-6 hours could be attributed to metabolite.

While one cannot go too high in the dosage of SKF 525A[2] and thus cannot totally block metabolism of tetradymol, we performed two Cyt P-450 blocking experiments which gave similar results. The data in Figure 4 were obtained by giving varying doses of SKF 525A followed by 350 mg/kg doses of tetradymol. The results suggest a death time of 14-16 hours. In the second experiment (Figure 5), SKF 525A was held constant at 80 mg/kg and the

---

[2]Doses of SKF 525A greater than 100 mg/kg alone cause some fatalities.

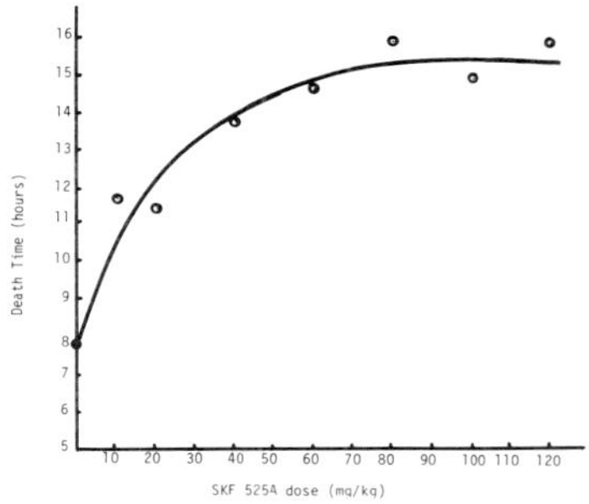

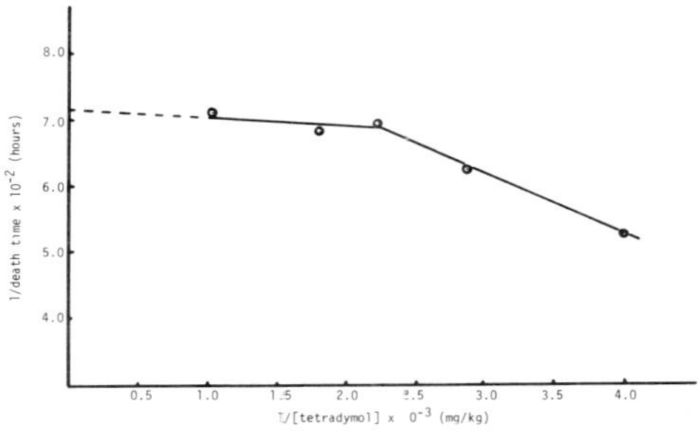

Fig. 4. *Death time as a function of SKF 525A dose.*
Fig. 5. *Death time due to tetradymol.*

concentration of tetradymol varied. These data, shown as a double reciprocal plot, also suggest a death time near 14 hours. Since SKF 525A is not high enough to totally prevent metabolism, I would guess the death time due to tetradymol would be greater than 14-16 hours. These three experiments taken together suggest that the phenobarbital produced metabolite is at least 2-7 times more potent in killing the animal than tetradymol.

V. MODE OF TOXIC ACTION

It was clear from the earliest results that animals poisoned by *T. glabrata* suffered from hepatodysfunction. Details as to why or how the liver is damaged shall be the subject of this section (11).

A few selected results garnered from drugged animals are shown in Table 2.

TABLE 2

Clinical Chemistry Results

Test	Result in Percent Change from Normal
Blood Serum Levels	
SGPT	+63
Indirect Billirubin	+72
Glucose	-42
NH_4^+	+800
Liver Characteristics	
ATP	-75
Liver Glycogen	Depleted
BSP	+400

From the BSP, indirect bilirubin, and serum glutamic-pyruvic transaminase levels in the blood serum, there is no doubt that the liver metabolism is malfunctioning. The high ammonia level suggests that the Urea Cycle also is not functioning. With glycogen stores depleted and blood glucose nearing hypoglycemic levels, the animal is out of energy. Finally, the reduced adenosine triphosphate (ATP) level in the liver means very few functions will be operable.

To counteract these depletions, the following experiments were tried. Administration of glucose for energy and Arginine or N-carbonyl-L-glutamate with Arginine to spark the urea cycle prolonged the animal's life to 10 1/2 hours after toxin administration, but did not protect it entirely. Prevention of toxic metabolite formation by blocking the MFO system using SKF 525A or ethanol is the best counteractive measure to date (see data in Table 1 of Section IV).

Initially, it was felt that the drugged animals were dying of high concentrations of blood ammonia. However, in additional experiments using NH_4^+ administered via IP injection, mice survived blood ammonia levels which exceeded measured amounts in tetradymol-poisoned mice by a factor of 5. Thus, we are not convinced that blood ammonia level is the major death-causing factor.

At the present time, we feel that the primary effect of the toxin is the reduction of liver ATP levels. This action would reduce the efficiency of a number of liver functions including the Urea Cycle which results in high blood ammonia levels. Furthermore, if the toxin acts as an uncoupler of the oxidative phosphorylation-electron transport system, then glycogen stores, glucose levels in the blood, and liver ATP levels would be lowered. The following discussion will elucidate the deatils of this mode of action.

The data shown in Table 3 clearly indicates tetradymol is an uncoupler of the mitochondrial oxidative phosphorylation-electron transport system.

TABLE 3

*Effect of Tetradymol on State 4 Respiration**

Condition	ngm-atom O/min
1 μM Tetradymol	0
5 μM Tetradymol	0
10 μM Tetradymol	9.80±4.5
25 μM Tetradymol	17.70±7.8
50 μM Tetradymol	24.58±3.4
100 μM Tetradymol	58.00±13.3
200 μM Tetradymol	94.40±33.5
350 μM Tetradymol	108.00±10.0
500 μM Tetradymol	88.10±10.9

*Succinate was used as substrate.

It is relatively weak in its action compared to other uncouplers such as 2,4-dinitrophenol, dicoumarol or hydrazones.

Albeit primary, enhanced oxygen uptake by mitochondria, as shown in Table 3, is only one of five criteria to be met by a compound prior to classification as an uncoupler. The other criteria are to: reduce respiratory control, restore oxygen uptake of inhibited ATPase, inhibit reverse electron flow, and have a pKa between 3-9. Except for the last item, all of the uncoupling criteria were verified for tetradymol. The fact that tetradymol does not have hydrogens acidic enough to fit the criteria caused both concern and interest. All known uncouplers such as 2,4-dinitrophenol and dicoumarol are weakly acidic. Tetradymol has a pKa around 18.5.

Without other criteria on which to disprove tetradymol[3] as an uncoupler, we conclude that the pKa requirement is not necessary. In Table 4, data is collected on a number of compounds which are similar to tetradymol.

TABLE 4

Relative Uncoupling Ability of Tetradymol-like Compounds

Condition 500 μM each	Increase of rate over State 4	Rate Relative to Tetradymol
Tetradymol I	303.0±4.24	1.00
Tetradymadiol Monoisobutyrate II	192.0±0	0.63
Tetradymadiol III	36.0±4.24	0.12
Tetradymadiol V	4.5±0	0.015
Tetradymol Ketone IV	15.0±0	0.05
Tetradymol Reduced VII	54.0±4.24	0.18
Tetradymol Reduced VII	66.0±4.24	0.22
Tetradymol Reduced VII	63.0±0	0.21
Oxidized Tetradymol VIII	28.5±6.36	0.09
Menthofuran	399.0±38.2	1.12
Benzofuran	33.0±0	0.11
Peperic Acid	15.0±0	0.05

Most of the compounds exhibit weaker uncoupling ability except for menthofuran. It is slightly more effective and has a pKa near 25. Thus, it appears that a new class of natural uncouplers may exist which do not fit the pKa criterion.

VI. REFERENCES

1. Kingsbury, J. M., "Poisonous Plants of the United States and Canada," Prentice-Hall, Englewood Cliffs, New Jersey, 1964.
2. a. Fleming, C. E., *Univ. Nev. Agric. Exp. Stn. Bull.*, No. 95, 27-30 (1918).

[3]Tetradymol does not exhibit its uncoupler effect by acting as a detergent.

b. Fleming, C. E., Miller, M. R., and Vawter, L. R., *Univ. Nev. Agric. Exp. Stn. Bull.*, No. 95 (1922).

3. Clawson, A. B., and Huffman, W. T., *Nat. Wool Grower* 20 (January 1936) and 14 (March 1934).
4. Huffman, W. T., Personal records on file at the USDA, Poisonous Plant Research Laboratory, Logan, Utah.
5. Reeder, S. K., Ph.D. Thesis, Montana State University, March 1971.
6. a. Jennings, P. W., Reeder, S. K., Hurley, J. C., Caughlan, C. N., and Smith, G. D., *J. Org. Chem.* 39, 3392 (1974).

   b. Jennings, P. W., Hurley, J. C., Reeder, S. K., Holian, A., Lee, P., Caughlan, C. N., and Larsen, R. D., *J. Org. Chem.* 41, 4078 (1976).
7. Holian, S. K., Master's Thesis, Montana State University, June 1975.
8. Roth, J. A., and Neal, R. A., *Biochemistry* 11, 955-961 (1972).
9. a. Conney, A. H., *et al.*, "Microsomes and Drug Oxidations," pp. 279-295. Academic Press, New York, 1964.

   b. Alvares, A. P., Schilling, G., Levin, W., and Kuntzman, R., *Biochem. Biophys. Res. Commun.* 29, 521-526 (1967).

   c. Hildebrandt, A. G., Speck M., and Roots, I., *Naunyn-Schmiedebergs Arch. Pharmacol.* 281, 371-382 (1974).

   d. Seawright, A. A., and Hrdlicka, J., *Br. J. Exp. Pathol.* 53, 242-252 (1972).

   e. Seawright, A. A., and O'Donahoo, R. H., *J. Pathol.* 106, 251-259 (1972).
10. Comai, K., and Gaylor, J. L., *J. Biol. Chem.* 248, 4947-4955 (1973).
11. Holian, A., Ph.D. Thesis, Montana State University, December, 1975.

LANTANA POISONING: A CHOLESTATIC DISEASE OF CATTLE AND SHEEP

Michael A. Pass, Alan A. Seawright, Trevor J. Heath,
and Robert T. Gemmell
Faculty of Veterinary Science and Department of Anatomy
University of Queensland

I. ABSTRACT

Lantana poisoning is a hepatotoxic disease of ruminants caused by the ingestion of Lantana camara L. *and is characterized by cholestasis. The toxic compounds are the triterpenes lantadene A and lantadene B. The toxins exert their effects on the hepatocytes and the canaliculi appear to be a major site of injury. Within a few hours after ingestion of the plant there is a decrease in canalicular ATPase activity and collapse of canaliculi. Although the secretory function of the hepatocytes is lost, their ability to metabolize compounds is retained to some extent: they are able to conjugate bilirubin. Toxicity is associated with an increase in the agranular endoplasmic reticulum in hepatocytes, but the significance of this change is not clear. Experiments have confirmed that lantana causes gallbladder paralysis but not intestinal paralysis.*

II. INTRODUCTION

Lantana camara L. is a plant which is poisonous to most domesticated ruminants and which grows in a number of countries including Australia, U.S.A., and Mexico. Although there are a number of varieties of the plant only some of them are toxic (1).

The disease is characterized by photosensitization, jaundice, and loss of appetite (2,3). The most signficant post-mortem findings are cholestatic injury to the liver, distension of the gallbladder, and necrosis of the renal tubules (2). Although many affected animals die, others survive and complete recovery of the liver lesion may occur. The deaths that occur have been attributed mostly to liver insufficiency and renal failure, but myocardial damage and intestinal paralysis have also been implicated in some animals (2,4).

Although the clinical and pathological findings of lantana poisoning have been well known for several years there has, until recently, been uncertainty about which compounds in the plant are toxic. In this paper we will review the recent evidence on the toxic principles of lantana and on the pathophysiological effects of the toxins on the liver, gallbladder, and intestinal tract.

III. TOXIC PRINCIPLES OF LANTANA

Although the disease related to ingestion of lantana has been recognized for many years it is only recently that the chemical nature of the toxins has been definitely established. Louw in 1948 suggested that the triterpene lantadene A was the toxic principle of lantana (5), but this was not confirmed in later experiments (6,7,8). More recently, however, it was demonstrated that both lantadene A and lantadene B (Fig. 1) are toxic to sheep when given by the oral route (9).

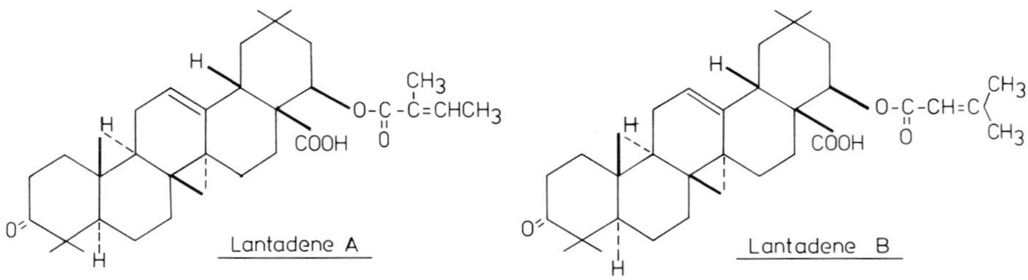

Fig. 1. *The chemical structures of lantadene A and lantadene B.*

The dose of lantadene A necessary to produce the clinical signs of lantana poisoning is about 60 mg per kg when given orally. Lantadene B appears to be less toxic than lantadene A and the reduced form of lantadene A slightly more toxic (9).

Recently we have investigated the toxicity of lantadene A given intravenously to sheep. Three syndromes were identified after lantadene A was injected and these were related to the dose of lantadene A and to the course of administration. When a single dose of lantadene A was given at 1-3 mg per kg mild liver injury occurred. Evidence for this included a rise in the levels of GOT and SDH in serum. However, the serum bilirubin levels did not increase and histological changes were not evident in the liver.

The second syndrome involved cholestasis and it occurred in some animals given lantadene A at 3 mg per kg and in animals given seven doses of lantadene A at 1 mg per kg over a period of 3 days. The evidence for cholestasis included elevation of serum GOT, SDH, and bilirubin. On gross examination the liver appeared green or ocher in color and vacuolation of hepatocytes and accumulation of bile pigments in Kupffer cells was apparent on histological examination. Other findings included an enlarged gallbladder, dry impacted feces in the rectum, and renal tubular necrosis.

The third syndrome involved hepatic necrosis and it occurred in some animals given lantadene A at 3 mg per kg and in all animals given it at 4-8 mg per kg. On histological examination three patterns of necrosis were seen: centrolobular, midzonal, and massive necrosis. In the most mildly affected cases, centrolobular and midzonal lesions were predominant but in some livers all types of zonal distribution of the injury were identified. In those animals which die from hepatic necrosis within a few hours of administration of the toxin, hemorrhage into the intestinal tract was common.

It was concluded that lantadene A is hepatotoxic and is capable of producing the clinical and pathological signs of lantana poisoning.

IV. EFFECT OF LANTANA ON THE LIVER

The criteria necessary for defining liver injury as cholestasis include an enlarged green liver; presence of bile plugs in canaliculi; and accumulation of bile pigments in Kupffer cells and hepatocytes (10). The ultrastructural changes compatible with cholestasis are canalicular dilation; blunting and loss of the canalicular microvilli; widening of the pericanalicular ectoplasm; enlargement of the Golgi zone; and an increase in the area of smooth endoplasmic reticulum (10). The clinical, postmortem, and histological changes observed in animals with lantana poisoning appear to be sufficient to justify classifying the liver lesion as cholestasis (2,11).

The rise in serum bilirubin level that occurs in lantana poisoning and the failure to secrete infused bile salts indicates impairment to bile secretion (12,13). Secretion of bile is attributed to three processes. A fraction of the bile secreted into canaliculi is dependent on the secretion of bile salts (14,15,16) whereas the second fraction of canalicular bile is secreted independently of bile salts. The second fraction is thought to be related directly with sodium secretion (17). The third component of bile is secreted by the ductular epithelial cells and its secretion is stimulated by the gastrointestinal hormone secretin (18,19,20,21,22,23,24). In sheep the bile salt dependent fraction of canalicular bile and the ductular component of bile are large (16,21).

In experiments in sheep it has been shown that lantana decreases the secretion of canalicular bile but not of the secretin-stimulated ductular bile (12). In these experiments taurocholic acid, the main bile salt in sheep, was infused intravenously into sheep at approximately 20 μmole/min. The bile salt output in bile increased by 26 ± 3.6 μmole/min. The sheep were then given lantana by stomach tube. The response to bile salt infusion was tested one day later and bile salt secretion increased by only 0.3 ± 0.16 μmole/min during the infusion. In a similar experiment it was found that the maximum rate of bile salt secretion by the liver was severely decreased by lantana poisoning (12).

Although the canalicular secretion of bile salts was decreased by lantana, the response of the ductular cells to secretin was slightly enhanced (12). When secretin was infused intravenously at 0.44 clinical units/min into sheep, bile flow increased by 0.26 ± 0.048 ml/min. One day after the sheep had been dosed orally with lantana, secretin elicited an increase in bile flow of 0.44 ± 0.082 ml/min.

A number of observations indicate that lantana injures the canaliculi. Firstly, lantana poisoning is associated with loss of canalicular ATPase which is distributed on the canalicular membrane of sheep (Fig. 2a) (24). It has been demonstrated that within six hours of dosing sheep orally with lantana, there is some loss of canalicular ATPase from the centrolobular region of the hepatic acinus; and within 24 hours, there is complete loss of canalicular ATPase from the acinus. In some cases however, the periportal region is spared (Fig. 2b) (13).

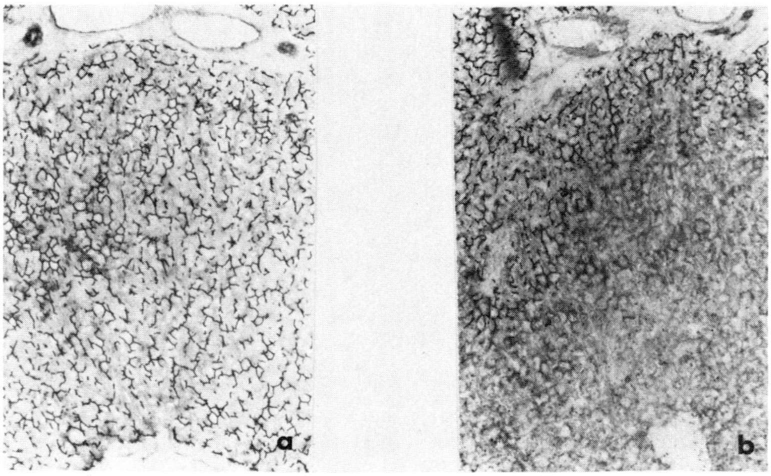

Fig. 2. *Effect of lantana on canalicular ATPase in sheep. (a) In normal liver there is an even distribution of ATPase activity throughout the hepatic acinus. (b) Twenty-four hours after lantana was given ATPase activity is present only in the periportal region of the hepatic acinus.*

A second observation supporting canalicular damage by lantana is collapse of the canaliculi (25). The normal canaliculus is an area approximately 1-5 μ in diameter between adjacent hepatocytes and its surface is lined by microvilli. Six hours after sheep were dosed orally with lantana the microvilli were fragmented and by 24 hours the canaliculi had collapsed (Fig. 3).

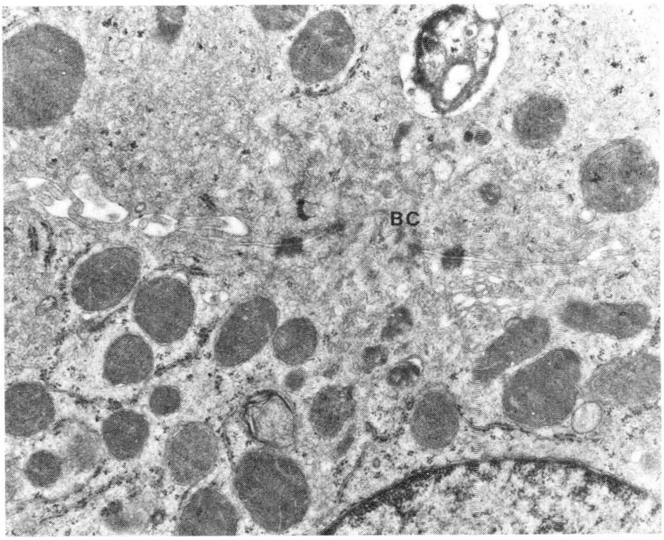

Fig. 3. *Collapse of a bile canaliculus (BC) is evident in the liver of a sheep 24 hours after lantana was given.*

Although bile secretion is reduced in lantana poisoning, it appears that the hepatocytes retain some of their metabolic functions. This is shown by the fact that in lantana-poisoned sheep about 60 percent of the retained bilirubin is conjugated (13). The total serum bilirubin level in poisoned sheep is several times that found in normal animals and, in normal sheep, only about 30 percent of the serum bilirubin is conjugated (13). Bilirubin is conjugated by the mixed function oxidase system of the agranular endoplastic reticulum of hepatocytes (26). It has been shown that lantana causes an increase in the area of agranular endoplasmic reticulum in hepatocytes (Fig. 4) (25) but whether there is an increase in the total enzymic capacity of these membranes has not been determined.

From the available evidence it appears that the hepatocytes are the liver cells affected by lantana and that damage to the canaliculi is an important injury which results in impairment to bile flow.

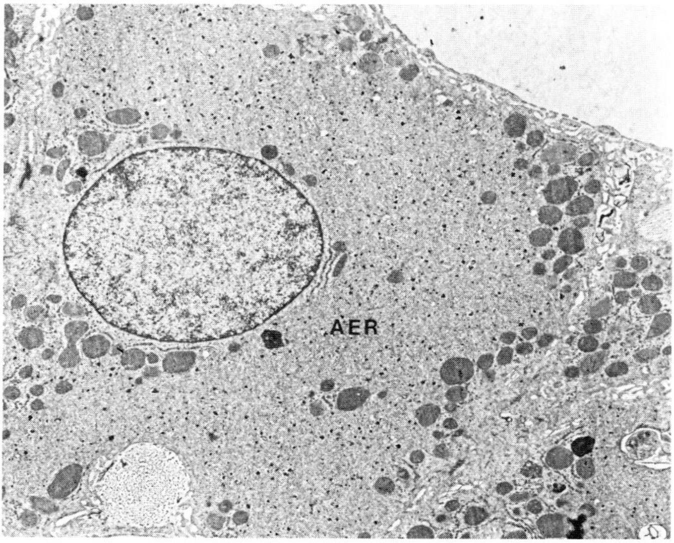

Fig. 4. *Large areas of agranular endoplasmic reticulum (AER) are evident in hepatocytes of a sheep 24 hours after lantana was given.*

V. EFFECT OF LANTANA ON THE GALLBLADDER

Distension of the gallbladder is a consistent finding in animals intoxicated with lantana and this has been attributed to paralysis of the gallbladder muscle (2). In a recent investigation the ability of the gallbladder of the sheep to contract during lantana poisoning was estimated (27). The sheep's gallbladder contracts in response to the intravenous administration of cholecystokinin, pentagastrin or pilocarpine and to the intraduodenal infusion of hydrochloric acid (28,29). After lantana was given to sheep there was a significant reduction in the maximum pressure developed in response to the administration of each of these agents (Table 1). This is taken to indicate that the gallbladder in a poisoned sheep is less able to respond to these stimuli: it is paralyzed.

Some years ago it was demonstrated that the triterpene, icterogen, paralyzed isolated rabbit duodenal muscle (30). In more recent experiments the triterpene lantadene A was shown to inhibit the response of isolated gallbladder muscle to cholecystokinin but

TABLE 1

Gallbladder Contractions in Sheep before and Four Days after Lantana Poisoning in Response to Various Stimuli

Stimulus	No. of sheep	Gallbladder pressure increase (mm mercury) Before poisoning	After poisoning
0.29 u cholecystokinin/kg I.V.	3	8 ± 0.3	2 ± 1.0[1]
1.79 ug pentagastrin/kg I.V.	3	6 ± 1.4	0[1]
60 ug pilocarpine/kg I.V.	4	4 ± 1.1	0.5[2,3]
20 ml hydrochloric acid intraduodenally	4	3 ± 0.7	1.0[2,3]

[1]$P<.05$ by the Wilcoxon two-sample test.
[2]$P<.025$ by the Wilcoxon two-sample test.
[3]Only one sheep responded.
(Reprinted by permission of J. Comp. Pathol.)

not the responses to acetylcholine or pentagastrin (27). During lantana intoxication a number of substances including bile salts are retained and it has been shown that taurocholic acid, the main bile salt in sheep, paralyzes isolated strips of sheep gallbladder (27). This indicates that endogenous substances retained during hepatic insufficiency, together with lantadene A, may contribute to paralysis of the gallbladder.

Hepatic bile enters the gallbladder and its organic components become concentrated by absorption of sodium, chloride, and water (28). In our experiments in sheep with lantana poisoning, the gallbladder became distended with bile which had an average bile salt concentration of 33 ± 5.3 μmole/ml (seven sheep). This was significantly lower ($P<.001$) than the average bile salt concentration of 78 ± 6.4 μmole/ml (eight sheep) found in normal gallbladder bile (13). However, when hepatic bile samples from a normal sheep with bile salt concentrations of 49 ± 3.2 μmole/ml were placed in the gallbladders of four sheep with lantana poisoning and left for three hours, the bile salt concentration increased to 105 ± 17.6 μmole/ml: the bile becomes concentrated (13). It is not known why the gallbladders of sheep with lantana poisoning do not concentrate the bile which normally accumulates.

VI. EFFECT OF LANTANA ON INTESTINAL MOTILITY

It has been considered for a number of years that intestinal paralysis is an important contributor to death in animals with lantana poisoning (2). Except for the demonstration of a reduction in the frequency of ruminal contractions in affected buffalos

(31) there has been no investigation of intestinal motility in animals with lantana poisoning, until recently (32). Contractions of the duodenum in response to pentagastrin given intravenously and to hydrochloric acid given intraduodenally was recorded in four sheep. Lantana was then given to the sheep and the responses to the same agents were tested four days later. There was no difference in the frequency in which these agents stimulated contractions of the duodenum before and during lantana intoxication (32).

In another experiment, vinyl tubes were placed into the jejunum, caecum, and spiral colon of sheep. Spontaneous motility and motility stimulated by subcutaneous injection of bethanechol chloride were recorded before and several times up to 11 days after lantana was given. At each of these times contractions of the jejunum, caecum, and spiral colon, either as spontaneous contractions or as those stimulated by bethanechol chloride, were recorded (32).

The results of these experiments were taken to indicate that intestinal paralysis does not occur in lantana poisoning (32) and that the failure to pass feces which often occurs in this intoxication has some other explanation.

VII. ACKNOWLEDGEMENTS

Part of this work was supported by grants from the Australian Meat Research Committee.

VIII. REFERENCES

1. Seawright, A. A., *Aust. Vet. J.* 41, 235 (1965).
2. Seawright, A. A., *Aust. Vet. J.* 39, 340 (1963).
3. Seawright, A. A., Ph.D. Thesis, University of Queensland, 1965.
4. Seawright, A. A., *Pathol. Vet.* 1, 504 (1964).
5. Louw, P. G. J., *Onderstepoort J. Vet. Sci. Anim. Ind.* 23, 233 (1948).
6. Brown, J. M. M., Rimmington, C., and Sawyer, B. C., *Proc. R. Soc. B* 157, 473 (1963).
7. Seawright, A. A., *J. Comp. Pathol.* 75, 215 (1965).
8. Brown J. M. M., *J. S. Afr. Vet. Med. Assoc.* 39, 35 (1968).
9. Seawright, A. A., and Hrdlicka, J., *Aust. Vet. J.* 53, 230 (1977).
10. Magnenat, P., *Helv. Med. Acta* 37, 175 (1973).
11. Gopinath, C., and Ford, E. J. H., *J. Pathol.* 99, 75 (1969).
12. Pass, M. A., Seawright, A. A., and Heath, T., *Biochem. Pharmacol.* 25, 2101 (1976).
13. Pass, M. A., Ph.D. Thesis, University of Queensland, 1977.
14. Klaassen, C. D., *J. Physiol. London* 224, 259 (1972).
15. Wheeler, H. O., Mancusi-Ungaro, P. L., and Whitlock, R. T., *J. Clin. Invest.* 39, 1039 (1960).

16. Heath, T. J., Caple, I. W., and Redding, P. M., *Q. J. Exp. Physiol.* 55, 93 (1970).
17. Erlinger, S., and Dhumeaux, D., *Gastroenterology* 66, 281 (1974).
18. Mellanby, J., and Suffolk, S. F., *Proc. R. Soc. B* 126, 287 (1938).
19. Preisig, R., Cooper, H. L., and Wheeler, H. O., *J. Clin. Invest.* 41, 1152 (1962).
20. Jones, R. S., and Grossman, M. I., *Am. J. Physiol.* 217, 532 (1969).
21. Caple, I., and Heath, T., *Aust. J. Biol. Sci.* 25, 155 (1972).
22. Wheeler, H. O., *in* "The Biliary System" (W. Taylor, Ed.), p. 481. Blackwell Scientific Publications, Oxford, 1965.
23. Wheeler, H. O., and Mancusi-Ungaro, P. L., *Am. J. Physiol.* 210, 1153 (1966).
24. Gemmell, R. T., and Heath, T., *J. Anat.* 115, 221 (1973).
25. Pass, M. A., Gemmell, R. T., and Heath, T. J., *Toxicol. Appl. Pharmacol.*, In press.
26. Arias, I. M., *in* "Handbook of Physiology" (C. F. Code, Ed.), Section 6, Vol. V, p. 2347. American Physiological Society, Washington, D.C., 1968.
27. Pass, M. A., and Heath, T., *J. Comp. Pathol.*, 87, 301 (1977).
28. Caple, I., and Heath, T. J., *Q. J. Exp. Physiol.* 56, 197 (1971).
29. Pass, M. A., and Heath, T. J., *Comp. Biochem. Physiol.* 56C, 127 (1977).
30. Rimmington, C., Quin, J. I., and Roets, G. C. S., *Onderstepoort J. Vet. Sci. Anim. Ind.* 9, 225 (1937).
31. Dhillon, K. S., and Paul, B. S., *Indian J. Anim. Sci.* 41, 945 (1971).
32. Pass, M. A., and Heath, T. J., *J. Comp. Pathol.*, In press.

V. PLANT CARDIO/PULMONARY TOXINS

Chairman: L. F. James

TOXICITY OF *MYOPORUM SPP*. AND THEIR FURANOSESQUITERPENOID ESSENTIAL OILS

A. A. Seawright, J. S. Lee, J. G. Allen, and J. Hrdlicka
Veterinary School, University of Queensland

I. ABSTRACT

Myoporum spp. *are common causes of poisoning in livestock in Australasia. The plants contain toxic sesquiterpenoid essential oils, the best known of which is ngaione. The intoxication is characterized mainly by liver necrosis, the zonal location of which in any particular animal may be either centrolobular, periportal, or midzonal. Suppression of the activity of the hepatic microsomal mixed function oxidases by pretreatment with drugs or toxins such as SKF525A or* CS_2 *reduces the toxicity of ngaione for the male rat but reduction in the level of these enzymes by means of dietary protein depletion or adrenalectomy does not. The liver lesion observed in all cases is centrolobular necrosis. When the microsomal enzymes are enhanced by pretreatment with phenobarbitone, DDT, or high protein diets the toxicity for ngaione is not altered but the liver lesion is always periportal necrosis. In the intermediate, control state the location of the liver lesion is midzonal. Hepatic microsomal mixed function oxidative metabolism appears to be involved in toxicity of these compounds in animals, but details of the mechanism are not understood.*

II. DISTRIBUTION OF THE PLANTS

The plant family Myoporaceae contains 4 genera, the main toxic representative of which is *Myoporum*. The latter is confined mainly to Australasia and the islands of the South West Pacific, but it is also found in Japan, China, and Mauritius (1). Reports of toxicity of *Myoporum spp*. for livestock have so far come only from Australia (2,3) and New Zealand (4).

The main toxic species are *M. deserti* (Ellangowan Poison Bush) and *M. acuminatum* in eastern Australia (3), *M. tetrandrum* (Boobialla) in Western Australia (5), and *M. laetum* (6) (Ngaio) in New Zealand, while *M. crassifolium* is potentially toxic to livestock in New Caledonia (7).

III. THE TOXIC PRINCIPLES

The toxic principles of these plants are found in the leaves and fruits and are furanosesequiterpenoid (FST) essential oils, the best known of which is ngaione (8). The essential oils of

M. deserti have been most thoroughly investigated chemically and at least 11 different FST have been isolated that are similarly toxic for laboratory animals (9) (Fig. 1).

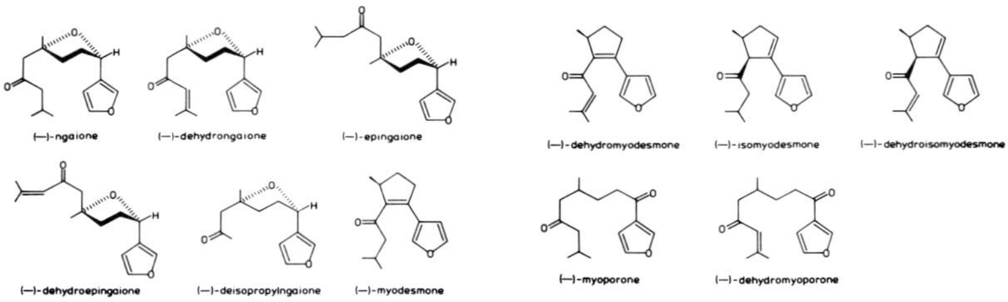

Fig. 1. *The structures of the 11 toxic furanosesquiterpenoids isolated from the various chemical races of* Myoporum deserti *growing in eastern Australia.*

In fact *M. deserti* contains some 9 distinct races within the species depending on the particular compounds present, and not all of them are toxic for livestock (10). For example *M. deserti* containing the FST myoporone and plants of this species not containing FSTs but monoterpenoids such as myodesertin are not toxic for sheep. These different races within *M. deserti* are not distinguishable morphologically. *M. tetrandrum* consistently contains mainly dehydrongaione (5) and *M. laetum* contains solely ngaione (11) as their respective toxic constituents while *M. crassifolium* contains mainly dehydroepingaione (12).

IV. POISONING OF LIVESTOCK

Poisoning of cattle, sheep, horses, and pigs due to consumption of *M. laetum* leaves has been reported in New Zealand (6) and is characterized mainly by acutely developing extensive liver necrosis. Comprehensive descriptions of experimental intoxications of sheep with *M. deserti* (13,14,15) and sheep and calves with *M. tetrandrum* leaves and *M. deserti* FST consisting mainly of hydrongaione (5) have been reported. Lesions noted include photosensitization, jaundice, pale and reddish mottled liver with edema of the gall bladder, excessive clear serous fluid in all the body cavities, free blood in the small and large intestines, intestinal stasis, and dehydration. Pulmonary edema with hydrothorax causing death within a few hours of dosing with the plant or FST oils is often seen in sheep. Microscopically there is either centrolobular, midzonal, or periportal hemorrhagic necrosis of the liver (Figs. 2, 3, and 4) with generalized fatty degeneration of the

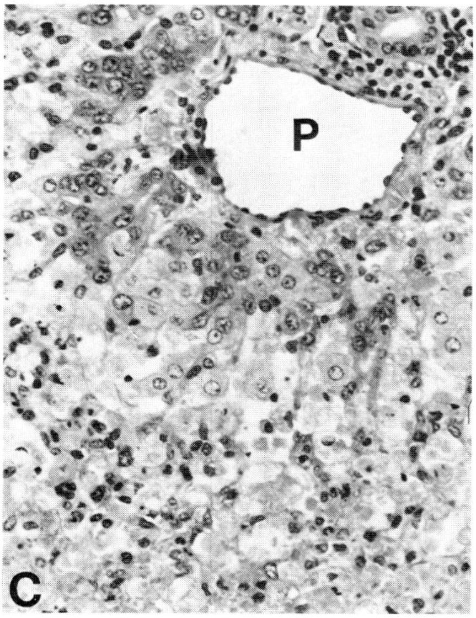

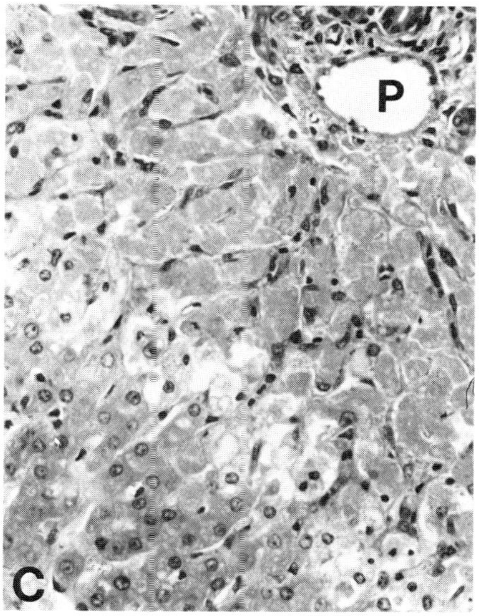

Fig. 2. *Hepatic hemorrhagic centrolobular necrosis in a calf poisoned with* M. tetrandrum.

Fig. 3. *Periportal coagulative necrosis in the liver of a sheep poisoned with* M. tetrandrum. *C = central vein, P = vein H and E x 240.*

parenchyma and fatty infiltration of the uriniferous tubular epithelium and of the myocardium.

V. EXPERIMENTAL HEPATIC LESIONS CAUSED BY FST

Experimental studies of rats and mice dosed with ngaione (6, 11,16) have shown that this oil consistently produces a regular pattern of midzonal necrosis of the hepatic parenchymal cells although centrolobular or periportal necrosis may be observed in some animals. All other known FSTs present in *M. deserti* behave similarly at the same oral dose rate of about 200 mg/kg with the exception of deisopropylngaione which is nephrotoxic as well (9). This apparent lability of the location of the zone of injury to the hepatocytes in FST poisoning of rats and mice also characterizes the pathology of natural *M. deserti* poisoning of sheep and

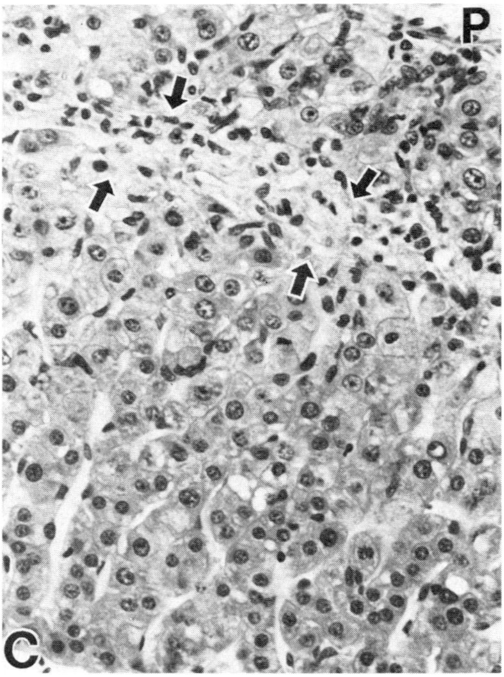

Fig. 4. *Injury to the midzonal hepatocytes of a sheep 5 days after dosing with* M. tetrandrum. *C = central vein, P = portal vein, arrows point to band of injury to parenchyma. H and E x 240.*

cattle (15,5), and provides difficulties for veterinary pathological diagnosis of this intoxication.

Preliminary investigations in mice (17) of the mechanism of this lability of the zone of hepatic parenchymal injury indicated that the location of the hepatocytes affected by these oils could be varied predictably by pretreatment with SKF 525A or phenobarbitone, agents which suppress and enhance respectively the hepatic microsomal mixed function oxidases (MMFO). For example phenobarbitone pretreatment prior to ngaione dosing consistently caused periportal necrosis while dosing with SKF525A before ngaione consistently resulted in centrolobular necrosis. Moreover, the latter pretreatment protected against the overall toxic effects of the oil for the animal by increasing the oral LD50 from 280 to 530 mg/kg. Susceptibility to ngaione at the control level, as well as return of the liver lesion from centrolobular to midzonal necrosis occurred when the suppressed MMFO returned to the initial levels. These findings suggested that ngaione required metabolism in the liver by the MMFO in order to be toxic for the animal. In this respect the compound forms a type I difference spectrum when added to oxidized rat liver microsomes and examined in a double beam recording spectrophotometer (18).

A valid criticism of this explanation of the protective effect afforded by SKF 525A pretreatment is that this compound rapidly causes an outpouring of excessive amounts of gastrointestinal fluids, causing dilution of the orally administered FST thus slowing down its absorption from the gut, and thereby reducing its toxic effect on the liver. Notwithstanding any transient effect SKF525A might have in reducing hepatic MMFO activity, the oil, more slowly absorbed from the gut seems nevertheless to be rapidly eliminated without harm to the animal. Preliminary experiments (19) have shown in fact that pretreatment with SKF525A reduces uptake of an orally administered LD50 of ngaione by about 50% over that of controls within the first hour but that the oil is completely eliminated from the animal by 24 hours. In control mice the ngaione is rapidly absorbed after dosing, but some 25% of the dose is always retained in the gut at the time of death due to liver necrosis 24 to 48 hours later.

VI. SOME FACTORS INFLUENCING THE TOXIC EFFECT OF NGAIONE IN RATS

A. Effect of Pretreatment with Drugs

More extensive investigations of factors which may affect susceptibility to the toxic effects of ngaione and other FSTs have recently been carried out using male rats fed synthetic diets high in carbohydrate with casein as the protein source (20). In order to eliminate variation in absorption from the gut as a factor in the overall toxicity the essential oil was given by the intraperitoneal route. Pretreatments used included phenobarbitone and DDT (20) to enhance the hepatic MMFO, and SKF525A and oral carbon disulphide (CS_2) (21) to reduce the latter enzymes.

As for the mice in previous studies, both SKF525A and CS_2 reduced the toxicity of ngaione for the rats and the lesions again were consistently centrolobular necrosis while in the controls they were midzonal. Induction with phenobarbitone and DDT did not alter the susceptibility of the rats to the ngaione but in both, the liver lesions were again consistently periportal (Table 1). These induced effects in rats subsided in the same way demonstrated in mice in a previous study (17).

B. Effect of Dietary Protein

McLean and McLean (20) showed that low protein diets protected rats against carbon tetrachloride hepatotoxicity through reduction of the hepatic MMFO. In similar experiments in which rats were fed for 10 days on nonprotein, 15% and 30% protein diets, ngaione appeared slightly more toxic for the nonprotein rats than for the

TABLE 1

Effect of Drug Pretreatment[1] *on Hexobarbitone Sleeping Time and Hepatic p-nitroanisole Demethylation* in vitro *and on Toxicity and Liver Lesions due to Ngaione in the Male Rat*

Parameter	Control	SKF525A	Treatment CS_2	Phenobarbitone	DDT
Hexobarbitone sleeping time[2] (minutes)	55±12	448±143	200±12	14±6	13±3
p-nitroanisole Demethylation by liver homogenates[2] (umoles product formed/g liver/ 40 min.)	1.63 ±0.21	0.90 ±0.28	0.26 ±0.09	3.36 ±0.17	2.51 ±0.17
Intraperitoneal LD50 for ngaione (mg/kg and 95% confidence limits)	166 (96-287)	386 (217-684)	413 (213-978)	145 (67-312)	196 (140-274)
Zone of hepatic injury[3]	MZ	CL	CL	PP	PP

[1]Controls were given no treatment, SKF525A was given as an intraperitoneal injection of 40 mg/kg one hour, CS_2 as a 1:1 solution in arachis oil by gavage at 0.5 ml/kg 24 hours, phenobarbitone as 3 consecutive daily intraperitoneal injections of 80 mg/kg the last one 24 hours, and DDT as a 1:10 solution in arachis oil by gavage at 100 mg/kg one week before the experiment respectively.

[2]For hexobarbitone sleeping time and p-nitroanisole demethylation 6 and 4 animals were used respectively. Results are expressed as mean and standard deviation. LD50 determinations were by the method of Weil, R. Biometrics 8, 249 (1952).

[3]CL, MZ, and PP are abbreviations for centrolobular, midzonal, and periportal respectively.

other groups even though the MMFO levels measured both *in vivo* and *in vitro*, were significantly reduced. Again the liver lesion produced in the nonprotein rats was centrolobular necrosis. There was no difference in the hepatic MMFO activity nor in the susceptibility to ngaione in the two protein supplemented groups, but in the 15% protein rats there was an even mixture of centrolobular, midzonal, and periportal liver lesions while in the 30% protein group the liver lesion due to ngaione was periportal (Table 2).

TABLE 2

Effect of Dietary Protein Level on Hexobarbitone Sleeping Time, and Hepatic p-nitroanisole Demethylation in vitro *and on Toxicity and Liver Lesions due to Ngaione in the Male Rat*

Parameter[2]	Protein content of diet[1]		
	Nonprotein	15%	30%
Hexobarbitone sleeping time (minutes)	112±21	24±5	19±4
p-nitroanisole demethylation by liver homogenates (umoles product formed/g liver/ 40 minutes)	0.75±0.16	1.39±0.23	1.20±0.23
Intraperitoneal LD50 for ngaione (mg/kg and 95% confidence limits)	124 (82-189)	185 (126-273)	166 (96-287)
Zone of Hepatic injury (centrolobular, midzonal, periportal)	centrolobular	centrolobular, midzonal and periportal	periportal

[1]Purified diets as described in reference 19.
[2]As for Table 1.

C. Effect of Adrenalectomy

Remmer (22) and Kato and Gillette (23) demonstrated that hepatic MMFO levels in rats are also reduced following adrenalectomy. In an experiment to study the effects of ngaione 7 days after adrenalectomy is was shown that while the LD50 was not significantly increased over that of controls despite the reduction in MMFO activity, the liver lesion in the test rats was centrolobular while in the controls the injury occurred in the midzonal hepatocytes.

D. Effect of Prefeeding *Eucalyptus caleyi*

It had been shown that when rats were fed the basic purified nonprotein diet (19) but supplemented with 10% powdered *Eucalyptus caleyi* (Ironbark) leaf for 7 to 21 days there was an enhancement of their hepatic MMFO (24). The component of the plant which is responsible has been found subsequently to be present in the essential oil fraction consisting mostly of cineol. Cineol itself is able to induce hepatic MMFO activity in rats without increasing the concentration of cytochrome P450 (25). Oral dosing of rats with 500 mg/kg of *E. caleyi* essential oil for 3 consecutive days caused a marked increase in the hepatic MMFO activity. As for previous induction procedures, the sensitivity of the rats to ngaione was unaltered while the liver lesions following ngaione dosing were always periportal.

The effects of the various pretreatments on the toxicity of subsequent administered ngaione are shown in Table 1.

VII. THE MECHANISM OF INDUCED CHANGES TO THE ZONE OF NECROSIS

The various experimental studies in the several species examined support the observation that the activity of the hepatic MMFO at the time of ngaione dosing influences the location of injury to the hepatic parenchyma following administration of the toxin and sometimes also the overall toxicity of the compound for the animal. It has been proposed (17) that ngaione and the other FST oils from *Myoporum spp.* require metabolism by the MMFO to a toxic intermediate compound for injury to occur in the liver cell. Since MMFO activity is low in the periportal hepatocytes then insufficient metabolism of ngaione would normally occur in these cells to cause injury and so they remain unaffected. Enzyme activity in the centrolobular hepatocytes on the other hand is high and since these cells also are unaffected, then the metabolism of ngaione that occurs in them represents an effective detoxication. The midzonal cells in which the enzyme activity is of an intermediate level are damaged and it is therefore proposed that in these cells a toxic intermediate forms and is permitted to accumulate.

With induction, the MMFO increase in all hepatocytes. The detoxicating activity in the midzonal cells is raised to that formerly in the centrolobular cells and they remain unaffected. In the periportal cells, the MMFO activity is raised to that formerly in the midzonal cells, thus permitting incomplete or toxic metabolism of the compound and so cell injury occurs. With suppression of the MMFO, the level of metabolism becomes reduced in all cells until even in the normally resistant centrolobular cells only incomplete detoxication of the FST occurs and cell injury and necrosis occur in this zone. The midzonal and periportal cells contain insufficient functional MMFO and so remain unaffected.

VIII. THE MECHANISM OF OVERALL TOXICITY

At higher dose rates of the FST death occurs too rapidly for the cause to be due simply to liver damage, and this in any case can be prevented by drug induced inhibition of the hepatic MMFO, especially that caused by hepatotoxic agents such as CS_2 (21). Ngaione itself does not appear to be intrinsically injurious to organs other than the liver, suggesting that its hepatic metabolism gives rise to the formation of a toxic metabolite which can leave the liver to affect vital tissues at distant sites. The well-known hepatic MMFO metabolism of largely inactive phosphorothionates to active choline esterase inhibitors is such an effect. In this respect it is of interest that inhibition of the hepatic MMFO in the mouse protects the kidneys from the nephrotoxic effects of deisopropylngaione (26). Moreover, it has been shown that with the synthetic 3-(N-diethylcarbamoyloxymethyl)-furan (DCMF), which causes liver lesions similar to that of ngaione (27), prior inhibition of the hepatic MMFO prevents the liver, lung, and kidney lesions which are also caused by the compound in mice. There is no evidence that inhibitors for the hepatic MMFO are necessarily similarly effective on MMFO in extrahepatic tissues. The more likely explanation of the protective effect described above is that these organs which are normally damaged by a metabolite of the DCMF formed in the liver by MMFO activity escape injury when the latter are inhibited because the proposed toxic metabolite formed is not produced and/or released from the liver in sufficiently large amounts.

IX. CONCLUSION

The findings of the various experimental studies with ngaione- and FST-containing plants in mice, rats, and sheep suggest that the degree of hepatic MMFO activity alone at the time of dosing with FST does not completely explain the pathogenetic mechanisms of toxicity caused by these compounds. For example, reducing the hepatic MMFO activity by means of protein depletion or adrenalectomy rather than by the use of drugs does not render ngaione less toxic for the animals as these procedures do in CCl_4 toxicity (20). Moreover, enhancement of the hepatic MMFO by any means does not increase the toxicity of the FST for the animal (15) but may even also reduce it (17). While it appears that inhibition or induction of the enzymes may consistently alter the zone of injury to the hepatocytes, they do not predictably determine the <u>amount</u> of the liver parenchyma that is damaged nor necessarily prevent the possible formation of toxic metabolites that may be released from the liver to damage remote vital tissues. In other words, qualitative as well as quantitative changes in the MMFO metabolism in the liver of animals exposed to toxic myoporaceous plants or their oils are almost certainly involved in any proposed mechanism of an hepatic MMFO mediation of FST intoxication.

X. REFERENCES

1. Hutchinson, J., "Families of Flowering Plants," Vol. 1, 2nd Ed., p. 503. Clarendon Press, Oxford, 1959.
2. Hurst, E., "Poison Plants of New South Wales," p. 383. New South Wales Poison Plants Committee, Sydney, 1942.
3. Everist, S. L., "Poisonous Plants of Australia," p. 379. Angus and Robertson, Sydney, 1974.

4. Connor, H. E., "The Poisonous Plants in New Zealand," p. 102. Bulletin No. 99, D.S.I.R., 1951.
5. Allen, J. G., Seawright, A. A., and Hrdlicka, J., *Aust. Vet. J.*, In press (1977).
6. Cunningham, I. J., and Hopkirk, C. S. M., *N. Z. J. Sci. Tech.* A26, 333 (1945).
7. Seawright, A. A., unpublished observations.
8. McDowall, F. H., *J. Chem. Soc.* 127, 2200 (1925).
9. Hamilton, W. D., Park, R. J., Perry, G. J., and Sutherland, M. D., *Aust. J. Chem.* 26, 375 (1973).
10. Sutherland, M. D., and Park, R. J., *in* "Terpenoids in Plants" (J. B. Pridham, Ed.), p. 147. Academic Press, London and New York, 1967.
11. Denz, F. A., and Hanger, W. G., *J. Pathol. Bact.* 81, 91 (1961).
12. Sutherland, M. D., personal communication.
13. Legg, J., and White, C. T., *Aust. Vet. J.* 17, 104 (1941).
14. Johnstone, L., and Allen, G. A., *Aust. Vet. J.* 20, 227 (1944).
15. Allen, J. G., and Seawright, A. A., *Res. Vet. Sci.* 15, 167 (1973).
16. Seawright, A. A., and O'Donahoo, R. M., *J. Pathol.* 106, 251 (1972).
17. Seawright, A. A., and Hrdlicka, J., *Br. J. Exp. Pathol.* 53, 242 (1972).
18. Remmer, H., Schenkman, J., Estabrook, R. W., Sasame, H., Gillette, J., Narasimhulu, J., Cooper, D. Y., and Rosenthal, O., *Mol. Pharmacol.* 2, 187 (1966).
19. Seawright, A. A., and Mattocks, A. R., unpublished observations.
20. McLean, A. E. M., and McLean, E. K., *Biochem. J.* 100, 564 (1966).
21. Bond, E. J., and DeMatteis, F., *Biochem. Pharmacol.* 18, 2531 (1969).
22. Remmer, H., *Naturwissenshaften* 45, 522 (1958).
23. Kato, R., and Gillette, J. R., *J. Pharmacol. Exp. Therap.* 150, 285 (1965).
24. Seawright, A. A., Steele, D. P., and Menrath, R. E., *Aust. Vet. J.* 48, 488 (1972).
25. Jori, A., DiSalle, E., and Pescador, R., *J. Pharm. Pharmacol.* 24, 464 (1972).
26. Lee, J. S., and Seawright, A. A., unpublished observations.
27. Seawright, A. A., and Mattocks, A. R., *Experientia* 29, 1197 (1973).

ACUTE RESPIRATORY DISTRESS OF RANGELAND CATTLE

Earl O. Dickinson and James R. Carlson
Oregon State University and Washington State University

I. ABSTRACT

Acute bovine pulmonary emphysema is a disease entity of adult cattle characterized by the sudden onset of acute respiratory distress shortly following a drastic change from dry, low-energy feed to relatively lush, rapidly growing forages. Incidence of the disease is influenced by climatic factors, range and water conditions, age and breed of cattle at risk, and management practices. Signs of increased respiration rate and severe dyspnea occur two to 10 days following the change in forage. Severe, diffuse pulmonary emphysema and edema are the predominant gross lesions. Microscopic changes are characterized by edema, thickening of interstitial tissues, and proliferation of alveolar lining epithelium. The disease may be caused by ruminal conversion of tryptophan, indoleacetic acid, or other indolic precursors to 3-methylindole. This conversion may be accelerated by increased rumen fermentation which occurs when a drastic change in type of forage is made. The lung changes are evidently initiated by extensive vascular leakage. Other edemogenic chemicals may account for the initiation of certain other forms of acute interstitial pneumonia.

II. INTRODUCTION

The subject of the present paper is different from that of most other presentations of this symposium. The plants commonly incriminated as the causative agents of the disease to be discussed are generally considered nontoxic and present a striking contrast to most of those that we characteristically classify as poisonous plants. In fact, the plants to be considered in this case are generally regarded as quite valuable forages and are commonly utilized as normal diets of livestock.

Acute bovine pulmonary emphysema (ABPE) is a disease of cattle characterized by a sudden onset of acute respiratory distress shortly following a change in feed or forage. The syndrome was described as early as 1830 in Europe and there have been numerous subsequent reports from many areas of the world (1). The disease has many synonyms but is generally referred to by the above terminology in the western regions of the United States. In other areas it is often referred to as bovine atypical interstitial pneumonia (2). Local terms often used by ranchers and veterinarians include cow asthma, green grass sickness, summer pneumonia, lungers, grunters, panters, and others. A recent report from Britain indicated that the classical form of fog fever of adult cattle is the same as that known as ABPE in the United States (3).

This paper will attempt to discuss features of the natural disease and report on some observations of field studies that have been conducted in the past few years. The paper to follow will present some of the recent experimental work that implicates the possible role of tryptophan and related indole-containing compounds in the causation of ABPE.

III. DIFFERENTIAL DIAGNOSIS

Acute bovine pulmonary emphysema should be regarded as a distinct entity of adult cattle that is associated with a sudden change from rather dry, low energy ration to a relatively lush, highly digestable forage. Several other forms of acute interstitial pneumonia may cause clinical signs and post mortem lesions that are superficially similar to ABPE (4). These include diseases caused by ingestion of moldy feeds (5,6), ingestion of certain poisonous plants such as *Zieria arborescens* (7,8) or *Perilla frutescens* (9), inhalation of organic allergens (10,11,12), migration of nematode larvae through the lungs (13,14,15), inhalation of noxious gases (16,17), or infection with some viruses (18). Similarities of these diseases to ABPE have led to the unfortunate tendency to attempt to categorize the latter entity as the same as one or another or the others. However, careful evaluation of the case history, epizootiology, signs, and lesions will generally permit a differential diagnosis.

IV. INCIDENCE

Disease incidence varies considerably from year to year and from one region to another (19,20). Its occurrence is quite unpredictable and causes for this variation are not always clear.

Morbidity in affected herds is reported to range from one to one hundred percent (19,21). Case fatality usually varies from zero to fifty percent, although some outbreaks have noted case fatalities up to ninety percent (19,20,21).

The disease occurs at any time of the year but is observed most commonly in the late summer or early fall (20,21,22). Seasonal incidence is apparently due to the practice of transferring cattle from dry summer range to improved pastures in the late summer. With less frequency, it may be observed at any time of the year following drastic changes in feed such as in rotational grazing or when cattle are changed from low energy to high energy rations.

A factor probably involved in variation in annual incidence is the variation in climatic conditions which affect either the summer range, the meadows onto which the cattle are transferred, or both (23,24). Generally speaking, the incidence is increased following exceptionally dry summers which contribute to adverse feed and water conditions of the summer range.

Marked differences in incidence occur between various ranges and water drainages (unpublished observations, 1974). Reasons for these differences are not clear. Range conditions and management practices between "problem" and non-problem" areas often appear quite similar. These observations suggest there may be subtle differences in soil and water factors which affect plant growth and physiology. Some preliminary work on our project demonstrated that soil samples taken from inciting areas were generally lower in phosphorous, potassium and zinc content than those taken from "non-trouble" areas (unpublished observations, 1974). These findings were not statistically significant; however, the trend was apparent and the influence of soil and water conditions should be studied further.

Disease incidence is much more prevalent in cattle over two to three years of age and quite rare in animals less than a year old (20,25,26,27). This feature of epizootiology is quite consistent. Generally speaking, when a high incidence of acute respiratory distress is observed in cattle less than two years of age, other causes such as migrating nematode larvae, ingestion of moldy feed or pulmonary viral infection should be suspected. Causes for the increased incidence in older animals are unknown. Experimental evidence suggests that young animals are affected to a minor degree but that the changes are subtle and not readily observed by casual examination (28). A possible explanation for the increased incidence in older cattle may be that repeated insults caused by this and other respiratory diseases result in a progressive decrease in pulmonary reserve. Consequently, older animals may lose their capacity to resist the disease. Experimental evidence tends to support this hypothesis (29), and increased susceptibility to the acute manifestations of the natural disease has been associated with the presence of chronic, pre-existing lung damage (30).

The disease has been reported in both dairy and beef animals and probably no breed is entirely resistant (20,31). However, variation in breed susceptibility has been suggested (32). Evidence suggests that among the beef breeds, Herefords are probably the most susceptible breed and that Angus cattle are more resistent. Another report indicated that among dairy animals, the Channel Island breeds are more susceptible (22).

The disease is observed most commonly in adult cows; however, bulls are affected and are probably equally susceptible (20,31). Increased observation in cows is probably a result of differences in management practices between the cow and bull herds.

Management practices play an important role in the incidence of the disease. As previously stated, the highest incidence occurs following a very sudden or drastic change in feed or forage. If efforts are made to avoid these sudden changes, disease incidence is minimized. Evidence for this is provided by the observation that one of the most effective methods for prevention of the disease is by controlled management of cattle at the time a change of forage is made (20,22,31). In this procedure, the cattle are moved to dry lot, fed hay, and placed in the new pasture for gradually increasing periods each day. This adjusts them gradually to the new forage so that a sudden or drastic change does not occur. In some instances a "new" outbreak has been reported following a change in ownership of a ranch (unpublished observations, 1974). Investigation sometimes reveals that the previous owners had been familiar with the disease but had "managed around" the situation to minimize the effects of a sudden change in forage. The new owner, unaware of the previous history, fails to take the precautions and a "new" outbreak is observed.

V. CLINICAL SIGNS

Antemortem signs of ABPE are fairly characteristic (19,20,21, 22,31,33). Onset usually becomes apparent between two and ten days after a change in feed or forage. The most obvious clinical sign is an increased rate of respiration accompanied by severe dyspnea. An audible expiratory grunt is commonly observed and is a useful diagnostic aid. The body temperature is generally normal or only slightly elevated.

Affected cattle stand with the head lowered. As the disease progresses, there is mouth breathing and the tongue is protruded. The animals will generally remain standing because it is easier for them to breath in that position.

The course may vary from a few hours to a few days after onset of clinical signs. It is often difficult to predict which cattle in an affected group will die because some that have severe clinical signs will recover, whereas others that have less obvious signs will die unexpectedly. Forced exercise and exertion often result in death.

VI. POST MORTEM LESIONS

Gross lesions at necropsy are quite striking and are generally limited to the respiratory system (4,34). Lesions in other tissues and organs are considered secondary to respiratory decompensation.

The lungs are very large and fail to collapse when the thorax is opened (4,15,23,31,33). Also, they are quite heavy due to the presence of considerable quantities of edematous fluid.

Interstitial pulmonary emphysema is quite striking (4,20,22, 31,33,34). Accumulations of air in the form of bubbles, clefts, and irregular spaces are prominent. Large bullae are often observed.

Pulmonary edema is a prominent and consistent feature (4,20, 22, 31,33,34). Thick gelatinous fluid is present throughout the lung lobules and interstitial areas. The lobules are dark red, firmer than normal and exude watery fluid when cut. White frothy fluid is generally observed in the trachea and branches of the bronchial tree.

Emphysema and edema may also be observed in the bronchial and mediastinal lymph nodes and other mediastinal and pericardial tissues (4,20,22). Severe cases are likely to have emphysema of the perirenal areas and subcutaneous tissues of the neck, shoulders, and back.

Microscopic changes are characterized by severe pulmonary edema, marked thickening of interstitial tissues and alveolar septa, and striking proliferation of alveolar lining epithelium (4,20,31,34). The swollen epithelial cells often detach from the alveolar linings to lie free in the alveolar lumina. Scattered inflammatory cells are present, but these are minimal.

VII. CAUSE AND PATHOGENESIS

The specific causes and pathogenesis of the disease remain unknown. A great variety of plant types have been associated with onset of the disease. Onset has been correlated with ingestion of both native and improved grass types (4,19,20,24,30,31,35,36,37), legumes (20,31,37,38,39), cruciferous plants such as rape and kale (31,33,40), some weeds (7,8,9,41), and others. No single plant type, dietary ingredient or combination of plants or ingredients have been consistently associated as the cause. The wide variety of plants that have been incriminated suggests that a change or sudden change to any lush forage, regardless of type, might precipitate an outbreak of the disease.

Other than the association with sudden change from dry to relatively lush forage, the specific cause and mechanism of the disease remains unknown. Numerous hypotheses have been proposed and extensive experimental work has been conducted. However, to date, none has conclusively demonstrated the cause and mechanism.

An allergic phenomenon associated with ingestion or inhalation of a sensitizing antigen or infection with *Dictyocaulus viviparous* has often been proposed as the basic mechanism of the disease (10, 42,43,44,45,46). Another popular proposal has been that the lung changes were induced as the result of inhaled gases or other volatile substances which act as irritants to the lung tissues (47,48, 49). Another proposal regarding pathogenesis has been that the respiratory disease represents a manifestation of indigestion, gastrointestinal intoxication, or enterotoxemia that is precipitated by change in feed (19,33). Each of the above points can be argued with some justification. However, no conclusive evidence to substantiate any of the hypotheses has been demonstrated.

Some recent experimental work has provided promising leads into the possible causes and mechanisms of the natural disease. It has been demonstrated that when cattle are given large intraruminal doses of tryptophan or indoleacetic acid, a disease is produced which has many similarities to naturally occurring ABPE

(50,51,52). Other work has demonstrated that ruminal microorganisms convert these compounds to 3-methylindole (3MI) and that both intraruminal and intravenous administration of 3MI cause acute pulmonary edema and emphysema in cattle (53,55). Onset, clinical signs, and post mortem changes of the experimental disease are essentially the same as those observed in the natural disease. Other interesting correlations between the experimental and natural diseases include similarities in the age, breed, and species susceptibilities.

The definitive link between the experimental disease and naturally occurring ABPE remains to be conclusively demonstrated. The working hypothesis is that tryptophan, indoleacetic acid, or similar indolic compounds are present in certain feeds or forages; that these are converted to 3MI by the action of rumen bacteria; that 3MI is transferred to the lungs by vascular transport; and that progressive damage occurs in the lung as a result of the effect of 3MI. Further, it is assumed that ruminal conversion of the precursors of 3MI is accelerated under appropriate conditions (increased rumen activity and fermentation) precipitated by sudden changes in feed or forage.

The observation that severe diffuse pulmonary edema is present as an early and consistent change in both the natural and experimental diseases suggests that the mechanism at the lung level is associated with increased vascular permeability. Alterations in the hemodynamic balance could come about as a result of increased capillary pressure, endothelial changes, epithelial damage, alteration of alveolar surfactant, or combinations of these changes. Regardless of the precise mechanism resulting in the edematous change, other lung lesions (interstitial emphysema, interstitial thickening, proliferation of alveolar epithelial cells) could develop as a result of severe edema as the initiating change.

VIII. SUMMARY

Acute bovine pulmonary emphysema represents a distinct entity of adult cattle which has certain features of epizootiology, clinical manifestations, and post mortem changes that serve to differentiate it from other forms of acute interstitial pneumonia of cattle. The disease is not caused by ingestion of classical types of poisonous plants. Instead, it is manifested as a result of ruminal conversion of non-toxic precursors to a toxic compound. Recent experimental work indicates that tryptophan or related indolic compounds may be responsible for the forage related disease as presently described.

It should also be emphasized that the authors make no attempt to propose that indolic compounds are factors in the causation of other forms of interstitial pneumonia. If there is a unifying concept between ABPE and certain other types of interstitial pneumonia, it might be that there are a number of chemical agents that are capable of inciting pulmonary edema of sufficient quantity and quality to induce a series of subsequent lung changes that once triggered, provide an end result that appears quite similar, i.e.; there may be more than one beginning to a commen end. We would like to propose that there may be certain chemicals in moldy feeds, certain toxic weeds, or other rations that serve as edemogenic agents that incite a pulmonary response characteristic of acute interstitial pneumonia. The validity of this hypothesis remains to be tested.

IX. ACKNOWLEDGMENTS

This project was supported in part by grants supplied through the Pacific Northwest Forest and Range Experiment Station, Portland, Oregon (FS-PNW-Grants 11, 16, and 31) and the Oregon Agricultural Experiment Station, Corvallis, Oregon (Project 256).

X. REFERENCES

1. Maki, L. R., and Tucker, J. O., *in* "Proceedings Symposium Acute Bovine Pulmonary Emphysema," p. 1. University of Wyoming, Laramie, Wyoming, 1963.
2. Blood, D. C., and Henderson, J. A., *in* "Veterinary Medicine,' 4th Ed., p. 915. Bailliere, Tindall, and Cassell, London, 1974.
3. Selman, I. E., Wiseman, A., Breeze, R. G., and Pirie, H. M., *Vet. Rec.* 99, 181-184 (1976).
4. King. J. M., *West. Vet.* 8, 42-50 (1961).
5. Monlux, W. S., Fitte, J., Kendrick, G., and Dubuisson, H., *Southwest. Vet.* 6, 267 (1953).
6. Peckham, J. C., Mitchell, F. E., Jones, O. H., and Doupnik, B., *J. Am. Vet. Med. Assoc.* 160, 169 (1972).
7. Stephens, W. H., *Tasmanian J. Agric.* 38, 84-86 (1967).
8. Munday, B. L., *Aust. Vet. J.* 44, 501-502 (1968).
9. Peterson, D. R., *in* "Proceedings Symposium Acute Bovine Pulmonary Emphysema and Related Respiratory Diseases," p. R1. University of Wyoming, Laramie, Wyoming, 1965.
10. Jenkins, P. A., and Pepys, J., *Vet. Rec.* 77, 464-466 (1965).
11. Pirie, H. M., Dawson, C. O., Breeze, R. G., Wiseman, A., and Hamilton, J., *Vet. Rec.* 88, 346-351 (1971).
12. Wiseman, A., Selman, I. E., Dawson, C. O., Breeze, R. G., and Pirie, H. M., *Vet. Rec.* 93, 410-417 (1973).
13. Allen, G. W., *Can. J. Comp. Med.* 26, 241-243 (1962).
14. McIntyre, W. I. M., *in* "Proceedings Symposium Acute Bovine Pulmonary Emphysema," p. 54. University of Wyoming, Laramie, Wyoming, 1963.
15. Mackenzie, A., *in* "Proceedings Symposium Acute Bovine Pulmonary Emphysema and Related Respiratory Diseases," p. E1. University of Wyoming, Laramie, Wyoming, 1965.
16. Haynes, N. B., *J. Am. Vet. Med. Assoc.* 143, 593-594 (1963).
17. Brightwell, A. H., *Can. Vet. J.* 13, 224-225 (1972).

18. Omar, A. R., *Vet. Bull.* 36, 259-273 (1966).
19. Tucker, J. O., and Maki, L. R., *Am. J. Vet. Res.* 23, 821-823 (1962).
20. Condensed Minutes of Meeting on Acute Bovine Pulmonary Emphysema, Sheridan, Wyoming, 1959, *in* "Proceedings Symposium Acute Bovine Pulmonary Emphysema," p. 71. University of Wyoming, Laramie, Wyoming, 1963.
21. Maki, L. R., and Tucker, J. O., *in* "Proceedings Symposium Acute Bovine Pulmonary Emphysema and Related Respiratory Diseases," p. Al. University of Wyoming, Laramie, Wyoming, 1965.
22. Hyslop, N. St. G., *Can. Vet. J.* 10, 251-257 (1969).
23. Railsback, G. A., *Vet. Med.* 40, 369-370 (1945).
24. Klussendorf, F. C., *North Am. Vet.* 35, 745-746 (1954).
25. Gibbons W. J., *Mod. Vet. Pract.* 43, 34-38 (1962).
26. Moulton, J. E., Cornelius, C. E., and Osburn, B. I., *J. Am. Vet. Med. Assoc.* 142, 133-137 (1963).
27. Blake, J. T., and Thomas, D. W., *J. Am. Vet. Med. Assoc.* 158, 2047-2052 (1971).
28. Dickinson, E. O., Ph.D. Thesis, p. 89. Washington State University, Pullman, Washington, 1970.
29. Dickinson, E. O., Ph.D. Thesis, p. 155. Washington State University, Pullman, Washington, 1970.
30. Gils, J. H. J. van, *Tijdschr. Diergeneeskd.* 76, 833-839 (1951).
31. Blood, D. C., *Can. Vet. J.* 3, 40-47 (1962).
32. Monlux, W. S., Cutlip, R. D., and Estes, P. C., *Cornell Vet.* 60, 547-551 (1970).
33. Schofield, F. W., *J. Am. Vet. Med. Assoc.* 112, 254-259 (1948).
34. Griner, L. A., *in* "Proceedings Symposium Acute Bovine Pulmonary Emphysema," p. 26. University of Wyoming, Laramie, Wyoming, 1963.
35. Begg, H., and Whiteford, W. A., *Vet. Rec.* 60, 135 (1948).
36. Maki, L. R., and Tucker, J. O., *Am. J. Vet. Res.* 23, 824-826 (1962).
37. Bennell, D. G., *N. Z. Vet. J.* 140, 73 (1966).
38. Moore, G. R., *North Am. Vet.* 33, 418 (1952).
39. Juin, A. H., *Can. Vet. J.* 2, 80 (1961).
40. Cote, F. T., *Can. J. Comp. Med.* 8, 38-41 (1944).
41. Rainey, J. W., *Vet. Rec.* 70, 167-168 (1958).
42. Mackey, D. R., *Southwest. Vet.* 5, 342-344 (1952).
43. Michel, J. F., *Nature* 171, 940 (1953).
44. Michel, J. F., *Vet. Rec.* 66, 381-384 (1954).
45. Mackenzie, A., *Proc. R. Soc. Med.* 59, 1008-1012 (1966).
46. Aitken, M. M., and Sanford, J., *J. Comp. Pathol.* 79, 131 (1969).
47. Hull, M. W., *in* "Proceedings Symposium Acute Bovine Pulmonary Emphysema and Related Respiratory Diseases," p. Hl. University of Wyoming, Laramie, Wyoming, 1965.
48. Hull, M. W., *in* "Proceedings Symposium Acute Bovine Pulmonary Emphysema and Related Respiratory Diseases," p. Ll.

University of Wyoming, Laramie, Wyoming 1965.
49. Cutlip, R. C., *Pathol. Vet.* 3, 474-485 (1966).
50. Johnson, R. J., and Dyer, I. A., *Life Sci.* 5, 1121-1124 (1966).
51. Dickinson, E. O., Spencer, G. R., and Gorham, J. R., *Vet. Rec.* 80, 487-489 (1967).
52. Dickinson, E. O., Ph.D. Thesis, p. *iv-vi*. Washington State University, Pullman, Washington, 1970.
53. Yokoyama, M. J., and Carlson, J. R., *Appl. Microbiol.* 27, 540-548 (1974).
54. Carlson, J. R., Dickinson, E. O., Yokoyama, M. J., and Bradley, B. J., *Am. J. Vet. Res.* 36, 1341-1347 (1975).

TRYPTOPHAN-INDUCED PULMONARY EDEMA AND EMPHYSEMA IN RUMINANTS

James R. Carlson and Earl O. Dickinson
Washington State University and University of Nebraska

I. ABSTRACT

Intraruminal doses of tryptophan cause acute pulmonary edema and emphysema in cattle (ABPE), and the time course, clinical signs and pulmonary lesions are similar to those observed in naturally occurring ABPE which develops after an abrupt change in pasture conditions. Tryptophan is converted to indoleacetic acid by ruminal microorganisms and indoleacetic acid is decarboxylated to 3-methylindole (3MI) by a recently identified Lactobacillus *organism. Three-methylindole is the ruminal fermentation product of tryptophan which causes the characteristic pulmonary lesions in cattle. Metabolism of 3MI rapidly clears the blood and results in the urinary excretion of 10 metabolites, primarily oxindole derivatives. The formation of metabolites may be related to pulmonary toxicity of 3MI. It appears that high intake of lush, green forage could provide adequate amounts of tryptophan to cause ABPE under field conditions. Ruminal fermentation conditions can effect the conversion of tryptophan to 3MI and may influence the incidence and severity of ABPE. Antibiotics and inhibitors decrease the formation of 3MI from tryptophan and prevent the onset of experimentally-induced ABPE. Ruminal fluid and plasma of cows given access to lush, green pasture contain 3MI. The results support the hypothesis that 3MI, formed from tryptophan in the rumen, is associated with the development of ABPE.*

II. INTRODUCTION

Acute bovine pulmonary edema and emphysema (ABPE) or fog fever, as it is referred to in Britain is a naturally-occurring disease of cattle and the clinical signs and pulmonary lesions associated with this syndrome have been reported (1-5). The disease occurs in cattle of both sexes but it is most frequent in cows over 2 years of age. It usually develops in late summer or early fall within a few days after cattle are changed from dry range grass to lush, green pasture (4,6,7).

The specific cause of ABPE has not been determined, but previous theories have generally involved some form of hypersensitivity or intoxication. Aitken and Sanford (8) have shown that experimental anaphylaxis results in pulmonary lesions which are similar to those observed in fog fever, including pulmonary congestion, edema, and interstital emphysema. But the anaphylactic response differed from fog fever by a more rapid onset and the lack of alveolar epithelial hyperplasia and hyaline membranes, suggesting that these syndromes were not the same (9). Breeze *et al.* (10) and Pirie *et al.* (11) have shown that fog fever does not result from hypersensitivity to lung worms (Dictyocaulus viviparus) or to moldy hay containing *Micropolyspora faeni* which results in extrinsic allergic aveolitis similar to farmers lung disease. In general, there is little convincing evidence that ABPE results primarily from a hypersensitivity reaction (9).

Specific forages have not been implicated as causative agents even though affected cattle have often been consuming alfalfa, kale, rape, turnip tops, rapidly growing pasture grasses, or other feeds (1,7,12). Moldy sweet potatoes have been shown to cause similar pulmonary lesions resulting from the presence of a toxin, 4-ipomeanol (13,14), but it is unlikely that this toxin is present in the lush, green pastures where most cases of ABPE occur. Attempts to show that ABPE resulted from Clostridial exotoxins were unsuccessful (15). The most consistent observation associated with the development of naturally occurring ABPE is the recent change to better quality pasture. This suggests that some component of the forage may be the causative agent and that excessive intake and/or altered ruminal fermentation resulting from the abrupt change in grazing conditions may contribute to the development of ABPE.

II. TRYPTOPHAN-INDUCED ACUTE PULMONARY DISEASE IN CATTLE

Intraruminal doses of L-tryptophan and indoleacetic acid (IAA) cause acute pulmonary edema and emphysema in cattle (16-20) and the time course, clinical signs, and pulmonary lesions appear to be identical to those seen in naturally occurring ABPE. D-tryptophan does not cause pulmonary disease (21).

The typical clinical signs of respiratory distress appear within 24 to 36 hours after L-tryptophan dosing and by 4 days the predominant pulmonary lesions include edema, interstitial emphysema, hyaline membranes, and hyperplasia of alveolar lining cells (18,20). A dose of 0.35 g L-tryptophan/kg body weight (BW) has been routinely used to induce pulmonary lesions and this dose usually results in the development of severe respiratory distress and/or death in approximately one-half of the cows within 4 days after dosing (18,20,22). Less severe clinical signs and pulmonary lesions may develop in some animals given the same dose of tryptophan. Slightly lower doses, equivalent to 0.26 - 0.3 g L-tryptophan/kg BW (0.51 - 0.60 g D,L-tryptophan/kg BW) have been used with similar incidence and severity of animal response (18) and higher doses do not necessarily increase the severity of response (R. G. Breeze, personal communication). Although tryptophan obviously induces pulmonary lesions in cattle, the results suggest that within the limits of the doses tested, the incidence and severity of pulmonary disease is not necessarily dependent on the size of the dose.

The minimum effective dose of tryptophan has not been established but the data indicate that a single dose of 0.26 - 0.35 g L-tryptophan/kg BW is sufficient to cause experimentally-induced ABPE. Parenteral administration of tryptophan or indoleacetic acid does not cause the characteristic pulmonary lesions indicating that ruminal fermentation of these compounds is required (16, unpublished observations). As will be discussed later, metabolism of tryptophan in the rumen can vary, suggesting that variations in fermentation could explain the somewhat variable response of cows to the same dose of tryptophan. If ruminal fermentation of tryptophan can be enhanced, it is possible that tryptophan doses, lower than those previously used, may induce ABPE in some cattle. In addition, if the tryptophan in the forages is the major substrate related to naturally-occurring ABPE, and if ruminal fermentation is variable; it is not essential that the tryptophan content of pastures be higher where ABPE occurs than where ABPE does not occur. Mackenzie (23) observed that the tryptophan contents of 2 control pastures and 3 pastures where fog fever occurred were not significantly different (mean concentration was 0.37% tryptophan, dry matter basis).

The amount of tryptophan consumed in the forage during naturally-occurring ABPE is not known. Cattle have been observed to readily consume the highly digestible lush, green grass after being moved from poor quality forage. This probably results in a higher than normal feed intake during the first few days after pasture change and during the time when drastic changes in ruminal flora may be occurring to accommodate increased amounts and a different type of forage than previously consumed. A reasonable estimate of tryptophan consumption can be calculated by assuming a dry matter intake of 3.5% of BW/day for a 450 kg cow (24) and tryptophan content of 0.37% (23). This estimate of 0.13 g tryptophan/kg BW/day is approximately one-half of the single oral dose used in experimental trials and indicates that amounts of tryptophan equivalent to those used in experimental doses can be ingested from forages if consumption continues for 2 or 3 days.

As described later, 3-methylindole (3MI) is the ruminal fermentation product of tryptophan which has been shown to cause pulmonary lesions. Infusion of 0.03 to 0.04 g 3MI/kg BW to goats (approximately 1/4 to 1/3 of the estimated daily tryptophan intake of cattle) causes severe pulmonary lesions suggesting that lower doses of 3MI are effective and that the percentage conversion of tryptophan to 3MI in the rumen may be important in development of ABPE. Since the minimum amount of tryptophan required to cause pulmonary lesions is not known, it appears that adequate amounts could be consumed in the forage under the rather unusual grazing conditions associated with ABPE.

III. TRYPTOPHAN FERMENTATION BY RUMINAL MICROORGANISMS

Results obtained from tryptophan administration to cattle

indicated that a product of ruminal fermentation was responsible for the experimentally-induced pulmonary disease (16). The fermentation of tryptophan by ruminal microorganisms was investigated both *in vitro* and *in vivo*. Incubation of tryptophan [containing L-(U-benzene ring-^{14}C) tryptophan] for 24 hours with ruminal fluid obtained from cattle fed hay, resulted in 39, 7, and 4% of the added radioactivity being converted to 3-methylindole, indole, and indoleacetic acid respectively (22,25). Incubation of IAA resulted in the formation of 3MI indicating that the major pathway of 3MI formation was the conversion of tryptophan to IAA and subsequent decarboxylation of IAA to 3MI. The major *in vitro* fermentation product of tryptophan was 3MI with smaller amounts of indole. D-tryptophan was not converted to any of these metabolites.

The next objective was to determine whether 3MI or indole was the cause of experimentally-induced ABPE. Three cows were each given an intraruminal dose of indole (0.35 g/kg BW). Clinical signs of respiratory distress were not observed in any of these animals during the 4-day experimental period and there were no significant pulmonary lesions at necropsy. Internal hemorrhage, bloody feces and renal damage were noted at necropsy in these cattle (unpublished observations).

Three-methylindole was given to cattle as a single intraruminal dose (0.2 and 0.1 g/kg BW) and by intravenous infusion (0.06 g/kg BW) over 12 hours. Characteristic clinical signs and pulmonary lesions developed in all of these cattle (26). All 3 of the cattle given an oral dose of 0.2 g 3MI/kg BW and 1 cow given the infusion died within 72 hr after dosing. The 2 cattle given an oral dose of 0.1 g 3MI/kg BW and the remaining 2 cows given an infusion developed severe pulmonary lesions. These results demonstrate that 3MI may be effective in lower doses and that the animal response is more uniform compared to tryptophan. Also, in contrast to tryptophan and IAA, 3MI is effective when given by intravenous infusion which indicates that 3MI is the fermentation product responsible for the development of pulmonary lesions in cattle. This was confirmed by giving L-tryptophan to 5 cows and measuring the 3MI in ruminal fluid and plasma after dosing (20). Three cows developed severe clinical signs, 1 developed moderate signs, and 1 developed mild clinical signs. At necropsy, 4 days after dosing, the severity of pulmonary lesions appeared to be related to the severity of clinical signs. Cows exhibiting a severe response had higher concentrations of 3MI in ruminal fluid and plasma and maintained these concentrations for a longer time than cows with a mild or moderate response. 3MI was not present in ruminal fluid or plasma of 3 control cows. The results of this study provide evidence that ruminal fermentation conditions in individual animals may alter the conversion of tryptophan to 3MI and the severity of pulmonary lesions.

The unusual grazing conditions associated with ABPE often involve cattle which have been grazing on sparse, poor quality forage and which have been moved, with little access to feed for a period of time, before being given access to high quality forage.

It is conceivable that these conditions contribute to greater ruminal 3MI formation when the cattle consume large amounts of lush forage. This contention is supported by the observation that the incidence and severity of ABPE may be less during years when higher quality forage is available on the summer ranges and when the degree of change in forage quality is less when cattle are moved.

The factors affecting the conversion of tryptophan to 3MI in the rumen are not completely understood but progress has been made in elucidating the reactions and the microorganism involved in 3MI formation. The *in vitro* studies demonstrating the formation of 3MI from tryptophan suggested that this is a two step process: (1) conversion of tryptophan to IAA, and (2) decarboxylation of IAA to 3MI (25). Protozoa are not involved. Recently, a bacterium was isolated from ruminal fluid which is capable of decarboxylating IAA to 3MI, but it does not metabolize tryptophan (27). This organism is a gram positive, non-motile, non-spore forming bacillus. It is a strict anaerobe and produces lactic acid, predominately D (-) lactate. This is apparently the first demonstration of IAA decarboxylation to 3MI in pure culture and the organism has been assigned to the genus, *Lactobacillus*. Factors affecting the growth and 3MI production by this organism are currently under investigation.

IV. METABOLISM OF 3MI IN CATTLE AND GOATS

For metabolic studies, goats have proven useful because of their smaller size and because both intraruminal doses and infusion of 3MI causes qualitatively similar clinical signs and pulmonary lesions compared to cattle (28,29). A remarkable feature of 3MI metabolism in both of these species is the relatively low plasma concentrations and the rapid clearance of 3MI from the plasma after dosing. We have often noted that the plasma 3MI concentrations have decreased to low levels by the time significant clinical signs of respiratory distress appear (20,26,28,29,30). Jugular infusion of 0.06 g 3MI/kg BW over 12 hr in cattle or 0.03 - 0.04 g 3MI/kg BW over 2 hr in goats resulted in a maximum of about 8-10 μg 3MI/ml plasma and the total estimated blood volume contained approximately 1 - 1.5% of the dose during infusion (26,29). After infusion, 3MI is cleared from the blood with a half-life of approximately 0.3 - 0.4 hr (29,31). These results demonstrate that 3MI is rapidly removed from the blood and suggest that it is either accumulating in the tissues or excreted.

For metabolic studies, [methyl-^{14}C] 3MI was prepared microbiologically from [2-^{14}C]-indoleacetic acid. Goats given 0.03 - 0.04 g 3MI/kg BW by infusion over 2 hr excreted 25% of the infused radioactivity by one-half hr and 90% of the total radioactivity by 72 hr. Less than 1% of the radioactivity appeared in the expired air and negligible amounts were excreted in the feces (32). As anticipated from these results, 3MI did not accumulate in the lung, liver, kidney, or other tissues from one-half to 24 hr following start of infusion, but equivalent radio-activity levels were 3-50 times higher than 3MI in these tissues at one-half hr indicating the presence of metabolites (29). Pulmonary alveolar epithelial cell damage and mild pulmonary edema were observed using transmission electron microscopy by one-half hr after beginning the infusion. These results demonstrate that during the development of early pulmonary lesions, 3MI is being rapidly metabolized and excreted in the urine, and that it does not accumulate in high concentrations in the tissues.

The nature of the urinary metabolites was investigated using ion-exchange chromatography for separation and charcoal filtration, thin-layer chromatography, enzymatic hydrolysis, gas chromatography and mass spectrometry for characterization (33). The urine contained 10 radioactive metabolites but 3MI was not present. Approximately 60% of the radioactivity was 3-methyloxindole and its hydroxylated derivatives. Smaller amounts were glucuronide conjugates of indole carboxylic acid and other compounds. From these observations it is clear that the major pathway of 3MI metabolism involves formation of oxindoles and that these compounds are rapidly excreted in the urine. Evidence is accumulating that the mixed function oxidase system is responsible for metabolism of 3MI and that this metabolism is also responsible for the development of pulmonary lesions (31). Under these conditions the metabolism of 3MI would be more closely related to development of pulmonary lesions than the absolute concentration of 3MI in the plasma.

V. PLASMA 3MI CONCENTRATION AND EXPOSURE TO 3MI

Ruminal fluid and plasma 3MI concentrations have been determined after tryptophan and 3MI administration. The primary factors affecting plasma 3MI concentration appear to be formation of 3MI from tryptophan in the rumen, absorption from the gastrointestinal tract, and metabolism by the animal resulting in the excretion of urinary products.

Cattle given radioactive tryptophan excrete 16 radioactive metabolites in the urine (34) whereas 10 radioactive peaks are observed after 3MI administration. At least 3 of the tryptophan metabolites can be recognized as 3MI excretion products and amount to approximately 35-40% of the urinary radioactivity of cows given tryptophan. This indicates that a significant fraction of tryptophan may be converted to 3MI when plasma and ruminal 3MI concentrations are usually low and suggests that absorption, metabolism, and excretion of 3MI are rapid processes compared to the rate of 3MI production. Ruminal 3MI concentrations reach a peak of approximately 4 to 10 μg/ml within 12 to 18 hr after giving a tryptophan dose which reflects the time necessary for the microorganisms to carry out the conversion of tryptophan to 3MI (20). The plasma 3MI concentrations are similar and follow the same time course. In addition, peak 3MI concentrations appear within 1.5 - 3 hr after giving 3MI in gelatin capsules to goats. This also suggests rapid absorption considering time for mixing in the rumen and the limited aqueous solubility of 3MI. The site and mechanism of 3MI absorption is not known. In view of the rapid clearance of 3MI from plasma, these results clearly indicate that 3MI absorption is rapid and that 3MI does not accumulate in ruminal fluid or plasma. Therefore, the plasma 3MI concentration reflects the balance between absorption and metabolism and it does not necessarily represent the total exposure to 3MI. This idea is reinforced by repeated observations that 3MI metabolites appear quantitatively in the urine after gram quantities are administered but the maximum plasma 3MI concentrations rarely account for more than 1% of the total dose or exceed 10 μg 3MI/ml (26,29). These results demonstrate that plasma 3MI concentrations may be useful as an indication of the presence of 3MI, but they may not necessarily be proportional to the total 3MI exposure since they are significantly affected by the relative rates of 3MI production, absorption, metabolism, and excretion. Measurement of the quantitative conversion of tryptophan to 3MI in cattle or goats by assay of the accumulated urinary excretion products of 3MI has not been feasible.

VI. 3-METHYLINDOLE AND FIELD CASES OF ABPE

A field trial was conducted to determine whether 3MI was present in the ruminal fluid and plasma of cows given access to lush, green pasture. Nineteen cows were removed from dry mountain range in central Oregon and placed on a lush meadow (35). Plasma and ruminal fluid samples were collected at intervals over a 7-day period in an attempt to obtain samples prior to the development of clinical signs. After about 102 hr, 7 cows developed clinical signs of respiratory distress. At the end of the trial, one cow with severe signs and one with moderate signs were killed and necropsy confirmed the development of ABPE in these cows.

The mean ruminal fluid 3MI increased from less than 0.01 μg/ml to 1.8 μg/ml at 78 hr and then slowly decreased to about 0.5 μg/ml at 174 hr. Peak 3MI concentration in individual cows ranged from 1.6 to 4.1 μg/ml and occurred between 30 and 174 hr. Cows which developed ABPE tended to maintain 3MI concentrations for a longer time than other cows but this difference was not significant. The 3 cows with the highest peak concentration in ruminal fluid (3.0 - 4.1 μg/ml) all developed clinical signs of respiratory distress. Plasma samples contained lower 3MI concentrations (0.01 to 0.27 μg/ml) but 3MI was present for nearly the entire experimental period in most cows. The interruption caused by sample collections may have reduced the severity of response and 3MI concentrations. Ruminal fluid was innoculated into media containing tryptophan and IAA and incubated for 24 hr. All cultures produced 3MI from these substrates indicating that the microorganisms which produce 3MI from tryptophan were present in the ruminal fluid of these cows.

The results indicate that the 3MI concentration increases in the ruminal fluid and plasma of cows after changing pasture conditions. The 3MI concentrations were lower than those observed after a single intraruminal dose of tryptophan but they were present for a much longer time.

Another field trial was conducted in Scotland in which 11 cattle were given access to newly seeded, heavily fertilized, parasite free, ryegrass pasture (36). All cattle developed clinical signs within 3 to 14 days after being given access to the pasture. The cattle were slaughtered after 15 to 18 days and pulmonary lesions including edema, hyperplasia of alveolar epithelial cells, and hyaline membranes were present in 7 cattle. Three-methylindole was present at slaughter in ruminal fluid of all cows and ranged in concentration from 3.5 to 9.5 μg/ml. No 3MI was detected in the plasma of these cattle. Although these samples were obtained after pulmonary lesions were present, the concentrations were similar to those observed in ruminal fluid of experimental animals given tryptophan (20). This experiment also demonstrated that 3MI was present in the ruminal fluid of cattle which developed ABPE after a pasture change.

Considering the rapid absorption and metabolism of 3MI, the results of these two field trials are consistent with the hypothesis that 3MI, a ruminal fermentation product of tryptophan, is associated with the development of naturally-occurring ABPE.

VII. VIEWPOINTS ON 3MI FORMATION AND ABPE

The formation of 3MI from tryptophan by ruminal microorganisms results in acute pulmonary lesions under experimental conditions and may also be the cause of naturally-occurring ABPE. Effective inhibition of this process may therefore result in prevention of this syndrome.

Ranchers report that the affected cattle are often those which appear to have consumed excessive amounts of lush, green forage. The sudden change in pasture conditions undoubtedly results in unbalanced ruminal fermentation for at least several days and this situation may be worsened by excessive intake. If the unbalanced fermentation conditions were more favorable for the organisms producing 3MI, then the probability that ABPE may develop is enhanced. Ranchers appear to have been partially successful in reducing the incidence of ABPE by using management procedures such as removing cattle from the pastures or supplemental hay feeding which may reduce the consumption of lush forage. Presumably, this could moderate the fermentation conditions during the grazing transition and also reduce the substrate load.

Another approach to reducing 3MI formation is to directly alter the fermentation by administration of particular compounds or inhibitors. An experiment was conducted in which 18 cows were divided into 3 groups of 6 cows (unpublished observations). All cows were given 0.35 g L-tryptophan/kg BW, to induce pulmonary disease. One group was pretreated with chlortetracycline (8 g at -1 day and 5 g/day for 3 days); one group was given molasses (1.4 kg every 12 hr from -1 to 3 days), and one group served as controls. Ruminal fluid 3MI was measured at intervals after dosing. Clinical signs were observed in 3 control and 2 molasses treated cows. One control and 2 molasses treated cows died of acute pulmonary disease. No clinical signs were observed in the group given a large dose of chlortetracycline.

Ruminal 3MI concentrations were similar in control and molasses treated cows (peak concentration of 15 μg/ml) but much lower in antibiotic treated cows (peak concentration of 0.7 μg/ml). It is clear that antibiotic treatment reduced the formation of 3MI from tryptophan and prevented the development of pulmonary disease in these cows. Molasses had no effect on the animal response or on 3MI concentrations in ruminal fluid. These results demonstrate that reducing the formation of 3MI prevents the onset of pulmonary disease in experimental cattle. The amounts of antibiotic used were large which would make field testing more difficult.

Inhibition of amino acid degradation in the rumen has been reported for the iodonium compounds, diphenyliodonium chloride and 4,4'-dimethyl-diphenyliodonium chloride (37). Also, monensin has been reported to have some bacteriostatic effects and to reduce feed consumption when given to cattle (38,39). The effects of monensin, chlortetracycline, and two iodonium compounds on 3MI formation from tryptophan was tested in an *in vitro* trial. The iodonium compounds and monensin were generously supplied by Smith Kline Corp., West Chester, Pa., and Eli Lilly & Co., Indianapolis, Indiana respectively. Ruminal fluid was collected and incubated with tryptophan according to previously reported procedures (25). After 24 hr, the presence of 3MI in the *in vitro* mixture was determined by gas chromatography (40). Control cultures converted approximately 43% of the tryptophan to 3MI which was similar to previous findings (25). All inhibitors and particularly the iodonium compounds greatly reduced the formation of 3MI. Monensin, chlortetracycline and iodonium compounds reduced 3MI formation to about 9.3, 3.0, and 0.3% of the control cultures respectively. These promising observations indicate that 3MI formation by ruminal fluid can be effectively inhibited. Animal testing is in progress to determine the most effective and economical way to reduce 3MI formation in the rumen.

VIII. SUMMARY AND CONCLUSIONS

(a) Intraruminal doses of tryptophan cause acute clinical signs and pulmonary lesions which appear to be identical to those observed in naturally-occurring acute pulmonary edema and emphysema of cattle.

(b) Ruminal fermentation of tryptophan results in the formation of 3-methylindole (3MI) by a 2 step process involving formation of indoleacetic acid (IAA) and subsequent decarboxylation to 3MI. A new species of *Lactobacillus* has been identified as the organism responsible for the formation of 3MI from IAA.

(c) Three-methylindole causes the characteristic pulmonary disease when given by either intraruminal or intravenous infusion. This indicates that 3MI is the ruminal metabolite of tryptophan responsible for the development of pulmonary lesions.

(d) It appears that high intake of lush, green forage by cattle could provide adequate amounts of tryptophan to cause ABPE. Ruminal fermentation conditions affecting conversion of tryptophan to 3MI are apparently more important than the specific dose of tryptophan that is consumed by cattle.

(e) Three-methylindole is rapidly absorbed, metabolized, and excreted in the urine primarily as oxindole derivatives. The mixed function oxidase system may be involved in metabolism of 3MI and accumulating evidence suggests that this metabolism may also be related to the pulmonary toxicity.

(f) Plasma 3MI concentrations are useful as an indication of the presence of 3MI after doses of tryptophan or 3MI, or after abrupt changes in pasture conditions; but they may not necessarily be proportional to the total 3MI exposure since the relative rates of 3MI production, absorption, and metabolism significantly affect the plasma 3MI concentrations.

(g) Three-methylindole is present for at least 7-15 days in ruminal fluid of cattle after being moved from summer range to lush, green pasture. The concentrations may be lower than those observed after a single tryptophan dose but 3MI is present for a longer time. The results are consistent with the hypothesis that 3MI, formed from tryptophan fermentation in the rumen, is associated with the development of ABPE.

(h) Antibiotics and inhibitors decrease 3MI formation and can prevent the onset of experimentally-induced ABPE. Field testing is necessary to develop an effective means of prevention of ABPE.

IX. ACKNOWLEDGMENTS

This work was supported in part by grant No. HL-13645 from National Institutes of Health to J. R. Carlson.

Scientific paper No. 4844. College of Agriculture Research Center, project 1893. Washington State University.

X. REFERENCES

1. Schofield, F. W., *J. Am. Vet. Med. Assoc.* 112, 254 (1948).
2. Breeze, R. G., Pirie, H. M., Dawson, C. O., Selman, I. E., and Wiseman, A., *Folia Vet. Lat.* 5, 95 (1975).
3. Breeze, R. G., Pirie, H. M., Selman, I. E., and Wiseman, A., *J. Comp. Pathol.* 85, 147 (1975).
4. Breeze, R. G., Pirie, H. M., Selman, I. E., and Wiseman, A.,

Vet. Bull. 46, 243 (1976).
5. Pirie, H. M., Breeze, R. G., Selman, I. E., and Wiseman, A., *Vet. Rec.* 95, 479 (1974).
6. Blake, J. T., and Thomas, D. W., *J. Am. Vet. Med. Assoc.* 158, 2047 (1971).
7. Selman, I. E., Wiseman, A., Pirie, H. M., and Breeze, R. G., *Vet. Rec.* 95, 139 (1974).
8. Aitken, M. M., and Sanford, J., *J. Comp. Pathol.* 79, 131 (1969).
9. Selman, I. E., Wiseman, A., Breeze, R. G., and Pirie, H. M., *Vet. Rec.* 99, 181 (1976).
10. Breeze, R. G., Pirie, H. M., Selman, I. E., and Wiseman, A., *J. Comp. Pathol.* 84, 577 (1974).
11. Pirie, H. M., Dawson, C. O., Breeze, R. G., Wiseman, A., Hamilton, J., *Vet. Rec.* 88, 346 (1971).
12. Hyslop, N. St. G., *Can. Vet. J.* 10, 251 (1969).
13. Wilson, B. J., Yang, D. T. C., and Boyd, M. R., *Nature (London)* 277, 521 (1970).
14. Boyd, M. R., Burka, L. T., and Wilson, B. J., *Toxicol. Appl. Pharmacol.* 32, 147 (1975).
15. Maki, L. R., and Tucker, J. O., *Am. J. Vet. Res.* 23, 824 (1962).
16. Carlson, J. R., Dyer, I. A., and Johnson, R. J., *Am. J. Vet. Res.* 29, 1983 (1968).
17. Dickinson, E. O., Spencer, G. R., and Gorham, J. R., *Vet. Rec.* 80, 487 (1967).
18. Dickinson, E. O., Ph.D. Thesis, Washington State University, 1970.
19. Pirie, H. M., Breeze, R. G., Selman, I. E., and Wiseman, A., *Vet. Rec.* 98, 259 (1976).
20. Yokoyama, M. T., Carlson, J. R., and Dickinson, E. O., *Am. J. Vet. Res.* 36, 1349 (1975).
21. Carlson, J. R., Yokoyama, M. T., and Dickinson, E. O., *Science* 176, 298 (1972).
22. Husby, F. M., Ph.D. Thesis, Washington State University, 1974.
23. Mackenzie, A., Ford, J. E., and Scott, K. J., *Res. Vet. Sci.* 19, 277 (1975).
24. Church, D. C., and Pond, W. G., "Basic Animal Nutrition and Feeding," p. 212. D. C. Church, Corvallis, Oregon, 1974.
25. Yokoyama, M. T., and Carlson, J. R., *Appl. Microbiol.* 27, 540 (1974).
26. Carlson, J. R., Dickinson, E. O., Yokoyama, M. T., and Bradley, B. J., *Am. J. Vet. Res.* 36, 1341 (1975).
27. Yokoyama, M. T., Carlson, J. R., and Holdeman, L. V., *Appl. Environ. Microbiol.* (In press).
28. Dickinson, E. O., Yokoyama, M. T., Carlson, J. R., and Bradley, B. J., *Am. J. Vet. Res.* 37, 667 (1976).
29. Bradley, B. J., Ph.D. Thesis, Washington State University, 1977.
30. Horvath, H. A., Carlson, J. R., and Dickinson, E. O.,

J. Anim. Sci. 41, 404 (1975).

31. Bray, T. M., and Carlson, J. R., Presented at 2nd International Meeting on Tryptophan Metabolism: Biochemistry, Pathology and Regulation. International Study Group for Tryptophan Research. Madison, Wisconsin, August 10-12, 1977.
32. Hammond, A. C., and Carlson, J. R., *J. Anim. Sci.* 42, 1575 (1976).
33. Hammond, A. C., Carlson, J. R., and Willett, J. D., *Fed. Proc.* 36, 1116 (1977).
34. Yang, N. Y. J., and Carlson, J. R., *J. Nutr.* 102, 1655 (1972).
35. Terry, M. L., Bradley, B. J., Hammond, A. C., Cummins, K. A., Carlson, J. R., and Dickinson, E. O., *J. Anim. Sci.* 42, 1575 (1976).
36. Selman, I. E., Wiseman, A., Breeze, R. G., Pirie, H. M., and Bogan, J. A., International Congress on Diseases of Cattle, Paris, September 1976.
37. Chalupa, W., Patterson, J. A., Chow, A. W., and Parish, R. C., *J. Anim. Sci.* 43, 316 (1976).
38. Haney, M. E., Jr., and Hoehn, M. M., "Antibiotic Agents + Chemotherapy," p. 349, 1967.
39. Raun, A. P., Cooley, C. O., Rathmacher, R. P., Richardson, L. F., and Potter, E. L., *J. Anim. Sci.* 38, 1344 (1974).
40. Bradley, B. J., and Carlson, J. R., *Anal. Biochem.* 59, 214 (1974).

STUDIES ON THE TOXIC PRINCIPLE OF *Asclepias eriocarpa* AND *Asclepias labriformis*

J. M. Benson and J. N. Seiber
Department of Environmental Toxicology, University of California, Davis
R. F. Keeler and A. E. Johnson
Poisonous Plant Research Laboratory, Agricultural Research Service U.S. Department of Agriculture

I. ABSTRACT

Some milkweeds native to the western United States are extremely toxic to range animals. As little as 0.8 ounce of Asclepias labriformis *and 4 ounces of* Asclepias eriocarpa, *for example, can be lethal to a 100 pound sheep. The cardiac glycosides (cardenolides) in these species have been implicated as toxic principles. Experiments were conducted to verify this, and to determine the toxicity of three individual cardenolides common to both plant species. Four preparations were tested: dried, ground* A. labriformis *and* A. eriocarpa *plants, an ethanolic* A. eriocarpa *extract, and an extract from which pigments and fats had been removed. In addition, a purified cardenolide present in* A. labriformis *and* A. eriocarpa, *labriformin, and digitoxin, a clinically important cardenolide, were administered. Toxic symptoms and gross and histopathologic lesions were qualitatively similar in sheep regardless of whether plants, extracts, labriformin, or digitoxin were administered. Three cardenolides, labriformin, labriformidin, and eriocarpin, have been isolated from* A. labriformis *and* A. eriocarpa *and chemically characterized. They represent a new series of cardenolides similar, but not identical to those present in* A. curassavica, *a species whose cardenolides have undergone some toxicological investigation. Acute toxicity studies on these* A. labriformis *and* A. eriocarpa *cardenolides and uscharidin and calotropin from* A. curassavica *were performed using male Swiss Webster mice. Each* LD_{50} *is below 15 mg/kg. These cardenolides were also assayed for their ability to inhibit* Na^{+}-K^{+}-*ATPase, the proposed pharmacological receptor for cardiac glycosides in the heart. The milkweed cardenolides were comparable to ouabain in ability to inhibit lamb heart ATPase* in vitro. *Cardiac glycosides present in* A. eriocarpa *and* A. labriformis *represent a highly toxic group of compounds that account for the effects of these plants on sheep.*

II. *Asclepias eriocarpa* AND *A. labriformis* AS POISONOUS PLANTS

Some milkweeds (genus *Asclepias*) native to the western United

States are extremely toxic to range animals (1,2). Two examples that will be discussed in detail here are the California milkweed, *Asclepias eriocarpa* Benth. and *Asclepias labriformis* Jones., a milkweed occurring in Utah. As little as 4 ounces of *A. eriocarpa* and 0.8 ounce of *A. labriformis* may kill a 100 pound sheep (1). Due to their general unpalatability to range animals, these species usually represent a hazard only in times of drought, when the range has been overgrazed, when sheep are trailed, or when penned animals are fed milkweed contaminated hay.

The effects of *A. eriocarpa* on range animals, including toxic doses, clinical signs of poisoning, gross and microscopic organ lesions were reported in 1923 and 1924 by Marsh and Clawson of the U.S. Department of Agriculture (3,4), but the effects of *A. labriformis* have been described only briefly (5-7). Typical symptoms in sheep poisoned by *A. eriocarpa* include depression, weakness, labored respiration, alterations in body temperature, and sometimes diarrhea. Death is not preceded by convulsions or period of coma. Gross pathological lesions reported by Marsh and Clawson included congestion of the lungs, kidneys, and portions of the alimentary canal. Microscopic lesions occurred in the above organs and in liver, lymph nodes, and heart (4).

First attempts to characterize the toxic principle of *A. eriocarpa* were reported by Couch in 1929 (8). He isolated a non-alkaloidal, nonglucosidal resinoid from this species which was lethal to guinea pigs. The toxic dose and clinical signs of poisoning were not described. Roeske, however, found no evidence of material toxic to mice in *A. eriocarpa* using Couch's method of extraction and purification (9).

Certain *asclepiads*, including the neotropical milkweed, *A. curassavica* L. have cardioactive compounds called cardenolides. Roeske (9) has found a positive correlation between the cardenolide content of four milkweed species, *A. labriformis, A. eriocarpa, A. speciosa* Torr. and *A. fascicularis* Done. and their toxicity to mice. The order of cardenolide content and toxicity of the plants was *A. labriformis* > *A. eriocarpa* > *A. speciosa* > *A. fascicularis*. In addition, after extracting *A. eriocarpa* and subjecting the extract to solvent partition cleanup and column chromatography, the toxicity of the phases or column fractions to mice increased as the cardenolide concentration increased.

A. eriocarpa and *A. labriformis* contain approximately 5-8 mg digitoxin equivalents per gram of dried plant material, as determined by the spectroassay method of Brower *et al.*, (10,11). In addition, their qualitative cardenolide content, as determined by thin layer chromatography, is almost identical. Two cardenolides, called labriformin and labriformidin have been isolated from both plant species. A third compound, eriocarpin, has been isolated from *A. eriocarpa* (9,12). Preliminary structures for these compounds have been proposed based on data from wet chemical analyses, infrared, nuclear magnetic resonance, and mass spectral studies and are shown in Figure 1 (12).

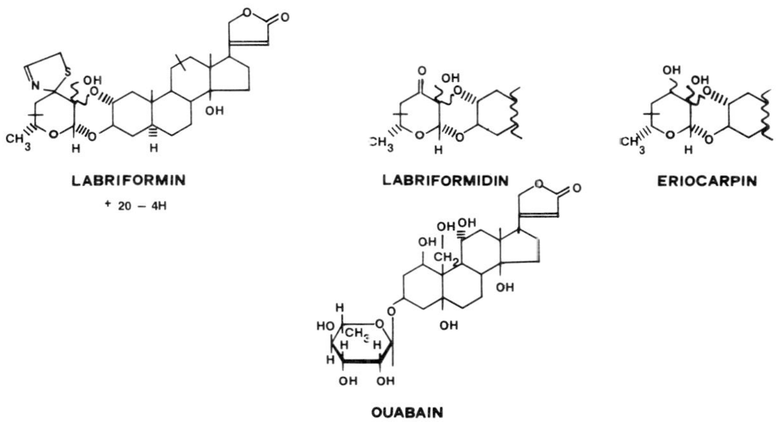

Fig. 1. *Structure of labriformin, labriformidin, eriocarpin, and ouabain.*

These cardenolides differ structurally from those used in clinical medicine such as digitoxin, digoxin, and ouabain in several respects. The major differences are in the stereochemistry of the A/B ring fusion (*cis* in digitoxin, *trans* in the milkweed cardenolides), in the types of sugars, and in the binding of sugars to the cardenolide genin. In the therapeutically useful compounds, a chain of one or more sugar moieties may be bound to the steroid nucleus through an ether linkage with a hydroxyl group at C_3 of the genin. Only one sugar moiety is found in the milkweed cardiac glycosides and it is attached to the steroid nucleus through hydroxyl groups at both the C_2 and C_3 positions of the genin. Compounds isolated from *A. labriformis* and *A. eriocarpa* are structurally similar to uscharin, uscharidin, and the isomers, calactin and calotropin, isolated from the milkweed *A. curassavica*, also known for its toxicity to cattle (13). There are, however, major distinctions in the structures of the new cardenolides of *A. eriocarpa* and *A. labriformis* and the previously characterized ones of *A. curassavica* (14,15).

III. EFFECTS OF MILKWEEDS AND CARDENOLIDES IN SHEEP

A. Experimental

Although a positive correlation was found between the cardenolide content of *A. eriocarpa* and *A. labriformis* and their toxicity to mice, more studies were needed before cardenolides could be positively identified as the principles responsible for the effects of these plants on range animals. An experiment was designed to compare the effects of both milkweed species, cardenolide-containing extracts *A. eriocarpa*, and pure cardenolides on two year old white face Columbia-Rambouillet-cross female sheep. The cardenolide content of the milkweeds and extract preparations were determined by spectroassay (10,11). Extracts were prepared by the scheme presented by Roeske *et al.* (16). "Crude extract" was obtained by subjecting the ethanolic extract of *A. eriocarpa* to a minimal solvent partition cleanup. "Cleaned extract" was prepared by subjecting "crude extract" to an extensive solvent partition cleanup.

TABLE 1

Cardenolide Content of Milkweed Plants and Extract Preparations

Material	Cardenolide content mg/gm dry material	Cardenolide enrichment
A. labriformis	7.2	--
A. eriocarpa	5.6	--
"crude extract"	38.1	6
"cleaned extract"	110.2	20

Toxic and lethal doses of dry *A. eriocarpa* and *A. labriformis* were estimated during a preliminary study employing four sheep. Twenty sheep were used in the principle experiment, with 3 controls and 17 animals dosed with experimental materials. Dried, ground *A. labriformis* and *A. eriocarpa* were each administered orally to 3 sheep at 3 dosages, (1.2-6.2 mg digitoxin equivalents/kg) so that moderate to severe signs of poisoning would be observed in at least one animal in each group and so that one or more from each group would survive long enough for blood and tissue pathology to develop. *A. eriocarpa* extracts were administered in doses containing approximately the same amount of total cardenolide as was present in the doses of *A. eriocarpa* plant. Labriformin, the purified milkweed cardenolide, was administered to 2 animals at arbitrarily selected doses of 1.1 and 2.4 mg/kg because of its limited availability. Digitoxin was dosed at levels of 1.1, 1.8, and 6.0 mg/kg.

Prior to administration and twice each day after administration of experimental preparations, sheep were observed for changes in ambulation, recumbancy, alertness, respiration, heart rate, appetite, or micturition. They were also observed for evidence of convulsions, weakness, distress or pain, vomiting, and for commencement of "raleing" sounds on expiration. Clinical observations on control sheep were used as a basis for comparison.

In addition, each animal was bled prior to being administered the experimental material and normal blood values were established for: erythrocyte and leukocyte numbers (RBC, WBC), packed cell volume (PCV), hemoglobin (Hgb), serum glutamate oxaloacetic transaminase (SGOT), lactate dehydrogenase (LDH), creatine phosphokinase

(CPK), gamma glutamyl transpeptidase (GGTP), and blood urea nitrogen (BUN). Each animal, then, served as its own control in addition to the blood values obtained from the control animals.

All sheep that died from the acute effects of cardenolides or cardenolide-containing materials were necropsied as soon as possible after death, the longest delay being 1 1/2 hours. Remaining animals, except controls, were euthanized by electrocution and exsanguination within 5 days after dosing and were necropsied. Control animals were not euthanized because gross lesions found in treated animals were quite pronounced. The condition of the lungs and organs of the gastrointestinal tract differed remarkably from the normal state.

Gross pathology was noted and portions of lung, kidney, heart, brain, rumen, abomasum, and intestine were taken for histopathological analysis. Tissues were fixed in buffered 10% formalin, processed for paraffin embedding, and stained with H&E.

B. Results

Before the experiment began, the behavior of all sheep was "normal." However, within 10 hours to one day following administration of the preparations, clinical signs of illness were observed in several of the experimental animals. The degree of change was related to dose level, being most pronounced in animals receiving the high doses. The signs of illness were similar in all animals regardless of the identity of the experimental preparation administered.

Affected sheep had a marked slowing of respiratory rate. The rate decreased from an average of about 60/min prior to treatment, to about 30/min. Expiration was very forced, and in severely affected animals, expiration produced "raleing" sounds. Cyanosis of mucous membranes was also observed in severely affected animals. These sheep were depressed and not alert, weakened, unsteady, ambulated with difficulty, and prior to death, some could not stand unassisted. They appeared to be in considerable distress and pain. There was no evidence of vomiting. Animals died without experiencing convulsions or a period of coma.

The sheep that received the high dose of "crude extract," high dose of *A. eriocarpa*, and the intermediate dose of *A. labriformis* showed severe signs of illness and died within two days after dosing. The sheep on the high doses of *A. labriformis*, "cleaned extract," labriformin, and digitoxin were showing pronounced signs of illness prior to being euthanized. Cardenolide doses causing illness or death were approximately 2 mg/kg for digitoxin and labriformin, and 4-6 mg/kg digitoxin equivalents/kg for milkweed preparations.

Significant increases in BUN levels were seen in animals fed high doses of labriformin, *A. eriocarpa*, *A. labriformis*, digitoxin, and cleaned *A. eriocarpa* extract. Notable CPK changes occurred in sheep fed high levels of labriformin, digitoxin,

A. labriformis, and cleaned *A. eriocarpa* extract; in those receiving intermediate doses of *A. eriocarpa* and *A. labriformis*, and in those administered low doses of labriformin and *A. eriocarpa* "crude extract." However, similar CPK changes occurred in the control animals, indicating that increases may have been due to skeletal muscle trauma induced by the method of capture and restraint used to obtain blood samples. SGOT changes occurred in animals receiving the intermediate dose of *A. labriformis*, the high dose of digitoxin, and the high dose of labriformin. Significant LDH changes were seen only in animals fed the high dose of labriformin and intermediate dose of *A. labriformis*.

Lesions were observed at necropsy of treated animals in the lungs, gastrointestinal system, kidneys, brain, heart, and mucous membranes. They were similar in type regardless of the identity of the material administered. Severity was related to the dose or to the time elapsed between dosing and death in some cases.

Brief descriptions of gross lesions follow. Lesions involving the lungs were the most obvious and included congestion, atelectasis, petechial and also very massive hemorrhages. Renal lesions included pale surfaces with or without diffuse reddened areas; congestion, and a darkening of the medullary region. Lesions of the gastrointestinal system were found generally in the abomasum, duodenum, small intestine, and occasionally in the omasum and cecum. They varied from mild to severe inflammation of the mucosa; edema of the gastrointestinal wall and surrounding tissues; petechiation of the mucosa, and areas of hemorrhage on the serosa, or in the associated connective tissue. Lesions on the heart varied from a few petechia to multiple echymoses, and were found on the epicardium or the endocardium. The brain lesion was congestion of the cerebral vessels. Four animals had a mild, diffuse redness on the surface of the cerebrum, but this did not appear to extend into the deeper tissues. Livers appeared occasionally to be slightly swollen, but there was little other evidence of pathologic change. Lymph nodes and lymphatic systems were unaltered except for some areas of hemorrhage in the thymus of one sheep, and mild edema of a few lymph nodes of some individuals. The gross appearance of lesions was similar among all sheep regardless of treatment.

Preliminary histologic survey was performed on 8 organs (brain, liver, kidney, heart, lung, rumen, abomasum, and intestine) from 6 of the 17 dosed sheep. No pathologic changes were found in brain or rumen, and small changes of a non-specific character in liver, heart, abomasum, and intestine were observed in some animals. Only kidney and lung from these sheep had lesions of potential significance with regard to experimental treatment.

Lung and kidney from all treated animals were examined because of these preliminary findings. Kidney lesions of an acute, non-inflammatory, necrotizing glomerulopathy occurred with moderate-to-marked severity in 11 and with lesser severity in 3 of the 17 sheep. In lung tissue, atelectasis, congestion, and focal intra-parenchymal and peribronchial hemorrhage were evident in all but

2 sheep. All changes were of an acute character and occurred with moderate-to-marked severity in 10 sheep and with lesser severity in 5 sheep. The lesions will be described elsewhere.

IV. STUDIES ON INDIVIDUAL *A. eriocarpa* AND *A. labriformis* CARDENOLIDES

A. Median Lethal Doses of Milkweed Cardenolides Determined in Mice.

Median lethal doses ($LD_{50}s$) of eriocarpin, labriformidin, and labriformin, isolated from *A. eriocarpa* of uscharidin and calotropin from *A. curassavica*, and of ouabain were determined using 15-25 gram male Swiss Webster mice. Compounds were dissolved or suspended (labriformin and uscharidin) in Emulfor 719 (17) (GAF Corporation, South San Francisco, CA 94080) -H_2O-EtOH (1:8:2) and administered ip. Four dose groups were used for each compound and there were usually four animals per dose group. In certain instances, when the amount of available compound was a limiting factor, three animals were used per dose group. The animals that died within 24 hours of being dosed were counted in the determination of the LD_{50} value. Results were analyzed by the statistical method of Spearman and Kärber as described by Finney (18).

Mice were observed for symptoms of poisoning. Autopsies were performed on some animals within 10 minutes after they died. Survivors at all dose levels were euthanized by decapitation and examined at two-day intervals following administration of compounds to determine if organ damage had occurred.

The median lethal doses of ouabain and a *A. eriocarpa* and *A. curassavica* cardenolides are given in Table 2. A threefold range

TABLE 2

Median Lethal Doses ($LD_{50}s$) of Cardenolides

Cardenolide	LD_{50}	LD_{50} ouabain
Ouabain	6.8(4)[1]	1.0
Labriformin	9.2(1)	1.35
Labriformidin	3.1(4)	0.46
Eriocarpin	6.5(2)	1.03
Uscharidin	11.8(2)	1.74
Calotropin[2]	9.8(2)	1.44

[1]Numbers in parentheses refer to the number of times an experiment was carried out. LD_{50} values are an average of the results obtained in all experiments with a given compound.

[2]Calotropin contained approximately 20% of its isomer, calactin, as quantitated by High Speed Liquid Chromatography.

in toxicity is seen in the LD_{50}s of labriformidin and labriformin from *A. eriocarpa*, but this range encompasses the LD_{50} of ouabain. The *A. curassavica* cardenolides calotropin and uscharidin appear to be slightly less toxic than the *A. eriocarpa* cardenolides and ouabain.

Affected animals became quiet and ataxic. Respiration became rapid, but labored, and animals lay flat on their abdomens, with their limbs spread. There was some trembling and severely affected animals convulsed. Symptoms appeared within a few minutes after the mice were dosed; and death, accompanied by clonic convulsions, usually occurred within 1 to 2 hours. Mice that exhibited symptoms of poisoning, but that did not die, did not appear ill on the days following treatment.

No lesions were seen in mice that died within 24 hours of being dosed. Hemorrhages were seen in the lungs of animals euthanized on the days following treatment, but the incidence of this lesion was not significantly greater than the incidence in the control group.

B. Effects of Milkweed Cardenolides on Sheep Cardiac Na^+-K^+-ATPase

Na^+-K^+-ATPase present in cardiac muscle has been proposed as the pharmacological receptor for cardiac glycosides (19,20) and much experimental evidence has been obtained to support this concept. Inhibition of this enzyme system is thought to be responsible for the therapeutic or for toxic effects of cardiac glycosides on the heart (21-23). Ability of natural and semi-synthetic cardiac glycosides to inhibit Na^+-K^+-ATPase preparations has also been used to predict the extent of their effect on the myocardium (24).

The ability of milkweed cardenolides to inhibit Na^+-K^+-ATPase isolated from lamb myocardium was determined in order to obtain an indication of the cardiac potency of these compounds. Na^+-K^+-ATPase was isolated and purified according to the procedure of Schwartz *et al.* (25). The enzyme was assayed in 1 ml of reaction mixture containing 2.5 mM Tris ATP, 5 mM $MgCl_2$, 1 mM EDTA-tris, 50 mM Tris HCl buffer (pH 7.4), 41 μg enzyme protein, 100 mM NaCl and 10 mM KCl. The volume was brought to 1 ml with water or aqueous solutions of cardiac glycoside or both. Inorganic phosphate released by the enzymatic hydrolysis of Tris ATP was assayed by the method of Martin and Doty (described in 25). Absorption of the reduced inorganic phosphate-ammonium molybdate complex was measured at 625 nm and compared to the absorbance given by inorganic phosphate standards also carried through the Martin and Doty procedure.

Each cardenolide was assayed three times at five different concentrations (0.1, 0.5, 0.8, 1.0, and 10.0 μM). Ouabain was used as a control in each assay and the I_{50} value (concentration of cardenolide resulting in 50% inhibition of enzymatic activity) obtained for each cardenolide was compared to that obtained for ouabain during the same assay (I_{50} ouabain).

The Vmax of the freshly prepared enzyme was 12.5 μM Pi/mg

protein/hour. The K_s (Michaelis constant) for potassium was 1.75 mM and the K_i's for ouabain, determined using 0.5, 0.8, and 1.0 μM ouabain were 0.18, 0.11, and 0.13 μM, respectively. The I_{50} and I_{50} ouabain values for labriformin, labriformidin, eriocarpin, calotropin, uscharidin, digitoxin, and ouabain are reported in Table 3.

TABLE 3

Cardenolide I_{50} Values,[1] Inhibition of Lamb Cardiac Na^+-K^+-ATPase

Cardenolide	Experimental mean I_{50} μM ± S.D.	Cardenolide I_{50} relative to ouabain I_{50} (I_{50} cardenolide/ I_{50} ouabain) mean (n=3) ± S.D.
Ouabain	0.89 ± 0.2	1.00
Labriformidin	0.78 ± 0.07	0.75 ± 0.09
Eriocarpin	0.81 ± 0.24	0.77 ± 0.18
Labriformin	0.96 ± 0.18	0.92 ± 0.10
Uscharidin	0.77 ± 0.20	0.92 ± 0.17
Calotropin	0.68 ± 0.16	1.04 ± 0.18
Digitoxin	0.36 ± 0.12	0.94 ± 0.13

[1]Values for ouabain are an average of 6 determinations, while those for the remaining cardenolides are an average of 3 determinations.

V. DISCUSSION AND CONCLUSIONS

A. labriformis and *A. eriocarpa* were acutely toxic at doses of 1 and 1.8 ounces of dry plant per 100 pound sheep, respectively. Assuming fresh plant loses approximately 2/3 of its weight when dried, the corresponding toxic doses of fresh plant would be approximately 3 and 6 ounce per 100 pound sheep. These values are somewhat higher than those previously reported (1).

The effects of *A. labriformis* were identical to those of *A. eriocarpa*. More significant, however, is the fact that the clinical signs of illness, blood parameter changes, gross and histopathology induced by labriformin and digitoxin were the same as those produced by both *A. eriocarpa* and *A. labriformis*. Toxic doses of pure cardenolides were somewhat lower than the cardenolide dose producing illness or death in animals administered milkweed materials. These differences may be attributed to differences in rates of absorption of pure cardenolides *vs* those contained in plant or extracts. The toxicity of the mixture of cardenolides present in the plant or extracts may also be different from that of an equivalent amount of a single highly toxic compound.

Cardenolides isolated from *A. eriocarpa* appear to be very

similar to ouabain in their effects on mice and Na^+-K^+-ATPase preparations. The median lethal doses of labriformin, labriformidin and eriocarpin were all less than 10 mg/kg. Labriformidin was the most toxic at 3.1 mg/kg and labriformin the least toxic at 9.2 mg/kg but this range encompasses the LD_{50} of ouabain. The I_{50} values for the inhibition of lamb heart Na^+-K^+-ATPase by the *A. eriocarpa* cardenolides were also very similar to the I_{50} of ouabain. It appears then, that the large structural differences between the milkweed cardenolides and those used in clinical medicine have little effect on the pharmacological activity of these compounds. These results are consistent with the findings of Parsons and Summers (27) and Kupchan *et al.*, (28) who also found that a *cis* configuration about the A/B rings of the steroid nucleus is not essential for biological activity (Figure 1).

Clinical signs of poisoning and the time course of poisoning were vastly different in mice and sheep. A possible explanation for the difference may be that the experimental materials were administered by different routes. The lack of organ lesions, expecially in the lungs and gastrointestinal tracts of mice surviving several days after administration of cardenolides should also be noted. One possible source for this difference may lie in differences in the sensitivity of the two species to direct effects of cardiac glycosides, or in the effects of cardenolide metabolites produced by sheep and mice. Westermarck has reported microbial degradation of cardenolides within the reductive environment of sheep rumen (29,30). Production of these metabolites in sheep, but not in mice, may be a possible explanation for the discrepancy in effects seen.

In conclusion, the results of experiments described here strongly suggest that *A. eriocarpa* and *A. labriformis* are poisonous to range animals because of the cardenolides they contain. The individual major cardenolides of these species are similar to ouabain in their effects on mice and isolated Na^+-K^+-ATPase, but more work is required to determine the potential therapeutic usefulness of these compounds. Further work is also needed in order to explain the large differences in effects of cardiac glycosides on ruminant and non-ruminant animal species.

VI. ACKNOWLEDGMENTS

The authors are grateful to Drs. C. V. Bagley, and Stuart Young for their interpretation of the gross and histopathologic lesions in sheep. We are also grateful to Joyce Johnson and Lew Dell Balls for their technical assistance, and to Carolyn Roeske and Robert I. Krieger for their help in preparing this manuscript.

Research was funded in part by NIH ES00125, NSF BMS 75-14266, and the U.S. Department of Agriculture.

VII. REFERENCES

1. Kingsbury, J., "Poisonous Plants of the United States and Canada," pp. 267-270. Prentice-Hall, Englewood Cliffs, New Jersey, 1964.
2. Muenscher, W., "Poisonous Plants of the United States," pp. 195-199. Collier Books, Macmillan Publishing Company, New York, 1975.
3. Marsh, C. D., and Clawson, A. B., *U.S. Dep. Agric. Dep. Cir.* 272 (1923).
4. Marsh, C. D., and Clawson, A. B., *U.S. Dep. Agric. Dep. Bull.* No. 1212 (1924).
5. Holmgren, A., *Utah Exp. Stn. Farm Home Sci.* 6, 11 (1945).
6. Huffman, W. T., Moran, E. A., and Binns, W., *in* "U.S. Department of Agriculture Yearbook of Agriculture 1956," p. 118. U.S. Government Printing Office, Washington, D.C., 1956.
7. Stoddart, L., Holmgren, A., and Cook, C., *Utah Agric. Exp. Stn. Spec. Rep.* 2 (1949).
8. Couch, J., *Am. J. Pharm.* 101, 815 (1929).
9. Roeske, C., Masters Thesis, University of California, Davis, 1971.
10. Brower, L., McEvoy, P., Williamson, K., and Flannery, M., *Science* 177, 426 (1972).
11. Brower, L. P., and Moffitt, *Nature* 246, 280 (1974).
12. Seiber, J., Benson, J., Roeske, C., Brower, L., "Qualitative and Quantitative Aspects of Milkweed Cardenolide Sequestering by Monarch Butterflies," presented at the 170th Meeting American Chemical Society Division of Pesticide Chemistry, Chicago, Illinois, August 28, 1975.
13. Tokernia, C., Dobereiner, J., and Cannella, C., *Pesqui. Agropecu. Bras. Ser. Vet.* 7, 31 (1972).
14. Brüschweiler, F., Stockel, L., and Reichstein T., *Helv. Chim. Acta* 52, 2276 (1969a).
15. Brüschweiler, F., Stocklin, W., Stockel, L., and Reichstein, T., *Helv. Chim. Acta* 52, 208 (1969b).
16. Roeske, C. N., Seiber, J. N., Brower, L. P., and Moffitt, C. M., *in* "Recent Advances in Phytochemistry: (J. W. Wallace and R. L. Mansell, Eds.), Vol. 10, p. 93. Plenum Press, New York, 1976.
17. Mention of a trade name, proprietary product, or specific equipment does not constitute a guarantee or warranty by the U.S. Department of Agriculture and does not imply its approval to the exclusion of other products that may be suitable.
18. Finney, D., "Statistical Methods in Biological Assay," Griffin, London, 1964.
19. Repke, K., *Proc. 2nd Int. Pharmacol. Meet.* 4, 65 (1963).
20. Repke, K., and Portius, H., *Sci. Pharm. Proc. 25th Congr. Pharm. Sci.*, Prague, 1965.
21. Akera, T., Larsen, F., and Brody, T., *J. Pharmacol. Exp. Ther.* 170, 17 (1969).

22. Smith, T., and Haber, E., *N. Engl. J. Med.* 289, 954 (1973).
23. Besch, H., Jr., Allen, J., Glick, G., and Schwartz, A., *J. Pharmacol. Exp. Ther.* 171, 1 (1970).
24. Beard, N., Rouse, W., and Somerville, A., *Br. J. Pharm.* 54, 65 (1975).
25. Schwartz, A., Nagano, K., Nakao, M., Lindenmayer, G., Allen, J., and Matsui, H., *in* "Methods in Pharmacology" (A. Schwartz, Ed.), Vol. 1, p. 361. Appleton-Century-Crofts Education Division, Meredity Corp., New York, 1971.
26. Barnes, C., and Eltherington, L., "Drug Dosage in Laboratory Animals, a Handbook," pp. 82 and 163. University of California Press, Berkeley and Los Angeles, 1966.
27. Parsons, J. A., and Summers, R. J., *Br. J. Pharmacol.* 42, 143 (1971).
28. Kupchan, S. M., Mokotoff, M., Sandha, R. S., and Kokin, L. E., *Med. Chem.* 10, 1025 (1967).
29. Westermarck, H., *Zentralbl. Veterinaermed.* 3, 727 (1956).
30. Westermarck, H., *Acta Vet. Scand.* 1, 67 (1959).

THE INTERACTION OF PATHOGENETIC MECHANISMS IN BOVINE HIGH MOUNTAIN (BRISKET) DISEASE

A. F. Alexander
Department of Pathology
College of Veterinary Medicine and Biomedical Sciences
Colorado State University

I. ABSTRACT

High Mountain (Brisket) Disease refers to the syndrome of congestive right heart failure in cattle, particularly associated with residence at high altitude. Overwhelming evidence has shown that the chronic alveolar hypoxia of high altitude and the resulting pulmonary hypertension are the underlying factors in the pathogenesis of this disease under these environmental conditions. However, a wide variety of modifying conditions may play an important role in the epidemiology of this disease. These conditions in some instances may bring about the failure syndrome without the existance of an altitude hypoxia component, but are of particular importance in the development of the disease in animals which have only a moderate altitude induced pulmonary hypertension. These modifying or contributing factors include cardiomyopathies, alveolar hypoxia from causes other than altitude, primary pulmonary parenchymal disease, and pulmonary vascular disease or functional alterations. In some instances plant toxins or allergens, both known and unknown, may be significant contributing factors or agencies in the development of this syndrome.

II. THE DISEASE

The term "Brisket Disease" is in many ways an unfortunate one that has led to some confusion. It is first, of course, not a disease of the "Brisket" but one of the circulatory system. More important, however, the use of the term has caused difficulty in the indentification of a wide variety of etiological conditions or situations. The term is generally used to identify the syndrome of congestive right heart failure in the bovine species, historically associated with residence at high altitude. The term "High Mountain Disease" probably best identifies the failure syndrome when it is associated with high altitude environments but as we shall see, even that situation may have a variety of contributing factors in addition to environmental hypoxia.

The syndrome was originally described in 1912 by Glover and Newson (1) as it occurred in the mountainous areas of Colorado. It has been recognized by ranchers of that region for the last quarter of the 19th century and there is hearsay information of its occurrence in the cattle of the Spanish Conquistidors (2,4). The identification of the disease in association with mountainous environment has since been made in Central America, the Andes of South America, and the highland country of East Africa. The syndrome undoubtedly occurs wherever domestic cattle are resident for long periods at elevations above 1,200 - 1,500 meters.

The importance of the disease at the lower elevations of 1,200 - 1,500 meters has recently been established by Jensen *et al.* (3) who documented that 6% of the death loss in a Colorado feedlot was due to this condition. Incidence in cow-calf operations above about 2,200 meters in Colorado and Wyoming varies from 0.5% - 2% (2,4,5,6). The incidence rises with an increase in resident altitude and in cattle newly imported from low elevations (2,4,5,6). The greatest occurrence under these conditions is in cattle under one year of age with no sex prediliction noted. A greater incidence in older cattle has been reported from Montana where resident altitudes are lower. The incidence and occurrence in East Africa is similar to that seen in Colorado while observations from the Andes indicate high incidences, especially among newly imported animals.

The syndrome is one of congestive right heart failure with all the clinical signs and lesions attributable to that condition (2, 4,5,6,8). Included are right ventricular hypertrophy and dilatation, subcutaneous edema, ascites, hydrothorax, profuse fluid diarrhea, chronic passive congestion of the liver, and hypervolemia with hemodilution. Pulmonary hypertension has repeatedly been documented both before and after the onset of the altitude dependent failure with the hypertension attributed to an increased resistance to flow at the precapillary level (8,9,10,11,12). Medial thickening of the small pulmonary arteries and arterioles may be prominent (13,14,15).

The underlying genesis of congestive right heart failure in any species results from the overwork of the right side of the heart, particularly the right ventricle. The cause of the overwork may lie within the heart itself or within the peripheral circulation, in this case the pulmonary vascular bed. Included in the pathogenesis may be the factors of an increased volume of blood to be pumped, an increased resistance to flow, or intrinsic weakness or disease of the myocardium, i.e. the pump itself. Many disease conditions may generate these possible components of failure. Likewise there may be a single cause or there may be multiple factors acting in consort or with an additive effect resulting in eventual failure of the pump. The clinical result is that of an animal in congestive heart failure with the signs and postmortem lesions so overwhelmingly of that condition that the basic pathogenesis may be hidden, overlooked, or misinterpreted. The remainder of this discussion will consider some of the specific factors that individually, or acting with others, may result in this clinical picture of failure, particularly in the bovine species.

Primary cardiac disease, usually considered as being either

congenital or acquired, may readily cause congestive failure. Failure from congenital disease results from volume overload of the heart, stenosis of outflow tracts, or increased pulmonary vascular resistance from induced pulmonary vascular sclerosis. Acquired valvular disease, not an uncommon entity in cattle, may result in failure from valvular incompetence or stenosis. Likewise traumatic pericarditis usually terminates in congestive heart failure.

Acquired myocardial disease may weaken the heart to that point that failure ensues. The causes may be infectious, toxic, or nutritional in nature. Toxic cardiomyopathy of drug origin is recognized (16) and one can speculate that certain plant toxins in addition to the cardiac glycosides, may also act in this manner. The myocardial lesions of nutritional origin are well recognized in cattle (17). Moderate nutritional myopathy occurring concommitantly with other causes of failure such as altitude induced pulmonary hypertension, could conceivably be of significance in the pathogenesis of cardiac failure in some instances.

The term "cor pulmonale" refers to right ventricular hypertrophy and failure occurring as the result of pulmonary disease. The increased cardiac workload is primarily the result of an increased pulmonary vascular resistance. The most thoroughly documented conditon of cor-pulmonale in cattle is the altitude related Brisket or High Mountain Disease (4,5,6,8,9,10,11). Following the initial work of von Euler and Liljestrand (18), the pulmonary hypertensive response to alveolar hypoxia has been demonstrated in essentially all mammalian species. Cattle are well recognized as having a particularly reactive pulmonary vascular bed to this stimulus and are used as an animal model of the phenomena (5). Alveolar hypoxia, i.e. lowered alveolar PO_2, appears to be the primary stimulus but the precise mechanism of response remains unknown. Chronic hypoxia causes an increased pulmonary vascular resistance at the precapillary level resulting in pulmonary hypertension, increased right ventricular workload and failure (9,10,11). Increasing the altitude, i.e. decreasing the alveolar PO_2, shortens the time necessary to develop severe pulmonary hypertension (11,15). Medial thickening with luminal restriction of the small pulmonary arteries and arterioles is a prominent morphologic feature which may be the result of maintained vasotonus and yet subsequently contribute to the increased resistance (13,14,15,19).

A variability exists in the pulmonary hypertension that develops in response to chronic hypoxia, with some cattle developing severe pulmonary hypertension while in others only a moderate increase is elicited (9,10,11,20,21). The exact basis for the difference in response is at present unclear but it has been shown to be a strongly inherited trait (5,20,23,24,25). Based on this knowledge selective culling in high altitude resident herds has resulted in a significant decrease in the incidence of High Mountain Disease. All work to date has supported the fact that chronic alveolar hypoxia and the resultant pulmonary hypertension remain the underlying mechanism in the pathogenesis of "Brisket

Disease" in cattle at high altitude.

Alveolar hypoxia may exist, however, from situations other than high altitude residence and through the same mechanisms cause some degree of pulmonary hypertension. These causes may be of particular significance when superimposed upon moderate high altitude induced pulmonary hypertension. The pulmonary hypertension in pneumonia may partially be due to this mechanism and indeed the precapillary vasoconstriction may be beneficial in diverting blood flow to non-pneumonic areas. The production and accumulation of fluids in the distal airway may likewise result in alveolar hypoxia. The feeding of iodine or the administration of organophosphate insecticides may be of importance in this way. The organophosphate insecticides may in addition cause alveolar hypoxia by means of airway constriction. The possibility that certain plant toxins may cause either airway constriction or the production and accumulation of fluid with resultant alveolar hypoxia and pulmonary hypertension may be a distinct possibility. The significance of this effect would be particularly important in animals which already had a mild pulmonary hypertension due to high altitude residence.

In man, extreme obesity is on occasion accompanied by alveolar hypoxia, pulmonary hypertension, polycythemia, cor-pulmonale and right heart failure. This condition has been given the name of the "Pickwickian Syndrome" based on Charles Dickens' description of the fat boy in "The Pickwick Papers" (26,27,28,29). Lowered alveolar PO_2 results from hypoventilation associated with the extreme obesity. I believe a similar phenomena exists in cattle which have become highly conditioned in feedlot situations. Right heart failure may occur in these animals and the pulmonary vascular changes appear identical to those seen at high altitude. Hypoventilation in feedlot animals may also result from increased intra-abdominal pressure associated with forestomach engorement and recumbancy. These factors may contribute to the cause of the rather surprisingly high incidence of right heart failure in feedlots located at moderate altitudes of about 1,600 meters (3). It is also conceivable that certain plant toxins may depress respiration at the central nervous system level with resultant alveolar hypoxia and significant pulmonary hypertension.

Primary pulmonary parenchymal disease, in most cases pneumonia of all types, may also cause pulmonary hypertension and increased right ventricular work by direct impingement of the process on the pulmonary vasculature. Lung damage in recovered cases of bovine asthma may account for the frequent development of right heart failure in those individuals that are returned to mountainous pastures. Metabolic products of plant origin have been implicated in bovine asthma and thus may play a role in the pathogenesis of this type brisket disease (30). Alveolar septal thickening, and the hypertrophy of air passage musculature which is frequently observed in older cattle may also increase pulmonary vascular resistance, cause alveolar hypoxia or both, and thus contribute to pathogenesis of right heart failure seen in this age group of cattle at mountainous elevations.

Disease or functional processes which directly affect the pulmonary vasculature may cause increased vascular resistance and cardiac workload. Inspiration of cold ambient air has now been shown to have a pulmonary vasoconstrictive effect resulting in a significant increase in pulmonary vascular resistance and pressure (31). This phenomena may partially explain the high incidence of High Mountain Disease in the higher elevations after onset of cold weather and during the winter months.

Metastatic calcification which is occasionally observed in cattle may result in congestive failure if the affected animal is resident at high altitude. This condition has been observed in the intermountain area where the cause has not been determined but plants with properties similar to *Solanum malocoxylon* in Argentina where the disease "enteque seco" is a problem cannot be discounted (32).

The effects of some of the pyrrolizidine alkaloids, particularly those from the Crotalaria genus, upon the pulmonary circulation are well documented (33,34,35,36). Although Crotalaria *per se* are not a factor in areas where "Brisket Disease" is a problem other pyrrolizidine bearing plant species, most notably the Senecios, are present. Pyrrolizidine toxicity is well known, with most of the attention having been focused upon hepatotoxic aspects. The effect of these alkaloids upon pulmonary vessels and the pulmonary circulation in cattle has not been investigated, but could be of significance in this animal species with an apparent hyperreactive pulmonary vasculature.

In Australia, St. George Disease is an entity of proven plant toxin etiology that in many aspects parallels High Mountain or Brisket Disease, or at least congestive right heart failure (37, 38,39,40,41). Although possibly acting on the distal side of the pulmonary vascular bed (40), the fundamental effect upon the workload of the right heart would be similar to an increased resistance at the precapillary level. Again the possible susceptibility of the pulmonary circulation to plant or other toxins is apparent and one can speculate that there are many more unknown than known.

In final analysis, Brisket or High Mountain Disease of cattle remains a syndrome of congestive right heart failure. Chronic alveolar hypoxia and the resulting pulmonary hypertension are the underlying factors in the pathogenesis of this disease at higher altitudes. The importance of alveolar hypoxia in the pathogenesis can be illustrated by the fact that surgical constricture of the pulmonary artery in calves at sea level does not lead to failure, but when these animals are moved to the moderate high altitudes of 1,500 meters failure ensues (42). Similarly, experimental verminous pneumonia at sea level rarely results in the failure syndrome whereas it frequently occurs at an elevation of 1,500 meters.

What must be kept in mind is that there are a wide variety of factors that may increase the workload of the right heart. Some of these factors, i.e. the alveolar hypoxia of high altitude, may in themselves result in a magnitude of increased work that causes failure. On the other hand other factors may not be sufficiently strong in their own right to cause failure but failure may occur when they act in consort with other conditions that increase the cardiac workload. These additive effects may be of particular significance in some occurrences of High Mountain Disease and must be factored out if a true understanding of the problem is to be obtained. Lastly, the effect of plant toxins, known and unknown can no longer be ignored as being possible contributing agents in some instances to this disease syndrome.

III. REFERENCES

1. Glover, G. H., and Newson, I. E., *Colo. Agric. Exp. Stn. Bull.* 204 (1915).
2. Alexander, A. F., and Will, D. H., "Biometerology," 2, p. 161. Pergamon Press, 1967.
3. Jensen, R., Pierson, R. E., Braddy, P. M., Saari, D. A., Benitez, A., Horton, D., Lauerman, L. H., McChesney, A. E., Alexander, A. F., and Will, D. H., *J. Am. Vet. Med. Assoc.* 169, 515 (1976).
4. Alexander, A. F., *Ann. N. Y. Acad. Sci.* 127, 640 (1965).
5. Alexander, A. F., Card, C. S., Jaenke, R. S., Hicks, J. L., and Will, D. H., "Research Animals in Medicine," (L. T. Harmison, Ed.), p. 193, NIH, Washington, D.C., 1974.
6. Alexander, A. F., and Will, D. H., *in* "Disease of Cattle" (W. J. Gibbons, Ed.), 2nd Ed., p. 110. American Veterinary Publications, Wheaton, Illinois, 1973.
7. Ryff, J. F., *J. Am. Vet. Med. Assoc.* 131, 425 (1957).
8. Hecht, H. H., Kuida, H., Lange, R. L., Thorne, J. L., and Brown, A. M., *Am. J. Med.* 32, 171 (1962).
9. Alexander, A. F., Will, D. H., Grover, R. F., Reeves, J. T., *Am. J. Vet. Res.* 21, 199 (1960).
10. Will, D. H., Alexander, A. F., Grover, R. F., and Reeves, J. T., *Cir. Res.* 10, 172 (1962).
11. Grover, R. F., Reeves, J. T., Will, D. H., and Blount, S. G., Jr., *J. Appl. Physiol.* 18, 567 (1963).
12. Alexander, A. F., and Jensen, R., *Am. J. Vet. Res.* 24, 1094 (1963).
13. Alexander, A. F., and Jensen, R., *Am. J. Vet. Res.* 24, 1098 (1963).
14. Alexander, A. F., and Jensen, R., *Am. J. Vet. Res.* 24, 1112 (1963).
15. Jaenke, R. S., and Alexander, A. F., *Am. J. Pathol.* 73, 377 (1973).
16. Jaenke, R. S., *Lab. Invest.* 30, 292 (1974).
17. Jubb, K. V. F., and Kennedy, P. C., "Pathology of Domestic Animals," Vol. 2, p. 484. Academic Press, New York, 1970.
18. Euler and Lilljestrand, *Acta Physiol. Scand.* 12, 301 (1946).
19. Tucker, A., McMurtry, I. F., Reeves, J. T., Alexander, A. F., Will, D. H., and Grover, R. F., *Am. J. Physiol.* 228

762 (1975).
20. Tucker, A., Reeves, J. T., McMurtry, I. F., Alexander, A. F., Will, D. H., and Grover, R. F., *Fed. Proc.* 33, 308 (1974).
21. Grover, R. F., Vogel, J. H. K., Averill, K. H., and Blout, S. G., *Am. Heart J.* 66, 1 (1965).
22. Will, C. H., Hicks, J., Card, C. S., and Alexander, A. F., *Physiologist* (1970).
23. Will, D. H., Hicks, J. L., Card, C. S., and Alexander, A. F., *J. Appl. Physiol.* 38, 491 (1975).
24. Grover, R. F., Will, D. H., Reeves, J. T., Weir, E. K., McMurtry, I. F., and Alexander, A. F., *in* "Progress in Respiration Research," (Proceedings International Symposium on Pulmonary Circulation II held in Prague, Czechoslovakia), S. Kerger, Basel, Switzerland, 1975.
25. Grover, R. F., Will, D. H., Reeves. J. T., Weir, E. K., McMurtry, I. F., and Alexander, A. F., *Prog. Respir. Res.* 9, 112 (1975).
26. Dickens, C., *in* "The Posthumous Papers of the Pickwick Club," Chapman and Hall, London, 1837.
27. Burwell, C. S., Robin, E. D., Whaley, R. D., and Bickelmann, A. G., *Am. J. Med.* 21, 811 (1956).
28. Hasleton, P. S., Heath, D., and Brewer, D. B., *J. Pathol. Bacteriol.* 95, 431 (1968).
29. Addington, W. W., Pfeffer, S. H., and Gaensler, E. A., *Respiration* 26, 214 (1969).
30. Dickenson, E. O., Spencer, G. R., and Gorham. J. R., *Vet. Rec.* 80, 457 (1967).
31. Will, D. H., McMurtry, I, F., Reeves, J. T., and Grover, R. F., *Physiologist* (Abstr.) 18, 450 (1975).
32. Jubb, K. V. F., and Kennedy, P. C., *in* "Pathology of Domestic Animals," Vol. 1, p. 108. Academic Press, 1970.
33. Kay, J. M., and Heath, D., "*Crotalaria spectabilis*, the Pulmonary Hypertension Plant," Charles C. Thomas, Springfield, Illinois, 1969.
34. Butler, W. H., Mattocks, A. R., and Barnes, J. M., *J. Pathol.* 100 (1969).
35. Allen, J. R., and Chesney, D. F., *Exp. Mol. Pathol.* 17, 220 (1972).
36. Atkinson, B. F., Katz, A. S., Knight, D., Pietra, G. C., and Fishman, A., *Lab. Invest.* (Abstr.) 36, 330 (1977).
37. Seawright, A. A., and Francis, J., *Aust. Vet. J.* 47, 91 (1971).
38. McClure, T. J., and Farrow, B. R. H., *Aust. Vet. J.* 47, 100 (1971).
39. Clark, I. A., *Aust. Vet. J.* 47, 285 (1971).
40. Clark, I. A., *Res. Vet. Sci.* 14, 341 (1973).
41. Kelly, W. R., *Aust. Vet. J.* 51, 233 (1975).
42. Vogel, J. H. K., McNamara, D. G., Hallman, G., Rosenberg, H., Jamieson, G., and McCrady, J. D., *Cir. Res.* 21, 661 (1967).

PIMELEA SPP. POISONING OF CATTLE

W. R. Kelly and A. A. Seawright
Department of Veterinary Pathology and Public Health
University of Queensland

I. ABSTRACT

Pimelea spp. *poisoning of cattle usually presents as a chronic syndrome of diarrhea, wasting, anemia, and progressive circulatory embarrassment. The circulatory disease appears to be related to constriction of pulmonary venules, and the anemia is caused by spectacular expansion of the plasma volume; blood loss and bone marrow depression seem not to be important factors in this regard. Livers of affected animals develop a form of peliosis hepatis, with marked distension of sinusoids with blood. Expansion of vascular spaces occurs in other organs with sinusoidal circulation. The toxic principle is a phorbol-type compound and is remarkably potent for cattle, much less so for other species, and is very stable and can persist in dead plants for many months.*

II. INTRODUCTION

This condition was originally known as "St. George disease," after the district in Queensland, Australia, where it was first recognized. Recently it was shown to be due to intoxication of species of *Pimelea* (1, 2, 3). The disease is limited in distribution and incidence but can cause heavy losses on extensively managed beef cattle properties when seasonal and other factors combine to increase exposure of cattle to the plant. So far as is known the disease is restricted to Australia.

III. THE TOXIC PLANT

The genus *Pimelea* (Fam. Thymelaeaceae) is mainly restricted to Australia, and shares with other genera of this family the property of very irritant fruit, bark, and leaves. Although there are about 80 species in the genus, only a few have been implicated in field intoxication of cattle (4). This is probably due to the unpalatable nature of the genus as a whole, rather than to variations in toxic concentration between species; however, detailed comparative studies have not been made. In the field the most important determinant of *Pimelea* toxin assimilation is the fact that the toxin is very stable and will persist in dead weathered fragments of some annual species for many months (5,6), at which stage the plant has lost some of its unpalatability. These

Pimelea species (*P. simplex*, *P. trichostachya*, *P. continua*) are restricted in distribution by preference for somewhat restricted soil types and climatic requirements, which fact allows preventive management on properties with varied soils.

Another major factor predisposing cattle to intoxication is food restriction during drought, which increases the animals' intake of the plant during close grazing.

IV. THE TOXIC PRINCIPLE

It was established early that the toxic component of *Pimelea* was insoluble in water (7) and was present in the alcohol-soluble component of the plant (8), but it was not until 1975 that a pure substance was isolated from *P. simplex* which could produce in cattle most of the more characteristic features of the field disease (9).

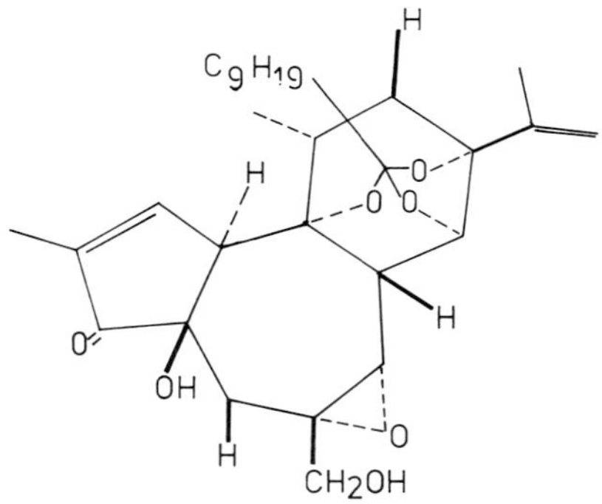

Fig. 1. *Structure of active component of* Pimelea simplex *(9). This probably is the same as that of huratoxin (10).*

These workers determined that the structure of this substance (Fig. 1) was similar, if not identical, to a phorbol compound huratoxin, whose structure was identified by Sakata *et al*. (10) who isolated it from *Hura crepitans*, a member of the Euphorbiaceae. A coumarin glycoside has been isolated from *Daphne mezereum*, but there is no evidence for its toxicity in cattle or other species (11).

V. THE DISEASE IN CATTLE

All classes and ages of cattle appear to be equally susceptible to *Pimelea* intoxication. The earliest sign is usually diarrhea which may progress to dysentery. With the onset of diarrhea, affected cattle rapidly lose condition and become depressed. Severe acute intoxication may be fatal before more specific "classical" signs develop, but it is more usual for naturally occurring cases to develop a prominent jugular pulse, together with subcutaneous ventral edema, which begins at the intermandibular space and may progress to a striking degree, reaching as far as the umbilicus and down the front legs (Fig. 2).

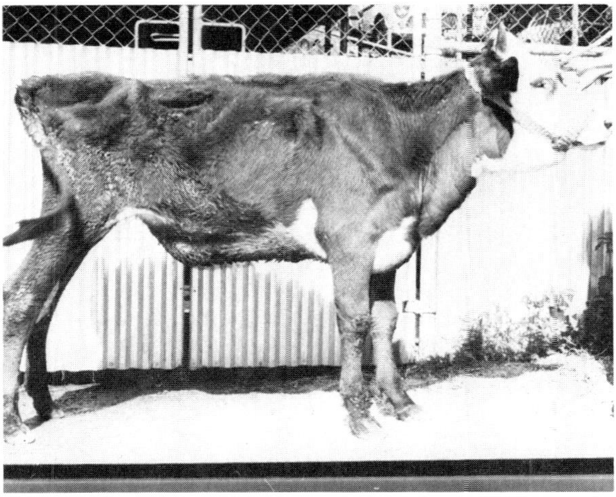

Fig. 2. *Heifer chronically intoxicated by daily oral administration of* Pimelea trichostachya *over a 31-day period. Severe ventral edema and wasting are apparent.*

Mucous membranes become pale and marked exercise intolerance develops. Affected animals often die suddenly during exertion. In fact the syndrome clinically very much resembles "Brisket disease" (pulmonary hypertension due to hypoxia of high altitudes (12).

It is rare to see signs of circulatory disease within three weeks of commencement of intoxication, although diarrhea usually begins within a few days. The toxin is very potent for cattle; daily oral dosage of 40 to 60 mg whole dried plant per kg body weight is sufficient to produce the complete spectrum of the field disease within 3 to 10 weeks. The syndrome is most reliably reproduced by lowering the dose rate once diarrhea becomes severe, so that intoxicated animals survive long enough to develop the characteristic circulatory embarrassment (6).

Affected animals always develop a degree of normocytic normochromic anemia (6). This anemia is not accompanied by any evidence of hemolysis and there is no compensatory erythropoietic response until the anemia becomes very severe (packed cell volume of 13% or less), when brisk erythropoiesis may supervene. There is moderate blood loss from the bowel, but ferrokinetic studies suggest that this is insufficient to produce the anemia (13).

There is usually a panleukopoenia in severely intoxicated animals, lymphocyte counts often being reduced more than neutrophils, but there is no evidence that such animals are significantly compromised immunologically.

At autopsy, sub-acutely intoxicated cattle are wasted, the lungs are moderately congested and the liver is slightly enlarged, but there is little in the way of specific pathology, apart from periportal sinusoidal dilatation and mononuclear cell sequestration in the liver (6). Microscopic examination of the gut shows surprisingly little pathology when one considers the severe diarrhea suffered by such animals.

Chronically intoxicated cattle, in addition to the severe subcutaneous ventral edema, have severe hydrothorax with notable absence of concomitant ascites. The liver is often very large, deep purple in color, and contains a vast excess of blood which runs freely from the sponge-like parenchyma on section. This hepatic change is consistent with some forms of peliosis hepatis, as it consists of distended large sinusoids and lakes of blood lined by stretched hepatocyte plates (Fig. 3). The blood lakes are largest just beneath the capsule, where they may become thrombosed.

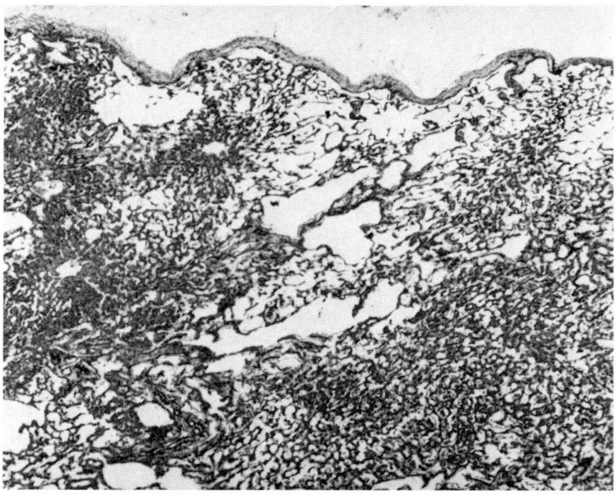

Fig. 3. *Section of subcapsular hepatic parenchyma of calf chronically intoxicated with* Pimelea trichostachya. *There is marked distension of sinusoids and stretching of hepatocyte plates. H and E x 160.*

Corrosion casts of severely affected livers (Fig. 4) show that there is ready communication between portal and hepatic veins via the enlarged vascular spaces (Kelly, unpublished observation).

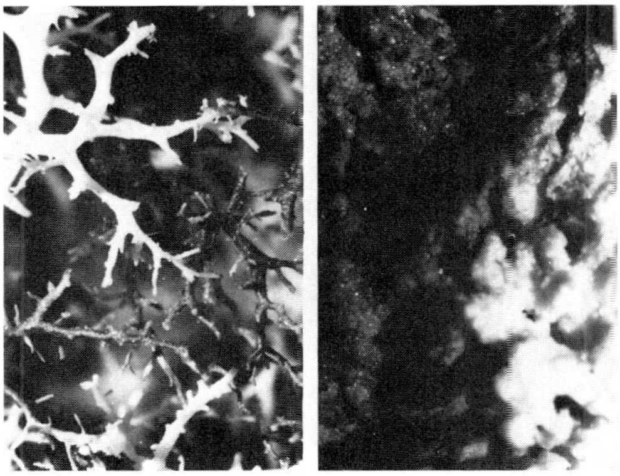

Fig. 4. *Vinyl acetate corrosion casts of hepatic and portal veins from a normal calf and from calf chronically intoxicated with* Pimelea trichostachya *and* P. continua. *The gray plastic represents branches of hepatic veins, the white the portal veins. Note the free intercommunication between the vessels in the affected liver, as opposed to the discrete branches in the normal liver.*

The liver lesion was described in detail by Seawright and Francis (14), who compared it to similar conditions in man and other species. Less spectacular vascular dilatation is also seen in other organs with sinusoidal circulations, such as spleen, bone marrow (Fig. 5), and adrenal renal cortex (11). The bone marrow shows not cytological abnormality to account for the anemia.

The lung and its vessels are histologically unremarkable in chronic cases, apart from atelectasis caused by the hydrothorax, and some alveolar septal thickening and siderosis in cases with prolonged severe circulatory embarrassment. There is no suggestion of the arteriolar lesions expected in "Brisket disease" (12). The right ventricle becomes dilated in chronic field cases which are forced to take some exercise, but myocardial hypertrophy seems never to be a feature of *Pimelea* poisoning. Myocardial necrosis is often seen and is attributed to the prolonged anemia combined with increased plasma volume (13).

VI. *PIMELEA* POISONING IN OTHER SPECIES

Pimelea spp. intoxication of sheep, horses, and cattle was recognized for many years before the association was recognized

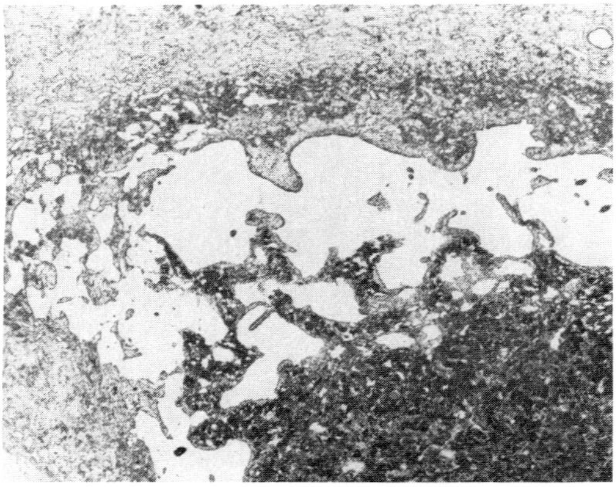

Fig. 5. *Section of femoral bone marrow showing sinusoidal dilation at the junction of hemopoietic and fatty marrow. H and E x 160.*

between this genus and "St. George disease" of cattle (4); the syndrome produced was invariably one of severe gastro-intestinal irritation, and none of the other features of chronic *Pimelea* poisoning in cattle have been recorded in field outbreaks of poisoning of other species.

Mice can be subacutely intoxicated by incorporating crude alcoholic extract of *Pimelea trichostachya* in their diet at levels of between 0.1 and 0.2% (Kelly, unpublished observations); in addition to diarrhea, the mice develop a moderate degree of hepatic sinusoidal dilation, but no other features of the bovine disease are produced.

VII. THE NATURE OF THE ANEMIA OF *PIMELEA* POISONING IN CATTLE

Severe anemia (PCV as low as 8%) can be produced in cattle by prolonged *Pimelea* intoxication; it is unique in that there is no compensatory erythropoiesis until the anemia is profound, however in some animals a brisk and effective erythropoietic response may then occur, bringing the animal's erythrocyte parameters close to normal (6).

Ferrokinetic studies have shown that there is no significant reduction of bone marrow erythropoiesis during *Pimelea* intoxication, but that the anemia is due to spectacular expansion of the plasma volume, coupled with greatly delayed erythropoietic response to the consequent hemodilution (13). There is some enhanced loss of blood from the bowel late in the intoxication, mostly from non-specific abomasal ulcers, but the total erythocyte mass is reduced comparatively little and may be within the expected range in cattle with obvious anemia. The total plasma volume may increase by as much as 178% and the total blood volume by as much as 100%, a phenomenon which is obviously related to the expansion of sinusoidal vessels throughout the body, and also to the development of cardiac failure. This degree of plasma and total blood volume expansion is apparently only paralleled by mice bearing certain transplantable gonadal tumors, in which increases in blood volume of up to 160% may occur (15).

The lack of compensatory erythropoiesis during the development of the anemia is unexplained.

VIII. THE EFFECT OF *PIMELEA* EXTRACTS ON PULMONARY VASCULATURE

Clark (16) emphasized the similarity between the clinical syndromes of *Pimelea* poisoning and "Brisket disease" of cattle, and showed in acute experiments in calves that intravenous injection of crude alcoholic *Pimelea* extract caused marked increase in pulmonary arterial pressure and increase in pulmonary vascular resistance. Because pulmonary congestion and edema followed these injections, Clark (16) suggested that the increase in pulmonary vascular resistance was due to constriction of pulmonary venules, and that this might be related to the heavy spiral muscle investment of these vessels (17).

This theory was tested by placing fresh spiral strips of bovine pulmonary vein in organ baths according to the method of Eyre (18) and exposing them to active extracts of *Pimelea trichostachya* (19). It was found that the extracts produced a slow, strong contraction of the spiral muscle which could not be effectively reversed by repeated washing of the strips or by application of substances such as methysergide or meclofenamate. Very slight reduction of the rate of contraction was achieved with papaverine. The response of these preparations to *Pimelea* extract was much slower than to serotonin or to histamine, and it is clear that the mechanism of the response to *Pimelea* is different to that mediated by pharmacologically active amines.

IX. REFERENCES

1. Clark, I. A., *Aust. Vet. J.* 47, 123 (1971).
2. McClure, T. J., and Farrow, B. R. H., *Aust. Vet. J.* 47, 100 (1971).
3. Roberts, H. B., and Healy, P. J., *Aust. Vet. J.* 47, 123 (1971).
4. Everest, S. L., "Poisonous Plants of Australia," p. 488. Angus and Robertson, Sydney, 1974.
5. Clark, I. A., *Aust. Vet. J.* 47, 285 (1971).
6. Kelly, W. R., *Aust. Vet. J.* 51, 233 (1975).
7. Hurst, E., "Poison Plants of New South Wales," p. 287. New South Wales Poison Plants Committee, Sydney, 1942.
8. Cantello, J. E., *Agric. Gaz. N. S. W.* 80, 418 (1969).

9. Roberts, H. B., McClure, T. J., Ritchie, E., Taylor, W. C., and Freeman, P. W., *Aust. Vet. J.* 51, 325 (1975).
10. Sakata, K., Kawazu, K., and Mitsui, T., *Agric. Biol. Chem.* 35, 2113 (1971).
11. Kingsbury, J. M., "Poisonous Plants of the United States and Canada," p. 386. Prentice-Hall, Englewood Cliffs, New Jersey, 1964.
12. Alexander, A. F., and Will, D. H., "Diseases of Cattle," Revised 2nd Ed. (W. J. Gibbons, Ed.), American Veterinary Publications Inc., Wheaton, Illinois.
13. Kelly, W. R., *Aust. Vet. J.* 51, 504 (1975).
14. Seawright, A. A., and Francis, J., *Aust. Vet. J.* 47, 91 (1971).
15. Furth, J., and Sobel, H., *J. Nat. Cancer Inst.* 7, 103 (1946).
16. Clark, I. A., *Res. Vet. Sci.* 14, 341 (1973).
17. Alexander, A. F., and Jensen, R., *Am. J. Vet. Res.* 24, 1083 (1963).
18. Eyre, P., *Br. J. Pharmacol.* 43, 302 (1971).
19. Kelly, W. R., and Bick, I. R. C., *Res. Vet. Sci.* 20, 311 (1976).

CYANOGENESIS, THE PRODUCTION OF HYDROGEN CYANIDE, BY PLANTS

Eric E. Conn

Department of Biochemistry and Biophysics
University of California

I. ABSTRACT

The production of HCN by higher plants is due to the presence, in the plants, of compounds which release HCN when acted upon by enzymes also usually found in the plant. The cyanogenic compounds, commonly glycosides of α-hydroxynitriles, are presumably located in one part of the plant cell (e.g. the vacuole) while the degradative enzymes are located in another. Numerous factors influence the potential toxicity of the cyanogenic compounds. These include: the concentration of the compound(s) in the plant; the amount of the toxic plant ingested; the size and kind of animal involved; the type of food ingested simultaneously; the possibility of the plant enzymes remaining active in the digestive tract of the animal; and the ability of the animal to detoxify the HCN which it encounters. Information on these factors, which is available in varying degrees, is summarized together with a description of the enzymatic process by which HCN is produced.

II. TOXICITY AND PRODUCTION OF HCN

The ability of plants to produce hydrogen cyanide (HCN) or prussic acid, a moderately toxic substance, was first described in 1803 (1). Today approximately 1000 species representing 250 genera and 80 families are known to be cyanophoric; that is, HCN is released when the tissues of the plant are crushed or otherwise disrupted. The production of HCN is usually attributed to the presence in the plant of one or more of the 21 known cyanogenic glycosides of α-hydroxynitriles (cyanohydrins). However, the parent glycoside has actually been identified in fewer than 100 plant species, and in at least one family (Sapindaceae) the HCN can arise from a cyanogenic lipid as well (2).

Knowledge of the manner in which cyanogenic glycosides give rise to HCN permits a better understanding and evaluation of the literature that is available on poisoning by these substances. The action of two enzymes, usually found in plants that contain cyanogenic glycosides, is illustrated in Figure 1 for prunasin, a cyanogen that occurs in many members of the Rosaceae, in *Eucalyptus cladocalyx*, and in *Pteridium aquilinum*. The initial reaction involves the hydrolysis by a β-glycosidase of the β-glycosidic bond between the sugar (usually glucose) and the

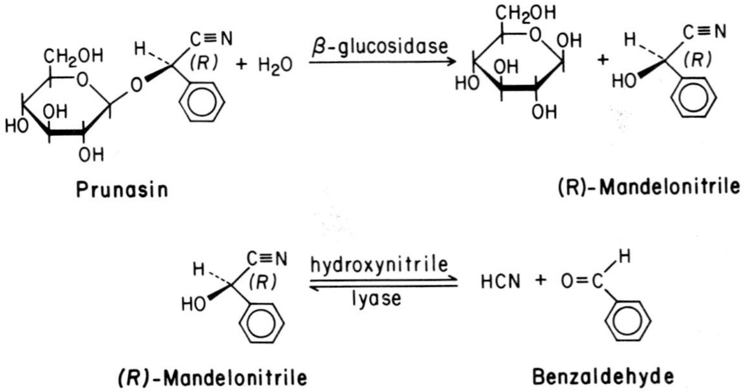

Fig. 1. *Conversion of Prunasin to HCN*

aglycone, in this case R-mandelonitrile (benzaldehyde cyanohydrin). β-Glycosidases catlyzing the hydrolysis of cyanogenic glycosides have been partially purified from almond (3), white clover (4), linen flax (5), and sorghum (6). These enzymes are highly specific for the β-glycosidic linkage that is found in the cyanogenic glycosides; the plant enzymes therefore differ from the α-glycosidases of the mammalian digestive tract that hydrolyze only α-glycosidic bonds.

Although the cyanohydrin can dissociate non-enzymically to produce HCN, plants contain enzymes called hydroxynitrile lyases that catalyze this facile equilibrium. In the presence of this enzyme, a α-hydroxynitrile dissociates to produce HCN and an aldehyde or ketone that is characteristic of the parent cyanogenic glycoside. The hydroxynitrile lyases of almond (7) and sorghum (8) have been extensively studied.

Being glycosides, the cyanogenic glycosides can be hydrolyzed by acid. This fact is apparently responsible for frequent references to hydrolysis of these compounds in the acidic environment of the stomach of monogastric animals. There are however no careful experiments establishing hydrolysis due to the acidic contents alone. Moreover the pH of the human stomach (approximately pH 2) is apparently not low enough to hydrolyze amygdalin, a cyanogenic glucoside common in the Rosaceae, since this glycoside is not hydrolyzed when incubated in 0.1 N H_2SO_4 at 37°C for 18 hours (9).

The literature on cyanogenic plants occasionally refers to the "HCN content" of a plant or plant tissue. However, it must be emphasized that HCN does not occur free within a plant but is produced, according to Figure 1, only after disruption of the plant cell has occurred and the glycoside and the degradative enzymes have been brought into contact with each other. Thus, this phenomenon is similar to the cellular hydrolysis that is initiated when animal cells are disrupted and lytic enzymes in the lysosome are exposed to their substrates. Recently, the cyanogenic glycoside that occurs in sorghum seedlings was shown to be located in the vacuoles of the tissue studied (10). This observation in turn suggests that the β-glycosidase of sorghum is located elsewhere in the plant cell and studies on the localization of the enzyme are awaited. It is of course possible that the enzyme exists in an inactive form in the vacuole as well. However, this seems unlikely since the hydrolysis of dhurrin is instantly initiated when the plant cell structure is disrupted and proceeds to completion within a short time.

During the past two decades, there has been a renewed interest in the production of HCN by plants. Thus, there are reviews on the chemistry (11), the isolation and characterization (2), and the biosynthesis (12) of the cyanogenic glycosides. Of greater interest to this audience are classical sources on poisonous plants (13,14) together with a recent book (15) which list species that have caused cyanide poisoning of animals including man. From these sources, from regional bulletins on poisonous plants (e.g. Ref. 16 and 17), and from current literature are assembled in Table 1 a list of some cyanogenic compounds occurring in some plants which have been indicted for poisoning of animals by cyanide. Useful as such sources are, what is also needed in this field are lists of the known cyanogenic species found in specific regions or areas of a country. Two such lists, for the northeastern United States (18) and for Oklahoma and Texas (19), have recently appeared and further publications covering other areas of this country are awaited. Two other important sources of information that should be consulted when determining if a given species has been reported as cyanogenic are the chemotaxonomic treatises of Hegnauer (20) and Gibbs (21).

As indicated in Figure 1 the release of HCN by a cyanophoric plant is a relatively simple process that depends on the cooccurrence of a cyanogenic glycoside and two enzymes in the plant under consideration. The question of whether a given plant will prove toxic to any animal that eats it is clearly more complicated. Probably of greatest importance is the amount of a cyanogenic glycoside which a given plant contains. Several methods are available for determining the amount of cyanogenic glycoside in plants (22-25). These are based on maceration and suspension of the tissue in H_2O or a buffer followed by hydrolysis by the enzymes that are usually present in the plant. If the enzymes are absent or low in activity, preparations of β-glucosidase (emulsin from almonds, linamarase from flax) can be added to accomplish the

TABLE 1

Cyanogenic Glycosides Occurring in Cyanophoric Plants Reported as Toxic to Animals

Glycoside	Sugar	Aglycone	Plant
Amygdalin	D-Gentiobiose	(R)-Mandelonitrile	Rosaceous species (foliage of wild cherry, choke cherry, mountain mahogany, apricot seeds, bitter almonds)
Prunasin	D-Glucose	(R)-Mandelonitrile	
Sambunigrin	D-Glucose	(S)-Mandelonitrile	*Sambucus nigra* (black elderberry); *Acacia cunninghamii*
Dhurrin	D-Glucose	p-Hydroxy-(S)-mandelonitrile	*Sorghum sp.* (grain and field sorghums, Johnson grass)
Taxiphyllin	D-Glucose	p-Hydroxy-(R)-mandelonitrile	*Taxus sp.* (Canadian and Japanese yew),[1] *Bambusa sp.* (bamboo)
Linamarin	D-Glucose	α-Hydroxyisobutyronitrile	*Trifolium repens* (white clover), *Linum sp.* (flax), *Lotus sp.*, *Manihot sp.* (cassava), *Phaseolus lunatus* (lima bean)
Lotaustralin	D-Glucose	α-Hydroxy-α-methylbutyronitrile	*Trifolium repens* (white clover), *Linum sp.* (flax), *Lotus sp.*, *Manihot sp.* (cassava) *Phaseolus lunatus* (lima bean)
Triglochinin	D-Glucose	Triglochinic acid[2]	*Triglochin sp.* (arrow grass)

[1]Toxicity due to an alkaloid
[2]Product obtained on hydrolysis of aglycone

hydrolysis. The HCN released can be determined in the hydrolysate by direct potentiometric titration or it can be removed by distillation, aeration, or diffusion and then determined. The HCN released can also be detected with filter paper impregnated with picric acid (13). This is the basis of a rapid, simple qualitative test that is conveniently performed in the field and has been used in a majority of the studies testing plants for cyanogenesis.

When the cyanogenic glycoside content of plants is determined as described above, it is observed that the amount in a given species can be influenced by a variety of factors including diurnal, seasonal, environmental, nutritional, and genetic factors. Thus the amount of linamarin in white clover is reported to fluctuate with the time of day, being higher in the morning and lower at the end of the day. The levels of prunasin in the California toyon, *Heteromeles arbutifolia* varies with the season, being higher in the spring and late fall (25a). Field sorghum that is grown widely for its grain and for silage, is reported to be especially toxic to livestock after a light frost or after being subjected to moisture stress (see Ref. 13 for discussion). There are also detailed studies on the effect of fertilizers on the cyanide producing potential of sorghum (26).

The ability to produce HCN is clearly polymorphic in two plant species, *Trifolium repens* and *Lotus corniculatus* (27), and is undoubtedly under similar genetic control in several other species including sorghum, almond, and macadamia. This is indicated since there are individual plants within a single species in these genera which are either strongly cyanogenic or only weakly so. Careful genetic analysis of the cyanophoric potential of *T. repens* has disclosed that two independent alleles are involved as follows (28):

$$\text{amino acid} \; \underset{\textit{Ac}\text{ gene}}{\rightarrow\rightarrow\rightarrow\rightarrow} \; \text{cyanogenic glycoside} \; \xrightarrow[\textit{Li}\text{ gene}]{\text{glycosidase}} \; \text{HCN} + \text{sugar and aldehyde or ketone}$$

The first of these, the *Ac* gene, controls the biosynthesis of the cyanogenic glycoside from its precursor amino acids. The second allele, *Li*, controls the level of the β-glucosidase enzyme in the plants. Thus for a plant to be cyanogenic when its tissues are disrupted, it must be dominant for both characters. The four phenotypes *AcAcLiLi*, *AcAclili*, *acacLiLi*, and *acaclili* can be obtained by selective breeding and those strains with little or no cyanogenic glycoside (*Ac* recessive) can be safely used for forage. The biosynthesis of cyanogenic glycosides in plants has been investigated extensively during the past decade and it is now possible to write a detailed biosynthetic pathway starting with a protein amino acid (12). Although there is evidence from studies with whole plants that one or more enzymatic steps in the pathway are lacking in *T. repens* plants recessive for the *Ac* gene, further work with isolated enzyme systems is necessary to ascertain whether a single enzyme step is missing (29).

While the potential of a plant to produce HCN is important in determining its toxicity, other factors must be considered; these include such factors as the size and kind of subject, the speed of ingestion, the type of food ingested simultaneously with the toxic plant, the possibility of the plant's degradative enzymes remaining active in the animal's digestive tract, and the ability of the animal to detoxify the HCN which it encounters. Unfortunately there are few if any detailed studies on any of these topics. Even so, there are general principles which bear repeating and may provide the stimulus for additional work.

A lethal dose of HCN taken orally for humans has been estimated at between 0.5 mg and 3.5 mg per kilogram body weight (30). These values compare with the figure of 2.0 mg per kilogram cited for cattle and sheep (31) and refer to single doses of HCN taken at one time. Obviously if an amount of plant material containing this concentration of HCN were consumed in an interval of a few minutes, the animal--man, sheep, or bovine--would probably die. On the other hand, if the time of ingestion is extended, the animal may suffer only mild symptoms. In either case, HCN will be rapidly absorbed from the gastrointestinal tract and produce recognizable symptoms at both fatal and non-fatal levels (13). With fatal doses, death results from the general anoxic state produced by the inhibition of cytochrome oxidase. With non-fatal doses, the inhibition of cellular respiration is reversed due to the removal of HCN by respiratory exchange or by metabolic detoxification. In the latter instance HCN is metabolized by the enzyme rhodanese which catalyzes the reaction shown in the following equation:

$$\underset{\text{thiosulfate}}{S_2O_3^{=}} + \underset{\text{cyanide}}{CN^{-}} \xrightarrow{\text{rhodanese}} \underset{\text{sulfite}}{SO_3^{=}} + \underset{\text{thiocyanate}}{SCN^{-}}$$

This process, incidentally, provides the basis for one of the treatments administered surviving animals suspected of suffering from cyanide poisoning; they are given intravenous injections of $Na_2S_2O_3$. A second compound often administered is sodium nitrite which oxidizes some of the blood hemoglobin to methemoglobin; this protein is capable of forming a stronger complex with HCN than is cytochrome oxidase. Consequently the HCN will dissociate from cytochrome oxidase and react with the methemoglobin, thereby allowing cellular respiration to proceed. Thiocyanate produced by detoxification is excreted in the urine. While the conversion of cyanide to thiocyanate catalyzed by rhodanese represents a detoxification of the HCN, it may be noted that thiocyanate in turn is a goitrogenic substance.

If the ingestion of cyanogenic plant material produces acute cyanide poisoning, it should be realized that the plant is probably providing both the cyanogenic glycoside and the enzymes responsible for the production of the lethal HCN. Moreover, the HCN production has to occur primarily within the short time between the mastication of the plant and its arrival in the stomach for, at least in man and the monogastric horse and pig, the normally acidic contents (pH 2) of the stomach would slow down if not prevent the action of the plant β-glucosidases that have an optimum pH of 5-6. (The enzymes of the mammalian digestive tract are α-glycosidases.) Then when the acidified stomach contents move into the duodenum and are mixed with the alkaline bile juice, the action of the plant enzymes may be restored. Presumably this situation will not exist in the case of ruminants where the food in the rumen will be at pH 6-7. This in turn may be one of the reasons that ruminants are considered more susceptible to poisoning by cyanogenic plants (31). Not only can the hydrolysis by plant enzymes continue uninhibited in the rumen, but the rumen bacteria are believed to be capable of hydrolyzing the cyanogenic compounds.

The risk of acute poisoning by cyanogenic plants is greatly diminished if the degradative enzymes (Fig. 1) are lacking or if they have been inactivated by heating or other treatment. An interesting example of the former situation was shown by Finnemore and Gledhill (32) to occur in several Australian acacias which contain a cyanogenic glycoside but not a β-glucosidase to hydrolyze the cyanogen. This finding was recently confirmed (33) for *Acacia cunninghamii* and shown to exist in three other Australian acacias. As an illustration of the latter situation, one of the standard procedures for making cyanogenic cassava tubers safe for human consumption is to cook the plant material thoroughly prior to its use for food. Alternatively, the cassava tuber is scraped or grated and then soaked in water to leach out the cyanogen and its hydrolysis products.

It has also been stated that the possibility of HCN poisoning is decreased if a large amount of starch-containing food is consumed simultaneously with the cyanogenic plant material (34). The rationale for this statement is not entirely clear but may be based on the suggestion that glucose, the hydrolysis product of starch, can bind HCN as a cyanohydrin to varying degrees. Glucose is also prescribed for the treatment of animals poisoned with HCN (34). However, there have been no clear-cut studies which have examined this suggestion by carefully controlling the other factors that can influence acute cyanide poisoning.

With this as background, one can then cite numerous examples of the acute poisoning of animals, including man, due to the ingestion of cyanogenic plant material. Thus there are reports of persons being poisoned by eating apricot kernals (35-37), choke cherry seeds (38), and bitter almonds (39). Young sorghum is frequently toxic to cattle which have inadvertantly been permitted to eat the tender, green leaves (40,41). Members of the rose family (apples, mountain mahogany, wild cherries, and choke cherries) have been cited for much loss of livestock in the United States (13). Arrow grass is a common culprit involved in livestock poisoning in the West (42), and cyanophoric species of acacia have been blamed for the death of sheep and cattle in Australia (43), South Africa (44), and the United States (13). While it was usually the leaf foliage of these plants that was consumed, it should be appreciated that the cyanogenic glycoside may occur in other parts as well. Thus the seeds (kernels) of the Rosaceae are also frequently cyanogenic. On the other hand, the seed of sorghum lacks the cyanogenic glycoside, and the concentration in flax seed is relatively low. Young seedlings of both species however exhibit a high level of glycoside so that a rapid synthesis of these compounds occurs in the first days of germination. Wild lima beans have a high cyanogenic glycoside content that remains essentially constant during germination, indicating either that translocation from the seed into the seedling occurs during germination or that simultaneous degradation in the seed and resynthesis in the young seedling tissue occurs.

The question arises as to whether the cyanogenic glycosides can be absorbed, transported within the body and ultimately degraded by intracellular enzymes. This possibility was considered by Coop and Blakley (45) who administered purified preparations of lotaustralin, a cyanogenic glucoside found in *Trifolium repens*, to sheep. Their studies clearly showed the compound to be toxic and they estimated the minimum lethal dose to be 4-5 mg lotaustralin per kilogram of body weight. More recently, linamarin, the other cyanogenic glycoside found in *T. repens* and also cassava, was administered orally by stomach tube to rats (48). A the high doses administered (500 mg/kg body wt) all animals died within 4 hours while at a somewhat reduced dose of 300 mg/kg body weight all animals survived. Analysis of the latter animals showed that about one-fifth of the linamarin was excreted in the urine while one-fourth was metabolized to thiocyanate. This last finding clearly demonstrates that intracellular enzymes can hydrolyze linamarin to produce HCN which then is detoxified to produce thiocyanate. The occurrence of a β-glucosidase in liver microsomes is well documented (47). Unfortunately the ability of this enzyme to hydrolyze cyanogenic glycosides was not examined.

The subject of intracellular hydrolysis of cyanogenic glycosides is directly relevant to the matter of chronic cyanide poisoning (48). There is extensive literature on the degenerative disease, tropical ataxic neuropathy, which implicates the high consumption of cassava with this disease in a group of Nigerians. Related neuropathies have been described in Jamaica and Malaya where cassava is consumed. Montgomery, in reviewing chronic cyanide poisoning, points out that cyanide in cassava has been blamed by others for the tropical amblyopia (blindness) that is common in West Africa (49). The blindness occurring in some heavy smokers (tobacco amblyopia) may be due to poisoning by the HCN that is a component of cigarette smoke (49,50). At least one report in the veterinary literature raises the question of whether chronic cyanide poisoning may not have occurred in horses (51) kept on sorghum pasture.

There is a need to carefully assess the potential for chronic cyanide poisoning, both in the livestock industry and in the human population. In the case of domestic animals, cassava chips and other cassava products are being increasingly employed as a starchy feed. Cassava apparently has a promising future as an animal food source and any disadvantages that may result from the cyanogenic potential of the plant therefore should be carefully evaluated (48). In the case of man, the increasing legalization of amygdalin as an anticancer agent, thereby overruling Food and Drug Administration regulations banning its use (52), urgently calls for careful scientific study of the possibility of chronic as well as acute poisoning by this cyanogenic glycoside.

III. REFERENCES

1. Schrader, J. C. C., *Gilbert Anallen* 13, 503 (1803).
2. Seigler, D. S., *Phytochemistry* 14, 9 (1975).
3. Haisman, D. R., and Knight, D. J., *Biochem. J.* 103, 528 (1967).
4. Hughes, M. A., *J. Exp. Bot.* 19, 427 (1968).
5. Butler, G. W., Bailey, R. W., and Kennedy, L. D., *Phytochemistry* 4, 369 (1965).
6. Mao, C. H., and Anderson, L., *Phytochemistry* 6, 473 (1967).
7. Becker, W., and Pfeil, E., *Biochem. Z.* 346, 301 (1966).
8. Seely, M. K., Criddle, R. S., and Conn, E. E., *J. Biol. Chem.* 241, 4457 (1977).
9. Dunn, J. E., and Conn, E. E., unpublished studies.
10. Saunders, J. A., Conn, E. E., Lin, C. H., and Stocking, C.R., *Plant Physiol.* 59, 647 (1977).
11. Eyjolfsson, R., *Fortschr. Chem. Org. Naturst.* 28, 74 (1977).
12. Conn, E. E., *Biochem. Soc. Symp.* 38, 277 (1973).
13. Kingsbury, J. M., "Poisonous Plants of the United States and Canada," Prentice-Hall, Englewood Cliffs, New Jersey, 1964.
14. Watt, J. M., and Breyer-Brandwijk, M. G., "The Medicinal and Poisonous Plants of Southern and Eastern Africa," 2nd Ed., E. & S. Livingstone Ltd., Edinburgh and London, 1962.
15. Everist, S. L., "Poisonous Plants of Australia," Angus and Robertson, Sydney, 1974.
16. Agricultural Extension Service, "Principal Livestock-Poisoning Plants of New Mexico Ranges," *Agric. Ext. Serv. Cir.* 274, New Mexico A&M College, 1957.
17. Agricultural Experiment Station, "Poisonous Plants and Live-stock Poisoning," *Wyo. Agric. Exp. Stn. Bull.* 324, 1953.
18. Seigler, D. S., *Econ. Bot.* 30, 395 (1976).
19. Seigler, D. S., *Proc. Okla. Acad. Sci.* 56, 95 (1976).
20. Hegnauer, R., "Chemotaxonomie der Pflanzen," Vol. I-VI, Birkhaüser-Verlag, Basel, 1963-73.
21. Gibbs, R. D., "Chemotaxonomie of Flowering Plants," McGill-Queen University Press, Montreal, 1974.
22. Winkler, W. O., *J. Assoc. Off. Agric. Chem.* 34, 541 (1951).
23. Akazawa, T., Miljanich, P., and Conn, E. E., *Plant Physiol.*

35, 535 (1960).
24. Hahlbrock, K., and Conn, E. E., *J. Biol. Chem.* 245, 917 (1970).
25. Blaedel, W. J., Easty, D. B., Anderson, L., and Farrell, T. R., *Anal. Chem.* 43, 890 (1971).
25a. Dement, W. A., and Mooney, H. A., *Oecologia* 15, 65 (1974).
26. Kriedeman, P. E., *Aust. J. Exp. Agric. Anim. Husb.* 4, 15 (1964).
27. Nass, H. G., *Crop Sci.* 12, 503 (1972).
28. Atwood, S. S., and Sullivan, J. T., *J. Hered.* 34, 311 (1943).
29. Hughes, M. A., and Conn, E. E., *Phytochemistry* 15, 697 (1976).
30. Montgomery, R. D., *in* "Toxic Constituents of Plant Food Stuffs" (I. E. Liener, Ed.), Academic Press, New York 1969.
31. Moran, E. A., *Am. J. Vet. Res.* 15, 171 (1954).
32. Finnemore, H., and Gledhill, W. C., *Aust. J. Pharm.* 9, 1974 (1928).
33. Secor, J. B., Conn, E. E., Dunn, J. E., and Seigler, D. S., *Phytochemistry* 15, 1703 (1976).
34. Couch, J. F., "Poisoning of Livestock by Plants that Produce HCN," *U. S. Dep. Agric. Leafl.* 88 (1932).
35. Sayre, J. W., and Kaymakcalan, S., *N. Engl. J. Med.* 270, 1113 (1964).
36. Gunders, A. E., Abrahamov, A., and Weisenberg, E., *J. Isr. Med. Assoc.* 76, 536 (1969).
37. "California Morbidity," No. 51, December 26, 1975.
38. Pijoan, M., *Am. J. Med. Sci.* 204, 550 (1942).
39. Pack, W. K., Raudonat, H. W., and Schmidt, K., *Z. Rechtsmed.* 70, 53 (1972).
40. "The Austin (Texas) American," p. 13, August 25, 1962.
41. Gibb, M. C., Carbery, J. T., Carter, R. G., and Catalinac, S., *N. Z. Vet. J.* 22, 127 (1974).
42. Marsh, C. D., Clawson, A. B., and Roe, G. C., *U. S. Dep. Agric. Tech. Bull.* 113, 1929.
43. Hurst, E., "The Poison Plants of New South Wales," Snelling Printing Works, Sydney, 1942.
44. Steyn, D. G., and Rimington, C., *Onderstepport J. Vet. Sci. Anim. Ind.* 4, 51 (1935).
45. Coop, I. E., and Blakley, R. L., *N. Z. J. Sci. Tech.* 32, 44 (1950).
46. Barrett, M. L., Hill, D. C., Alexander, J. C., and Zitnak, A., *Can. J. Physiol. Pharmacol.* in press (1977).
47. Patel, V., and Tappel, A. L., *Biochim. Biophys. Acta* 191, 86 (1969).
48. International Development and Research Center, "Chronic Cassava Toxicity: Proceedings of an Interdisciplinary Workshop" (B. Nestel and R. MacIntyre, Eds.), Ottawa, Canada, 1973.
49. Montgomery, R. D., *Am. J. Clin. Nutr.* 17, 103 (1965).
50. Anonymous, *Lancet ii*, 942 (1969).
51. Adams, L. G., Dollahite, J. W., Romane, W. M., Bullard, T. L., and Bridges, C. H., *J. Am. Vet. Med. Assoc.* 155, 518 (1969).
52. Holden, C., *Science* 193, 982 (1976).

PULMONARY TOXICITY OF NATURALLY OCCURRING 3-SUBSTITUTED FURANS

Benjamin J. Wilson, John E. Garst, and Robert D. Linnabary
School of Medicine, Vanderbilt University
Alan R. Doster
College of Veterinary Medicine, University of Georgia

I. ABSTRACT

Furans of various types are frequently encountered in the environment. The naturally occurring 3-substituted furans are of special interest because of their hepatic or pulmonary toxicity for several animal species including livestock. The sweet potato is capable of producing several hepatotoxic 3-substituted furans as stress metabolites when stimulated by various exogenous agents including fungus pathogens. Fusarium solani *infection results in accumulation also of three compounds with potent lung-toxic properties-- 4-ipomeanol, 1-ipomeanol, and 1,4-ipomeadiol. Experiments indicate these compounds are responsible for acute bovine pulmonary emphysema (ABPE) caused by consumption of* Fusarium-*infected sweet potato roots.*

Perilla ketone, egomaketone, and isoegomaketone are closely related pulmonary toxins occurring normally in the mint plant, Perilla frutescens. *These toxins are quite similar structurally to the sweet potato toxic metabolites.* P. frutescens *grows wild in much of the eastern United States and has been suggested as another etiological agent of ABPE. This speculation is supported by toxicity tests of perilla ketone in laboratory animals as well as in sheep and cattle. It seems probable that additional lung-toxic factors will be found in other plants grazed by livestock.*

II. OCCURRENCE OF FURANS

Compounds containing the furan moiety have been detected from a wide range of biological sources including plants and animal products used for foods. For example, coffee contains the three furans (1,2,3) below: 1, 2, 3:

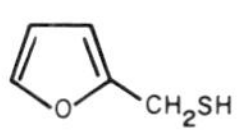

1

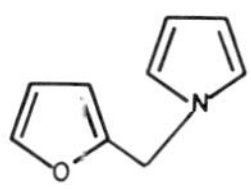

2

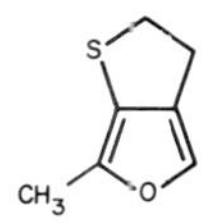

3

Cooked meat (4) may contain 2-methyl-3-sulfhydryl furan 4, milk (5) has yielded the furan amino acid 5, and cod and other fish (6) have been shown to contain a tetra-substituted furan 6.

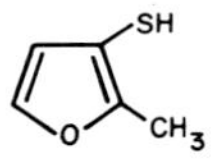

4

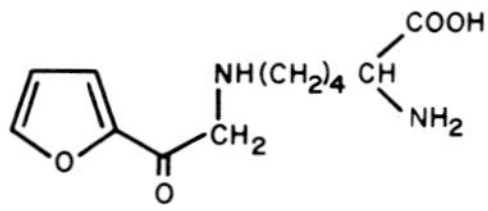

5

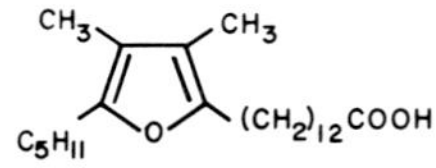

6

Examples of furans from fruits are 2-furaldehyde (7), 7, and limonin, 8, the latter found in the orange (8). Menthofuran, 9, from peppermint oil may occur in quantities equal to 8% of this product (9).

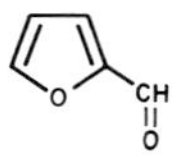

7

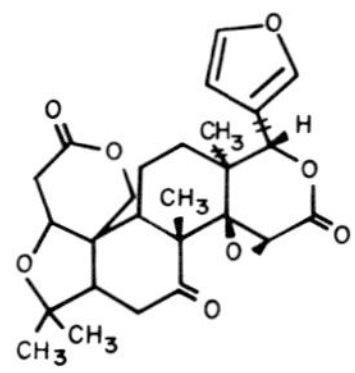

8

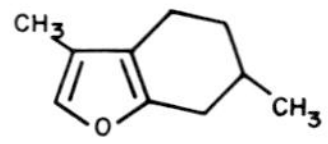

9

These are but a few of many such compounds occurring naturally or that can be generated during the course of food preparation. In addition, there are many 2-substituted furans prepared commercially for use as essences and flavor enhancers of foods. Few of these compounds have been adequately tested for possible toxicity in animals.

Furans can also arise from dehydration of sugars (10) as exemplified by the well-known conversion of fructose to hydroxymethylfurfural, 10. In this context it is interesting to note that normal adult urine (11) has been found to contain furan-2,5-dicarboxylic acid, 11.

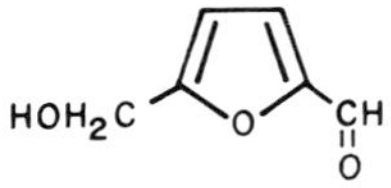

10

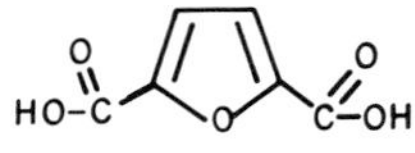

11

Among well-known therapeutic agents containing furans are furosemide, 12, a diuretic agent (12), and nitrofurantoin, 13, which is a frequently prescribed antibacterial agent for urinary tract infections (13).

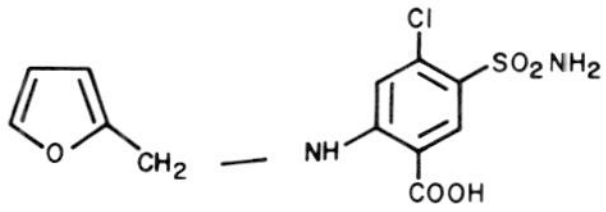

12

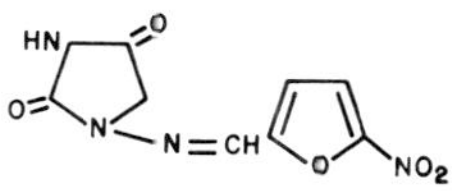

13

The 3-substituted furans are probably better known for their toxic properties. Among the more widely reported members of this class are several hepatotoxic, normal metabolites of the Ngaio tree and the Elangowan bush (*Myoporum laetum* and *M. deserti*, respectively) in Australasia (14). These plants produce several closely related hepatotoxic compounds which are chemical relatives of toxic stress metabolites of the sweet potato and of those occurring naturally in the essential oil of the mint plant, *Perilla frutescens*.

III. LUNG-TOXIC 3-SUBSTITUTED FURANS FROM THE MOLD-DAMAGED SWEET POTATO

Moldy sweet potato poisoning of cattle has been reported in Japan and the United States over several decades (15). Although a variety of names have been applied to the pulmonary disease, most descriptions fit the generally used term "acute bovine pulmonary emphysema" (ABPE), (16). This syndrome apparently can be caused by more than one agent, although evidence linking some of the purported toxic compounds and biological factors with ABPE is still quite tenuous.

Our interest in moldy sweet potatoes as a source of pulmonary toxins dates to 1969 when an outbreak of lethal bovine lung disease was encountered in Tift County, Georgia. This outbreak resulted in death of 69 Hereford cattle out of a herd of 275. Peckham *et al.* (17) described the pathological features of both the natural and experimentally induced disease as "atypical interstitial pneumonia." They were able to reproduce the condition by feeding sweet potato root slices inoculated with the fungus *Fusarium solani* which had earlier been demonstrated as the stimulating agent for toxin formation in the sweet potato (18).

Disease signs in moldy sweet potato poisoning in cattle, which may begin within 24 hours following consumption of the molded food, are usually confined to the respiratory tract. Afflicted animals will go off feed and soon begin to show dyspnea with rapid breathing which becomes more labored until death, due apparently to asphyxiation.

Postmortem opening of the thorax reveals lungs which are heavy, wet, and emphysematous (Fig. 1). There is usually marked vascular

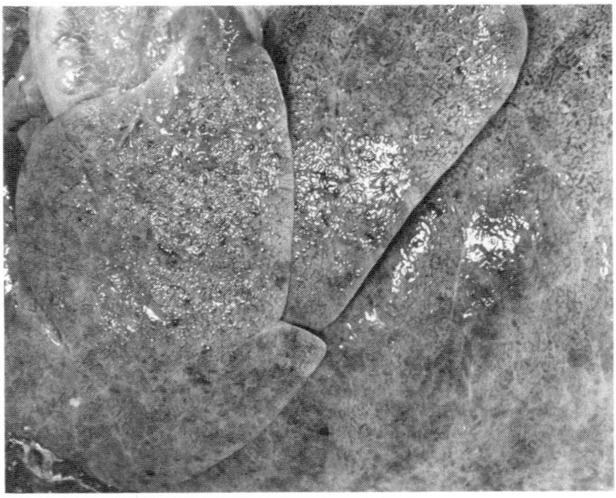

Fig. 1. *Diffuse pulmonary edema and emphysema in lung of cow dying of acute pulmonary emphysema.*

congestion giving the gross appearance of hepatization. At the microscopic level one sees congestion with alveolar edema and trapped air as well as several other phenomena to be mentioned.

Japanese investigators have isolated several 3-substituted furans mainly from sweet potatoes infected with the black-rot fungus pathogen *Ceratocystis fimbriata.* The most prominent compound is called ipomeamarone, a name that refers to the producing host, *Ipomoea batatas* (19).

Ipomeamarone, 14, is an oily compound which, like several other related stress metabolites of the sweet potato, such as 4-hydroxymyoporone, 15, is formed by the host tissues *per se* in response to several exogenous stimuli. These sesquiterpenoids are primarily hepatotoxic, causing hepatic cell necrosis in laboratory rats and mice at doses of around 200 to 300 mg/kg body weight (15). The lungs do not show significant damage. Ipomeamorone is the enantiomorph of ngaione, the hepatotoxic normal metabolite of *M. laetum* and *M. deserti* and other plants in Australasia (14).

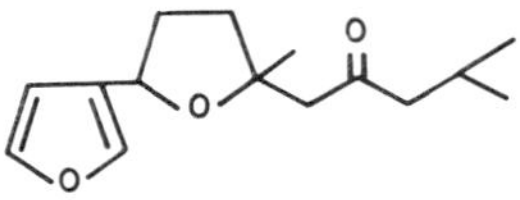

14

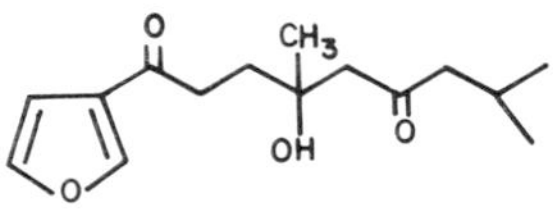

15

A search for the lung-toxic metabolites of moldy sweet potatoes by Dr. M. R. Boyd and myself finally led to separation and preparative isolation of two isomers with edemagenic properties for the mouse lung (20). They were given the trivial names 4-ipomeanol, 16, and 1-ipomeanol, 17, based on the respective position of the hydroxyl group in the side chain. 4-Ipomeanol is more abundant and more toxic than 1-ipomeanol. We postulated that the diketone, ipomeanine, 18, earlier reported by Kubota (21), would also be lung toxic, even though no reports of its toxicity had been published. It was also predicted that a diol, 19, would likely be found in the infected sweet potato. This compound, later named 1,4-ipomeadiol, was, in fact, detected in *Fusarium solani*-infected root tissue after obtaining authentic samples by chemical synthesis. Both ipomeanine and 1,4-ipomeadiol proved to be lung toxic (18).

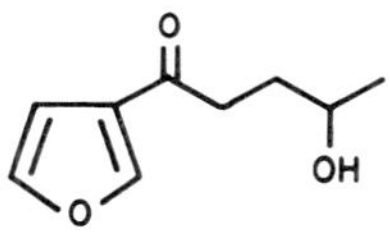

16

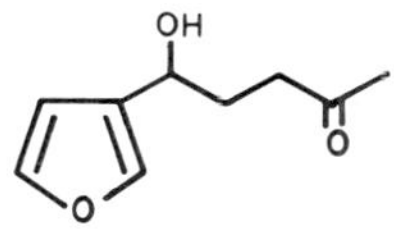

17

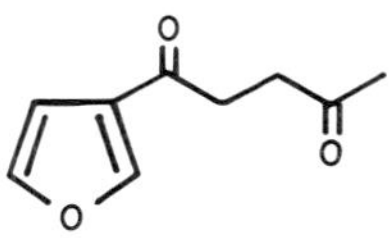

18

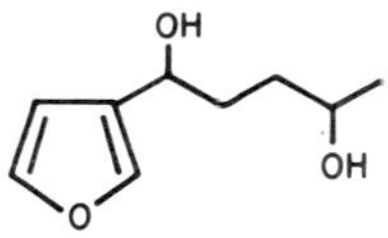

19

Although the diol occurs in significant quantities, we have no evidence indicating that ipomeanine accumulates in more than trace amounts in *Fusarium*-infected sweet potatoes. Therefore, the postulated lung edema factor of moldy sweet potatoes, at least at present, consists of three compounds--the two ipomeanols and the diol. The LD_{50}'s of the four compounds mentioned above are given in Table 1.

Prior to successful isolation and structural identification of the lung toxins, it was necessary to develop procedures for laboratory bioproduction of these metabolites from sweet potatoes. Only infection with *F. solani*, or closely related species, was capable of bringing about formation of lung toxins, 18, even though several other fungi and certain chemical agents could cause the sweet potato roots to form ipomeamarone and other hepatotoxic furans. For example, 1% mercuric chloride and the black-rot fungus, *C. fimbriata*, respectively, may be used for this purpose.

TABLE 1

LD_{50} Values (mg/kg) in Mice for Sweet Potato Lung-Edemagenic Agents[1]

	Intravenous	Oral	Intraperitoneal
Ipomeanine, 18	14	26	25
4-Ipomeanol, 16	21	38	36
1-Ipomeanol, 17	34	79	49
1,4-Ipomeadiol, 19	68	104	67

[1]The toxins were dissolved in 50% propylene glycol-water.

Further work has shown that *F. solani* growing on sweet potato root slices first stimulates host tissue to form ipomeamarone and 4-hydroxymyoporone, the latter is then converted to ipomeanine which is reduced to the three other lung toxins (22). Thus, the fungus is serving, not only as an initial stressing agent, but as a metabolic converter of host-formed precursors (hepatotoxins) to the shorter chain lung toxins.

We have significant but incomplete information on biochemical events leading to toxic action of 4-ipomeanol in lung tissue of laboratory animals. Synthetic toxin labeled with C^{14} in the side chain is apparently activated by microsomal P-450 oxygenase enzymes followed by covalent binding of the activated form of toxin to tissue macromolecules (23). The extent of binding to lung protein parallels the degree of pulmonary edema-genesis and lethality. Binding to lung protein normally exceeds that in the liver and other vital organs.

Several laboratory animals are quite susceptible to the pulmonary toxicity of 4-ipomeanol. These include the mouse, rat, guinea pig, and rabbit. The Assyrian golden hamster is the most resistant of all species studied. In the mouse, pleural fluid accumulation is a prominent feature. This animal is also unique in that near-fatal doses for pulmonary disease may cause delayed death due to extensive tubular necrosis of the kidneys (Fig. 2).

In recent unpublished experiments, Doster *et al.* have shown that 4-ipomeanol given intraruminally to seven cross-breed heifers caused the typical toxic lung syndrome seen in moldy sweet potato poisoning outbreaks in cattle. The doses given ranged from 6 to 14 mg/kg body weight with the severity of the reactions and survival times following a dose-response pattern. Deaths followed toxin administration within 8 days when a dose of 9 mg or more per kilogram body weight was given. Gross lesions were confined to the lungs and mediastinum with pulmonary edema and emphysema being prominent (Fig. 3).

In addition to disruptive changes noted within and around the lymphatics and blood vessels, the alveoli were often greatly distended with air, or ruptured, forming large emphysematous spaces.

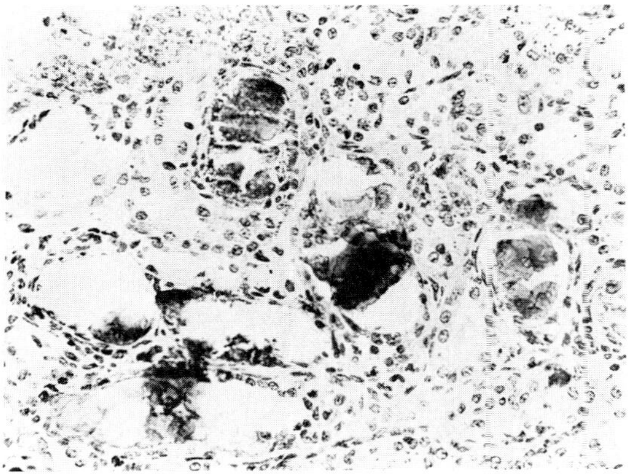

Fig. 2. *Photomicrograph of mouse kidney showing tubular necrosis and deposition of calcium.*

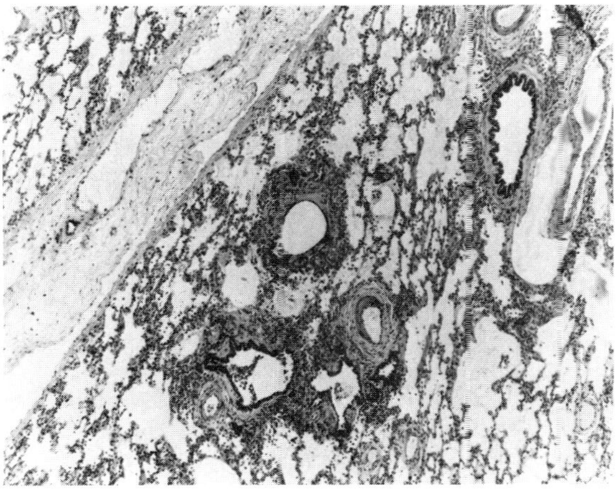

Fig. 3. *H&E stained section of lung from heifer showing interlobular, interstitial, and alveolar edema with emphysema; peribronchiolar reaction and fibrosis are also evident.*

The alveolar spaces also contained a homogenous eosinophilic residue which in some areas composed hyaline membranes. Variable numbers of cellular elements were present including neutrophiles, lymphocytes, eosinophiles, macrophages, and erythrocytes. Among other marked changes were thickened alveolar walls with edema, congestion and focal hemorrhages, terminal bronchioles lined with hyperchromatic, cuboidal epithelium; and peribronchiolar fibrosis. The heifer receiving 9 mg/kg, which was killed *in extremis* on the 8th day after dosing, had alveoli lined by hyperplastic epithelium in an adenomatous arrangement (Fig. 4).

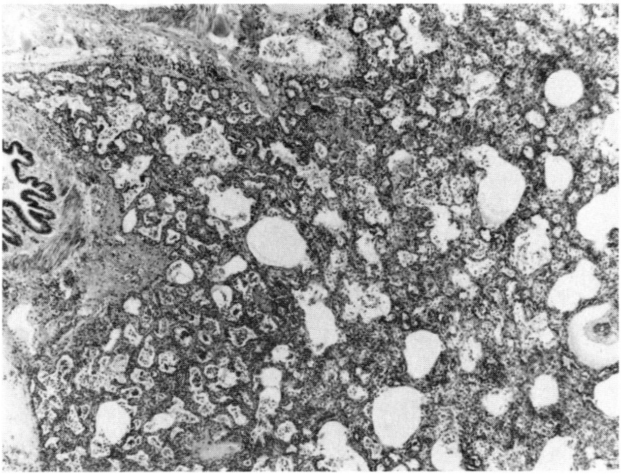

Fig. 4. *Microscopic section of cow lung showing diffuse interstitial fibrosis, alveolar edema and emphysema, and adenomatous appearance of hyperplastic epithelium.*

Two animals receiving 6 and 7.5 mg/kg initial doses had fewer pulmonary changes. However, the alveolar septa contained collagen fibers along with the cellular elements mentioned above. Hypertrophy of the alveolar epithelium was multi-focal and less extensive than in the higher dose animals. Both animals were classed as survivors and were sacrificed on the 11th and 54th day, respectively.

In another study a single Jersey heifer was given 32 mg/kg intraruminally. The animal died within 10 hours with extensive pulmonary edema. There were also infarcts in the kidneys and liver.

These bovine studies clearly show that 4-ipomeanol, and in all probability the other lung toxins of the *Fusarium solani*-infected sweet potato, are capable of producing the disease manifestations of naturally occurring sweet potato poisoning. The gross and microscopic pictures vary somewhat with toxin dose and the time of survival after dosing. Apparently the cow is the most susceptible species considered thus far, which may be due to marked covalent binding of activated toxin to lung microsomal protein observed for this species. The failure to observe liver damage in naturally occurring cases of sweet potato poisoning (17), where ipomeamarone and other liver-toxic 3-substituted furans are usually abundant in the infected root tissues, is possibly due to inherent resistance of bovine liver to the longer chain compounds.

IV. LUNG-TOXIC FURANS FROM *PERILLA FRUTESCENS*

In recent months we have become aware of another biological source of 3-substituted furans and one that in all probability is a major cause of bovine pulmonary emphysema. *Perilla frutescens* (Figs. 5a, 5b; 6a, 6b) is a plant commonly used in the Orient for a wide variety of purposes (24). Following importation into the United States it apparently garden-escaped and is now widely spread over much of the eastern half of the country.

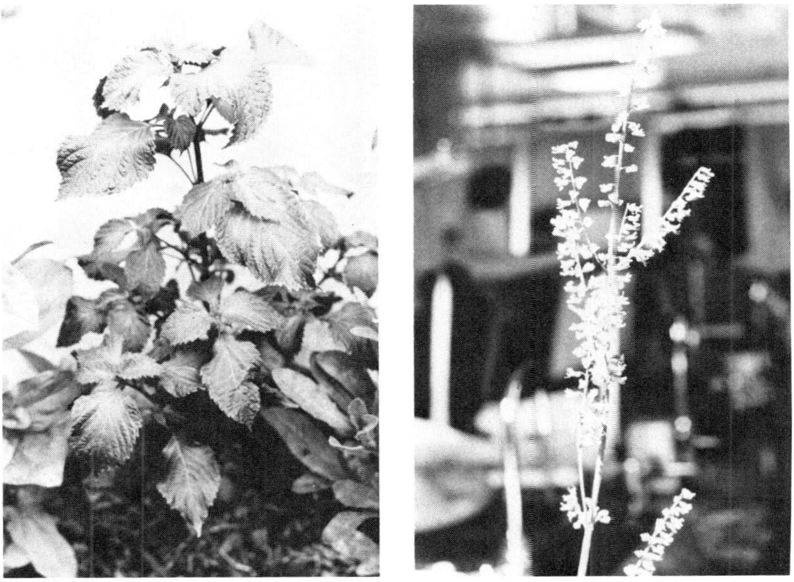

Fig. 5 (a, left). Perilla frutescens: *Cultivated plant approximately 12 weeks after planting (seeds from Oklahoma).* (b, right). *Leafless, dry stem with infructescences and intact calyces collected during winter in Tennessee. The dry stem contained detectable levels of perilla ketone.*

Our interest in perilla was based on Japanese reports describing closely related 3-substituted furans isolated from various parts of the plant. As shown below, three of these compounds are close relatives of 4-ipomeanol; perilla ketone, 20, differs only in having a methyl group in place of the hydroxyl of 4-ipomeanol. The other two, egomaketone, 21, and isoegomaketone, 22, additionally have a double bond in the side-chain (24).

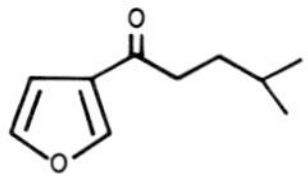

20

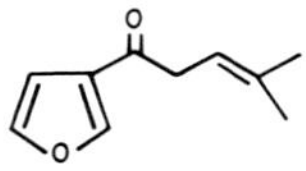

21

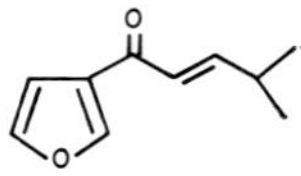

22

Dr. John Garst, in our laboratory, synthesized these compounds, and we determined their toxicity for laboratory animals. No reports on their toxicity had been found. As we suspected, all three are potent lung toxins for rats and mice. The only difference observed in the pathological responses of the mouse to these toxins and 4-ipomeanol is failure of the perilla metabolites to induce the kidney damage (Fig. 2) previously described for the sweet potato toxins. The intraperitoneal LD_{50}'s for mice are about one-fifth that of 4-ipomeanol.

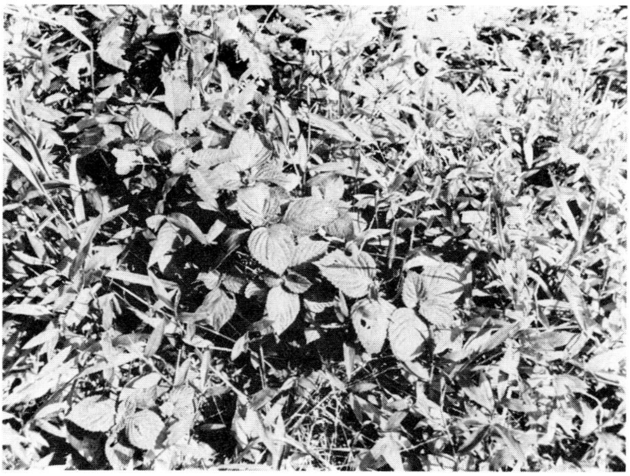

Fig. 6a. Perilla frutescens: *Young plants growing in Tennessee cow pasture.*

Our interest in perilla toxins was heightened further by belated discovery of a 1963 report by Dr. Duane Peterson, of Oklahoma State University, linking *P. frutescens* to several outbreaks of ABPE in Oklahoma. His findings suggested that losses of several thousand cattle earlier in neighboring Arkansas might also be attributable to this plant (25).

We carried out experiments with synthetic perilla ketone in Angus heifers when limited supplies of the toxin were available (29). The first two animals failed to respond when 3 and 9 mg/kg,

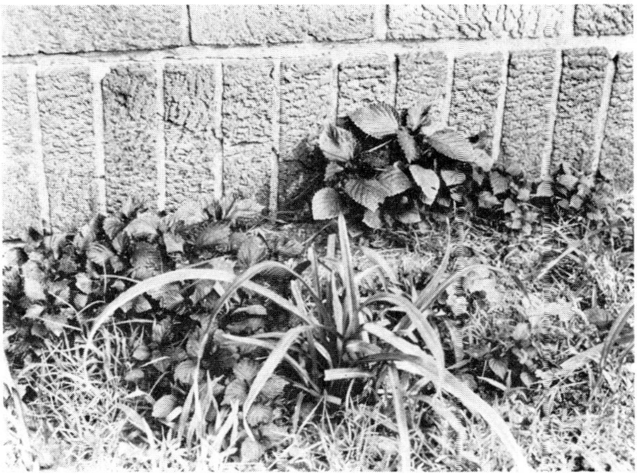

Fig. 6b. Perilla frutescens: *Young growth of purple colored variety in foundation plantings.*

respectively were injected directly into the rumen. However, another animal injected intravenously with 8 g (30 mg/kg) developed typical signs of pulmonary emphysema and died 3 days later. Postmortem examination revealed lungs that were extremely congested and had many other gross and microscopic lesions of ABPE. Unlike the cattle receiving 4-ipomeanol, there was an abundance of straw colored pleural fluid in the thorax with the typical minty odor of perilla ketone.

A male sheep injected with 19 mg/kg perilla ketone intravenously showed labored breathing after 72 hours. Signs lasted for about 48 hours at which time the animal began to show evidence of recovery and was killed for examination. The lungs showed patches of intraalveolar edema. No other organs were affected. Additional large animal toxicity tests are planned.

In summation, we believe we have identified two plant sources of 3-substituted furans that are capable of producing ABPE in cattle and perhaps similar conditions in other farm animals. These compounds offer us model lung edemagenic agents for further studies on their pathogenesis and mechanism(s) of action in susceptible animals.

It seems very likely that additional plant sources of similar pulmonary toxins will be found, plants which even now are responsible for losses of livestock in the United States and other countries of the world (26).

V. REFERENCES

1. Acheson, R. M., "An Introduction to the Chemistry of Heterocyclic Compounds," 3rd Ed., p. 151. Interscience, New York, 1976.
2. Gianturco, M. A., Giammarino, A. S., Friedel, P., and Flanagan, V., *Tetrahedron* 20, 2951 (1964).
3. Buchi, G., Degen, P., Gautschi, F., and Willhalm, J., *J. Org. Chem.* 36, 199 (1971).
4. Evers, W. J., Heinsohn, H. H., Jr., Mayers, B. J., and Sanderson, A., *in* "Phenolic, Sulfur, and Nitrogen Compounds in Food Flavors," (G. Charalambous and I. Katz, Eds.), American Chemical Society, Symposium Series No. 26, p. 184. Washington, D. C., 1976.
5. Finot, P. A., Bricout, J., Viani, R., and Mauron, J., *Experientia* 24, 1097 (1968).
6. Gunstone, F. D. R., Wijesundera, R. C., Love, R. M., and Rose, D., *Chem. Commun.* 630 (1973).
7. Hulme, A. C., "Biochemistry of Fruits and Their Products," Vol. 1, p. 242. Academic Press, New York, 1970.
8. Barbon, D. H. R., Pradham, S. K., Sternell, S., and Templeton, J. F., *J. Chem. Soc.* 255 (1961).
9. Krupski, E., and Fischer, L., *J. Am. Pharm. Assoc.* 39, 433 (1950).
10. Moye, C. J., *Aust. J. Chem.* 19, 2317 (1966).
11. Flaschenträger, B., Cagianut, B., and Meier, F., *Helv. Chem. Acta* 28, 1489 (1945).
12. Haussler, A., and Hajdú, P., *Arneimittel-Forsch.* 14, 713 (1964).
13. Dodd, M. C., and Stillman, W. B., *J. Pharmacol. Exp. Ther.* 82, 11 (1944).
14. Sutherland, W. D., and Park, R. J., *in* "Terpenoids in Plants" (J. B. Pridham, Ed.), p. 147. Academic Press, New York, 1964.
15. Wilson, B. J., *Nutr. Rev.* 31, 73 (1973).
16. Maki, L. R., and Tucker, J. O., *in* "Proceedings Symposium on Acute Bovine Pulmonary Emphysema (ABPE)," p. A1. Laramie, Wyoming, 1965.
17. Peckham, J. C., Mitchell, F. E., Jones, O. H., Jr., and Doupnik, B., Jr., *J. Am. Vet. Med. Assoc.* 160, 1969 (1972).
18. Boyd, M. R., Burka, L. T., Harris, T. M., and Wilson, B. J., *Biochim. Biophys. Acta* 337, 184 (1974).
19. Watanabe, H., and Iwata, H., *J. Agric. Chem. Soc. Jpn.* 26, 180 (1952).
20. Wilson, B. J., Boyd, M. R., Harris, T. M., and Yang, D. T. C., *Nature* 231, 52 (1971).
21. Kubota, T., and Ichikawa, N., *Chem. Ind.* 29, 902 (1954).
22. Burka, L. T., Kuhnert, L., Wilson, B. J., and Harris, T. M., *J. Am. Chem. Soc.* 99, 2302 (1977).
23. Boyd, M. R., Burka, L. T., and Wilson, B. J., *Toxicol. Appl. Pharmacol.* 32, 147 (1975).
24. Wilson, B. J., Garst, J. E., Linnabary, R. D., and Channel, R. B., *Science* 197, 573 (1977).

25. Peterson, D. R., *in* "Proceedings Symposium on Acute Bovine Pulmonary Emphysema (ABPE)," p. Rl, Laramie, Wyoming, 1965.
26. Selman, I. E., Wiseman, A., Breeze, R. G., and Pirie, H. M., *Vet. Rec.* 99, 181 (1976).

VI. PLANT NEUROTOXINS

Chairman: A. A. Seawright

CENTAUREA SPECIES AND EQUINE NIGROPALLIDAL ENCEPHALOMALACIA

D. R. Cordy
University of California, Davis

I. ABSTRACT

Prolonged ingestion of Centaurea solstitialis *or* C. repens *produces a nervous disease in horses called equine nigropallidal encephalomalacia with rather sterotyped lesions and signs. Only horses are affected by feeding. Younger animals are especially involved. There is an unexplained biphasic seasonal prevalence of the disease. While the actual toxin remains unknown, the circumstances of poisoning and the pathogenesis of the disease are becoming clearer. The onset of the disease is abrupt, following a feeding period of some weeks without signs. All lesions in any one horse are usually of the same age and do not enlarge. The initial lesions are simply foci of pannecrosis which subsequently undergo slow cleanup of the dead tissue. The signs appear to be due to a dopamine deficiency following the specific destruction of the nigrostriatal tract in the globus pallidus and substantia nigra of the brain.*

II. INTRODUCTION

The prolonged consumption of *Centaurea solstitialis* (yellow star thistle) (1) or of *C. repens* (Russian knapweed) (2) produces in horses a nervous disease called equine nigropallidal encephalomalacia (ENE). The entity is characterized by the abrupt onset of difficulties in eating and drinking, and by aimless walking or drowsy inactivity. These signs are the consequence of foci of necrosis and softening in the globus pallidus and substantia nigra of the brain. The offending toxin remains unidentified, but the circumstances of poisoning and the pathogenesis of the disease have become somewhat clearer.

III. EPIZOOTOLOGY

Since 1950 we have studied 126 field cases drawn from northern California. This is the area of greatest prevalence of *C. solstitialis* in the United States, but cases are also reported from southern California and southern Oregon (3). Abroad the disease is seen in subhumid areas of Argentina (4) and Australia (5). Similar lesions in horses due to ingestion of *C. repens*, the related Russian knapweed of the intermountain region, have been reported in western Colorado and eastern Utah (6), and in eastern

Washington (7). Both species are of Old World origin, but strangely, there appear to be no reports of such a neurologic disease in the veterinary literature of that area.

Under the conditions of California's wet winter-dry summer climate, cases have occurred in pastured animals from March to December (Fig. 1). Two peaks of prevalence have consistently

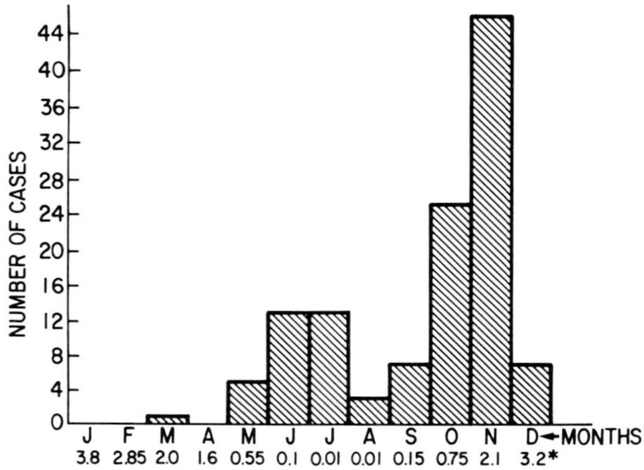

Fig. 1. *Month of onset of 118 documented cases. (*Average monthly precipitation in inches at Davis, California, for reference.)*

appeared, one in June-July (22% of cases) and a much larger peak in October-November (59%). This biphasic pattern is also reported in Argentina where Martin *et al.* (4) suggest that the first peak is due to regrowth of plants behaving as biennials while the second peak is due to those acting as conventional annuals. We do not think this is the case under California conditions where the plant behaves almost entirely as an annual.

Most of our cases have appeared on weedy paddocks or fallow fields, since the plant does not compete well with irrigated crops or established pastures.

There is a preponderance of cases among younger horses. While affected animals have ranged in age from 4 months to 18 years, 34% were aged 12 months or less and 56% were aged 2 years or less. The sexes have been about equally represented. Several breeds of horses and ponies have been affected, but no mules or burros have been presented. The disease is not known to occur in other species. Ruminants graze the same pastures with impunity.

IV. THE CLINICAL DISEASE

A. Nervous Signs

Clinical signs in this disease are rather stereotyped in their nature and development (1). The onset of signs is abrupt and essentially concurrent with the development of lesions. For the first day or two signs are erratic and often severe. These then subside to a static level which persists without much change for the duration of the disease. Signs of malnutrition may eventually be superimposed. Affected horses succumb to dehydration or starvation, die of intercurrent disease, or are killed. A few with very small lesions adapt to their neurologic deficiencies and survive.

Typically affected horses show hypokinesia, manifested as a somnolent state with meager spontaneous activity and a defect in the initiation of movement. Others walk aimlessly with the muzzle to the ground. Some animals retain for long periods awkward postures in which they chance to come to rest. Eating and drinking are severely impaired. Prehension and mastication are especially involved, but actual swallowing is unaffected. The mouth is often held half open with the tongue partly protruded. Hypertonia of the muscles innervated by the fifth, seventh, and twelfth cranial nerves appears to account for the difficulties in eating and drinking.

B. Dopamine Deficiency

An explanation of these signs is provided by rats in which the dopaminergic nigrostriatal pathway (Fig. 2) is specifically destroyed (8). These animals show signs essentially identical to those in horses, even to the initial erratic behavior. The initial signs are thought to result from massive release of the stored neurotransmitter, dopamine, from the nigrostriatal nerve endings in the striate, and the subsequent stabilized signs are thought to reflect the ensuing dopamine deficiency. Similar signs are seen with experimental bilateral nigral and pallidal destruction in monkeys (9).

V. LESIONS

Lesions are typically found in any of four sites in the brain, the globus pallidus and substantia nigra of left and right sides (Fig. 3). Bilateral lesions in both nuclei were seen in 58% of cases. In 26% only bilateral nigral lesions were found, and in 11% only bilateral pallidal lesions. No significant differences in signs were apparent among these groups, suggesting interruption of a single pathway at different levels. The severity of signs

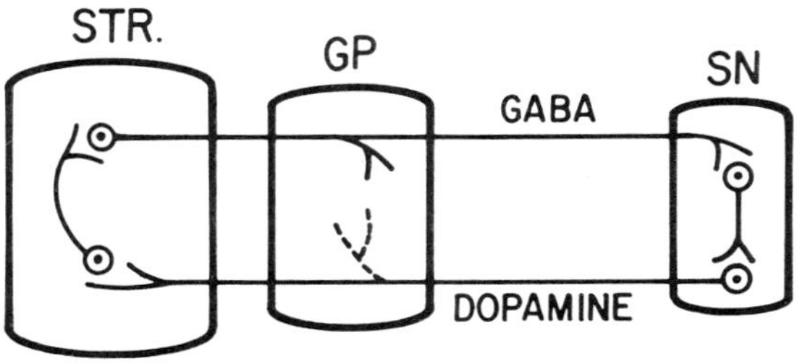

Fig. 2. *Diagram of presumed feedback loop in the basal ganglia. Other pathways are omitted. Dopamine is the neurotransmitter of the nigrostriatal tract, gamma-aminobutyric acid (GABA) of the striopallidonigral pathway, (STR-putamen and caudate, GP-globus pallidus, SN-substantia nigra).*

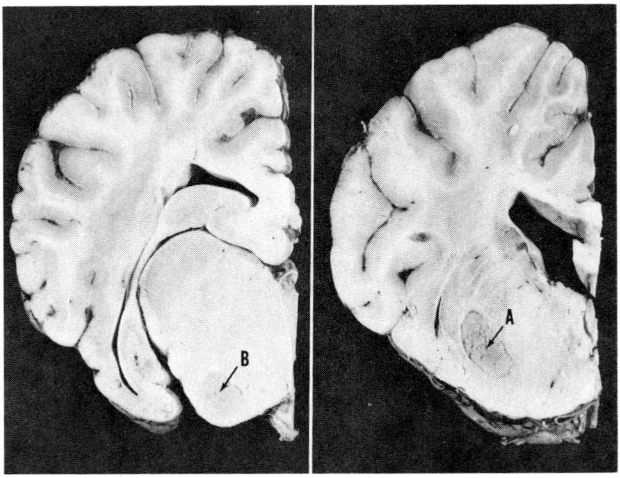

Fig. 3. *Gross lesions in globus pallidus (A) and substantia nigra (B) of 2 weeks' duration. (Reprinted with the permission of the Journal of Neuropathology and Experimental Neurology.)*

seems to correlate more with the size of lesions than with their numbers of sites.

The remaining 5% of horses had an odd number of lesions or had unilateral foci in both nuclei. Sidedness of signs was seen in some of these asymmetric cases.

Foci elsewhere than in the four typical sites have been reported in experimentally fed horses (10), and we have observed similar small atypical lesions in 3 of 13 brains recently reexamined. These unusual sites include the nucleus of the inferior colliculus, the dentate nucleus, and the mesencephalic nucleus and tract of the fifth cranial nerve. It must be admitted that brains from many of our more recent cases have not been exhaustively examined once diagnostic lesions were found in conventional sites.

All of the lesions in any individual animal were always of the same age with only two exceptions. In both of these horses, small older lesions, commensurate in age with the duration of signs, were accompanied by much larger more recent lesions in other conventional sites. It is not known if these two animals continued to ingest unusual amounts of the plant.

In all cases, necrosis in the foci occurs suddenly and completely, and lesions do not enlarge beyond their initial size even in such horses as are able to ingest additional plant.

While gray substance is chiefly involved, white substance is not spared. Fiber tracts passing through the foci undergo total necrosis in the same manner as the gray substance. It is thought that many of these fibers are corticobulbar axons which descend to synapse on cranial nerve motor nuclei.

The lesions are typically rounded, with a smooth intact margin, an outline much as would be made by a drop of water falling on a blotter. Pallidal and nigral sites showing no gross lesions appear quite normal by light microscopy. Partial lesions, showing only selective neuron necrosis, are not seen among field cases.

Microscopically the initial lesions are simply foci of pannecrosis and all later changes are those of progressive removal of dead tissue. Examination of the earliest lesions (second day of signs) shows that, except for a few surviving vessels traversing the foci, all elements are necrotic--neurons, glia, and capillaries (Figs. 4, 5). Vessels in the foci are not distended and hemorrhage is rare. The margin between living and necrotic tissue is very sharply defined with only the narrowest of transition zones.

By the third or fourth day macrophages begin to accumulate as a thin line at the margin of the necrotic area. These phagocytes increase in number and move into the dead tissue as an advancing front. They form a broad zone about residual central necrotic tissue at 7-10 days. By two weeks the entire lesion usually consists of closely packed, debris-filled macrophages lying among a few vascular trabeculae (Fig. 6, 7). Lesions several months old appear as cysts containing only fluid and a few residual phagocytes.

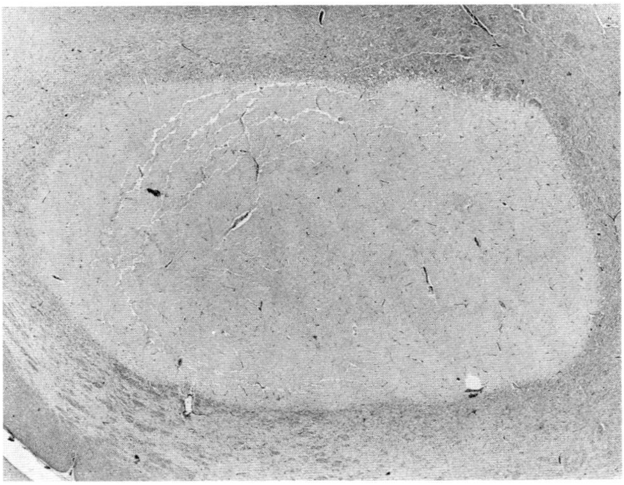

Fig. 4. *Nigral focus of acute necrosis about 2 days old. No macrophages have accumulated at the margin.*

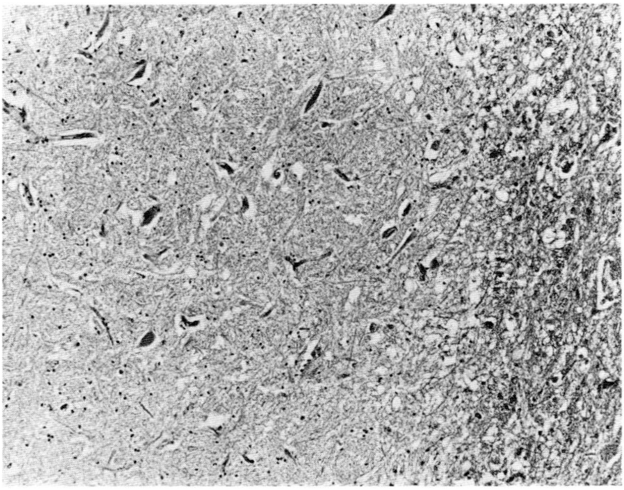

Fig. 5. *Margin of focus in Fig. 4 with normal tissue at right. The junction of necrotic and living tissue is quite distinct.*

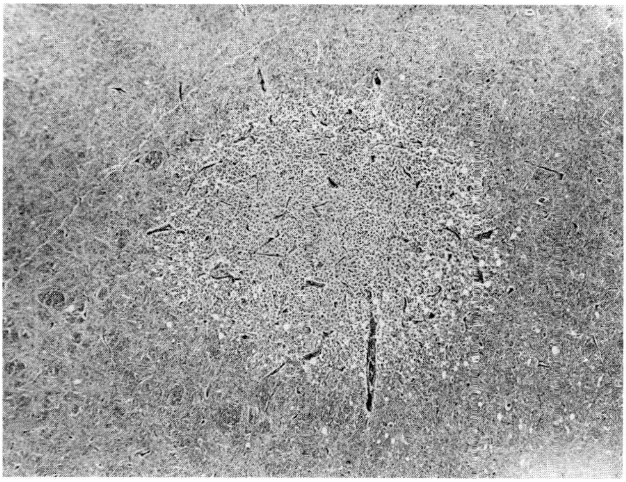

Fig. 6. *Small nigral focus of malacia nearly 2 weeks old.*

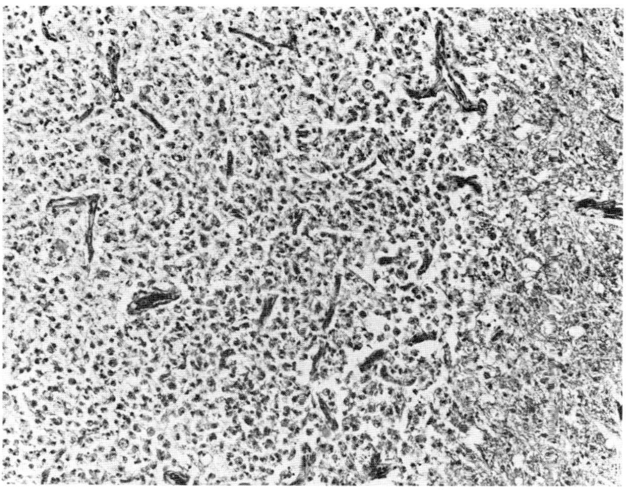

Fig. 7. *Margin of focus in Fig. 6 with normal tissue at right. Lesion consists chiefly of debris-filled macrophages.*

VI. TOXICITY TRIALS

A. Whole Plant Toxicity

Only the horse is affected by experimental feedings (1,6,10). In addition to earlier reported cases, we have produced bilateral pallidal lesions in two additional horses after feeding fresh *C. solstitialis* for 26 and 67 days. Young *et al.* (10) have calculated that an intake rate of 1.8-2.5 Kg/100KgBW/day is required for *C. repens* toxicity and 2.3-2.6 Kg for *C. solstitialis*. The horse must consume fresh *C. repens* equivalent to 59-71% of its body weight before signs appear, but with *C. solstitialis*, 86-200% is required. Feeding periods are also longer with *C. solstitialis*, 26-81 (average 54) days compared to 28-35 (average 30) for *C. repens*. Thus *C. repens* appears to be the more toxic. ENE has also been produced by feeding dried *C. repens* (6).

Earlier reports have showed no neurologic disease with prolonged feeding of fresh *C. solstitialis* to sheep (1), guinea pigs (11), rats (12), or monkeys (12), or of dried plant to rats (12) or guinea pigs (11). We have since fed fresh plant to three lots of rabbits for 51, 92, and 112 days without producing anything resembling the horse disease. We have also fed a meal-type ration containing one-third dried ground thistle to dogs, chicks, mice, and guinea pigs for periods of 56-84 days without ill effect. Rabbits and guinea pigs may starve on diets entirely composed of mature plants. Dried *C. solstitialis* at this stage contains 10.5% crude protein and 37% crude fiber.

B. Administration of Crude Extracts

Oral or parenteral administration of various crude extracts of *C. solstitialis* to several species, including the horse, have all failed to produce a disease resembling ENE (personal communications, F. A. Mettler; M. E. Fowler). Subcutaneous injection of aqueous or alcoholic extracts at a high dosage produced convulsions and death within a few hours in mice and rats, while a low dosage level was innocuous over a two-week period (12). Intermediate levels given over more prolonged periods have not been investigated, although such a regimen might more closely approximate the horse's daily intake of plant over several weeks.

VII. DISCUSSION

Although the toxin in *Centaurea* species has not been isolated and identified, the disease is clearly associated with prolonged ingestion of the plant. It appears that the thistle is eaten without apparent ill effect until some critical threshold is exceeded, at which time lesions and signs abruptly appear. While accumulation of a toxin or progressive depletion of a nutrient have been suggested as mechanisms (1), the disease may well be due instead to the summative effects of small daily injuries to cell structures. In effect, the lesions appear to result suddenly and completely from a final daily dose in itself too small to be toxic.

We have no explanation for the unique susceptibility of the horse, but wonder if it may be more related to the intestinal microbiota than to any peculiarity of the host itself. Possibly some innocuous plant substance is converted by a microorganism to a toxin or antimetabolite, or perhaps plant chemicals disturb the microbial population balance with consequent ill effects.

Signs appear to result from damage to the nigrostriatal tract with a consequent dopamine deficiency. How much of the difficulty in eating and drinking is due to nigrostriatal damage and how much is due to damage to passing corticobulbar or other fibers is uncertain.

It is quite obscure why these particular sites are so specifically affected. In seeking clues to pathogenetic mechanisms, we have reviewed a number of naturally occurring and experimental conditions in various species characterized by bilateral basal ganglia necrosis. Some of these have lesions very suggestive of the pattern seen in ENE. Included are such diverse agents as cyanide (13,14), azide (15), carbon disulfide (16), carbon monoxide (13), manganese (17), ammonium compounds (18), hyperbaric oxygen (19), and chronic hypothiaminosis (20). In most of these examples an ultimate hypoxic condition is postulated, but this fails to explain the unique site vulnerability. Morphologic and biochemical studies of these nuclei give no substantial clues to their selective liability to injury.

Before we can begin to answer the many questions posed by this disease, we must isolate the specific toxin and find a small animal test system which will fully reproduce the horse disease.

VIII. REFERENCES

1. Cordy, D. R., *J. Neuropathol. Exp. Neurol.* 13, 330 (1954).
2. Larson, K. A., and Young, S., *J. Am. Vet. Med. Assoc.* 156, 626 (1970).
3. Fowler, M. E., *J. Am. Vet. Med. Assoc.* 147, 607 (1965).
4. Martin, A. A., Yanarella, F. G., Maurel, R. A., and Ruager, J., *Analecta Vet.* 3, 43 (1971).
5. Gard, G. P., de Sarem, W. G., and Ahrens, P. J., *Aust. Vet. J.* 49, 107 (1973).
6. Young, S., Brown, W. W., and Klinger, B., *J. Am. Vet. Med. Assoc.* 157, 1602 (1970).
7. Farrell, R. K., Sande, R. D., and Lincoln, S. D., *J. Am. Vet. Med. Assoc.* 158, 1201 (1971).
8. Ungerstedt, U., *Acta Physiol. Scand. Suppl.* 367, 95 (1971).
9. Denny-Brown, D., "The Basal Ganglia and their Relation to Disorders of Movement," p. 105. Oxford University Press, London, 1962.
10. Young, S., Brown, W. W., and Dlinger, B., *Am. J. Vet. Res.* 31, 1393 (1970).

11. Cordy, D. R., *Proc. Am. Vet. Med. Assoc.* p. 149 (1954).
12. Mettler, F. A., and Stern, G. M., *J. Neuropathol. Exp. Neurol.* 22, 164 (1963).
13. Hurst, E. W., *Aust. J. Exp. Biol. Med. Sci.* 20, 297 (1942).
14. Haymaker, W., Ginzler, A. M., and Ferguson, R. L., *Mil. Surg.* 111, 231 (1952).
15. Mettler, F. A., *Fed. Proc.* 31, 1504 (1972).
16. Richter, R., *J. Neuropathol. Exp. Neurol.* 4, 324 (1945).
17. Mella, H., *Arch. Neurol. Psychiatry* 11, 405 (1924).
18. Ishii, T., *Psychiatr. Neurol. Japonica* 65, 667 (1963).
19. Balentine, J. D., and Gutsche, B. B., *Am. J. Pathol.* 48, 107 (1966).
20. Blank, N. K., Vick, N. A., and Schulman, S., *Acta Neuropathol.* 31, 137 (1975).

CYCAD POISONING IN AUSTRALIA - ETIOLOGY AND PATHOLOGY

P. T. Hooper
Arid Zone Research Institute

I. ABSTRACT

This paper describes the circumstances and pathologic changes resulting from poisonings in livestock in Australia by the cycad palms, Cycas spp., Bowenia spp., *and* Macrozamia spp. *In cattle, the most common disorder is ataxia and paralysis mainly affecting the hind limbs. This is caused by axonal degeneration similar to the "dying-back syndrome" seen with other neurotoxins. In sheep, there is more commonly an hepatic syndrome, either acute necrosis or in longer term cases, hepatocyte hypertrophy interpreted as a form of megalocytosis, and veno-occlusive disease.*

Poisons which have been isolated include glucoside derivatives of methylazoxymethanol (MAM), and an amino acid α amino β methylaminoproprionic acid. Recently, there has been evidence of a neurotoxic compound with a molecular weight exceeding 1000. Most experimental work has been done with MAM and its derivatives which in addition to being the hepatotoxic components of cycads, are radiomimetic because of their carcinogenic, teratogenic, and mutagenic properties. The teratogenic effects include abnormalities of the brains in fetuses and newborn animals but these are probably unrelated to the ataxic and paralytic diseases seen in domestic animals.

II. INTRODUCTION

Early information on cycad poisoning has been comprehensively reviewed by Whiting (1) who summarized information on field and experimental disease throughout the world in both man and animals. There have been reviews on later experimental work (2,3,4) and a more recent series of short papers published from a cycad research conference (5).

III. THE CYCADS

Cycads are easily recognized by their palm-like appearance. Their botanical descriptions are given elsewhere (1,6,7). They occur in tropical and subtropical environments throughout the world with fairly well defined geographical locations for the genera, for example, *Encephalartos spp.* in Africa, *Diion spp.* and *Zamia spp.* in central America, and *Cycas spp.* in Oceania. In Australia, there are 5 species of *Cycas* representing the family

Cycadaceae and 18 species of the 3 genera, *Bowenia, Lepidozamia,* and *Macrozamia,* representing the family Zamiaceae and all these are commonly called "zamias," "zamia palms," or "burrawangs" (7).

Cycas spp. are mostly found in Australia in tropical areas, in the north Kimberley area of Western Australia, northern end of the Northern Territory, and north Queensland. *Bowenia spp.* occur along the northeast coastal region of Queensland and *Lepidozamia spp.* along the coast of Queensland and northern New South Wales. Most *Macrozamia spp.* occur in eastern New South Wales and eastern Queensland but *M. riedlei* (also frequently spelled *M. reidlei*) occurs in southwest Western Australia, and *M. macdonnellii* in central Australia (Northern Territory). Everist (7) lists the species found in Australia. So far, the following have been associated with toxicity, *C. media* and *C. angulata* in northern Northern Territory and north Queensland, *C. circinalis* in Torres Strait, *B. serrulata* and possibly *B. spectabilis, M. moorei, M. miquelii* (also *M. douglasii*), *M. communis, M. lucida, M. spiralis, M. heteromera,* and *M. pauli-guilielmi* in Queensland and/or New South Wales, and *M. riedlei* in Western Australia. Everist believes that many of the poisonings reported in early literature attributed to *M. spiralis* could have been other species such as *M. moorei, M. lucida, M. heteromera,* and *M. diplomera.* Many other untested cycads could also be toxic.

IV. THE DISEASE SYNDROME

Cycads have been known to be poisonous for centuries (1). Sailors employed by Captain Cook, the discoverer of eastern Australia in 1770, were made ill by eating the nuts. There has been evidence also of 2 distinct field disease syndromes for a long time (8).

One syndrome is characterized by hepatic and gastrointestinal disease and the other by ataxic signs consistent with disease in the central nervous system (CNS). An additional third syndrome is that produced as experimental radiomimetic and/or carcinogenic effects of the group of the cycad toxins that cause the hepatic and gastrointestinal syndrome. The disease changes seen are variations caused by altering dosages, animal species, times, and routes of administrations. Even though the hepatic and radiomimetic toxins caused neural disease in fetuses and newborn animals, the ataxic syndrome in domestic animals is probably caused by a different toxin or group of toxins.

The animal species most frequently affected are cattle and sheep but horses and pigs have also been affected (1). Cattle are more frequently affected by the CNS disease while sheep are more frequently affected by the hepatic and gastrointestinal disease. There are numerous occurrences of disease in man with symptoms corresponding to the hepatic/gastrointestinal syndrome and there is evidence that a paralytic or ataxic syndrome, similar to amyotrophic lateral sclerosis, occurs in people who consume the plant in a number of tropical areas, for example, Guam (9).

A. The Hepatic and Gastrointestinal Syndrome

Massive outbreaks of disease have been described in sheep consuming nuts of *Macrozamia sp.* (10) in which there is acute disease with post mortem changes of hepatitis, gastroenteritis, and hemorrhages. Extensive experiments have been described (11) of the feeding of *Cycas circinalis* to rats, pigs, horses, cattle, and calves in which all species develop, among other visceral lesions, liver cirrhosis with occlusion of central and hepatic veins, and proliferative gastroenteritis. Rats developed progressive tumors in their livers, kidneys, and pancreas. The feeding of *C. circinalis* also caused confluent, hemorrhagic necrosis of a periacinar pattern in laboratory animals (12).

Thus, there can be 2 forms of liver disease, acute and chronic. Both forms have been seen in sheep poisoned by *Macrozamia riedlei* (13,14) and by *Cycas media* (Hooper and McEwan, unpublished observations). Chronic disease arose in sheep poisoned by *M. riedlei* after they had consumed total quantities of between 4.1 kg and 4.5 kg of the nuts over a period of 3 to 11 months (13). There was a fairly precise dose-response effect irrespective of the duration of feeding. The only significant clinical sign was progressive loss of appetite and each sheep developed liver cirrhosis and mild nephrosis. Both nuts and leaves could cause acute disease (14).

The microscopic appearance of sheep poisoned by *C. media* was that of both acute necrosis and chronic hepatocyte hypertrophy interpreted as a form of megalocytosis and veno-occlusive disease (Hooper and McEwan, unpublished data). Sheep were poisoned by a mean of 2.08 g of dried flour made from the nuts per kg body weight (BW) compared with 85.5 g of leaves/kg BW. This is consistent with chemical analyses of the toxin cycasin by S. Baseden (personal communication) showing about 2% in dried flour and 0.1% in wet leaf. The principal hepatic lesions in the liver were megalocytosis, well developed necrosis of a periacinar pattern of distribution, fibrosis around central veins consistent with the term venous occlusion, fat infiltration, accumulations of bile in Kupffer cells and other macrophages, and very moderate bile duct proliferation. The megalocytes were diffuse although the larger cells were periportal. One sheep showed quite large nucleoli while other sheep showed more diffusely hyperchromatic nuclei. Cytoplasmic invaginations were rare as were cytosegrosomes. The kidneys were less severely affected. There was, consistently, heavy brown pigmentation of proximal tubules. More severely affected kidneys showed dilated distal tubules and loops of Henle, protein casts, some enlarged and proliferating epithelial cells of Bowman's capsules, periglomerular and interstitial fibrosis, and some regenerating epithelial cells.

"Gastroenteritis" is a frequent observation in field outbreaks of this syndrome although there have been few details described of the microscopic appearance of the lesions. Mickelsen (11) used the term "proliferative gastroenteritis." It is possible that these lesions develop in larger animals when consuming quantities of cycads sufficient to cause acute intoxication. Intestinal lesions have been produced in rats by methylazoxymethanol (15) the active metabolite of the hepatic toxin. Extracts of *C. media* given orally to guinea pigs caused very severe gastric ulcerations of the glandular mucosa. Focal necrosis and ulceration occurred in the abomasum in some sheep after dosing with about 20 g of flour made from *C. media* nuts/kg BW (Hooper and McEwan, unpublished observations).

B. The Neural Syndrome

A series of papers by Hall have described the clinical signs quoting his own experiences and those of earlier workers. A local Australian name for the disease is "rickets," a name which does not refer to bone abnormalities or to vitamin D metabolism. Hall (16) quoted T. L. Bancroft, "The chief symptom of the disease is loss of proper control over the movements of the hind limbs. Affected animals seem never to recover completely, the weakness of the hind quarters continuing throughout life. Although their infirmity handicaps them in obtaining food, they are capable of being fattened if placed on good feed, and the flesh of those animals in good condition appears to be quite sound." Later, Hall (17) wrote that the signs were "those of uncontrolled extension and flexion of the hind limbs. This causes dropping of the hind quarters, which may swing to either side. In the early stages there is over extension of the lower hind limbs, and a 'goose stepping' gait. Later there is incomplete extension, and the beast 'knuckles over' on its phalanges. Affected animals become worse when exercised, and very severe cases will fall with the hind legs extended behind them dragging themselves along with their forelimbs which are apparently never affected. There is never complete recovery."

Hall and McGavin (18), and Mason and Whiting (19) were the first to describe microscopic changes in the central nervous system (CNS) of cattle consistent with the clinical signs. These observations (18) were on steers poisoned by *Macrozamia lucida* and *Bowenia serrulata*. They did not report changes visible under normal hematoxylin and eosin stains. However, staining by the Marchi method revealed bilateral symmetrical degeneration of nerve fibers in the fasciculus gracilis up to the nucleus gracilis, and the dorsal spinocerebellar tract and possibly the ventral spinocerebellar tract up to the cerebellum through the posterior cerebellar peduncle. There was also degeneration in an area probably corresponding to the corticospinal tract [Hall, cited by Mason and Whiting (19)]. Hall and McGavin believed that the abnormality in the fasciculus gracilis could be appreciated grossly by a depression in the cervical spinal cord. Mason and Whiting (19) confirmed that there was evidence of myelin degeneration, "even in hematoxylin eosin stained slides" by the "presence of large round holes sometimes with swollen axons," in cattle poisoned by *Zamia spp.*

More distinct axonal degeneration was seen in steers poisoned by *Cycas media* (20). The affected axons developed spheroids, pink staining masses inside of their cylinders, 10u to 50u in diameter, with a defined pattern of distribution similar to that described earlier (18). The spheroids were most frequent in the superficial dorsolateral areas of the white matter of the cervical and thoracic spinal cords particularly between C_3 and T_4. Further down the cords, they were present in the ventromedial areas, probably the corticospinal tracts. There was also histological evidence of degeneration in dorsal root ganglia of affected steers.

Little histological work has been done with other species. J. B. Armstrong (personal communication) produced paralysis in a sheep very similar to that in cattle by feeding the freshly collected tips of old fronds of *M. riedlei*. These sheep showed demyelination histologically. It is clear, however, that the hepatic syndrome is far more important in this species. Goats and buffalos have been affected (21), but horses probably not (2).

Some animals with hepatic disease may show clinical signs of hepatic encephalopathy. Sheep poisoned by *Cycas media* have shown nervous signs and CNS spongy degeneration associated with hepatic disease (22) but these neurologic signs and lesions were secondary effects to hepatic disease only.

V. THE TOXINS IN THE CYCADS

Data to date from chemical and toxicological studies have suggested 3 groups of toxins in cycads. These are methylazoxymethanol and its glucoside derivatives, an amino acid(s), and a higher molecular weight compound(s) whose nature is as yet unidentified.

Cooper (23) isolated a glucoside from *M. spiralis* and called it macrozamin. This compound was toxic by mouth but seemed to be non-toxic by subcutaneous injection. The active component of the glucoside was recognized as methylazoxymethanol (MAM) (24,25). There is a range of MAM based glucosides with varying attached carbohydrate groups, the neocycasins (26), which all depend on their MAM content for toxicity. Well-known carbohydrate links to MAM include that in macrozamin to primeverose (27) and in cycasin to glucose (28). There can be little doubt that MAM and its derivatives are responsible for the hepatic and gastrointestinal diseases produced by cycads.

Experimental work must take into account routes of administration. The MAM derivatives require conversion to MAM for activation, by removal of the glucoside by the enzyme glucosidase. Glucosidase is normally present in bacteria in the gastrointestinal tract (29) or in the skin of newborn animals (30). The net effect is that except for newborn animals, oral dosage is required for experimental reproduction of hepatic and radiomimetic lesions using plants, plant extracts, or purified toxins such as cycasin.

An amino acid, α - amino β methylaminoproprionic acid has been isolated from the seeds of *C. circinalis* and proved to be neurotoxic in rats and chicks (31,32). The neurotoxic effects include convulsions and paralysis which could occur soon after injection. Further studies have shown that the compound is present in a free or bound form in a wide variety of cycads (33). There is little likelihood that it is the cycad toxin causing neural disease in the field because it is probably in too low a concentration in the plants (33) and is not present in all neurotoxic cycads (34).

Work by Louw and Oelofsen (35) with *Encephalartos altensteini* suggests that there could be in cycads, a compound with a molecular weight exceeding 1000 which could produce incoordination then paralysis in guinea pigs. These paralyses followed single dosages after a latent period of 15-30 days. The experimental material consisted of the retentate left after ultrafiltration at a molecular retentivity of 1000. The diffusate contained macrozamin. Another effect of the retentate in the guinea pigs was "swelling of the eyes" within 1 day of dosage. Similar results have been obtained with *C. media* in guinea pigs (Hooper, Hamdorf, and McEwan, unpublished observation) and work is continuing with *E. altensteini* (Louw, personal communication) and *C. media* (Hamdorf and McEwan, personal communication) with a view to identifying the compound(s) and reproducing the disease in domestic animals.

VI. OTHER EXPERIMENTAL DISEASES CAUSED BY METHYLAZOXYMETHANOL AND ITS DERIVATIVES

Although hepatic disease is the principal disease in domestic animals caused by MAM and its derivatives, these compounds have radiomimetic effects on tissues. One such effect is on the neural tissues of fetuses and newborn animals.

A. Experimental Disease in the Central Nervous System Caused by Methylazoxymethanol and its Derivatives

Neurotoxicity characterized by ataxia and hind limb paralysis was produced by single, subcutaneous injections of cycasin into newborn but not adult mice (36). The neurologic signs followed necrosis of cells in the external granular layer of the cerebellum (37). A similar necrotic effect was induced by cycasin in the retinas of newborn mice and rats (38). Teratogenic CNS lesions were also produced by the active aglycone of cycasin, MAM, in the brains and retinas (39,40,41) particularly microencephaly in rats (4).

The inhibition of development in the CNS, particularly microencephaly, is now known as a common feature of a number of animal species given prenatal or perinatal treatments of MAM (42). The actual effect depends partly on the species and partly on the stage of development of the CNS (43,44,45). The part of the brain which is rapidly growing is the most sensitive, for example, the cerebellum in the newborn and cerebrum in the fetus. This effect is a form of "granuloprival cerebellar hypoplasia" (43,44) similar to that caused by radiation and radiomimetic viruses and poisons. This CNS effect seems more closely related to the carcinogenic and hepatogenic effects of MAM and its derivatives than the neurotoxic effects of cycads seen in field diseases.

B. Other Experimental Radiomimetic Syndromes in Laboratory Animals

Methylazoxymethanol and its derivatives are readily carcinogenic in some laboratory animals. For example, cycasin causes mainly renal and intestinal tumors in rats and hepatic tumors in mice, hamsters (46), and rabbits (47). A delayed effect of treatment of newborn rats is the appearance of CNS tumors (4).

Other radiomimetic effects are teratogenesis in the neural syndromes mentioned above (40), mutagenesis (48,49), chromosomal aberrations (50), karyorrhexis and irregular and enlarged cells in crypt nuclei of the intestines, decrease in hemopoiesis in the spleen, slight irregularities in the thymus, and testicular damage (51).

The radiomimetic efforts are probably caused by methylation of DNA (52) in a manner similar to dimethylnitrosamine (DMN). It is possible that MAM and DMN have very similar properties and both could exert their effects after metabolism to an alkylating agent, diazomethane (53). The radio protective compound cysteamine gives some protection against MAM (54).

VII. CIRCUMSTANCES RELATED TO TOXICITY

In the Northern Territory, Australia, although there are very pronounced wet and dry seasons, the neural disease in cattle caused by *C. media* occurs throughout the year, irrespective of season. Sickness can occur in the rainy season even though there is an alternative abundance of green feed. There seems to be an individual animal preference for the plant. There can be a particularly dangerous circumstance in the dry season because bushfires are common in the area denuding the ground of other feed material and there is rapid regrowth of the cycad after fire. All that remains in some pastures is the palm with its attractive looking green fronds.

Cattle in both good and poor nutritional condition seem equally susceptible. The disease occurs commonly in cattle newly introduced to an area but also in stock born in the area. Not all cycad infested areas seem toxic. In some areas, there is apparent freedom of disease although there is abundance of plant which seems to be readily eaten.

Probably most species of cycad can be toxic. However, proof requires prolonged experimental support. Until recently, pastures containing *C. angulata* in the Northern Territory seemed safe, but in 1977 there were reports of "cycad staggers" in an area where the plant was the probable cause.

The results of experimental reproduction can vary depending on which species is being tested, what part of the plant is used and how it is processed. Both nuts and fronds of the cycads can be either hepatotoxic and enterotoxic, or neurotoxic. Sheep and cattle are the animal species most frequently affected, sheep developing hepatic disease while cattle develop ataxia. Sheep, however, develop spinal disease (Armstrong, personal communication) and cattle also can develop the hepatic disease after being fed comparatively low quantities of fresh *M. pauli-guilielmi* but ataxia when fed larger quantities of dried plant (17).

It seems that the hepatotoxic components of the cycads are the least stable and often do not survive storage, particularly in the leaves. Multiple washings of cycad flour render it safer because of the instability of MAM derivatives in the plants and their solubility in water. These techniques have been employed by many people in different tropical regions (1). The instability of the toxins could also explain the wide disparities in results of different experimental feeding trials. Care in experimental work is also required with routes of administration. The MAM derivatives require enzymic metabolism to MAM in the intestines.

Wesley-Smith (55) has summarized techniques used for the control of *C. media*. Chemical control is practical although he warns that care must be taken for at least 2 years as regeneration is possible within that time. He believed that frequent fires which are a common feature of the area reduce the plant populations but on the other hand, cause immediate problems because of prompt regeneration of fronds on the stumps. Kelly (56) emphasized the importance of treating stumps with poisons, for example arsenic. More specific preventative measures directed at the neurotoxin of cycads await elucidation of its chemical nature.

VIII. DISCUSSION

A most important task remaining in cycad research is to determine what is the neurotoxic principle(s). Much of the experimental work has been with MAM and its derivatives, but there is no evidence that the compounds cause ataxic syndromes in older domestic animals. The animo acid, α amino β methylproprionic acid, seemed to be too low in concentration and not always present in toxic plants.

Future work with the higher molecular weight compound (35) isolated from *E. altensteini* and from *C. media* must show that it is capable of inducing in cattle clinical signs of ataxia and histological evidence of axonal degeneration then demyelination in spinal cords, particularly in the spinocerebellar tracts of the cervical cord and corticospinal tracts further down. The degeneration in the spinocerebellar tracts is in a cranial direction while that in the corticospinal tracts is in a distal direction. This is consistent with a "dying back" degeneration process (57) of nerve fibers starting in their axons at their most distinct extremities away from the nerve bodies. This process has also been recognized in other intoxications including those induced by some organophosphorus compounds in man (58), cattle (59,60), and some pigs (61) and by some poisonous plants, *Solanum esuriale* (62,63) and in part by coyotillo (*Karwinskia humboldtiana*) (64).

The derivatives of MAM almost certainly cause the hepatic and gastrointestinal syndromes. The enlargement of cells which I have called megalocytosis has been discussed by Zedeck and Sternberg (65). Compared with the megalocytes induced by pyrrolizidine alkaloids, the duration of megalocytes is short-lived. However, the latent effect on cells is long-lived, as megalocytes developed in rat livers regenerating after partial hepatectomy, 26 weeks after MAM administration (65). Venous-occlusion is consistent with the similarity of cycasin and related compounds to dimethylnitrosamine (53) and probably occurs because there is severe hepatic insult over a sufficient length of time.

Other than "gastroenteritis," there have been few reports of radiomimetic effects caused by cycads in domestic animals. Certainly there have been no reports of unusual prevalences of cancer similar to the bladder tumors associated with consumption of *Pteridium aquilinum* (66). There is as yet nothing to suggest why cattle are more likely to develop the ataxic syndrome and sheep the hepatic disease.

The question of the diseases in man is still unresolved. There does not seem to be any increased prevalence of cancers in areas where there is cycad consumption (67), presumably because of adequate treatment of cycad flour. There is, however, an increase in prevalence of neural disorders, a varient of amyotrophic lateral sclerosis and a parkinsonis - dementia complex, but this again is difficult to relate to cycad consumption (44).

IX. ACKNOWLEDGMENTS

Special thanks are due to Mrs. P. Newman for her assistance in the preparation of this paper.

X. REFERENCES

1. Whiting, M. G., *Econ. Bot.* 17, 271 (1963).
2. Whiting, M. G., Spatz, M., and Matsumoto, H., *Econ. Bot.* 20, 98 (1966).
3. Laqueur, G. L., and Spatz, M., *Cancer Res.* 28, 2262 (1968).
4. Spatz, M., *Ann. N. Y. Acad. Sci.* 163, 848 (1969).
5. Various authors in *Fed. Proc.* 31, 1465 (1972).

6. Birdsey, M. R., *Fed. Proc.* 31, 1467 (1972).
7. Everist, S. L., "Poisonous Plants of Australia" p. 165. Angus and Robertson, Sydney, 1974.
8. Cleland, J. B., *Third Rep. N. S. W. Gov. Bur. Microbiol.* 187, (1914).
9. Mickelsen, O., *Fed. Proc.* 31, 1465 (1972).
10. Seddon, H. R., Belschner, H. G., and King, R. O. C., *N. S. W. Dep. Agric. Vet. Res. Rep.* No. 6, p. 70 (1931).
11. Mickelsen, O., Campbell, E., Yang, M., Mugera, G., and Whitehair, C. K., *Fed. Proc.* 23, 1363 (1964).
12. Laqueur, G. L., Mickelsen, O., Whiting, M. G., and Kurland, L. T., *J. Nat. Cancer Inst.* 31, 919 (1963).
13. Gardiner, M. R., *Aust. J. Agric. Res.* 21, 519 (1970).
14. Gabbedy, B. J., Meyer, E. P., and Dickson, J., *Aust. Vet. J.* 51, 303 (1975).
15. Zedeck, M. S., Sternberg, S. A., Poynter, R. W., and McGowan, J., *Cancer Res.* 30, 801 (1970).
16. Hall, W. T. K., *Queensl. Agric. J.* 79, 173 (1954).
17. Hall, W. T. K., *Queensl. J. Agric. Sci.* 14, 41 (1957).
18. Hall, W. T. K., and McGavin, M. D., *Pathol. Vet.* 5, 26 (1968).
19. Mason, M. M., and Whiting, M. G., *Cornell Vet.* 58, 541 (1968).
20. Hooper, P. T., Best, S. M., and Campbell, A., *Aust. Vet. J.* 50, 146 (1974).
21. Commonwealth of Australia, Northern Territory Administration, *Ann. Rep. Anim. Ind. Branch* 1961/62, 30 (1962) and 1962/63, 26 (1963).
22. Hooper, P. T., *Acta Neuropathol. (Berl.)* 31, 343-351 (1975).
23. Cooper, J. M., *Proc. Linn. Soc. N. S. W.* 74, 450 (1941).
24. Matsumoto, H., and Strong, F. M., *Arch. Biochem. Biophys.* 101, 299 (1963).
25. Matsumoto, H., Nagahama, T., and Larson, H. O., *Biochem. J.* 95, 13c (1965).
26. Nishida, K., *Jpn. J. Chem.* 13, 730 (1959).
27. Lythgoe, B., and Riggs, N. V., *J. Chem. Soc.* 4, 2716 (1949).
28. Nishida, K., Kobayashi, A., and Nagahama, T., *Bull. Agric. Soc. Jpn.* 19, 77 (1955).
29. Spatz, M., Smith, D. W. E., McDaniel, E. G., and Laqueur, G. L., *Proc. Soc. Exp. Biol. Med.* 124, 691 (1967).
30. Spatz, M., *Proc. Soc. Exp. Biol. Med.* 128, 1005 (1968).
31. Vega, A., and Bell, E. A., *Phytochemistry* 6, 759 (1967).
32. Nunn, P. B., Vega, A., and Bell, E. A., *Biochem. J.* 106, 15p (1967).
33. Polsky, F. I., Nunn, P. B., and Bell, E. A., *Fed. Proc.* 31, 1473 (1972).
34. Dossaji, S. F., and Herbin, G. A., *Fed. Proc.* 31, 1471 (1972).
35. Louw, W. K. A., and Oelofsen, W., *Toxican* 13, 447 (1975).
36. Hirono, I., and Shibuya, C., *Nature* 216, 1311 (1967).
37. Hirono, I., Shibuya, C., and Hayashi, K., *Proc. Soc. Exp. Biol. Med.* 131, 593 (1969).
38. Fushimi, K., and Hirono, I., *Acta Pathol. Jpn.* 23, 307 (1973).
39. Spatz, M., Dougherty, W. J., and Smith, D. W. E., *Proc. Soc.*

Exp. Biol. Med. 124, 476 (1967).
40. Spatz, M., and Laqueur, G. L., *Proc. Soc. Exp. Biol. Med.* 129, 705 (1968).
41. Shimada, M., and Langman, J., *Teratology* 3, 119 (1970).
42. Haddad, R. K., Rabe, A., and Dumas, R., *Fed. Proc.* 31, 1520 (1972).
43. Jones, M., Yang, M., and Mickelsen, O., *Fed. Proc.* 31, 1508 (1972).
44. Kurland, L. T., *Fed. Proc.* 31, 1540 (1972).
45. Hirono, I., Laqueur, G. L., and Spatz, M., *J. Nat. Cancer Inst.* 40, 1003 (1968).
46. Hirono, I., *Fed. Proc.* 31, 1493 (1972).
47. Watanabe, K., Iwashita, H., Muta, K., Hamada, Y., and Hamada, K., *Gann* 66, 335 (1975).
48. Smith, D. W. E., *Science* 152, 1273 (1966).
49. Teas, H. J., and Dyson, J. G., *Proc. Soc. Exp. Biol. Med.* 125, 988 (1967).
50. Teas, H. J., Sax, H. J., and Sax, K., *Science* 149, 541 (1965).
51. Zedeck, M. S., Sternberg, S. S., Poynter, R. W., and McGowan, J., *Cancer Res.* 30, 801 (1970).
52. Matsumoto, H., and Higa, H. H., *Biochem. J.* 98, 20c (1966).
53. Shank, R. C., and Magee, P. N., *Biochem. J.* 105, 521 (1967).
54. Miwa, T., *Acta Sch. Med. Gifu Univ.* 23, 495 (1975).
55. Wesley-Smith, R. N., *J. Aust. Inst. Agric. Sci.* 39, 233 (1973).
56. Kelly, T. K., *Queensl. Agric. J.* 93, 184 (1967).
57. Cavanagh, J. B., *Int. Rev. Exp. Pathol.* 3, 219 (1964).
58. Johnson, M. K., *Arch. Toxicol.* 34, 259 (1975).
59. Williams, J. F., Dade, A. W., and Benne, R., *J. Am. Vet. Med. Assoc.* 169, 1307 (1976).
60. Beck, B., Wood, C. D., and Whenham, G. R., *Vet. Pathol.* 14, 128 (1977).
61. Kruckenberg, S. M., Strafuss, A. C., Marsland, W. P., Blauch, B. S., Marsh, T. R., Vestweber, J. G., and Winter, W. A., *Am. J. Vet. Res.* 34, 403 (1973).
62. O'Sullivan, B. M., *Aust. Vet. J.* 52, 414 (1976).
63. McMeniman, N. P., *Aust. Vet. J.* 52, 433 (1976).
64. Charlton, K. M., Pierce, K. R., Storts, R. W., and Bridges, C. H., *Pathol. Vet.* 7, 435 (1970).
65. Zedeck, M. S., and Sternberg, S. S., *Cancer Res.* 35, 2117 (1975).
66. Evans, I. A., and Mason, J., *Nature* 203, 913 (1965).
67. Hirono, I., Kachi, H., and Kato, T., *Acta Pathol. Jpn.* 20, 327 (1970).

THE TOXIN OF *Lolium rigidum* (ANNUAL RYEGRASS) SEEDHEADS ASSOCIATED WITH NEMATODE-BACTERIUM INFECTION

C. C. J. Culvenor, J. L. Frahn, M. V. Jago, and G. W. Lanigan
CSIRO Division of Animal Health

I. ABSTRACT

Aqueous acetone extraction of toxic seedheads of Lolium rigidum *infested with the nematode* Anguina lolii *and* Corynebacterium sp., *probably* C. rathayi, *leads to a toxic precipitate, insoluble in water at pH 3.5. Partial purification of the toxin, which is retained on an XM-300 membrane with nominal cut-off at 300,000 mol. wt., is described. Despite a similarity in some properties, the concentrate at present available differs from known bacterial toxins, including the phytotoxins of plant pathogenic* Corynebacterium sp., *in having very low peptide and carbohydrate contents.*

II. INTRODUCTION

Lolium rigidum, Annual or Wimmera Ryegrass, is a dominant pasture species and a weed in crops in the 14 to 16 inch rainfall areas of southern Australia. First known to poison sheep about 20 years ago in a small area of South Australia, it is now toxic over areas of about 100 km radius in both South and Western Australia. Toxicity is associated with infestation of the seedheads by a nematode, *Anguina lolii* and a bacterium, *Corynebacterium sp.*, probably *C. rathayi* (1). Nematode larvae climb young ryegrass plants, remain on the growing tips, then bore into the developing flower, carrying the bacterium with them. The seed does not develop normally, becoming instead a gall containing either nematodes or bacteria, rarely both.

Sheep grazing toxic grass at the seeding stage may, when disturbed show a stiff-legged, staggering gait and collapse with convulsions. Pathological findings include a pale, friable liver, congestion of the lungs, and hemorrhage in various organs (2,3). Mortalities are commonly about 40-50% and can approach 80%. The parasitization and associated toxicity closely resemble those reported from Oregon where *Festuca rubra commutata* is infested by *Anguina agrostis* and a bacterium thought to be a *Corynebacterium sp.* (4,5). The disease is being investigated by the CSIRO Division of Animal Health and the Department of Agriculture, Western Australia. We are looking primarily at the source of toxicity and identification of the toxic principle, and the Department of Agriculture at biological and control aspects.

III. ORIGIN OF TOXICITY

Hand separation of bacterial and nematode galls has enabled demonstration that the bacterial galls, but not the nematode galls are toxic (6). However cultures of *C. rathayi* on various artificial media have not developed toxicity and it is still unclear whether the toxin is of bacterial origin or produced by the grass in response to infection.

IV. BIOASSAYS AND TOXIC EFFECTS

The fractionation of extracts was followed initially by toxicity in guinea pigs that died with marked loss of weight, tremor, and spasms after receiving extracts equivalent to 35 g. toxic grass over a period of 5 days. Two week-old chickens were later used, being about twice as sensitive on a body weight basis, although they do not show tremors. More recently, 2-week-old rats were found to be very sensitive to toxic extracts given by intraperitoneal injection. The rats exhibit incoordination and convulsions and die 2-7 days after injection. There is widespread focal necrosis in the brain, hemorrhage in the brain, spinal cord, and sometimes in the stomach and duodenum. The peripheral circulation rate is greatly reduced after 3 days and gangrene of the tail and hind legs may develop. Thus the toxin appears to have a long-acting vasoconstrictive effect (7). Young and old rats show immediate inhibition of gastric motility, persisting for a day or more.

A toxic extract shows no pyrogenic effect when injected into rabbits (Buttery and Jago, unpublished results).

V. PROPERTIES OF THE TOXIN

Toxic extracts were obtained from toxic seedheads by extraction with aqueous acetone (1:1) but not with cold water, ethanol, or acetone. Concentration of the aqueous acetone to a small volume and adjusting the aqueous residue to pH 3.5 gave a precipitate containing all the toxicity. A base-grade concentrate was prepared by extracting the precipitate with aqueous butanol, removing solvent and dissolving the residue in dilute NaOH, removing non-toxic material by washing with ether and filtering through a Diaflo XM-300 membrane. The retentate is toxic; the filtrate is discarded.

The toxin is soluble in water above pH 7.5, but insoluble or very sparingly soluble at pH 3 and below. The high pH form is insoluble in acetone and ethanol whereas the low pH form is soluble in these solvents. At low pH, the toxin is slightly soluble in chloroform and can be extracted from aqueous solution or slurry with butanol or a mixture of tetrahydrofuran and diisopropyl ether. The failure of the toxin in aqueous solution at pH 8.5 to pass an XM-300 membrane (nominal cut-off at molecular weight 300,000) may be due to micelle formation or binding to a high molecular weight carrier. When the pH 3 precipitate is dissolved in ethanol-water (3:1), the toxin passes through the membrane. It is fairly stable to heat, being unaffected when dried at 100° for 3 hr. On paper electrophoresis at pH 9.2, it binds to the paper and does not move from the starting line.

Substantial purification of the toxin has been achieved by means of chromatography on Sephadex LH20 and silica gel. The most toxic fraction achieved so far is lethal to 2-week-old rats at the level of 0.8 mg/kg. The toxin appears to be associated with UV absorption at about 260 nm and has a low R_F on silica TLC plates run in an acidified mixture of chloroform, ethanol, and methanol. If sufficiently concentrated, the spot can be visualized by lightly spraying the plate with water, when a white spot appears on a translucent background. This effect has been reported for certain steroids and other compounds which are not water-wetting (8,9). Smaller amounts are detected by spraying with 20% ammonium sulphate and heating at 140° for 1 hr, when almost all the organic material present becomes fluorescent.

VI. COMPARISON WITH KNOWN BACTERIAL TOXINS

Although no evidence has been obtained for formation of the toxin in cultures of the *Corynebacterium sp.* on artificial media, it is of interest to compare its properties with those of the known bacterial toxins. Those from bacteria pathogenic to animals are either proteins - the exotoxins of gram-positive bacteria and certain cytoplasmic endotoxins of gram-negative bacteria - or high molecular weight lipopolysaccharide-protein complexes from the cell wall of gram-negative bacteria (10). Like other gram-positive bacteria, *Corynebacterium spp.* do not produce classical endotoxins but some plant pathogenic species are known to produce extracellular phytotoxins which resemble the endotoxins in being lipopolysaccharide-peptide or glycopeptide in nature. Those from *C. sepedonicum* and *C. insidiosum* have molecular weight 21,400 and 5,000,000, respectively, and the former, for example, contains 4.6% peptide, 62% sugars and 9.9% keto-deoxysugar acids of the type found in endotoxins (11,12). Similar glycopeptides are found in *C. michiganense* and probably in *C. nebraskense* and other plant pathogenic bacteria.

The annual ryegrass toxin is clearly not a protein but in some respects it resembles the lipopolysaccharide-peptide toxins - e.g. in a degree of lipid solubility, stability to heat and apparent high molecular weight (under some conditions). A classical endotoxin structure is ruled out for the ryegrass toxin by the failure to induce fever in rabbits. A correlation with the phytotoxic lipopolysaccharide-or glycopeptides was an attractive prospect, but it has not been supported by analysis of the best available concentrates. Amino-acids and sugars are found after hydrolysis but in amounts representing less than 1% of the concentrate. Ketodeoxysugar acids were not detected, a faint color obtained with the thiobarbituric acid test having the properties of a deoxyribose derivative (13,14). Solutions of the toxin also show no reduction in toxicity when incubated with pronase or emulsin (which has β-glycosidase activity). Thus in its present form, the toxin does not appear to be a glycopeptide. There remains a possibility that, as initially extracted, it was bound to glycopeptide material which was not essential for toxicity and was removed during fractionation.

VII. REFERENCES

1. Price, P. C., "Investigation of a nematode-bacterium disease complex affecting Wimmera ryegrass," Ph.D. Thesis, University of Adelaide, 1973.
2. McIntosh, G. H., and Thomas, M. R., *Aust. Vet. J.* 43, 349 (1967).
3. Berry, P. H., and Wise, J. L., *Aust. Vet. J.* 51, 525 (1975).
4. Shaw, J. N., and Muth, O. H., *J. Am. Vet. Med. Assoc.* 114, 315 (1949).
5. Galloway, J. H., *J. Am. Vet. Med. Assoc.* 139, 1212 (1961).
6. Lanigan, G. W., Payne, A. L., and Frahn, J. L., *Aust. Vet. J.* 52, 244 (1976).
7. Peterson, J. E., and Jago, M. V., *Aust. J. Exp. Biol. Med. Sci.*, In press.
8. Gritter, R. J., and Albers, R. J., *J. Chromatogr.* 9, 392 (1962).
9. Bang, H. O., *J. Chromatogr.* 14, 523 (1964).
10. Raynaud, M., and Alouf, J. E., *in* "Microbial Toxins," (S. J. Ajl, S. Kadis, and T. C. Montie, Eds.), Vol. 1, p. 67. Academic Press, New York, 1970.
11. Strobel, G. A., *Proc. Int. Conf. Plant Pathol. Bact.*, 3rd, p. 357-365, 1971,
12. Strobel, G. A., Talmadge, K. W., and Albersheim, P., *Biochim. Biophys. Acta* 261, 365 (1972).
13. Warren, L., *J. Biol. Chem.* 234, 1971 (1959).
14. Weissbach, A., and Hurwitz, J., *J. Biol. Chem.* 234, 705 (1959).

PERENNIAL RYEGRASS STAGGERS IN NEW ZEALAND

P. H. Mortimer
Ruakura Agricultural Research Centre

I. ABSTRACT

A brief review is given on perennial ryegrass staggers, a neurotoxic disease of unknown etiology affecting sheep, cattle, and horses with a high prevalence in New Zealand summers. Trials relating its incidence to pasture composition and to high rates of stocking are reviewed.

Recent appraisals of the clinical manifestations have recognized that, underlying the overt forms showing incoordination and collapse, basic tremors exist.

Its relationship to staggers produced experimentally by cultures of Penicillium spp. *containing known tremorgens (e.g. penitrems) and by tremorgen-containing sclerotia of* Claviceps paspali *has been extensively studied.*

The striking similarities between perennial ryegrass staggers and the two experimental disorders strongly support the hypothesis that ryegrass staggers is also caused by a tremorgenic mycotoxin.

Pretreatment of sheep with hexachlorobenzene, a known stimulant of microsomal drug metabolizing enzymes, afforded significant protection from penitrem-induced staggers but not from C. paspali*-induced staggers. Sheep similarly pretreated with hexachlorobenzene and grazed throughout the summer on perennial ryegrass staggers-prone areas showed a similar significant degree of protection.*

II. INTRODUCTION

Ryegrass staggers, as commonly seen in New Zealand, appears to be a neuromuscular disorder affecting sheep most frequently, but in some localities also affecting cattle and horses (1). The disease has also been reported in Australia (2), in the United States (3), and in England (4).

III. OCCURRENCE

The disorder generally occurs in livestock grazing permanent pastures in which there is a predominance of perennial ryegrass (*Lolium perenne*) although at least one outbreak reportedly occurred on short-rotation ryegrass (1). The disease occurs under a wide range of pasture conditions; on short-grazed dried-up ryegrass pastures with little green leaf, on ryegrass stubble shortly after removal of haycrop, on ryegrass pastures with short fresh regrowth, and on predominantly stemmy pastures (5). We have also seen the disorder in sheep grazing and uprooting short ryegrass crowns.

The occurrence of the disease often follows a close seasonal pattern, milder outbreaks often commence in early January, may then disappear or continue in a low key until the late summer or autumn (March-April) when the highest incidence and severity is likely to occur. Weather conditions may alter this pattern.

IV. INCIDENCE AND DURATION

Sheep, cattle, and horses of all ages may be affected and most breeds of sheep and cattle appear to be susceptible. Within a flock or herd there is strong evidence that differences in susceptibility exist, for the same individuals often show clinical signs in most summers while others in the group are never affected.

In the field, morbidity can be high in both dairy and beef cattle herds, and especially high in flocks of sheep where an incidence of 80% may be reached. Mortality is generally low and is rarely from the disease *per se*. Losses may result from drownings in watercourses or troughs during tetanic spasms, or from fractured limbs, falls, or related misadventure. Loss of production may occur but is generally not great. Rams are joined with the ewe flock during the staggers season but conception rates are believed to be little affected.

It often becomes difficult or impossible to muster and move livestock safely so routine management procedures and rotational grazing practices have to be abandoned until recovery is well advanced. Generally both sheep and cattle recover completely in one to four weeks if they can be moved or are allowed to slowly migrate onto safe pastures or crops, or when toxic conditions spontaneously regress.

V. CLINICAL SIGNS

In an outbreak clinical signs develop gradually over a few days: experimental feeding of toxic grass to penned sheep usually requires from seven to twelve days for onset of signs (M. Byford, personal communication).

Cunningham and Hartley (1) have given a clear account of the overt clinical signs seen in severe staggers outbreaks in sheep, cattle, and horses. Since that time R. G. Keogh has made detailed observations of clinical signs in sheep in field outbreaks and his findings are germane to our subsequent studies. From his observations he established a system of assessing severity of ryegrass staggers in sheep for use in interpreting effects of experimental treatments (5). Recourse to these descriptions is most enlightening for it recognizes that the disorder is from the onset and throughout a tremoring syndrome upon which may be superimposed head shaking, degrees of incoordination, abnormal staggering gait, eventual stumbling, and collapse to the ground sometimes to be followed by severe muscular spasms after which the sheep will regain its feet after a variable time and walk away. Keogh's severity score is also related to the amount of exercise (running) required to produce the maximal clinical signs that the sheep can express at a particular degree of neurotoxic involvement.

In clinical cases it is our observation also that the clinical component of tremors is either present, or is capable of being immediately promoted by disturbance or excitement of the animal.

VI. MORBID ANATOMY

Neither at the stage of acute incoordination nor in chronically affected animals are clearcut neuropathologic changes to be found. Histologic changes sometimes detected in the cerebellum, mainly of Purkinje cell degeneration and white matter rarifaction resembling status spongiosus, are not regarded as pathognomonic of ryegrass staggers. It is stated that they may probably arise from a number of factors such as insults or anoxia occurring during convulsive seizures (6,7). After prolonged recumbency focal pale areas of muscle dystrophy may be present in hind or forelimbs, but again these are held to be non-specific secondary changes (1).

Our observations on pathologic changes in staggers induced by tremorgen-producing *Penicillia* and on staggers induced by *Claviceps paspali* sclerotia, to be discussed later, are limited but in agreement with findings reported for ryegrass staggers (1,6).

VII. ETIOLOGIC CONSIDERATIONS

For a number of years opinion has been held that a toxin present in ryegrass was responsible for the disorder (1). Ergots of *Claviceps purpurea*, parasitizing ryegrass seedheads, failed to reproduce the syndrome of ryegrass staggers (8).

It is commonly recognized that sclerotia of *C. paspali*, parasitizing *Paspalum dilatatum* seedheads, produces paspalum staggers (dallis grass poisoning) a neurotoxic condition similar if not identical to ryegrass staggers (9). However paspalum staggers is differentiated from ryegrass staggers by reference to the offending pasture where the presence of rank ergotized paspalum seedhead confirms the origin of the disorder. In ryegrass, Aasen *et al.* (2) suggested that the alkaloids perloline and halostachine may be responsible for the disorder but their efforts were inconclusive.

A. Associations with Pasture Composition and Grazing Pressure

Recent experiments have shown that when sheep were forced to graze the base (bottom 2.5 cm) of ryegrass dominant pasture plots and ingest significantly more dead material, the incidence of staggers was high, whereas sheep moved whenever the herbage in plots was grazed down to a level about 2.5 cm above ground level did not develop staggers (5). A similar result has been obtained at Ruakura (M. Byford, personal communication) in trials involving both sheep and cattle grazed at three rates of stocking on either original unimproved pasture plots (average ryegrass composition 28%) or on plots renovated by thorough cultivation and sown with Ellet's (Mangere) ryegrass to establish a sward with an average ryegrass content of 63%. The incidence of severe staggers was very high on the renovated ryegrass dominant plots but low on the white clover/weed dominant original plots. Furthermore, there was a stepwise increase in incidence and severity of staggers through the low to the medium to the high stocking-rate plots.

B. Associations with Tremorgenic *Penicillia*

In 1974 the growing incidence of outbreaks of ryegrass staggers in New Zealand prompted intensification of Government-sponsored research towards recognition of the causal factors and hopefully towards establishment of suitable control measures. Speculation at this time was leaning towards a mycotoxic etiology.

Although the connection appeared extremely tenuous, attention was focused on *Aspergillus* and, especially, *Penicillium spp.* fungi previously shown to produce neurotoxic tremorgens (10,11,12 13,14) which are remarkably tremorgenic when dosed to mice and other laboratory animals. A previous survey had shown that neither of these fungal spp. are common on staggers prone pastures in the North Island of New Zealand (15) although tremorgen-producing *Penicillium spp.* were known to occur in New Zealand soils (16,17).

Isolates of *P. cyclopium*, taken from the top 1 cm of soil on staggers prone paddocks at this Research Centre, were cultured in the laboratory (18). A few mg of this mycelial material given intraperitoneally to mice caused within minutes severe tremors identical to those described by Wilson *et al.* (11). Solvent extracts of three Ruakura isolates of *P. cyclopium* prepared on chromatograms (11) yielded fractions which contained components identified as penitrems A and B (11,19,18). Homogenized mycelium of several New Zealand strains of *P. cyclopium* have now been dosed to more than 150 sheep and six steers. Dosing regimes ranged from repeated oral daily doses (to sheep) of 50 mg air-dried mycelium per kg body weight for up to three weeks to single doses of 600 mg per kg. Proportionally higher doses were given to steers.

The clinical syndromes produced in these sheep and cattle were closely compared with those seen in concurrent field outbreaks of ryegrass staggers in the locality (18). They were strikingly similar in all respects ranging from initial mild head tremors extending to the neck, shoulder, flank, and hind limb muscle groups, to the onset of incoordinated limb movements, limb abducted stance, unsteadiness, and rocking. The severe patterns of abnormal stilted gait seen in running and the attitudes of collapse were all mimicked. Both groups displayed the brief phase of tetanic spasms in recumbency and the quick recovery to regain their feet and walk off to join other groups. The total recovery phase from the overall neurotoxic effects took a similar number of days when cases of similar severity were compared.

Generally there was little difference in the susceptibility of sheep and cattle to *P. cyclopium* tremorgens, although within-species variations were noted.

C. Comparisons Between *P. Cyclopium* and *C. paspali*-Induced Staggers

Attention was recently drawn to the close similarities between paspalum staggers (dallis grass poisoning) in cattle and experimental poisoning of calves with tremortins (penitrems) isolated from *P. palitans* (13). Sclerotia of *C. paspali* also contain non-alkaloidal mycotoxic tremorgens (20) which produce the neurotoxic symptoms of paspalum staggers seen mainly in cattle but occasionally in sheep and horses (Mantle, Mortimer, and White, in press). The field disease has been recorded in New Zealand (9), in the United States (21), in Australia (22), and also in several Mediterranean countries.

The staggers syndrome produced by oral doses of *C. paspali* sclerotia was concurrently compared with *P. cyclopium*-induced staggers in both sheep and cattle. In general the clinical signs produced by both types of fungal material were indistinguishable. On a body weight basis sheep required two to three times more *C. paspali* tremorgens than did cattle to produce comparable effects. The higher dose level required for sheep considerably prolonged their recovery period.

The tremorgens of *C. paspali*, while insufficiently separated to allow structures to be proposed, appear to be allied structurally to known tremorgens containing one indolic N, such as the penitrems and other *in vitro* metabolites of *Penicillia* (Mantle, Mortimer, and White, in press).

VIII. MODIFICATION OF RESPONSES OF SHEEP TO TREMORGENIC AGENTS

A. Liver Microsomal Enzyme Stimulation by Hexachlorobenzene (HCB): Protection Against Effects of Penitrems

The fungicide hexachlorobenzene (HCB) has been shown to induce drug-metabolizing enzymes in rat liver (23) and in sheep liver (24). A protective effect had been noted in sheep previously dosed with HCB [M. Avrahami, quoted by Turner and Green (23,24)].

To gain further information on relationships between penitrem-induced and *C. paspali*-induced staggers, and information on metabolism of tremorgens by sheep, a pilot trial was conducted involving 24 sheep (Mortimer and Mantle, unpublished work). Twelve sheep were pretreated with intraperitoneal injections of HCB in arachis oil on four consecutive days (total dose approximately 15 mg per kg body weight). Commencing three days later, six of the group and six of the non-injected sheep were orally dosed with a total of 0.38 g air-dried mycelium of *P. cyclopium* cultures per kg, divided over five days. The remaining two groups of six sheep were orally dosed with a total of 4.0 g of paspalum ergot sclerotia per kg over five days. Assessments of clinical responses were made daily from the first day of dosing to the time when recovery was complete.

Comparing the two *P. cyclopium*-dosed groups, the HCB group showed a high degree of protection from the tremorgenic effects. However in the other groups HCB treatment gave no protection against *C. paspali*-induced staggers (Mortimer and Mantle, unpublished results).

These sheep were then slaughtered at intervals up to 28 weeks after HCB stimulation and liver microsomes were assayed *in vitro* for evidence of stimulation. At 16 weeks a high level of stimulation was still apparent.

The *P. cyclopium*/HCB component of the above experiment was then repeated using 20 sheep per group and the clinical signs were scored on the scale devised by Keogh (5). The total dose of *P. cyclopium* mycelium given was 0.53 g per kg, given over six days. Highly significant protection against tremors and incoordination was afforded over the period of the experiment (Mortimer and Manns, unpublished findings).

B. Liver Microsomal Enzyme Stimulation by Hexachlorobenzene: Protection Against Field Outbreaks of Ryegrass Staggers

Our most recently completed trials (Mortimer and Manns, unpublished findings) were planned with the object of utilizing the established liver microsomal enzyme stimulatory effect in an attempt to augment detoxification and afford protection to sheep throughout the summer and autumn grazing period when there is risk of ryegrass staggers outbreaks. Facial eczema is another mycotoxic disease of grazing ruminants in which serious hepato-biliary lesions are produced by the mycotoxin sporidesmin. This mycotoxicosis has the same seasonal incidence as ryegrass staggers. The trials could, therefore, test protection by HCB against both diseases. Nine trial sites with a known high probability for the occurrence of one or both diseases were chosen at sites spread over the North Island. In January 1977, 450 sheep were placed into nine groups of 50 which, in turn, were equally divided and matched for weight into two sub-groups. Half the sheep (25) of each group received a series of six injections of HCB on alternate days. The other nine sub-groups of 25 served as non-injected controls. The 9 original groups of 50 were reformed and a group was placed on each trial site and grazed as one group throughout the season. The controlling staff on sites were unaware of the identity of the treated and control animals.

In relation to these mycotoxic diseases the season was generally disappointing to us but kind to the sheep. At two widely separated sites severe extensive outbreaks of ryegrass staggers developed. Thrice weekly both the incidence and the individual severity of the disease was assessed and recorded. At the end of May, when all danger had abated and recovery was complete, the recorded scores were returned for analysis, in the event a remarkable degree of protection from ryegrass staggers had been afforded over the whole season to the HCB pretreatment groups. At one site the degree of protection was statistically significant throughout a period of 27 days both with regard to overall incidence and severity in individual animals. At the other site the outbreak was somewhat less severe but was also statistically significant at the height of the outbreak.

The statistical strength of these results fully confirms the observation of M. Avrahami [quoted by Turner and Green (24)] that HCB affords sheep considerable protection from perennial ryegrass staggers.

Although not directly related to this topic, it is also reassuring to report that HCB also gave, over the same season, a degree of protection against facial eczema liver damage (sporidesmin poisoning) that was statistically viable at three trial sites.

IX. DISCUSSION

The recent investigations of Keogh (5) and Byford (personal communication) emphasize the close association between high incidence of ryegrass staggers and management systems which allow tight grazing of short ryegrass pastures in the traditional danger season. Avoidance of this and the use of strategic crops for *in situ* grazing are obvious measures for disease control. Byford's investigations using renovated ryegrass plots again stress the close association of staggers with ryegrass dominance in pasture swards.

The recognition that tremors are the earliest and most consistent, though least spectacular, clinical signs in staggers gives great impetus to the role of mycotoxic tremorgens as the neurotoxic principle(s) acquired during grazing. The multiplicity of causal fungi and neurotoxic agents also needs to be considered. The tremorgenic *Penicillia* which are readily isolated from superficial soil layers in staggers-prone locations are not conspicuous components of the microbial flora of pasture leaf or litter, the major component ingested by grazing stock. Thus the acquisition of mycotoxic material by grazing stock in quantities sufficient to initiate and maintain neurologic symptoms sometimes over several weeks requires further examination. In this respect, under certain conditions, soil intake can reach 400 g per day for ewes and up to 179 kg per month for cows (25,26). Furthermore, the regularity with which large numbers of viable propagules of tremorgenic *Penicillia* can be isolated from feces of animals with staggers (di Menna, Mantle, and Mortimer, unpublished findings) lends further support to the possible involvement of tremorgenic *Penicillia*.

The close similarity of clinical signs in perennial ryegrass staggers, in paspalum staggers and in penitrem-induced staggers strongly suggests that the neurotoxic agents involved have a common pharmacologic action. In this category may be mentioned the penitrems, fumitremorgens, paxalline, verruculogen, and at least two tremorgens in *C. paspali* sclerotia yet to be characterized.

In this preliminary report of our recent work it appears that the penitrems and the so-far unidentified neurotoxins of ryegrass staggers, but not the tremorgens of *C. paspali*, are metabolized and detoxified at microsomal sites in the liver. It suggests that the tremorgens are toxic *per se*. Prior augmentation of certain liver microsomal enzymes by HCB has proved to be sufficiently long lasting to afford a high degree of protection to sheep grazing throughout the length of a "toxic" season of many weeks.

The persistence of HCB in tissues of food animals would clearly present an unacceptable health hazard to man, so our findings are not likely to have any early impact on prevention of the disease. There may be a place for the use of HCB for prevention of staggers in horses.

With the availability of harvested toxic pasture material, known methods for safe storage, the use of sheep as definitive test animals for feeding bulk material, the use of mice for rapid microscale assays for neurotoxins, together with increasing information on the source and chemical nature of a growing number of tremorgen candidates, there is now every likelihood of an early breakthrough in understanding the etiologies of staggers syndromes in livestock. Unfortunately it does not follow that such enlightment will immediately enhance the implementation of further economically viable control measures.

X. REFERENCES

1. Cunningham, I. J., and Hartley, W. J., *N. Z. Vet. J.* 7, 1 (1959).
2. Aasen, A. J., Culvenor, C. C. J., Finnie, E. P., Kellock, A. W., and Smith, L. W., *Aust. J. Agric. Res.* 20, 71 (1969).
3. Shaw, J. N., and Muth, O. H., *J. Am. Vet. Med. Assoc.* 114, 315 (1949).
4. Clegg, F. G., and Watson, W. A., *Vet. Rec.* 72, 731 (1960).
5. Keogh, R. G., *N. Z. J. Exp. Agric.* 1, 55 (1973).
6. Munday, B. L., and Mason, R. W., *Aust. Vet. J.* 43, 598 (1967).

7. Mason, R. W., *Aust. Vet. J.* 44, 428 (1968).
8. Thornton, R. H., *N. Z. Vet. J.* 12, 13 (1964).
9. Hopkirk, C. S. M., *N. Z. J. Agric.* 53, 105 (1936).
10. Wilson, B. J., and Wilson, C. H., *Science* 144, 177 (1964).
11. Wilson, B. J., Wilson, C. H., and Hayes, A. W., *Nature (London)* 220, 77 (1968).
12. Ciegler, A., *Can. J. Microbiol.* 17, 599 (1969).
13. Cysewski, S. J., *J. Am. Vet. Med. Assoc.* 163, 1291 (1973).
14. Ciegler, A., *Lloydia* 38, 21 (1975).
15. di Menna, M. E., and Parle, J. N., *N. Z. J. Agric. Res.* 13, 51 (1970).
16. Thornton, R. H., *N. Z. J. Agric. Res.* 1, 922 (1958).
17. Thornton, R. H., *N. Z. J. Agric. Res.* 3, 203 (1960).
18. di Menna, M. E., Mantle, P. G., and Mortimer, P. H., *N. Z. Vet. J.* 24, 45 (1976).
19. Ciegler, A., and Pitt, J. I., *Mycopathol. Mycol. Appl.* 42, 119 (1970).
20. Brook, P. J., and White, E. P., *Annu. Rev. Phytopathol.* 4, 171 (1966).
21. Simms, B. T., *Auburn Vet.* 8, 22 (1951).
22. Langdon, R. F. N., *Aust. J. Sci.* 26, 55 (1964).
23. Turner, J. C., and Green, R. S., *Biochem. Pharmacol.* 23, 2387 (1974).
24. Turner, J. C., and Green, R. S., *Res. Vet. Sci.* 20, 155 (1976).
25. Healy, W. B., *Proc. N. Z. Soc. Anim. Prod.* 27, 109 (1967).
26. Healy, W. B., *N. Z. J. Agric. Res.* 11, 487 (1968).

A COMPARATIVE STUDY OF DARLING PEA (*SWAINSONA SPP.*) POISONING IN AUSTRALIA WITH LOCOWEED (*ASTRAGALUS* AND *OXYTROPIS SPP.*) POISONING IN NORTH AMERICA

W. J. Hartley
The University of Sydney

I. ABSTRACT

Swainsona spp. *poisoning is a chronic progressive neurologic disorder seen in extensively grazed cattle, sheep, and horses in Australia. There are no macroscopic lesions but microscopically the entity is characterized by widespread neurovisceral 'watery' cytoplasmic vacuolation, and in more protracted cases also neuroaxonal dystrophy and pigment deposition. The stored substance is thought to be contained in lysosomes, but its nature is not known.*

The lesions in this entity are closely similar to those caused by locoweeds in the U.S.A., except that congenitally deformed lambs and calves have not been seen in Australia.

The effects of experimental A. lentiginosus *intoxication in the pregnant ewe are summarized.*

II. INTRODUCTION

A nervous disease of sheep, cattle, and horses associated with the ingestion of several species of *Swainsona* (Darling Pea) has been recognized in eastern Australia for at least 100 years. The early field reports and feeding trials up to 1940 have been reviewed by Hurst (1). Since that time further investigations have been carried out in New South Wales (N.S.W.) (2,3,4,5,6,7,8, 9,10), in Queensland (11), and in Western Australia (12).

This contribution will summarize the clinical, pathological, and experimental findings in *Swainsona spp.* poisoning and briefly compare them with those seen in *Astragalus* and *Oxytropis spp.* toxicity.

III. THE GENUS *SWAINSONA*

There are over 50 species of *Swainsona* in Australia of which *S. galegifolia, S. luteola, S. greyana, S. canescens, and S. procumbens* are considered to be the main ones poisonous to livestock (13). *S. canescens* is largely confined to Western Australia and the Northern Territory, the other species occur through South Australia, Victoria, and N.S.W. to Queensland. These species are now largely confined to open range country, hills, and plains where livestock are extensively grazed the year round.

Swainsona spp. are perennials and are the first plants to develop after early spring or autumn rains and, on heavily infested country, they are the predominant pasture species available to stock at these times. The plant is considered to be toxic at all stages of growth.

IV. CONDITIONS OF TOXICITY

Large areas of northern N.S.W. and southern Queensland are heavily infested with Darling Pea. Fortunately most property-bred cattle and sheep either develop a tolerance to the plant or they largely avoid it when other vegetation is available. Outbreaks of poisoning tend to occur following rains in early spring or autumn following long periods of drought or food shortage.

Young stock, particularly weaned calves and introduced stock, appear to be very susceptible. Some of these develop an apparent craving for the plant and will seek it out even when plentiful herbage of other pasture species is available. The disease is generally more severe in the cattle than in the sheep, but occasionally only sheep are involved.

V. CLINICAL SIGNS

A. Cattle

In N.S.W. young beef cattle grazing *S. galegifolia* (5) are noticed first to lose condition, they then develop neurologic signs which include staring eyes, head shaking, low head carriage, stiff-clumsy gait, incoordination, and hyperexcitability. If stressed, particularly in hot weather, the neurologic signs are intensified, the animal salivates and pants, and may collapse and die. If affected animals are removed from infested pastures early in the disease they usually improve in condition and, in most cases, the nervous signs gradually diminish. Most young animals will not survive for more than a few weeks once obvious neurologic signs are observed. In adult cattle the disease is not so severe and the neurologic signs not so pronounced, and they may survive as chronic cases for many months.

An additional feature of *Swainsona* toxicity in cattle, not observed in sheep flocks, is that affected animals have a very poor breeding performance. They conceive and maintain pregnancy for at least 5-7 months, but later either abort or the calves die at or shortly after a full term birth (5).

B. Sheep

Irrespective of the species of *Swainsona* involved the signs of poisoning in sheep seem to be similar. The disease appears to be less severe than in young cattle and appears to be more prevalent in young stock. Clinical signs consist of head tremors, staring eyes, high head carriage, high stepping stiff gait, disturbed vision, and incoordination. These signs are usually intensified when animals are driven, and the animal may then collapse. As the disease progresses there is gradual loss of condition. Affected animals may survive for several months, some become recumbent, and others die from misadventure.

A further entity seen in affected flocks is a progressive, irreversible loss of condition leading to emaciation and death, without neurologic signs.

There are no substantial reports of the association of *Swainsona spp.* with abortion, nor of congenital limb abnormalities.

C. Horses

Although there are reports from eastern and western Australia of suspected *Swainsona spp.* poisoning in horses, few contain detailed descriptions of clinical signs. Signs mentioned include difficulty in handling, incoordination, mania, and death.

VI. PATHOLOGY

A. Gross Lesions

The only significant post mortem finding in cases of *Swainsona* poisoning is seen in those animals showing acute signs and still grazing infested pastures and that is a rumen or stomach filled with *Swainsona*. No obvious lesions are detectable in the central nervous system (C.N.S.) or elsewhere in those animals showing neurologic signs. However, in the entity reported above in sheep with gradual emaciation, without nervous signs, there is a distinct focal symmetrical golden yellow discoloration of the anterior and mid brain stem (6).

B. Light Microscopic Lesions

The characteristic lesions present in all recent cases of *Swainsona* toxicity in cattle, sheep, and horses consist of widespread neurovisceral cytoplasmic 'watery' vacuolation (3,4,5,6, 11,12). These lesions, in the most severe cases, affect virtually all neurones from cerebral cortex to cord and autonomic ganglia. Similar cytoplasmic 'watery' vacuolation is seen in the renal convoluted tubules, hepatocytes, pancreatic exocrine parenchyma, thyroid acinar epithelium, and the choroid plexus (5,6). Lymph nodes contain many foamy macrophages in the sinusoids. Cytoplasmic vacuolation has not been observed in pituitary or adrenals, nor in cardiac, skeletal, or smooth musculature. The effect of the toxic agent on fetus and fetal membranes has not been examined.

In more protracted cases, in addition to neurovisceral cytoplasmic vacuolation, lesions of neuroaxonal dystrophy are seen. These consist of small eosinophilic, argyrophillic bodies or spheroids. These are seen at all levels of the C.N.S. and many, but not all, are in close proximity to nuclei of neurones (6). In old-standing or chronic cases spheroids are the only lesions observed.

Circumstantial evidence indicates that the neurovisceral cytoplasmic foamy vacuolation disappears shortly after the animals are removed from the offending pasture. However, the spheroids persist and these may represent residual prolonged effects of the intoxication.

In the sheep with emaciation and macroscopic pigmentation of the C.N.S. and in other sheep and cattle with prolonged signs of intoxication, variable amounts of small, orange granules are present in parenchymal and perivascular glial cells and as free aggregates. This pigment is periodic acid Schiff positive and Ziehl Neelson positive (6). A similar pigment is present in sinusoidal and cortical macrophages of lymph nodes.

C. Ultrastructural Lesions

Limited electron microscopy has been carried out on experimental *Swainsona* intoxication (8) and on field cases (Hartley, unpublished). The vacuoles seen by electron microscopy are bounded by a single unit membrane, are frequently empty, but some contain amorphorus material. They probably result from the accumulation of a soluble material in lysosomes.

VII. EXPERIMENTAL *SWAINSONA SPP*. POISONING

In the 50 years prior to 1940 numerous feeding trials had been carried out in an effort to elucidate the toxic properties of *Swainsona spp*. (1). In a number of these trials carried out in N.S.W. and Queensland clinical signs similar to those observed in the field were observed. Recently feeding trials with *S. luteola* and *S. galegifolia* in Queensland (11) with *S. canescens* in Western Australia (12), and with *S. galegifolia* in N.S.W. (7,10) have been carried out in sheep and/or laboratory animals. In these trials the *Swainsona spp*. were fed for periods from 4 to 8 weeks and neurologic signs in treated animals were mild or absent, but widespread neurovisceral cytoplasmic vacuolation was observed, spheroids were few or absent, and no abnormal pigment was demonstrated.

In guinea pigs fed *S. galegifolia, S. luteola,* and *S. greyana* vacuolated lymphocytes appeared in the circulation by 7 days (10). Similar cells were seen in naturally affected calves at the time of their removal from infested pastures. Ten days later the cells had disappeared, only to reappear 3 days after renewed access to *Swainsona* (10).

VIII. COMPARATIVE ASPECTS OF DARLING PEA AND LOCOWEED TOXICITY

Locoism, a neurologic disorder of sheep, cattle, and horses of the open range country of the western United States of America (U.S.A.) has been recognized for over a hundred years. It was later shown to be associated with the ingestion of certain members of the genera *Astragalus* and *Oxytropis* (14). Seventy-five years ago it was reported that there were clinical similarities between locoed sheep in the U.S.A. and pea-eating sheep in Australia (15). Subsequently locoweeds were shown to produce vacuolation of neurones (16) and later widespread neurovisceral cytoplasmic vacuolation and neuroaxonal dystrophy were demonstrated in field cases (17,18). These observations were confirmed in laboratory trials in sheep fed *A. lentiginosus, A. pubentissimus,* and *Oxytropis sericea* (19,20), and the lesions were compared directly with those produced by feeding *S. galegifolia* (20). These reports indicate that there are no obvious differences between the neurovisceral cytoplasmic storage lesions seen in *Astragalus spp.* and *Oxytropis spp.* intoxication and those seen in *Swainsona spp.* poisoning.

Additional field and experimental observations in the U.S.A. have demonstrated that the same *Astragalus spp.* can be responsible for abortions in sheep and cattle (16,21,22), and for congenital limb abnormalities in lambs and calves (21,22,23). In Australia *S. galegifolia* probably causes abortions and stillbirths in cattle (5) but there is no field or experimental evidence available to suggest that the same occurs in sheep. Likewise no association of limb deformities have been reported in lambs or calves.

IX. PATHOGENESIS OF NEUROVISCERAL CYTOPLASMIC VACUOLATION

The nature of the substance stored in the cytoplasmic vacuoles is not known; it is obviously soluble and appears to be contained in lysosomes. As there are distinct similarities between the lesions of both *Swainsona spp.*, locoweed poisoning and some of the known inherited lysosomal storage diseases of animals - e.g. mannosidosis of cattle, one can postulate that these plants may contain substances which cannot be fully degraded by the normal complement of tissue lysosomal enzymes (29). Support for this suggestion comes from the experimental studies in which 'watery' storage was induced by the injection of sucrose and dextran, substances which are not, or only slowly, hydrolyzed by lysosomal enzymes (30). A further possibility is that the storage substance inhibits lysosomal enzyme activity.

X. SUMMARY OF EXPERIMENTAL *A. LENTIGINOSUS* INTOXICATION IN THE PREGNANT EWE (WITH L. F. JAMES, LOGAN)

Abortions, stillbirths, and weakly lambs often result from ewes affected with locoism during pregnancy (22). To study the pathogenesis of this condition several experimental feeding trials have been carried out. Groups of ewes from 1-120 days pregnant were fed for 4-40 days with approximately 400 grams of dried *A. lentiginosus* (24,25,26,27,28). Ewes were killed sequentially up to full term and samples taken for pathologic examination. These trials have consistently produced lesions in the dam, fetus and fetal membranes, the extent and severity largely depending on the age of the fetus at, and the duration of, the exposure. The following changes have been seen in some or all of the test animals.

A. Gross Lesions

(a) abortion
(b) deformed lambs
(c) pallor of the uterus and fetal membranes
(d) fetal edema

B. Microscopic Lesions

(a) Cytoplasmic vacuolation of the stroma of the maternal caruncle, corpus luteum, and atretic ovarian follicles.
(b) Necrosis of the fetal elements of the placentome.
(c) Cytoplasmic vacuolation of the chorion and of the trophoblastic epithelium and the syncitial cells of the placentome.
(d) Neurovisceral cytoplasmic vacuolation of fetal neurones, thyroid acinar epithelium, renal convoluted tubular, and Bowman's capsular epithelium and hepatocytes. Pancreatic exocrine parenchyma and lymph nodes were not affected.
(e) Mild cerebral neuroaxonal dystrophy.

The lesions of neurovisceral cytoplasmic vacuolation and neuroaxonal dystrophy in the dam and fetus had greatly diminished within 15 days of cessation of feeding the locoweed and had virtually disappeared within 30 days (28). It would thus seem that unless abortion or limb deformities occur, prior exposure of the unborn fetus to the toxins of *Astragalus* has little effect on subsequent intrauterine fetal development.

XI. REFERENCES

1. Hurst, E., "The Poison Plants of New South Wales," p. 185. Snelling Printing Works, Sydney, 1942.
2. Diplock, P. T., *Vet. Insp. (N.S.W.)* 26, 55 (1962).

3. Kater, J. C., *Vet. Insp. (N.S.W.)* 28, 58 (1964).
4. Hartley, W. J., and Kater, J. C., *Aust. Vet. J.* 41, 107 (1966)
5. Hartley, W. J., and Gibson, A. J. F., *Aust. Vet. J.* 47, 300 (1971).
6. Hartley, W. J., *Acta Neuropathol.* 18, 342 (1971).
7. Huxtable, C. R., *Aust. J. Exp. Biol. Med. Sci.* 47, 339 (1969).
8. Huxtable, C. R., *Aust. J. Exp. Biol. Med. Sci.* 48, 71 (1970).
9. Huxtable, C. R., *Aust. J. Exp. Biol. Med. Sci.* 50, 109 (1972).
10. Huxtable, C. R., and Gibson, A., *Aust. Vet. J.* 46, 446 (1970).
11. Laws, L., and Anson, R. B., *Aust. Vet. J.* 44, 447 (1968).
12. Gardiner, M. R., Linto, A. C., and Aplin, T. E. A., *Aust. J. Agric. Res.* 20, 87 (1969).
13. Everist, S. L., "Poisonous Plants of Australia," p. 340. Angus and Robertson, Sydney, 1974.
14. Marsh, C. D., *U. S. Dep. Agric. Bur. Anim. Ind. Bull.* 112 (1909).
15. Maiden, J. H., "Plants Reputed to be Poisonous to Livestock in Australia," p. 10. Department of Agriculture N.S.W. Miscellaneous Publication 447, 1901.
16. Mathews, F. P., *Texas Agric. Exp. Stn. Bull.* 456 (1932).
17. Oehme, F. W., Bailie, W. E., and Hulbert, L. C., *J. Am. Vet. Med. Assoc.* 152, 271 (1968).
18. James, L. F., Van Kampen, K. R., and Staker, G. R., *J. Am. Vet. Med. Assoc.* 155, 525 (1969).
19. Van Kampen, K. R., and James, L. F., *Pathol. Vet.* 6, 413 (1969).
20. James, L. F., Van Kampen, K. R., and Hartley, W. J., *Pathol. Vet.* 7, 116 (1970).
21. James, L. F., Shupe, J. L., Binns, W., and Keeler, R. F., *Am. J. Vet. Res.* 28, 1379 (1967).
22. James, L. F., Keeler, R. F., and Binns, W., *Am. J. Vet. Res.* 30, 377 (1969).
23. Balls, L. D., and James, L. F., *J. Am. Vet. Med. Assoc.* 162, 291 (1973).
24. Van Kampen, K. R., and James, L. F., *Vet. Pathol.* 8, 193 (1971).
25. James, L. F., *Cornell Vet.* 61, 667 (1971).
26. James, L. F., *Am. J. Vet. Res.* 33, 835 (1972).
27. Hartley, W. J., and James, L. F., *Am. J. Vet. Res.* 34, 209 (1973).
28. Hartley, W. J., and James, L. F., *Am. J. Vet. Res.* 36, 825 (1975).
29. Jolly, R. D., and Hartley, W. J., *Aust. Vet. J.* 53, 1 (1977).
30. Lloyd, J. B., *in* "Lysosomes and Storage Diseases" (H. G. Hers and F. Van Hoof, Eds.), p. 173. Academic Press, New York, 1973.

ANALYSIS AND CHARACTERIZATION OF NITRO COMPOUNDS FROM *ASTRAGALUS* SPECIES

Frank R. Stermitz and Garold S. Yost
Colorado State University

I. ABSTRACT

Miserotoxin, 3-nitro-1-propyl β-D-glucopyranoside, is the acutely poisonous constituent of a number of Astragalus *species. A variety of 3-nitropropanoyl-D-glucopyranoses occur in other members of the* Astragalus *which are less toxic. No species have been found to contain both miserotoxin and the 3-nitropropanoic acid derivatives. Current methods of analysis, isolation, and characterization are presented along with a summary of the species from which these nitro compounds have been isolated. Suggestions regarding the biosynthesis of the two types of compounds are made.*

II. INTRODUCTION

Glucose derivatives of 3-nitropropanoic acid (called hiptagenic acid in the early literature) have been known for sometime (1) as constituents of *Indigofera* (Leguminosae). A number of *Indigofera* species were extensively investigated by Finnegan (2) who dubbed the nitropropanoylglucopyranoses "endecaphyllins."

Work on *Astragalus* species began when the identity of the toxic component of *A. miser* var *oblongifolius* was established (3, 4) as 3-nitro-1-propyl β-D-glucopyranoside and named miserotoxin. This discovery renewed interest in nitro compounds of the Leguminosae. Our published and some unpublished recent results on nitro compounds from *Astragalus* will be summarized in the present paper. Fig. 1 gives structures of the major nitro compound constituents found so far in these species. Miserotoxin has only been found in *Astragalus*, but nitropropanoic acid derivatives occur in several higher plant families. Table 1 lists these occurrences.

III. ISOLATION AND ANALYSIS

In our hands, multiple cold extraction with acetone has yielded the best results (4). Aqueous ethanolic extracts may give higher yields of total nitro compounds, but some hydrolysis of the sensitive esters occurs either during extraction or at the time of solvent evaporation. With ethanol extractions we have thus usually isolated considerably more 3-nitropropanoic acid and much less of the glucose derivatives. The crude acetone extract is

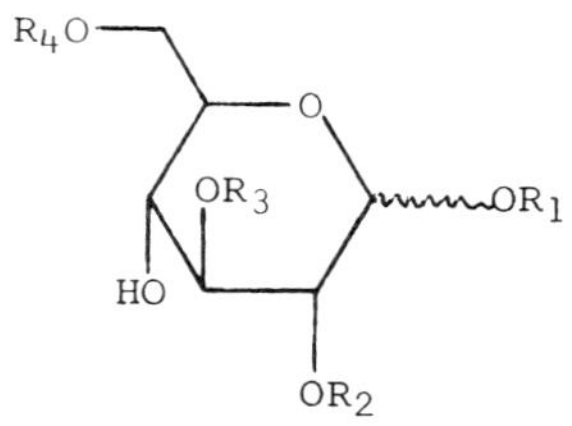

miserotoxin: R_1 = β-$CH_2CH_2CH_2NO_2$; R_2 = R_3 = R_4 = H

karakin: R_1 = β-NPA; R_2 = R_4 = NPA; R_3 = H

cibarian: R_1 = β-NPA; R_4 = NPA; R_2 = R_3 = H

coronarian: R_1 = α-H; R_2 = R_4 = NPA; R_3 = H

"6-mono": R_1 = α- and β-H; R_4 = NPA; R_2 = R_3 = H

(NPA = $-\overset{O}{\overset{\|}{C}}CH_2CH_2NO_2$)

Fig. 1. *Nitro compounds found in* Astragalus

TABLE 1

Occurrences of 3-Nitropropanoic Acid Derivatives in Higher Plants

Hiptage mandablota	(Malpighiaceae)
Hiptage benghalensis	(Malpighiaceae)
Heteropteris angustifolia	(Malpighiaceae)
Corynocarpus laevigata	(Corynocarpaceae)
Viola odorata	(Violaceae)
Indigofera spicata	(Leguminosae)
Indigofera endecaphylla	(Leguminosae)
Coronilla varia	(Leguminosae)
Astragalus sp.	(Leguminosae)

then chromatographed on a large silica gel column with $CHCl_3$-EtOH or $CHCl_3$-MeOH elution. Fractions which test positive for nitro compounds according to the Griess-Ilosvay method or a thin layer analysis are then rechromatographed. For the second purification, low pressure (80 psi) high performance preparative liquid chromatography on silica gel with 5:3 benzene-MeOH as eluting solvent has given the best results.

Thin layer chromatography can be employed for analytical purposes at any time during the extraction and isolation procedure. For maximum separation in one system, benzene-MeOH (5:3) is used as developing solvent with silica gel plates. Visualization of nitro compounds has best been accomplished with the diazotized *p*-nitroaniline spray of Majak and Bose (5,6). Table 2 lists our thin layer chromatography (tlc) results in this system for the nitro compounds we have found in *Astragalus*.

TABLE 2

Properties of Nitro Compounds from Astragalus

Compound	R_f Value[1]	Color[2]	m.p.
1. 3-Nitro-1-propanol	.58	red	oil
2. Karakin	.58	brown	122-123°
3. Coronarian	.50	brown	151-152°
4. Cibarian	.45	brown	121-122°
5. Unknown A	.42	brown	oil
6. Miserotoxin	.33	red	oil
7. Unknown B	.33	brown	oil
8. 6-Mono	.23	brown	oil
9. 3-Nitropropanoic acid	.17	red-brown	59-61°

[1]Silica gel, benzene-MeOH (5:3).

[2]Diazotized *p*-nitroaniline (Reference 5); only for fairly dilute samples.

Our earlier work (7,8) used a different visualization reagent based upon the Griess-Ilosvay color test for nitrite. This led to some incorrect data (see especially Reference 8) which must now be corrected. The Griess-Ilosvay spray gives identical colors for miserotoxin and unknown B and since the R_f values were identical, species which contained unknown B were listed (8) as containing miserotoxin. The identification was not based solely on tlc. We reported (8) the use of analytical high pressure liquid chromatography (HPLC) for the determination of nitro compound content as well as tlc. We have now found (unpublished results) that unknown B and miserotoxin have identical retention times in the HPLC analysis employed (8).

Unknown B is a nitropropanoic acid derivative, probably the 2-monosubstituted compound. Miserotoxin is easily distinguished from nitropropanoic acid derivatives by nuclear magnetic resonance (nmr) because it exhibits a quintet centered at δ 2.30 (d_6-acetone or D_2O solvent). This region is blank in the nmr spectra of the nitropropanoic acid derivatives and even crude extracts can be examined for miserotoxin. We reported (7) the presence of miserotoxin in *A. flexuosus* by tlc and HPLC and that its presence was checked by preparative tlc and subsequent nmr analysis. We have recently rechecked (unpublished results) the same collection of *A. flexuosus* and have found no miserotoxin. No supporting evidence or spectra can be found to support the contention (9) that *A. flexuosus* contains miserotoxin. The presence of unknown B was indeed detected (unpublished results) and it is evident that this work and much of that reported in Reference 8 is incorrect. We have reexamined most of the species of Reference 8 as well as others. Table 3 lists our corrected results for *Astragalus* nitro compound content to date.

TABLE 3

Nitro Compounds in Various Astragalus *Species*

Species	Compound[1]								
	1	2	3	4	5	6	7	8	9
atropubescens	+					+			
canadensis var. *brevidens*		+		+	+		+		+
canadensis var. *mortonii*		+		+				+	+
cibarius		+	+	+	+		+	+	+
convallarius var. *convallarius*						+			
diversifolius						+			
emoryanus var. *emoryanus*	+					+			
emoryanus var. *terlinguensis*	+					+			
falcatus		+	+	+	+		+	+	+
flexuosus		+	+	+	+		+	+	+
michauxii	+					+			
miser var. *oblongifolius*[2]	+					+			
pterocarpus	+					+			
tetrapterus						+			
toanus						+			

[1]The compounds are keyed to Table 2.

[2]Varieties *serotinus* and *hylophilus* also contain miserotoxin, while varieties *miser*, *tenuifolius*, *praeteritus*, *decumbens*, and *crispatus* contain no nitro compounds.

We encountered one contamination problem during investigation of the compounds of *A. falcatus*. Crude extracts showed a very strong test for a compound having very close to the same R_f value as miserotoxin and unknown B. This compound, however, gave a yellow spot when sprayed with NaOH solution, which is the first step in the Majak visualization method. No nitro compounds give such a color. Subsequent purification showed that the compound giving rise to this spot was astragalin, a common flavonoid of the Leguminosae. Astragalin gave a brown color when tested with the deazotized nitroaniline spray.

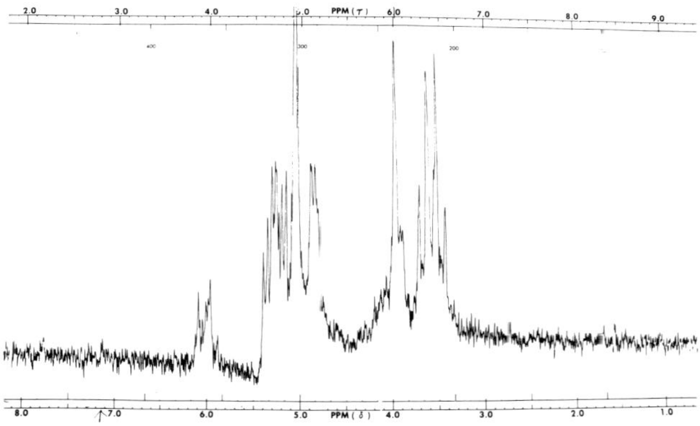

Fig. 2. *60 MHz ^1H Nmr of Cibarian.*

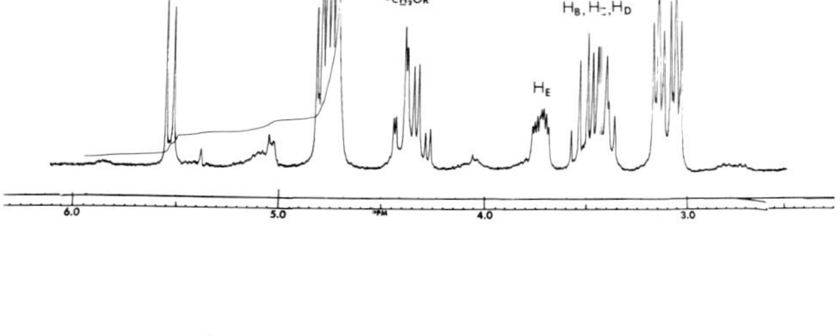

Fig. 3. *220 MHz ^1H Nmr of Cibarian.*

The spectral method of most value in determining structure or proving identity has been nmr. No discernible molecular ions could be found *via* mass spectrometry. Chemical ionization mass spectrometry can give considerable structural information (10), but even with this technique fragmentation is too facile and a molecular ion cannot be seen. Proton nmr at 60 MHz can distinguish miserotoxin (as mentioned above), but is relatively useless for much structure work (see Fig. 2). The use of 220 MHz nmr has been very valuable in our structure determinations (see Fig. 3), but is not commonly available. We have recently (unpublished results) obtained ^{13}C nmr spectra of most of the compounds of Table 2 and all are distinctive. All assignments of resonances have not yet been made, but the technique will certainly be a great aid in structure work on new compounds as well as for the proof of identity.

IV. STRUCTURE RELATIONSHIPS AND BIOSYNTHESIS

Biosynthetic studies have been reported on the formation of 3-nitropropanoic acid in bacteria where it is a common constituent. Shaw showed (11) that aspartic acid is an important precursor of 3-nitropropanoic acid in *Penicillium atrovenetum*. He also found that nitropropenoic acid could be converted by *P. atrovenetum* to 3-nitropropanoic acid. The nitropropenoic acid is not a normal constituent and so its position as an obligatory intermediate is not known:

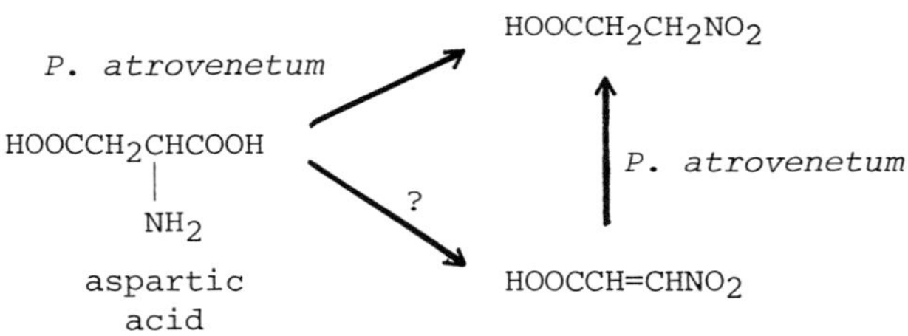

In higher plants, the only reported work is that of Unrau (12) who found that aspartic acid was <u>not</u> incorporated in 3-nitropropanoic acid in *Indigofera spicata*. Better incorporation was found (12) from malonate, but there was an unexplained labeling pattern in some feedings. Percentage incorporations were below 0.1% and the possibility that incorporations from malonate represent only a minor pathway is certainly a possibility.

The discovery (3,4) of 3-nitro-1-propanol as a constituent of *Astragalus* suggested that there might be an interconversion between it and 3-nitropropanoic acid. We synthesized ^{15}N-labeled 3-nitro-1-propanol, fed it to *A. falcatus*, and found 1.2% incorporation into cibarian (unpublished results). Thus, the alcohol can certainly be used as a precursor to the acid. An examination of our revised results of Table 3 indicates, however, that there is no known occurrence of both the alcohol and the acid. It therefore seems likely at this time that there is an independent synthesis of each in the specific plants that contain them and that one is not the precursor of the other. There is, of course, the possibility that plants which contain only the acid metabolize the alcohol so rapidly that it cannot be detected. Because of the sensitivity of the tlc visualization test we are using, this possibility seems less likely to us at the moment than the possibility of completely independent synthesis.

If 3-nitro-1-propanol is formed in plants independently of 3-nitro-1-propanoic acid, a possible precursor may be homoserine. Homoserine is known to undergo important transformations in legumes:

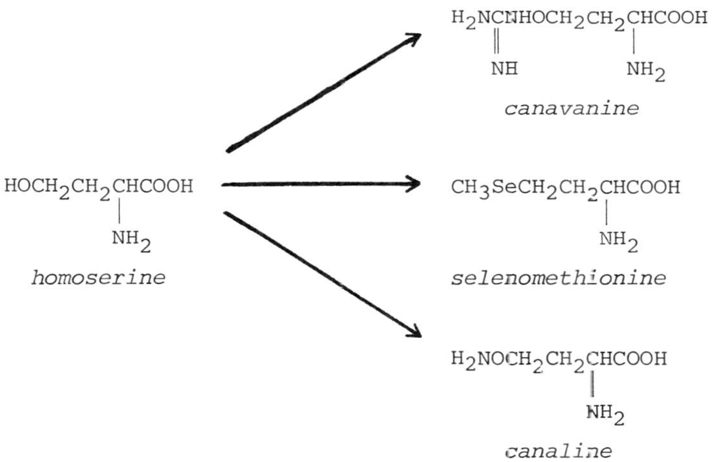

A biogenetic scheme for nitropropanol and nitropropanoic acid formation in legumes could also involve homoserine:

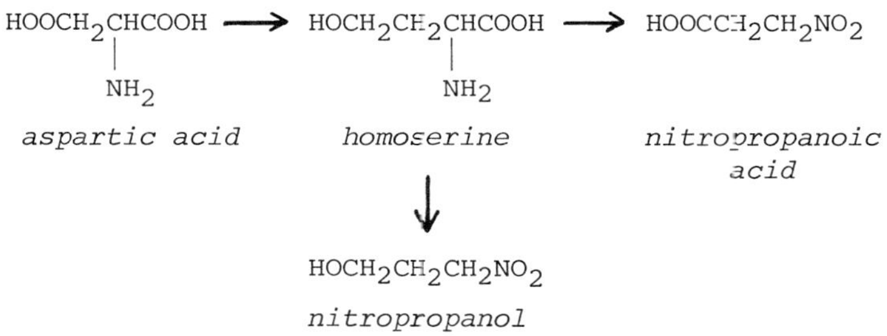

V. REFERENCES

1. Cooke, A., *Arch. Biochem. Biophys.* 55, 114 (1955).
2. Finnegan, R. A., and Mueller, W. H., *J. Pharm. Sci.* 54, 1136 (1965); Finnegan, R. A., and Stephani, R. A., *J. Pharm. Sci.* 57, 353 (1968).
3. Stermitz, F. R., Norris, F. A., and Williams, M. C., *J. Am. Chem. Soc.* 91, 4599 (1969).
4. Stermitz, F. R., Lowry, W. T., Norris, F. A., Buckeridge, F. A., and Williams, M. C., *Phytochemistry* 11, 1117 (1972).
5. Majak, W., and Bose, R. J., *Phytochemistry* 13, 1005 (1974).
6. Majak, W., and Bose, R. J., *Phytochemistry* 15, 415 (1976).
7. Harlow, M. C., Stermitz, F. R., and Thomas, R. D., *Phytochemistry* 14, 1421 (1975).
8. Williams, M. C., Stermitz, F. R., and Thomas, R. D., *Phytochemistry* 14, 2306 (1975).
9. Thomas, R. D., Ph.D. Thesis, Colorado State University, 1974.
10. Stermitz, F. R., Lowry, W. T., Ubben, E., and Sharifi, I., *Phytochemistry* 11, 3525 (1972).
11. Shaw, P. D., and McCloskey, S. A., *Biochemistry* 6, 2247 (1967).
12. Candlish, E., LaCroix, L. J., and Unrau, A. M., *Biochemistry* 8, 182 (1969).

LIVESTOCK POISONING FROM NITRO-BEARING *ASTRAGALUS*

M. Coburn Williams and Lynn F. James
Poisonous Plant Research Laboratory, Agricultural Research Service
U.S. Department of Agriculture

I. ABSTRACT

Aliphatic nitro compounds were found in 263 species and varieties of North American Astragalus. *Nitro compounds catabolize to 3-nitro-1-propanol (3-NPOH) and 3-nitropropionic acid (3-NPA) in the digestive tract of ruminants. Since 3-NPOH is more readily absorbed from the digestive tract than 3-NPA, 3-NPOH is more toxic per mg of NO_2 ingested.*

Animals chronically poisoned by nitro-bearing Astragalus *develop a general weakness in the hindquarters. Methemoglobin may reach 4 to 6% of total hemoglobin. Acutely poisoned animals die 4 to 20 hours after eating nitro-bearing* Astragalus. *The syndrome is characterized by general weakness, incoordination in the hindquarters, trembling, labored and audible breathing, collapse, and ultimately death from cardiac and respiratory failure. Methemoglobin usually surpasses 20% of total hemoglobin at time of death.*

Nitro-bearing Astragalus *that are closely related tend to synthesize the same form and concentration of nitro compounds. This chemotaxonomic character can be used to predict the occurrence of nitro compounds in* Astragalus, *assess the potential toxicity of the species, and identify foreign nitro-bearing species that would be unsuitable for importation because of their poisonous properties.*

II. INTRODUCTION

Poisonous *Astragalus* species are found throughout the world but are particularly prevalent in the western hemisphere. The genus achieves its greatest diversity and concentration on the deserts, foothills, and mountains of western North America. Major livestock losses occur yearly in the major grazing regions from British Columbia to Mexico.

The poisonous *Astragalus* are divided into three principal groups: (a) selenium accumulators, (b) locoweeds, and (c) species that synthesize aliphatic nitro compounds.

The selenium accumulators comprise about 25 species in the western United States. They occur on soil derived from selenium-bearing strata from which they absorb toxic amounts of selenium. The selenium replaces sulfur in sulfur-containing amino acids to form highly toxic organic selenium compounds. The seleniferous *Astragalus* have caused many livestock losses in the West (1).

The locoweeds produce an organic poison that affects the central nervous system of animals. The animals are affected after consuming locoweeds for several days, after which they may show an erratic or "loco" (crazy) behavior.

The third group of *Astragalus* synthesize aliphatic nitro compounds. The first of these compounds, miserotoxin, the β-D-glucoside of 3-nitro-1-propanol, was isolated from Wasatch milkvetch, *Astragalus miser* var. *oblongifolius* (Rydb.) Cron. (2). The compound is catabolized in the digestive tract of ruminants to the highly toxic 3-nitro-1-propanol (3-NPOH). Upon absorption into the circulatory system, this compound affects the central nervous system, particularly that area of the brain that controls coordination and automatic responses. The nitro functional group of some compounds complexes with ferrous hemoglobin to produce methemoglobin.

Other *Astragalus* species synthesize cibarian, hiptagin, and karakin (3). These nitro compounds catabolize to 3-nitropropionic acid (3-NPA). The 3-NPA is more slowly absorbed from the digestive tract than is 3-NPOH and is, therefore, considerably less toxic than 3-NPOH per milligram of NO_2 ingested (4). However, the 3-NPA species often synthesize 4 to 6 times more NO_2/g of plant than 3-NPOH species; therefore, the two types are about equal in toxicity per gram of plant.

Chronic poisoning occurs when ruminants graze for several days *Astragalus* species that contain low concentrations of nitro compounds. Methemoglobin levels reach 4 to 6% of total hemoglobin. Ruminants are acutely poisoned after grazing *Astragalus* that contains moderate to high concentrations of nitro compounds. Methemoglobin levels usually reach 20% of total hemoglobin or more within 4 hours and the animal dies 4 to 20 hours after the plant is consumed.

III. POISONING IN LIVESTOCK

Wasatch milkvetch has been responsible for livestock losses in Colorado, Utah, and Wyoming since the introduction of cattle and sheep to the western range (5). Chronically poisoned animals develop a condition known as "cracker heels" in which the fetlocks knuckle over and general weakness in the hindquarters causes the hooves to strike or rub together. The chronic state is further characterized by loss of motor control in the extremities, particularly in the hindquarters, so that the animal weaves or staggers when walking. Optical nerves are affected so that vision is impaired and the animal may fall over a small object or walk into objects in its path. Acutely poisoned animals die within a few hours after ingesting a lethal amount of plant.

We initiated biochemical and control research on Wasatch milkvetch in the late 1950's shortly after 39 cattle were acutely poisoned on a mountain meadow near Logan, Utah. Miserotoxin was subsequently isolated as the poisonous compound and the 3-carbon nitro-containing side chain, 3-NPOH, was identified as the specific agent of nitro-poisoning.

The metabolism of miserotoxin in ruminants was studied by adding the compound to ovine and bovine ruminal fluids and anaerobically incubating the mixture at 30° C for 4 hours in a constant temperature bath (6). Miserotoxin disappeared within 3 to 4 hours in both sheep and cattle ruminal fluid and was replaced by 3-NPOH as the only nitro compound present. The ruminal fluid was taken from animals that had been on a hay diet. Miserotoxin was completely metabolized to 3-NPOH in 1 hour in ruminal fluid taken from a grain-fed steer.

The toxicity of miserotoxin was investigated in cattle and rabbits (7). Rabbits given a lethal dose of miserotoxin (137 mg NO_2/kg of body weight) by intravenous injection exhibited symptoms of poisoning within 30 minutes. The eye changed from reddish pink to brownish red as methemoglobin formed. Within 1 to 1 1/2 hours the rabbits had developed respiratory dyspnea with abdominal respiratory effort and oral breathing. The hindquarters became paralyzed and death occurred 2 to 3 hours after treatment. Methemoglobin reached 33% of total hemoglobin in blood samples just before death.

Rabbits injected intravenously with a lethal dose of miserotoxin followed within 1 minute by an IV injection of methylene blue showed no toxic signs. Methemoglobin did not exceed 4% of total hemoglobin. Miserotoxin was apparently catabolized to inorganic nitrite in rabbits and the nitrite toxicosis was countered by proper medication with methylene blue.

A steer was gavaged Wasatch milkvetch at 25 mg NO_2/kg (compared with 137 mg NO_2/kg for the rabbit). This animal was immediately innoculated IV with methylene blue at 3 mg/kg. The animal developed respiratory dyspnea and muscular weakness 3 1/2 hours after treatment and died at 4 1/2 hours. Frothing at the nose and rapid heartbeat, normally seen in miserotoxin poisoning, did not occur. Methemoglobin did not exceed 0.5% at the time of death.

In the monogastric rabbit, death resulted from methemoglobinemia. Intravenous injection of methylene blue in a rabbit following a lethal dose of miserotoxin prevented the appearance of clinical symptoms. Methylene blue controlled methemoglobinemia in the steer, but the animal died as quickly as if no methylene blue had been given. Methylene blue proved to be no antidote for the 3-NPOH formed in the rumen.

The clinical signs of acute nitro poisoning are weakness, inability to place the hindlimbs properly and loss of proprioceptive awareness. The fetlocks knuckle over; the animal sways in the rear quarters. The neck becomes extended, the head is lowered and the tongue protrudes. Cyanosis is noted in the mucous membrane of the oral cavity and nasal passages. Respiratory effort is by abdominal lift. The animal urinates frequently; breathing is rasping and labored. Froth appears in the nose, and the animal grinds its teeth. Acutely poisoned animals collapse and soon die from cardiac and respiratory failure.

Lesions include severe pulmonary edema and hydrothorax, congested thyroid glands and paratid lymph nodes; petechiae underlie the tracheal mucosa. Microhemorrhages are found in the brain and hemorrhages separate the myocardial bundles. Methemoglobinemia is a constant toxic sign.

Chronically poisoned animals are often found on ranges infested with *Astragalus* species that contain 3 to 7 mg NO_2/g of plant. Although fewer animals die, losses can be severe due to the permanent damage inflicted on the vital organs in the animals.

An outbreak of poisoning due to nitro compounds from Emory milkvetch, *A. emoryanus* var. *emoryanus* (Rydb.) Cory, occurred in the spring of 1975 near Roswell, New Mexico (Williams, unpublished). Unusually favorable precipitation in the autumn of 1974 resulted in widespread germination and establishment of this winter annual. By March, the species carpeted vast tracts of range in densities not seen in the previous 35 years. Death losses among cattle and sheep reached 2 to 3%; 15 to 20% of the animals were chronically poisoned. Plants averaged 5 to 7 mg NO_2/g of plant as miserotoxin. Some affected animals appeared normal until excited. If startled, they often ran a few feet, then collapsed. Some cattle walked about on knuckled fetlocks. One group of cattle was observed in a corral where they had been confined for 6 weeks after becoming ill from eating Emory milkvetch. Dispite a diet of nutritious hay the animals remained unthrifty, depressed, and afflicted with diarrhea. The animals could not be sold at the slaughter house; they were permanently affected by the nitro-toxin. The loss to the rancher, for all practical purposes, would have been no less had the animals been acutely poisoned.

There is no known treatment for ruminants poisoned by nitro-containing *Astragalus*. Livestock losses can be reduced in two ways: reduce the density of the poisonous *Astragalus* with herbicides or avoid grazing livestock on infested areas when the plant is most poisonous. Many *Astragalus* species can be controlled with one of the phenoxy herbicides, but chemical control is not always feasible because of terrain, presence of other desirable species, or the size of the acreage that must be treated.

Wasatch milkvetch synthesized the greatest concentration of miserotoxin from bloom to immature pod stage of growth (Table 1) (8). While nitro compounds are found in all parts of the plant, they occur primarily in the leaves. Once the leaves have begun to dry and lose their green color, nitro compound levels drop rapidly. This pattern of metabolism of nitro compounds has been noted in other *Astragalus* species. Once Wasatch milkvetch has completely dried and bleached, it is virtually non-toxic (Table 2) (9). The herbicide silvex rapidly dries and bleaches the leaves of *Astragalus*; therefore, the chemical detoxifies as well as kills the plant (10). Silvex and 2,4,5-T have been used successfully in the control of Wasatch milkvetch (11).

Several tests are available to determine if nitro compounds are involved in livestock poisoning. The presence and concentra-

TABLE I

Seasonal Variation of Miserotoxin in Astragalus miser *var.* oblongifolius *Collected Near Logan, Utah during 1968*[1]

Date collected	Stage of growth	Percent miserotoxin 1968
May 31	Prebloom	2.3
June 13	Prebloom	2.5
June 20	Bloom	3.2
June 28	Bloom-early pod	3.1
July 5	Bloom-early pod	3.2
July 12	Immature pod	3.4
July 19	Immature pod	3.4
July 25	Immature pod	3.4
August 2	Immature pod	2.9
August 8	Past seed	3.0
August 16	Past seed	2.2
August 26	10% dry	1.3
August 30	20% dry	1.2
September 6	60% dry	1.0
September 13	75% dry	0.8
September 19	80% dry	0.8
September 27	100% dry	0.4

[1]After Williams and Norris (8).

TABLE 2

Grams of Timber Milkvetch (water extract) Required for LD_{50} in 1-week-old Chicks[1]

Date of sampling	Stage of growth	LD_{50}-- grams Whole plant	Leaflets	Petioles
May 27	Vegetative--bud	1	1	1
June 6	Early flower	1	1	1
June 13	Full flower	2	1	1
June 17	Full flower	2	1	2
June 24	Past flower	3	1	3
July 1	Past flower	3	1	3
July 8	Seed	3	1	3
July 15	Past seed	3	1	3
July 22	25% dry	4	2	4
July 29	50% dry	6	4	6
Aug. 5	75% dry	7	6	8
Aug. 12	90% dry	8	8	8
Aug. 19	Completely dry	26 (nontoxic)	25 (nontoxic)	25 (nontoxic)
Aug. 29	Completely dry	51 (nontoxic)	43 (nontoxic)	58 (nontoxic)

[1]After Williams and Binns (9).

tion of nitro compounds in plants can be determined by the Griess-Ilosvay test (12). This test can be completed in a few hours and requires only 0.5 g of plant. A shorter, qualitative test can detect small amounts of nitro compounds in 10 mg of leaf tissue (13). One-week-old chicks are quite susceptible to the poison. A water extract of the plant concentrated so that 1 ml = 1 g of plant can be given orally to chicks in graduated doses of 1 to 7 mg. Toxic signs are usually observed within 1 hour if the dose contains a toxic amount of nitro-toxin. When nitro-containing *Astragalus* is eaten, methemoglobin levels in the blood immediately increase (Figs. 1,2). A chronically poisoned animal that has consumed sublethal doses of nitro-toxins each day usually has a methemoglobin level of 4 to 6% of total hemoglobin. The methemoglobin level in an animal acutely poisoned by miserotoxin or 3-NPOH usually increases by 5% or more/hour. Methemoglobin levels in animals acutely poisoned by 3-NPA nitro-toxins increase much

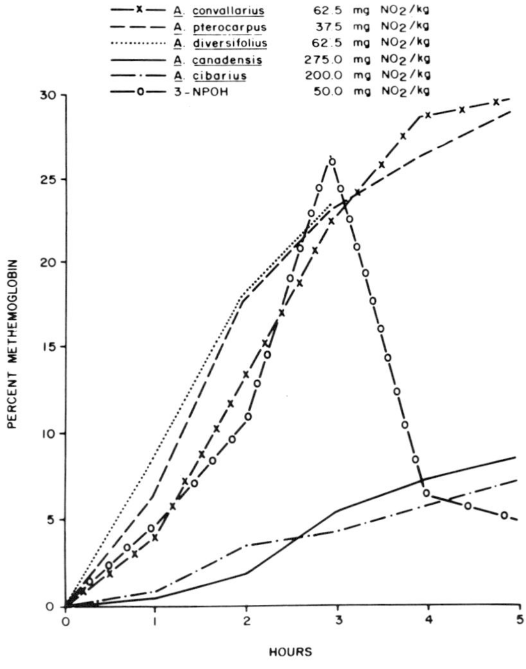

Fig. 1. *Percent methemoglobin in blood of sheep fed on minimum lethal dose (mg NO_2/kg of body weight) of five* Astragalus *species and 3-NPOH. The animal fed* A. diversifolius *died between 3 and 4 hours after treatment. [After Williams and James (4)].*

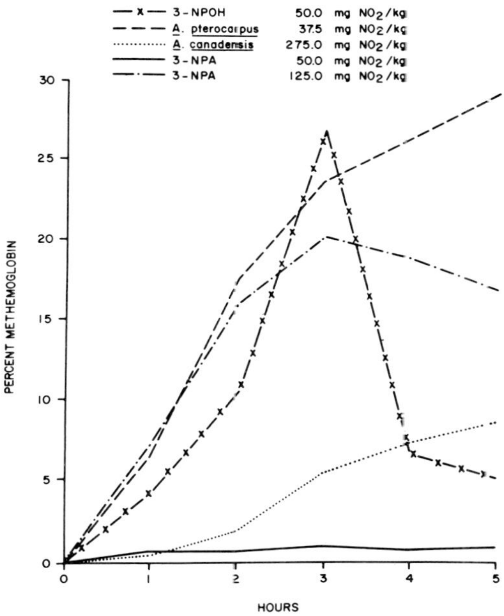

Fig. 2. *Percent methemoglobin in blood of sheep fed* Astragalus, *3-NPOH, and 3-NPA. All except 3-NPA at 50 mg NO_2/kg are minimum lethal doses. [After Williams and James (4)].*

more slowly. Once the methemoglobin level passes 20 to 22% of total hemoglobin, the animal nearly always dies (4).

IV. CHEMOTAXONOMIC CHARACTERISTICS OF NITRO-CONTAINING *ASTRAGALUS*

Species that are closely related morphologically often synthesize similar classes of compounds. The seleniferous *Astragalus*, related both morphologically and in their capacity to absorb and utilize selenium, are the best example in this genus. The nitro-containing *Astragalus* have also been found to have chemotaxonomic relationships.

Barneby (14) divided the North American *Astragalus* into 93 sections, 368 species, and 184 varieties. Since 1964, four additional species have been described to bring the total number of species and varieties to 556. Some sections are so unique that they contain only one species. Others contain numerous species and varieties.

Section *Genistoidei*, to which Wasatch milkvetch belongs, contains three species. Species *A. miser* is divided into eight varieties that are scattered throughout the Rocky Mountains from Colorado and Utah to British Columbia. Miserotoxin occurs in Wasatch, Yellowstone, and Columbia milkvetches (8). The other five varieties do not synthesize nitro compounds. The three varieties that synthesize nitro compounds are the most closely related taxonomically within the species. Subsequent investigations revealed that the other two species of section *Genistoidei*, *A. diversifolius* Gray and *A. convallarius* Greene, synthesize nitro compounds in approximately the same concentration as *A. miser* (15).

The discovery that nitro compounds occurred in these species suggested that nitro-toxins might occur in many other species of *Astragalus*. The problem confronting us was the task of analyzing for nitro compounds the majority of species and varieties found in North America and extending this work to include others of the estimated 2,000 species of *Astragalus* throughout the world. The answer lay in analyzing small leaf samples from herbarium specimens.

Nitro compounds were found to be very stable and to persist for long periods in plants (15) collected while green and carefully dried. Nitro compounds could be detected in concentrations as low as 3 mg NO_2/g of plant in leaves of herbarium specimens collected up to 100 years ago. The Griess-Ilosvay test for detection of nitro compounds was subsequently modified to accomodate a qualitative analysis for 10 mg of leaflet (13). Thus, large numbers of species and varieties from herbarium specimens could be analyzed in a few days. The herbarium specimen was not damaged since only one to four leaflets were removed for analysis. The nitro content was rated on a scale of T (trace) to 5. The ratings approximated the following equivalents in mg NO_2/g of plant: T = 2 to 3; 1 = 4 to 8; 2 = 9 to 13; 3 = 14 to 19; 4 = 20 to 25; and 5 = over 25.

The chemotaxonomic character of nitro-toxin synthesis can be used to: (a) predict the presence or absence of nitro-toxins in *Astragalus*, (b) predict the type of nitro compound present and subsequently predict the nitro-catabolite (3-NPOH or 3-NPA), (c) predict the concentration of nitro-toxin, and (d) predict the presence or absence of nitro compounds in widely geographically separated species within the same taxonomic section. Presence or absence of nitro compounds could often be predicted within groups of sections.

A study of *Astragalus* in the Intermountain Herbarium at Utah State University (15) showed that most species in sections 40 through 47 synthesized nitro-toxins. Only *A. michauxii* (O. Kze.) F. J. Hermann of section 43 was not examined because of the unavailability of this species that grows on the Atlantic coastal plain from North Carolina to Florida. Species in sections 40 through 42 and 44 through 47 were homogeneous in synthesizing nitro-toxins at levels 2 and 3. One would predict that *A.*

michauxii, in section 43, would also synthesize nitro-toxins at level 2 or 3. Further, since nitro-toxins synthesized at that level are nearly always miserotoxin, one would predict that miserotoxin would be found in this species. An analysis of leaflets from the New York Botanical Garden and freshly collected leaves from Georgia confirmed that miserotoxin was present and synthesized at level 2 (16).

Most nitro-containing *Astragalus* synthesize nitro-toxins at levels T to 3 (13). A few species synthesize nitro-toxins at levels 4 and 5. Section *Scytocarpi* is particularly homogeneous in this respect; all species and varieties that synthesize nitro-toxins do so at levels 4 and 5.

The *Uliginosi*, comprising the widespread *A. canadensis* L. and the rare *A. oreganus* Nutt. ex T. & G., synthesize nitro-toxins in excess of 25 mg NO_2/g of plant. *Astragalus canadensis* var. *brevidens* (Gand.) Barneby has been reported as being poisonous to cattle in Oregon. *A. canadensis* is important in the chemotaxonomy of *Astragalus* because of its relationship to other members of the section in Eurasia. About eight species are known in section *Uliginosi* world-wide. Of these, sicklepod milkvetch, *A. falcatus* Lam., was introduced into Washington for evaluation as a forage plant about 1920. By the 1930's, it had escaped to become an occasional weed in several counties in southeast Washington. For the past 25 years sicklepod milkvetch has been recommended for range seeding.

Since sicklepod milkvetch and Canada milkvetch occur in the same taxonomic section, sicklepod milkvetch became suspect as a nitro-synthesizing species. Subsequent investigations showed that sicklepod milkvetch contained 60 to 80 mg NO_2/g of leaf (17). The plant was toxic to cattle and sheep. Eradication of sicklepod milkvetch is now recommended.

Leaflets of three other species from section *Uliginosi* collected in Iran, India, and China were obtained from the New York Botanical Garden. All contained large amounts of nitro compounds (18). All species of section *Uliginosi*, therefore, are likely to be poisonous, and no Eurasian species from this section should be imported under any circumstances.

A study of 400 Old World and South American *Astragalus* showed that only about 8% were nitro-containing, compared with 52% in North America. Nevertheless, the foreign species tended to be chemotaxonomically related so that many of the nitro-containing species occurred within the same taxonomic section. Sections 2, 4, 5, and 6 of the North American *Astragalus* contain nitro-bearing species. Species from these sections that occur in Eurasia also tend to be nitro-bearing.

The majority of the nitro-containing *Astragalus* synthesize nitro-toxins at levels T to 3. In all species so far examined, miserotoxin has been the only nitro-toxin present. In species that synthesize nitro-toxins at levels 4 and 5, karakin, hiptagin, and cibarian have been the only nitro-toxins. Nearly all poisonings from nitro-containing *Astragalus* have been from the miserotoxin group.

The data obtained on nitro-toxin synthesis, distribution, and chemotaxonomy have provided valuable information that should reduce livestock losses from nitro-containing species.

A list is now available of the nitro-containing *Astragalus* in North America as determined from analysis of herbarium specimens (13). To date, all species that have given positive reactions for nitro compounds in herbarium specimens have also contained nitro compounds when collected fresh in the field. From this list we have identified nitro-toxins as the poisonous agent in *Astragalus* already on record as poisoning domestic livestock: *A. canadensis* L., *A. tetrapterus* Gray, *A. emoryanus, A. atropubescens* Coult. and Fish., and *A. miser*. An introduced species, *A. cicer* L., contained no nitro compounds and was found to be non-toxic to cattle and sheep. A species can be cleared as well as condemned of being poisonous.

Chemical or biological control of poisonous *Astragalus* is not always possible; therefore, grazing practices must be modified to avoid livestock losses where these species occur. If infestations can be avoided until seed maturation, livestock losses could be significantly reduced. Carefully managing range to preserve desirable vegetation and avoiding an increase in density and spread of poisonous plants also reduces losses.

Astragalus species that synthesize miserotoxin are especially to be avoided. These species account for the majority of range poisonings from nitro-containing *Astragalus*.

The chemotaxonomic character of nitro compound synthesis in *Astragalus* is international in scope. Analyses of specimens in herbaria throughout the world would pinpoint those species that synthesize nitro compounds. Such information could be used worldwide to reduce livestock losses, prevent the importation and exportation of toxic *Astragalus*, and greatly contribute to our understanding of this complex and interesting genus.

V. REFERENCES

1. Rosenfeld, I., and Beath, O. A., "Selenium: Geobotany, Biochemistry, Toxicity, and Nutrition." Academic Press, New York, 1964.
2. Stermitz, F. R., Norris, F. A., and Williams, M. C., *J. Am. Chem. Soc.* 91, 4599 (1969).
3. Williams, M. C., Stermitz, F. R., and Thomas, R. D., *Phytochemistry* 14, 2306 (1975).
4. Williams, M. C., and James, L. F., *J. Range Manage.* 28, 260 (1975).
5. Beath, O. A., Draize, J. H., and Eppson, H. F., *Wyo. Agric. Exp. Stn. Bull.* 189 (1932).
6. Williams, M. C., Norris, F. A., and Van Kampen, K. R., *Am. J. Vet. Res.* 31, 259 (1970).

7. Williams, M. C., Van Kampen, K. R., and Norris, F. A., *Am. J. Vet. Res.* 30, 2185 (1969).
8. Williams, M. C., and Norris, F. A., *Weed Sci.* 17, 236 (1969).
9. Williams, M. C., and Binns, W., *Weeds* 15, 359 (1967).
10. Williams, M. C., *J. Range Manage.* 23, 400 (1970).
11. Cronin, E. H., and Williams, M. C., *Weeds* 12, 177 (1964).
12. Cooke, A. R., *Arch. Biochem. Biophys.* 55, 114 (1955).
13. Williams, M. C., and Barneby, R. C., *Brittonia* 29, 310 (1977).
14. Barneby, R. C., "Atlas of North American Astragalus." Mem. New York Botanical Garden 13 (1964).
15. Williams, M. C., and Parker, R., *Weed Sci.* 22, 259 (1974).
16. Williams, M. C., Yost, G. S., and Stermitz, F. R., *Phytochemistry* 16, 1438 (1977).
17. Williams, M. C., James, L. F., and Bleak, A. T., *J. Range Manage.* 29, 30 (1976).
18. Williams, M. C., and Barneby, R. C., *Brittonia* 29, 327 (1977).

CHRONIC PHALARIS POISONING OR PHALARIS STAGGERS

W. J. Hartley
The University of Sydney

I. ABSTRACT

Phalaris *poisoning or* Phalaris *staggers is a progressive neurologic disorder of sheep and cattle not uncommonly encountered in Australasia in sheep grazing pastures containing new growth of* Phalaris tuberosa. *There is macroscopic focal bluish pigmentation of the brain stem, and this is due to granular pigmentation of the cytoplasm of nerve cell bodies. There are also variable lesions of demyelination of the white matter of the cord. There is also often a bluish-grey discoloration of the dorsal root ganglia, renal medulla, and liver. Occasionally a symmetrical skeletal myopathy may be present.*

II. INTRODUCTION

Three apparently distinct entities in sheep and cattle are associated with the ingestion of new growth of *Phalaris spp.* These are peracute *Phalaris* poisoning, or sudden death syndrome, acute *Phalaris* poisoning with transient neurologic signs (1,2,3), and chronic *Phalaris* poisoning, or *Phalaris* staggers, a slowly progressive usually fatal neurologic disorder (4,5,6,7,8,9).

The peracute and acute entities have been shown experimentally (10,11) to be caused by tryptamine alkaloids sometimes present in the plant at high levels. The cause of *Phalaris* staggers has not yet been eluciated, but it is presumed to be due to a toxin in or on the *Phalaris* plant. My remarks here will be restricted to *Phalaris* staggers.

III. DISTRIBUTION

Phalaris staggers has been reported from Australia (4,5,7,12), New Zealand (6,8,9), and South America (Hartley and McFarlane, unpublished) in sheep. It has also been seen in cattle in Australia.

IV. CONDITIONS OF OCCURRENCE

Most outbreaks of *Phalaris* staggers have occurred in the late summer and early autumn in sheep grazing on *Phalaris tuberosa*, an important pasture species in dry areas. One similar outbreak has been reported in New Zealand in the spring in sheep grazing *P. arundinacea* (13). Usually outbreaks are seen following warm autumn rains preceded by a hot dry spell and occur within a few weeks of grazing on the new growth.

V. CLINICAL SIGNS

The first clinical signs noticed are incoordination, a stiff stilted gait, muscle tremors, head nodding, and hyperexcitability. As the disease progresses and particularly following stress, these signs are exacerbated and the animal may go down into lateral recumbency with convulsions. After a rest the animal will regain its feet and walk away unsteadily. Later the neurologic signs become more pronounced and the animal may become recumbent and die. Sometimes stress will cause sudden death. In some outbreaks chronic cases move about on their knees - the animals apparently being unable to straighten their forelimbs.

The morbidity and mortality range considerably between outbreaks, from 5 to over 50 per cent. In some outbreaks clinical recovery of mild cases may occur if they are moved early to other pasture, in others fresh cases can occur after removal.

VI. LESIONS

Gross lesions are seen in the nervous system and elsewhere. There consist of obvious discoloration of certain tissues due to abnormal deposition of a grey/green/blue pigment (8,9,12,13,14). In the brain this is characteristically seen as focal symmetrical pigmentation of certain areas of the brain stem. The main sites involved are in association with the following nuclei - lateral geniculate, red, trigemminal, pontine, vagus, hypoglossal, and lateral cuneate. In the cord there is often pigmentation of the ventral horns and of the dorsal root ganglia. In addition to the nervous tissue, pigmentation is commonly seen diffusely affecting the renal medulla and less commonly the liver. (Following several weeks storage of affected tissues in formalin the pigment leaches into the fixative giving it a pale blue color.)

In several cases of advanced *Phalaris* staggers a symmetrical pallor of several hind limb muscles has been observed (Hartley, unpublished).

Microscopically the pigment occurs in variable amounts throughout the brain in the cytoplasm of nerve cell bodies (9,12,13,14). It is yellow brown and granular and does not stain with either the periodic acid Schiff stain or Luxol fast blue (Hartley, unpublished). The pigment apparently accumulates in and eventually destroys the affected neurones. Additional neurologic lesions consist of mild to moderate Wallerian type degeneration of nerve fibers in the white matter of the cord (4,12,13).

Ultrastructural examination of pigmented neurones suggests

that the pigment accumulates in and then destroys mitochrondria (14,15). It may then be taken up by lysosomes (15). The pigment has very little ultrastructure, being mostly amorphous, with some granules made up of electron dense areas and others containing 'finger print' patterns (Hartley, unpublished).

VII. PREVENTION

In the early investigations of *Phalaris* staggers in sheep it was found that frequent oral dosing with cobalt sulphate effectively prevented the development of the disease (7). Subsequently it was shown that the introduction of heavy cobalt pellets into the rumen was also effective (16).

VIII. REFERENCES

1. Moore, R. M., Arnold, G. W., Hutchings, R. J., and Chapman, H. W., *Aust. J. Sci.* 24, 88 (1961).
2. Moore, R. M., and Hutchings, R. J., *Aust. J. Exp. Agric. Anim. Sci.* 7, 17 (1967).
3. Gallagher, C. H., Koch, J. H., and Hoffman, H., *Aust. Vet. J.* 43, 495 (1967).
4. McDonald, I. W., *Aust. Vet. J.* 18, 119 (1942).
5. McDonald, I. W., *Aust. Vet. J.* 22, 91 (1946).
6. LeSoeuf, H. D., *Aust. Vet. J.* 24, 12 (1948).
7. Lee, H. J., and Kuchel, R. D., *Aust. J. Agric. Res.* 4, 88 (1953).
8. Milne, J. A., *N. Z. Vet. J.* 3, 119 (1955).
9. Hartley, W. J., and Kater, J. C., *N. Z. Vet. J.* 10, 128 (1962).
10. Gallagher, C. H., Koch, J. H., Moore, R. M., and Steel, J. D., *Nature* 204, 542 (1964).
11. Gallagher, C. H., Koch, J. H., and Hoffman, H., *Aust. Vet. J.* 42, 279 (1966).
12. Hartley, W. J., and Kater, J. C., *Aust. Vet. J.* 41, 107 (1965).
13. Simpson, B. H., Jolly, R. D., and Thomas, S. H. M., *N. Z. Vet. J.* 17, 240 (1969).
14. Gallagher, C. H., Koch, J. H., and Hoffman, H., *New Sci.* 31, 412 (1966).
15. Jolly, R. D., and Hartley, W. J., *Aust. Vet. J.* 53, 1 (1977).
16. Dewey, D. W., Lee, H. J., and Marston, H. R., *Nature (London)* 181, 1367 (1958).

VII. PLANT TERATOGENS AND TOXINS AFFECTING REPRODUCTION

Chairman: LeGrande Shupe

ALKALOID TERATOGENS FROM *LUPINUS, CONIUM, VERATRUM,* AND RELATED GENERA

Richard F. Keeler
Poisonous Plant Research Laboratory, Agricultural Research Service
U.S. Department of Agriculture

I. ABSTRACT

Certain naturally occurring congenital deformities in domestic livestock are produced by quinolizidine, piperidine, and steroidal alkaloid teratogens from members of the Lupinus, Conium, *and* Veratrum *genera when plants are ingested during gestation. The considerable structural and configurational specificity among the teratogens have allowed speculations about compounds from other plants that are probably teratogens. Some of the speculations have been verified.*

II. INTRODUCTION

Until twenty-five years ago studies on poisonous plants considered the direct effects on animals ingesting the plants. Then teratology was a young science and little thought was given to the possibility that range plants could be responsible for any of the common congenital defects of livestock. But during recent years it has become evident that many common congenital malformations are caused by plants ingested by the pregnant dam during gestation. We have actively investigated a number of livestock deformities and found plants to be responsible for some of them.

In this report I will review background and describe the state of our knowledge on quinolizidine, piperidine, and steroidal alkaloidal teratogens mainly from *Lupinus, Conium,* and *Veratrum*--the effects produced, compounds responsible, speculations about other compounds probably active, and certain related matters.

III. LUPINE

Maternal ingestion of certain lupines was suspected over 20 years ago (1) to cause congenital crooked calf disease. During the last 10 years experiments have shown (2) this to be true. The disease is marked (2,3) by twisted or bowed limbs (arthrogryposis), spinal curvature (scoliosis or kyphosis), twisted neck (torticollis), cleft palate, or a combination of these deformities. Over 30% of a herd may be affected but incidence varies with the year, area, and herd (3).

The disease causes serious economic problems so ranchers have sought ways to reduce incidence or eliminate the disease. Many considered it to be an hereditary condition and changed bulls and killed affected animals but could not reduce the incidence. Others advocated that mineral supplementation would reduce incidence; but when experiments were carefully designed and implemented, little success resulted (4).

The arthrogrypotic malformation is the most commonly observed manifestation (Fig. 1). Joints are flexed and cannot be extended,

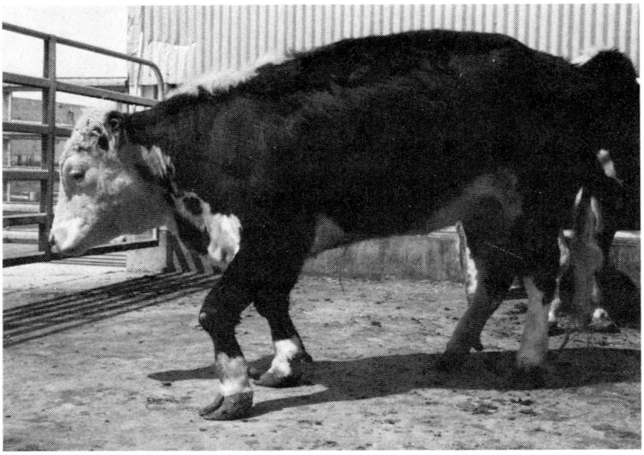

Fig. 1. *Calf with lupine-induced congenital arthrogryposis.*

even after the flexure tendons are cut. In crooked calf disease, the osseus changes are permanent and generally become worse as the calf matures and the limbs are subjected to greater load-bearing stress. The spinal curvature manifestation of the disease results from vertebral wedging or rotation of the vertebral column and, consequently, there is no spontaneous recovery.

Some 20 years ago Wagnon (1) reported that California ranchers believed that congenital deformities in calves was due to maternal ingestion of *Lupinus laxiflorus*. He said:

> "Deformed calves are most likely to be produced by cows bred in July then poisoned in late August. The incidence of congenital deformities has been highest with heifers at first calving, but has occurred with females at all ages. It has been reported that setting the breeding season ahead two months from July to May and moving cattle out of lupine areas are effective prevention procedures. Cattle apparently show no interest in this lupine until the seed pods are well formed, usually during later August. The seed pods and plant tops are extensively fed upon."

Wagnon (1) conducted feeding trials of lupine in pregnant cows but failed to produce the disease.

Our feeding trials of certain plants, including lupine and of other preparations, culminated in establishing that lupine did produce crooked calf disease. Pregnant cows fed *Lupinus sericeus* or *Lupinus caudatus* in 1964 and 1965 trials delivered calves with the disease. We established that the pregnant cows were most susceptible from the 40th to the 70th day of gestation (3). Only questionable or modest deformities resulted when the period did not include at least some of those days.

Most lupines are classed as poisonous plants because of their high content of toxic alkaloids. We considered alkaloids attractive as possible teratogens among the compound classes from the plant, and began a program to test that possibility. We had about two hundred lupine plant samples and records concerning their relationship to crooked calf disease. If an alkaloid were responsible, we speculated one might see a correlation between the presence or concentration of that alkaloid and its ability to produce crooked calf disease.

We compared by gas chromatography lupine alkaloid profiles among members of the *Lupinus* genus that produced crooked calf disease experimentally with those that did not. We compared those profiles to profiles from plants collected in areas where the disease is common and in areas where the disease is not known. There were profile similarities in all teratogenic plants not shared by non-teratogenic plants (5). Four major alkaloid peaks were generally present in profiles from teratogenic plants, but only peak 4 was invariably present in teratogenic plants and invariably absent or of low concentration in non-teratogenic ones (5). The compound of peak 4 was anagyrine based on mass, nuclear magnetic resonance, and infrared spectrometry analysis (6). Thus from an epidemiologic point of view, the teratogen was probably anagyrine.

For many years we prepared extracts and fractionated material of lupine plants and gavaged the preparations to pregnant cows in an effort to isolate and identify the teratogen. In recent years the experimental work was designed to test preparations containing the alkaloids. These experiments established (7) that alkaloid extracts from teratogenic lupines produced crooked calf disease when the extracts were gavaged to cows during the gestational period when they were susceptible. We believe that the alkaloid anagyrine is the teratogen because preparations rich in that alkaloid were teratogenic while other alkaloids present in the semipurified anagyrine preparations did not produce the disease when fed to other cows. The foregoing preparations were essentially devoid of non-alkaloidal contaminants. Consequently, both feeding trials and epidemiologic evidence ascribed the teratogenicity to anagyrine. Severity of malformations was directly related to the level of anagyrine present in the preparations gavaged.

The structures (6) of the alkaloids of peaks 1-4 are shown in Fig. 2. They bear considerable similarities. All have a carbonyl at carbon atom 2 in ring A, but anagyrine has 2 double bonds in ring A. Anagyrine is configurationally different at carbon atom 6 from lupanine and epimethoxylupanine. We conclude that either the

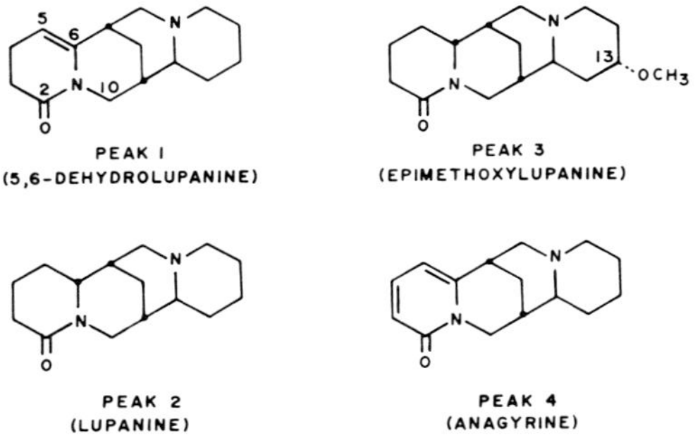

Fig. 2. *Structures of the four major quinolizidine alkaloids from teratogenic lupine.*

additional unsaturation of ring A or the configuration at carbon atom 6, or both, are important in conferring teratogenicity on the molecule.

If ring A functionality and A/B ring juncture are the essential features, then a number of other naturally occurring related quinolizidine alkaloids may also be teratogenic. They include cytisine that is devoid of ring D but otherwise identical to anagyrine, the 2 C_{13} alcohols baptifoline and (-)-epibaptifoline, the anagyrine epimer thermopsine, and rhombifoline, which is [N-(3-butenyl)-cytisine]. We are now testing some of these possibilities with plants or preparations rich in cytisine, thermopsine, and rhombifoline. We are using *Cytisus scoparius* as the source of cytisine, *Thermopsis montana* as the source of thermopsine, and an unidentified lupine from central Nevada which we believe contains rhombifoline as the source for that compound. Among lupines we have examined, *Lupinus laxiflorus* is the richest in anagyrine and we now use it as the source for anagyrine. Very few lupines contain significant amounts of anagyrine (5). Our analysis showed, however, that *L. sericeus, L. caudatus, L. laxiflorus*, and an unidentified lupine collected in Alaska do.

We believed that if plant concentration of anagyrine varied as a function of plant maturity, one might plan a grazing program to reduce incidence. Cows were principally susceptible only at a specific gestational period (40th-70th days). So to reduce incidence, one could prevent cows from grazing lupine if anagyrine content were high and cows were in the gestational period of susceptibility.

We collected *L. sericeus* and *L. caudatus* that we knew produced the disease from sites in four states. Various plant parts at various stages of plant maturity were collected during two separate yearly growing seasons. Concentrations of total and individual major alkaloids, especially anagyrine, were measured. Concentrations of all alkaloids, including anagyrine, in above ground parts were high early in growth and decreased markedly as plants matured. The concentration in mature, intact seeds was also very high (8). Thus, a pregnant cow in the 40th to 70th day gestation period is at greatest risk when grazing teratogenic lupine early in growth or during seeding. Hazard is low in early flowering and post-seeding stages of the plant.

We have followed, using ranch records and personal interviews with ranchers and public land managers, the experience on 6 ranches in Oregon, Montana, and Idaho with a history of crooked calf disease. We compiled a record of the incidence of crooked calf disease and various management programs related to the etiology of the disease.

Data collected from the ranches for lengthy periods (as many as 25 years) allowed the common conclusions that (a) incidence was highly variable from year to year, (b) variation in incidence was unrelated to various mineral supplementation programs, a commonly advocated practice, but (c) incidence was related to abundance of lupine (amount grazed), level of teratogen in the plant, and gestational stage of cows when they ingested it. Because mineral supplementation to reduce incidence of crooked calf disease is so widely practiced, we were particularly interested in the ineffectiveness of supplementation on the incidence. The supplements included in varying levels and ratios the following: Zn, Mg, Mn, Co, Fe, Cu, Na, P, Ca, I, vitamin A, vitamin E, protein, corn oil, molasses, barley, and flavoring. We believe that reports claiming that mineral supplementation programs reduced incidence of crooked calf disease can be traced to the level of teratogen ingested by the dam during the susceptible period and not to the supplements themselves.

We believe the best available strategy for reducing of the incidence of crooked calf disease lies in capitalizing on the knowledge of the stage of gestation at which cows are susceptible and variation of concentration of the teratogen in lupine as it matures. Hazard is maximum when young lupine or lupine in mature seed stage is grazed by cows whose average stage of gestation is between the 40th and 70th days. Hazard is minimum when lupine of either early flower or post-seed stage is grazed by cows whose average stage of gestation is either earlier than the 40th or later than the 70th day.

IV. *CONIUM MACULATUM*

Most crooked calf disease in western United States we have investigated was attributable to maternal ingestion of lupine plants during gestation. Some were not accounted for, and we published speculation that maternal ingestion of the plant *Conium maculatum*

(9) might be one of the causes. The speculation was based on field observations in 1971 of an outbreak of limb malformations in calves in northern Utah. The deformities were like those produced by ingestion of lupine and included limb rotation, permanent carpal or elbow joint flexure, spinal curvature or cleft palate and lip. No known teratogenic plants were found in the pastures where the deformed calves were observed, but considerable *Conium maculatum* was found. The pastures represented the principal source of feed for the cattle. They were grazed in summer months, and the harvested hay was fed to the cattle in winter months.

Edmonds, Selby, and Case (10) later reported that *Conium maculatum* might be the plant responsible for an epidemic of congenital deformities of swine in Missouri.

We speculated that if *Conium maculatum* was the teratogenic plant, one of its piperidine alkaloids might be the responsible compound. One of the alkaloids, coniine, was commercially available. Consequently, as a shortcut first trial we gavaged coniine to pregnant cows during the gestational period determined for similar deformities produced by lupine. Coniine was teratogenic. Calves with deformities like those of the field outbreak resulted.

To determine whether the plant could produce terata, pregnant cows were gavaged fresh, young plant. The plant produced congenital defects in calves when cows were gavaged during the 50th-75th day of gestation (Fig. 3). Both arthrogryposis and spinal curvature like the defects produced by the piperidine alkaloid coniine were produced.

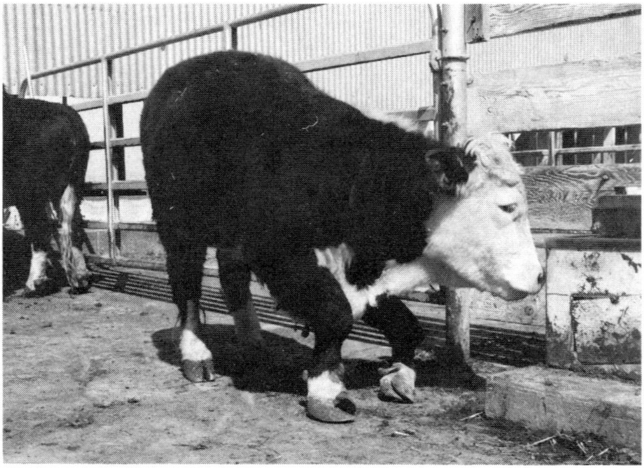

Fig. 3. *Calf with* Conium-*induced congenital arthrogryposis.*

The alkaloid coniine is 2-propylpiperidine and is similar to many piperidine compounds common to plants and therefore found in animal feed. We wondered whether they and related piperidine analogs were teratogenic.

The structures of the five principal alkaloids of *Conium maculatum* are shown in Fig. 4. We identified both coniine and

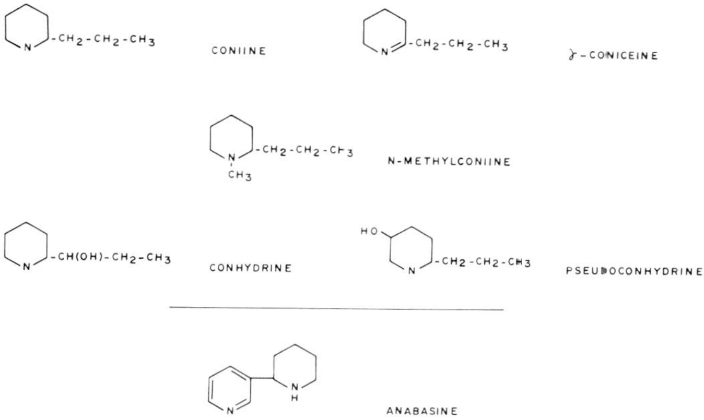

Fig. 4. *The five major piperidine alkaloids of* Conium maculatum *(top) and the tobacco alkaloid anabasine (below).*

γ-coniceine in *Conium maculatum* collections used in feeding trials (11). We also found three other piperidine alkaloids present that are probably those shown in Fig. 4. Over 98% of the total alkaloid of fresh vegetative *Conium maculatum* that was fed to cows that delivered calves with the disease was γ-coniceine. Evidently γ-coniceine and coniine are both teratogenic and introduction of a double bond in the ring between the nitrogen and the α carbon atom (i.e., producing a tertiary nitrogen) did not result in loss of activity. Whether introduction of a hydroxyl function in the ring (pseudoconhydrine) or in the side chain (conhydrine), or attaching a methyl group to the nitrogen (n-methylconiine) will change teratogenicity remains to be determined.

Returning to the question of whether other piperidines of more remote structure would be teratogenic, we wondered what changes could be introduced in the side chain and ring of coniine and still retain teratogenicity? We tested a number of piperidines to examine this question. The compounds were gavaged to cows at levels that were either as high as they appeared to be able to tolerate on the basis of clinical toxicity signs (no lower than 4gm/day) or were at a level of 10 gm/day. Levels were nearly three to seven times higher than teratogenic levels of coniine. None caused congenital deformities. Both chain length and degree of unsaturation in the ring appear to affect teratogenicity. Neither 2-ethylpiperidine nor 2-methylpiperidine was teratogenic, even though coniine (2-propylpiperidine) was. Coniine with a fully saturated ring and possibly γ-coniceine with one double bond were active, but the fully unsaturated ring coniine analog conyrine was not active. It is not likely that naturally occurring pyridines or piperidines that have a fully unsaturated ring, or chain length shorter than propyl will present a teratogenic hazard to grazing cows. But some may be teratogenic because the side chain α to the nitrogen is at least propyl in length and the ring is saturated. One of these is a naturally occurring piperidine alkaloid in tobacco that we speculate may be teratogenic and account for the effects of tobacco on pigs reported by Crowe and others.

Crowe (12) described 1967-69 observations of malformed pigs from five Kentucky farms. During gestation sows that delivered 64 litters with 300 skeletally deformed pigs had access to tobacco stalks during gestation. Crowe speculated that the tobacco produced the deformities. Subsequently, Menges and coworkers (13) reported a tobacco-related epidemic of congenital deformities of swine. Twisting of the fore or hind limbs and dorsal flexure of hind limb digits were common. In 1974 Crowe and Swerczek (14) produced congenital deformities in pigs by feeding tobacco leaf filtrates to pregnant sows. They did not determine whether the alkaloids were responsible, but they reported that negative results suggested that nicotine was probably not the active principle. Feeding trials in sheep and cows with free-base nicotine at our laboratory in cooperation with Dr. Crowe produced no congenital defects.

Among known tobacco alkaloids, the compound we believe might be teratogenic would be anabasine (Fig. 4). Unlike most tobacco alkaloids, it does have an α-substituted piperidine ring and the α group (pyridine) is certainly larger than propyl. We are conducting feeding trials now to test the hypothesis that anabasine is a teratogen.

V. *VERATRUM*

Until some 20 years ago epidemics of cyclopia and related cephalic congenital deformities in sheep had been reported in Idaho. Hundreds of lambs were afflicted with this disease each year.

Cephalic deviations included single or double globe cyclopia (Fig. 5). Animals had a shortened upper jaw and protruding lower jaw, sometimes with a peculiar skin-covered proboscis above the single eye. The double globe cyclopia gave rise to the common name for the condition, monkey face lambs, called that by ranchers. Animals mildly affected had normal eyes and a shortening of the upper jaw or cebocephaly. We established by feeding trials that *Veratrum californicum* caused the condition when pregnant ewes ingested plant on the 14th day of gestation (15). We wanted to isolate and characterize the active principle, and our early studies suggested that it was likely an alkaloid. We gavaged a variety of veratrum alkaloids to pregnant sheep to test their teratogenicity. Of these alkaloids, the compounds jervine and two others, to which we gave the names cyclopamine and cycloposine, were active and

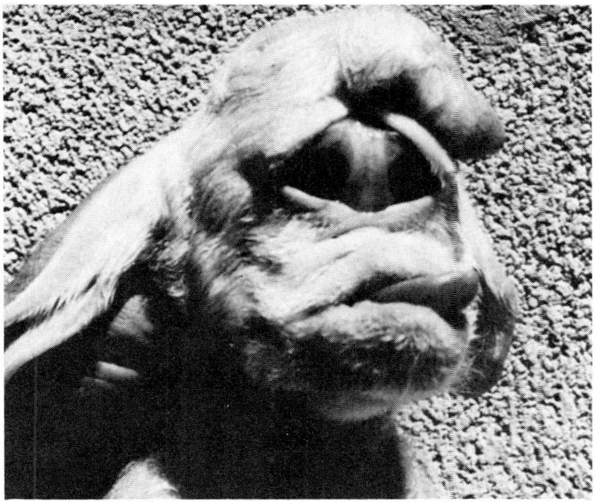

Fig. 5. Veratrum *induced congenital cyclopia*

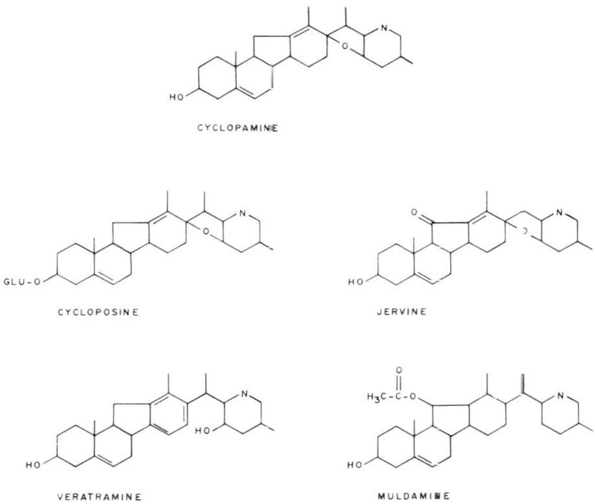

Fig. 6. *Five steroidal alkaloids from* Veratrum californicum.

produced deformities typical of natural cases (16). Other compounds were inactive.

By IR, NMR and MS analysis we showed (Fig. 6) that cyclopamine was 11-deoxojervine (17) and that cycloposine was 3-glucosylcyclopamine (18), the glucoside of cyclopamine. Thus the three active compounds were structurally similar to one another. We believe that cyclopamine is the teratogen of importance naturally because of its high concentration in the plant.

Accompanying these three active compounds (Fig. 6) are two of high concentration that did not produce cyclopia in sheep--veratramine and muldamine. Cyclopamine and veratramine differ slightly because the latter is devoid of the oxide bridge forming ring E, has a hydroxyl function on ring F, and a greater degree of unsaturation in ring D. Cyclopamine and muldamine (19) differ because the latter has no ether bridge, no unsaturation in ring D, and an O-acetate function on carbon 11. We believed that the fused furanopiperidine ring E/F arrangement of cyclopamine was essential for the activity (20) because compounds containing that ring arrangement were active in feeding trials in sheep, but others were not.

A variety of animals are susceptible to cyclopamine and a single oral dose of 20 mg on day 7 of gestation in hamsters (21) produces nearly 100% incidence in litters; 50% or more individuals are malformed. Consequently, we are using hamsters in many of our present studies.

The teratogenic steroidal alkaloids from veratrum are structurally related to a number of solanum alkaloids, and because of this we have had an interest for many years in the possible teratogenicity of solanum alkaloids (20). J. H. Renwick (22) hypothesized in 1972 that maternal blighted potato consumption by humans was responsible for congenital spina bifida and anencephaly. If a teratogen is present in potatoes as Renwick alleged, we wondered could it be of the steroidal alkaloid class? Potato alkaloids have not been isolated that have a fused furanopiperidine ring E/F arrangement like the veratrum teratogens. Spirosolane solanum alkaloids, by contrast, have a furan ring E that is fused to the steroidal end of the molecule, but in some cases, that feature confers upon them a configuration similar to the *Veratrum* teratogens. We compared (23) the teratogenicity of the configurationally similar solanum alkaloid solasodine and the teratogenic veratrum alkaloids cyclopamine and jervine in our hamster assay. Solasodine is not a potato alkaloid, but its glycosides are common in egg plant. Tomatidine, with a piperidine ring configuration opposite that of solasodine and closely related to Δ^5-tomatid-3β-ol the aglycone of certain potato glycosides, was also tested. All were compared with diosgenin, the non-nitrogen containing analog of solasodine.

Solasodine (Fig. 7) was teratogenic. Malformations were produced in hamster fetuses when dams were gavaged 1200 to 1600 mg/kg. Cyclopamine was active at doses 1/10 that amount. Tomatidine and diosgenin were not teratogenic at doses double that of solasodine. The nitrogen of the piperidine ring was essential because diosgenin, nitrogen-free but otherwise identical to solasodine, was not active. Importance of piperidine ring configuration is suggested by lack of activity of tomatidine; the nitrogen of the piperidine ring is β rather than α to the plane of the steroid as in solasodine and cyclopamine. Preliminary experiments showed that saturation at the 5-6 bond as in tomatidine (the only difference aside from the piperidine ring difference between tomatidine

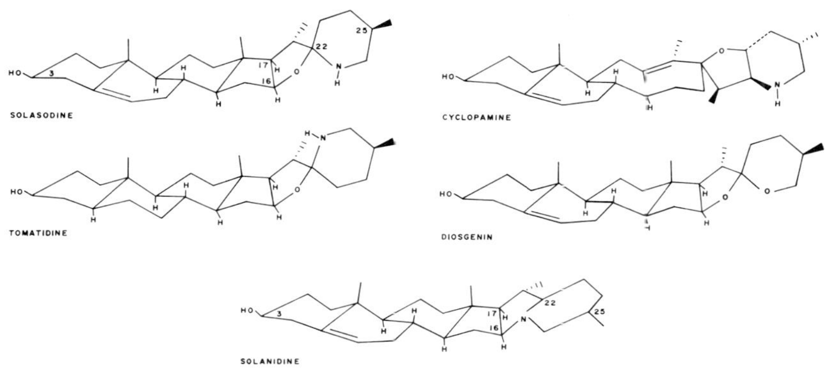

Fig. 7. *Projection drawings of solasodine, cyclopamine, tomatidine, diosgenin, and solanine.*

and solasodine) was not required for the molecule to be teratogenic. Solasodine, devoid of the C-nor-D-homo ring system, has a spirofuran/piperidine ring juncture rather than a fused furanopiperidine spiro to the steroid as in cyclopamine and is less basic. The nitrogen of solasodine, like cyclopamine, is on the α side of the molecule, but in cyclopamine it extends much more markedly in the α direction. Spirosolane alkaloids based on tomatidine or Δ^5-tomatidine-3β-ol and present in some potatoes and other food sources with nitrogen on the β side of the molecule are unlikely to be active in hamsters (22). Compounds based on solasodine or any as yet unidentified spirosolanes with α-piperidine ring configuration might be active. Activity would probably be governed by basicity and the extent of α projection of a rigidly positioned nitrogen.

The steroidal solanum alkaloid aglycone most common to potatoes is solanidine (Fig. 7). Unlike solasodine it has no furan ring E and has no spiro connection between rings D and E or rings E and F. The piperidine ring is not at right angles to the steroid system and so the tertiary nitrogen in solanidine is not α to the plane of the steroid. But solanidine is basic, the nitrogen is positioned with respect to overall molecular shape in about the right place, and it has a free electron pair on the tertiary nitrogen (24). My colleague Dr. D. Brown will present structure-activity evidence suggesting that steroidal alkaloids with a tertiary nitrogen whose lone electron pair is constrained toward the α side of the molecule are active (24).

We tested a variety of potato preparations and found that high alkaloid potato sprouts, but not tubers or peel from tubers, from certain potato cultivars are teratogenic in a particularly susceptible hamster strain (25). Spina bifida, exencephally, microphthalmia and encephalocele were the defects observed. We have not identified the teratogen. Either a spirosolane with a rigidly positioned basic nitrogen projecting in the α direction or a solanidane whose lone electron pair on the nitrogen projected in the α direction seem to be good possibilities.

VI. REFERENCES

1. Wagnon, K. A., *J. Range Manage.* 13, 87 (1960).
2. Shupe, J. L., Binns, W., James, L. F., and Keeler, R. F., *J. Am. Vet. Med. Assoc.* 151, 198 (1967).
3. Shupe, J. L., Binns, W., James, L. F., and Keeler, R. F., *Zuchthygiene* 2, 145 (1967).
4. Keeler, R. F., James, L. F., Shupe, J. L., and Van Kampen, K. R., *J. Range Manage.* 30, 97 (1977).
5. Keeler, R. F., *Teratology* 7, 23 (1973).
6. Keeler, R. F., *Teratology* 7, 31 (1973).
7. Keeler, R. F., *J. Toxicol. Environ. Health* 1, 887 (1976).
8. Keeler, R. F., Cronin, E. H., and Shupe, J. L., *J. Toxicol. Environ. Health* 1, 899 (1976).
9. Keeler, R. F., *Am. Coll. Vet. Toxicol.* (abstract) Detroit Meeting (1971).
10. Edmonds, L. D., Selby, L. A., and Case, A. A., *J. Am. Vet. Med. Assoc.* 160, 1319 (1972).
11. Keeler, R. F., *Clin. Toxicol.* 7, 195 (1974).
12. Crowe, M. W., *Mod. Vet. Pract.* 69, 54 (1969).
13. Menges, R. W., Selby, L. A., Marienfield, C. J., Aue, W. A., and Greer, D. L., *Environ. Res.* 3, 285 (1969).
14. Crowe, M. W., and Swerczek, T. W., *Am. J. Vet. Res.* 35, 1071 (1974).
15. Binns, W., Shupe, J. L., Keeler, R. F., and James, L. F., *J. Am. Vet. Med. Assoc.* 147, 839 (1965).
16. Keeler, R. F., and Binns, W., *Teratology* 1, 5 (1968).
17. Keeler, R. F., *Phytochemistry* 8, 223 (1969).
18. Keeler, R. F., *Steroids* 13, 579 (1969).
19. Keeler, R. F., *Steroids* 18, 741 (1971).
20. Keeler, R. F., *Teratology* 3, 169 (1970).
21. Keeler, R. F., *Proc. Soc. Exp. Biol. Med.* 149, 302 (1975).
22. Renwick, J. H., *Br. J. Prev. Soc. Med.* 26, 67 (1972).
23. Keeler, R. F., Young, S., and Brown, D., *Res. Commun. Chem. Pathol. Pharmacol.* 13, 723 (1976).
24. Brown, D., and Keeler, R. F., *Am. Chem. Soc.* Abst. MEDI 86 (1977).
25. Keeler, R. F., Brown, D., Douglas, D. R., Stallknecht, G. F., and Young S., *Bull. Environ. Contam. and Toxicol.* 15, 522 (1976).

STRUCTURE-ACTIVITY RELATION OF STEROIDAL AMINE TERATOGENS

Dennis Brown
Poisonous Plant Research Laboratory, Agricultural Research Service
U.S. Department of Agriculture

I. ABSTRACT

Derivatives of jervine and 11-deoxojervine were tested for teratogenic activity in the hamster. Interpretation of the results is based on structure-activity correlation. Testing derivatives altered in the steroid ring suggests that these compounds act as steroid hormone blocking agents. Testing muldamines suggests a rigid side chain portion of the steroid may not be required for potency. The substituent effects for N-substituted jervines were, in order of decreasing activity, $CHO \simeq H \simeq CH_3 > n\text{-}Bu > Ac > (CH_3)_2I^-$. *This order of activity indicates that an imino function was not required for substantial teratogenicity, and that a negative center such as an amide carbonyl may function similar to the amino group in teratogens. Two compounds having the (22S, 25R)-solanidanine configuration were about similarly active to jervine. Compounds of (22S, 25S) and (22R, 25S) configurations produced increases in resorption without a significant incidence of malformations. The conformation of nitrogen in these compounds was used to explain the differences in activity. Findings support the hypothesis that highly teratogenic compounds present a negatively charged center accessible to the steroid* α *face.*

II. INTRODUCTION

Research in our laboratory on nitrogen-containing steroids causing birth defects has comprised roughly two areas: (a) structural modification of teratogenic steroid alkaloids in an effort to determine the features essential to their activity, and (b) a search for new substances with a potential for activity based on those features. Corollary to these studies would be defining features causing the activity of known teratogens. Our laboratory is especially suited to such a study because of its experience in the study of the alkaloids of a western range plant, false hellebore (*Veratrum californicum*), which causes birth defects (1). Until recently, the teratogens jervine (1, Fig. 1) and 11-deoxojervine (2, Fig. 1) were the only steroid alkaloids[1]

[1]Cycloposine, the 3-glycoside of 11-deoxojervine, might be regarded as a third teratogen but aside from possible dose/response differences the activity of the glycoside stems directly from the activity of the aglycone.

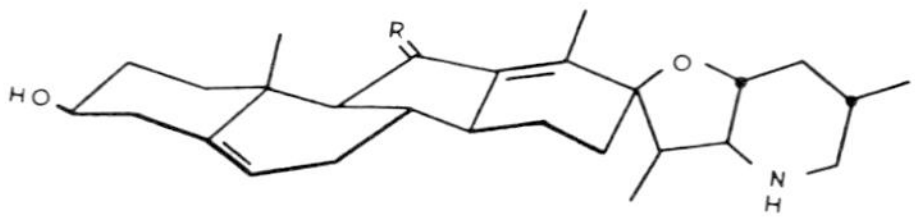

1. Jervine R = O
2. 11-Deoxojervine R = H_2

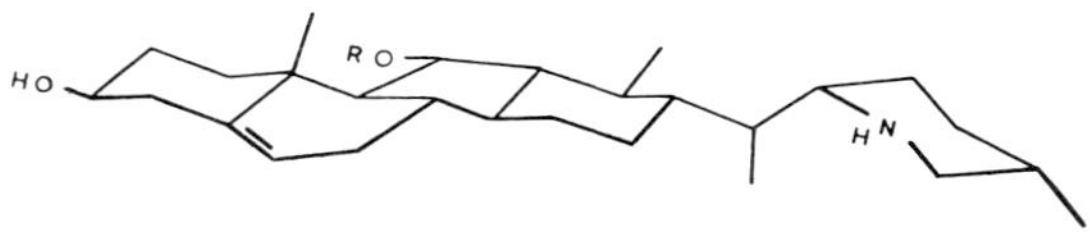

3. Muldamine R = Ac
4. Deacetylmuldamine R = H

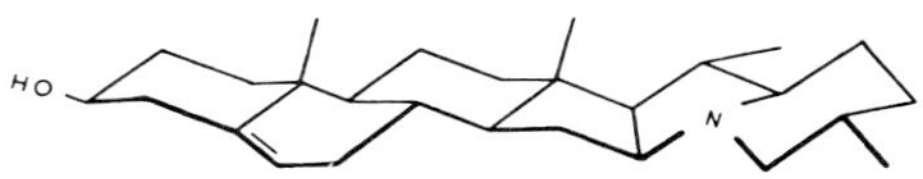

5. Solanidine ; (22R, 25S)-5-solanidenine-3β-ol

Fig. 1. *Steroid alkaloid structures.*

known to have such activity. A third compound, first reported teratogenic in rats (2) differs from the former two in that it is the first known active alkaloid that has a conventional steroid ring system. Keeler has already referred to this substance, solasodine with particular emphasis on our interpretation of the difference between its activity and that of tomatidine, a structurally similar compound (3).

Teratogenic amines were synthesized primarily from jervine, which also became our primary reference for activity. These derivatives can be arranged into roughly 2 groups, each intended to test several structure-activity questions.

Derivatives of the jervine ring system were synthesized to determine which, if any, functional groups present in the steroid system might be relevant to teratogenicity. We were also looking for (a) changes in polarity or conformation induced by altering functional groups, (b) evidence of the importance of a rigid furanopiperidine group in the side chain, and (c) support for the suggestion (4) that the alkaloid functions as a steroid hormone blocking agent.[2]

Derivatives of the jervine imino group were also directed at several questions. Most important of these perhaps was the question of whether a tertiary amino group can cause birth defects; and, if so, to what extent steric requirements limit that activity. Finally, we wanted to know to what extent a basic nitrogen, as was suggested by alkaloid studies (3), influences activity.

Structurally, jervine (1, Fig. 1) is a C-27 triterpene and thus is classed as a steroid. Beyond this, its resemblance to a steroid hormone is not great because of the several functional groups present plus a unique ring system referred to as "C-nor-D-homo." The molecule, nevertheless, has a general shape similar to conventional steroids, and for that reason (i.e. similar yet different) was of considerable interest to the drug industry for potential therapeutic use (5). One possible change induced by the atypical ring system is added flexibility of the side chain caused partly by the 6-member D ring and the C-12 double-bond. The side chain is itself quite rigid, of course, but the spiro bridge head (C-17) can swing perpendicular to the steroid plane. This freedom makes it impossible to predict with certainty the position of the imino function relative to the steroid plane which might be important to the activity of the system.

One point on chemical reactivity may also be worth pointing out. Both of the active parent alkaloids (1,2, Fig. 1) are sensitive to acid conditions. 11-Deoxojervine is particularly sensitive and reacts (resulting in an open C17-C23 oxygen bridge) to produce materials that are much less active, if not completely non-teratogenic. Ring opening of 11-deoxojervine was reported to occur (6) at acid concentration equivalent to that of a non-ruminant stomach. The property also poses a synthetic problem because 11-deoxojervine is also quite sensitive to hydrogenolysis of the oxygen bridge. So much so that a reduction of the 12,13 bond, to our knowledge, has not been reported for that compound. Fortunately the same bond in jervine itself can be reduced in good yield. Most compounds used in this study have been reported (7) and were selected because they provided products easily purified in high yield.

III. STRUCTURE-ACTIVITY RELATIONS

A. The Jervine Ring System

Table I shows results of gavaging Syrian Golden hamsters a number of derivatives of jervine and 11-deoxojervine. The table

[2]It is implicit in this argument that if the alkaloid functions as a hormone blocking agent, the atypical C-nor-D-homo jervine ring system has no direct bearing on activity.

TABLE 1

Data on Hamsters Fed Jervine Derivatives and Reference Compounds

Compound	Dams fed	Dose[1] mg/kg	Over-dose death	Resorbed %	Abnormal Off-spring %	Abnormal Litters %	Mean litter size
12β, 13 α-dihydro-jervine	5	150	4	46	100	100	6.00
	6	113	1	18	63	60	9.20
	5	75	1	9	26	25	8.75
12β,13α-dihydro-jervine-11α-ol	17	150	3	2	2	21	13.2
	4	113	0	25	0	0	11.0
12β,13α-dihydro-jervine-11β-ol	22	150	3	10	0	0	11.4
3-*O*-acetyljervine	3	225	0	77	100	100	3.00
	11	150	0	35	30	50	6.27
11-deoxojervine-4-en-3-one	17	150	7	52	52	83	5.60
	7	75	0	15	59	86	10.1
	7	38	0	19	70	83	7.71
	9	15	0	3	0	0	6.44
muldamine	11	600	2	38	16	29	6.44
	4	300	0	5	0	0	9.75
deacetylmuldamine	10	150	0	16	2	20	9.90
N-methyljervine	18	170	0	6	10	44	9.61
N-butyl-3-O-acetyl 12β,13α-dihydro-jervine	10	170	1	10	4	22	11.8
N-methyljervine methiodide	5	225	0	27	0	0	7.00
N-formyljervine	9	170	6	9	10	33	9.67
	11	85	1	14	13	60	10.4
N-acetyljervine	27	170	0	7	1	4	10.8
N,*O*-diacetyljervine	9	170	0	1	1	11	12.2
jervine	25	127	1	7.3	16	36	5.08
water	--	42	--	3.9	0.25	2.4	9.45

[1]Compound suspended in 4 ml water gavaged by stomach tube on day 7 or 8 of gestation.

also gives data on the alkaloids muldamine, included to show the relationship between that compound and its deacylated derivative, and jervine as a reference active compound. The upper portion of table 1 includes compounds testing structure-activity relations of the steroid system.

As shown, the most active teratogen in this study was 11-deoxojervine-4-en-3-one. Functional group changes as reduction of the 12,13 bond of jervine or acylation of the 3-hydroxyl group have an apparently negligible effect on activity. 11-Hydroxyl derivatives of jervine have greatly reduced but differing activities, and both muldamine (3, Fig. 1) and its deacetyl derivative (4, Fig. 1) apparently can cause birth defects.

These data tend to support the suggestion (4) that jervine alkaloids function as hormone blocking agents in the developing embryo as follows. The >2X increase in activity of 11-deoxojervine-4-en-3-one over that of jervine is not surprising because the former compound is structurally more hormone like.[3] Thus a more hormone like structure would be expected to reach and interact to a greater degree with hormone receptors. The several theories of steroid hormone/receptor interaction have been reviewed (8). Less hydrophobic substituents in the steroid nucleus would be expected to reduce activity. Thus, the relative activities of the 11-hydroxy derivatives also support a hormone blocking action. Further note that the 11α-ol retains a reduced activity relative to jervine and the 11β-ol gave no abnormal offspring at a similar dose level. These results also support the theory of hormone blocking action because the hydrophobic interaction of steroid and receptor is thought to be β to the C ring (8). A β hydroxyl group in the C ring would repel such an interaction or promote non-specific interactions that prevented the agent reaching an active site.

Previous observations suggested that a rigid furanopiperidine side chain was required for activity. Preliminary observations of the compounds not having an ether bridge, muldamine and deacetylmuldamine, indicate this may not be the case. Both of these compounds show reduced activity and coupled with the reduced activity of 11-hydroxy jervines it is possible that the C-11 function is more relevant to reduced activity of the muldamines than side chain rotation. Clearly, additional work is needed to determine which of these parameters is more important to activity. Present indications suggest that free rotation of the side chain does not reduce activity to as large an extent as the 11-hydroxyl.

One additional comment on the position of the side chain may also be in order. The 12β,13α-dihydrojervine is about as teratogenic as the parent molecule (jervine). As mentioned previously, jervine has a relatively flexible D ring, but flexibility is greatly impaired by hydrogenation of the 12,13-bond. Conformation of the derivative is undoubtedly a chair form of the D ring C-18 being equatorial and the C-17,20 bond also equatorial. The net effect is to fix the position of the side chain and incline it toward the steroid β face. The retention of substantial activity by the dihydro derivative indicates that such a position of the

---

[3]All steroid hormones except the estrogens have the 4-en-3-on A,B ring system.

side chain (and, thus, the imino group) does not substantially alter activity. Either minor alterations of the nitrogen position created by hydrogenation are unimportant to activity or the parent molecule (jervine) can accomodate such a position of its nitrogen.

B. *N*-Substituted Jervines

Table 1 also gives the results of hamster bioassay of teratogenic *N*-substituted jervines. The order of decreasing activity of these compounds was: CHO $\simeq$ H $\simeq$ CH_3 >n-Bu> Ac > $(CH_3)_2I^-$. This general trend suggests that a basic nitrogen, or better yet a negative center of some sort, is required for teratogenicity. Note that the methiodide salt of jervine does not have significant activity.

Data on alkyl jervines suggest that *N*-alkylation reduces activity in proportion to the steric bulk of the substituent. Thus *N*-methyljervine, about equal in activity to jervine, has only the relatively small methyl substituent. The reduced activity of the n-butyl derivative clearly must relate to the bulky four-carbon chain. These findings also support a contention that the nitrogen function is vital to the teratogenicity of the molecule.

The activity of acyl jervines is not so easily explained since these compounds are not particularly basic. A normal amide has a pK_a of 1-2, and protonation is generally thought to be at the carbonyl oxygen rather than at nitrogen. Nevertheless *N*-formyljervine is quite active and the acetyl derivatives have a persistent low activity that is difficult to ignore. We originally thought the activity of the formyl compound resulted from the following. The compound was absorbed into tissues more efficiently where its gradual decomposition to the parent compound released the active species. This conclusion was supported by the apparent increase in toxicity of the derivative relative to jervine. If it reached tissues more efficiently, it became also a more efficient toxin.

These data can, however, be interpreted in another way. The amide function's carbonyl oxygen could act as the center of negative charge for interaction with the active site, rather than nitrogen as proposed for amines. Amide nitrogen adds considerable double-bond character to the C-N bond, thus increasing the strength of the negative charge on the carbonyl oxygen. This effect is strong enough that rotationally non-equivalent (i.e. *cis*, *trans*) forms of a steroid alkaloid *N*-formyl derivative have been isolated (9). A similar effect is seen in the nmr spectrum of *N*-formyljervine for which two peaks are observed (δ 8.04 and 8.50) for the formyl-derivative proton. This indicates that two rotationally non-equivalent forms contribute to the signal, although the rapidity of the exchange rate prevents their isolation. Thus it is reasonable to assume that, rather than a nitrogen interaction with the active site, the negative center is in the case of acyljervines oxygen, functioning in a similar capacity.

Clearly the area should be investigated more fully to resolve this question.

C. Teratogenic Solanidanines

We have found a highly teratogenic steroid in a group of epimers related to the alkaloid solanidine (5, Fig. 1). Four possible C-22, C-25 epimeric compounds having this structure are known and easily synthesized from other alkaloids (10).

Until very recently all the steroid alkaloids having the indolizidine skeleton were known to have a (22*R*, 25*S*) configuration (11) with a *trans* conformation of the E,F ring juncture. They occur in both *Veratrum* and *Solanum* species and are perhaps best known as constituents of foods such as potatoes. A conformational analysis of the four possible epimers mentioned previously is given in Table II. The analysis predicts that all four epimers exist as *trans* conformers; the 22*R* epimers have nitrogen non-bonding electrons α and 22*S* epimers nitrogen non-bonding electrons β. Note particularly that this analysis predicts two compounds with axial methyl groups in the F ring.

TABLE II

Conformational Analysis of the Solanidanine E and F Rings

Configuration C-22	Configuration C-25	Nitrogen nonbonding electrons	C-27[1] methyl group	E,F ring juncture	Steric problems[2]
R	*S*	β	e	*trans*	None
		α	e	*cis*	C-18,C-23
R	*R*	β	a(β)	*trans*	None
		α	e	*cis*	C-18, C-26
S	*S*	β	e	*cis*	C-21, C-24
		α	a(α)	*trans*	None
S	*R*	β	e	*cis*	None
		α	e	*trans*	None

[1]Assume the F ring to be a chair form.
[2]Carbons indicated have hydrogens apparently falling within Van der Waals radii.

Figure 2 shows the result of inverting the (22*R*, 25*S*) and (22*S*, 25*R*) epimers. Conformational analysis is a simple means of predicting the most favorable configuration of a molecule that can exist in more than one shape. In the present case we are most concerned with the most favorable position of the nitrogen non-bonding electrons since these appear important to teratogenic activity. Table II, as well as Fig. 2, support the prediction

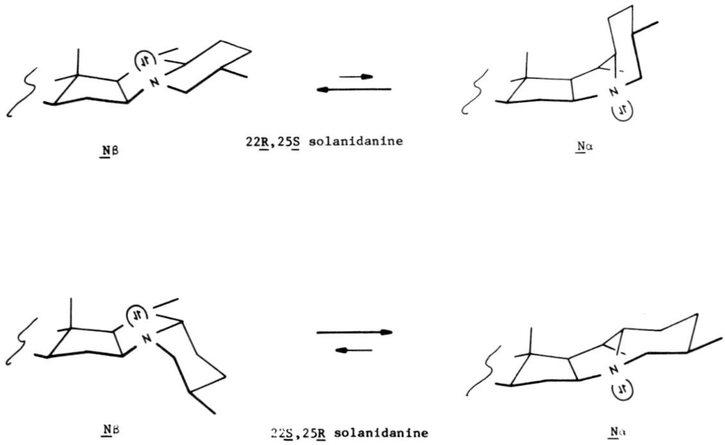

Fig. 2. *E,F ring conformations of solanidanines.*

that one of these compounds will present an unhindered nitrogen electron pair on the α face of the steroid, the (22*S*, 25*R*) epimer, and it can be predicted that it may be teratogenic on these grounds. Other epimers would be predicted less active but may retain some minor activity because the compounds can exist in an active conformation via inversion of the nitrogen. Recently the first steroid indolizidine with (22*S*, 25*R*) configuration was reported (12). The nmr evidence presented indicated that this compound was conformationally *trans* having its nitrogen non-bonding electrons α, in keeping with the conclusions reached above on conformational grounds.

The results of gavaging hamsters with epimeric solanidanines are given in Table III. The abnormalities produced were essentially similar to those in offspring of dams fed the control alkaloid, jervine (Table 1). This similarity suggests that the two types of compounds cause birth defects by fundamentally similar mechanisms. The abnormalities noted were, in order of decreasing frequency: harelip, cleft palate or both; cranial bleb; exencephaly; micropthalmia; and cebocephalia. Jervine differed only in producing an increased rate of cebocephalia.

The dramatic difference in activity of solanidanine epimers substantially supports the suggestion that an unhindered basic nigrogen, accessible to the α steroid face, is required for activity. Both of the compounds in Table III that have (22*S*, 25*R*)

TABLE III

Data from Hamsters Fed Solanidanines

Compound	Dams fed	Dose[1] mg/kg	Over-dose death	Resorbed %	Abnormal Offspring %	Abnormal Litter %	Mean litter size
(22*R*, 25*S*)-5α-solanidanine-3β-ol	4	343	1	67	0	0	2.67
	3	187	0	19	0	0	8.67
	4	150	0	20	3	25	8.25
(22*S*, 25*S*)-5α-solanidanine-3β-ol	3	312	0	67	0	0	3.33
	3	165	1	3	0	0	14.5
(22*S*, 25*R*)-5α-solanidanine-3β-ol	3	177	1	100	0	0	0.00
	4	81	0	19	25	50	8.00
	4	42	0	0	0	0	9.00
(22*S*, 25*R*)-5-solanidanine	4	184	0	75	75	100	4.00
	4	88	0	25	42	50	6.00
	4	39	0	0	5	25	9.75

[1]Compound suspended in 4 ml water gavaged by stomach tube on day 7 or 8 of gestation.

configuration are potent teratogens in the hamster. Their conformation suggests they are Nα and thus they agree with the proposed structural activity requirement. Because these compounds are conventional steroids, their activity also indicates that the activity of jervines is not exclusively a property of the C-nor-D-homo ring system, and that structural differences not interfering with the nitrogen/receptor interaction are relatively unimportant. Note the large differences in shape of the side-chain portions of the active molecules. In our limited trial the (22*S*, 25*S*) epimer did not produce birth defects (Table III), although fetal resorption rate significantly increased. On conformational grounds, this compound was predicted to place an axial methyl on the α face of the steroid plane. Fortuitously this methyl group is located in such a way to produce a strong 1,3-diaxial interaction with the nitrogen non-bonding electrons, thus sterically preventing the necessary interaction between nitrogen and receptor.

Also in the limited trial, the (22*R*, 25*S*) epimer was not found active. This compound also gave an increased resorption rate and in this case a single abnormal fetus was produced. It is tempting to postulate that the molecule shows a low-grade ability to interact with a receptor based on the conformational properties of nitrogen. The naturally occurring compound of this series, solanidine (5, Fig. 1), has for some time been suspected of causing birth defects (13). The structure-activity relationship shown by the present work suggests that this risk may indeed exist.

IV. REFERENCES

1. Keeler, R. F., *Lloydia* 38, 56 (1975).
2. Seifulla, Kh. I., and Ryzhova, K. E., *Mater. Vses. Kone Issled, Lek. Rast. Perspekt. Ikh Ispol'z. Proizvod. Lek. Prep.* 1970, 160 (1972). *Chem. Abstr.* 83, 22383t (1975).
3. Keeler, R. F., Young, S., and Brown, D., *Res. Commun. Chem. Pathol. Pharmacol.* 13, 723 (1976).
4. Keeler, R. F., *Teratology* 3, 169 (1970).
5. Wintersteiner, O., and Moore, M., *Tetrahedron* 21, 779 (1965).
6. Keeler, R. F., *Teratology* 3, 175 (1970).
7. Masmune, T., Sato, N., Kobayashi, K., Yamazaki, I., and Mori, Y., *Tetrahedron* 23, 1591 (1967).
8. Vida, J. A., "Androgens and Anabolic Agents: Chemistry and Pharmacology." Academic Press, New York, 1969.
9. Toldy, L., and Radics, L., *Tetrahedron Lett.* 4753 (1966).
10. Sata, Y., and Ikekawa, N., *J. Org. Chem.* 26, 1945 (1961).
11. Schreiber, K., *Pure Appl. Chem.* 21, 131 (1970).
12. Pakrashi, S. C., Chakravarty, A. K., and Ali, E., *Tetrahedron Lett.* 7, 645 (1977).
13. Kúc, J., *in* "Recent Advances in Phytochemistry," (V. C. Runeckles, Ed.), Vol. 9, p. 139. Academic Press, New York, 1975.

TOBACCO - A CAUSE OF CONGENITAL ARTHROGRYPOSIS

M. Ward Crowe
University of Kentucky

I. ABSTRACT

Epidemics of arthrogryposis in newborn pigs have occurred on more than 15 Kentucky farms since 1967. More than 1,100 newborn pigs have been malformed. In all instances the pregnant sows giving birth to these pigs had access to tobacco stalks and in several instances were observed consuming the stalks. Trials designed to reproduce the anomalies observed were conducted involving the feeding of tobacco and related chemicals to pregnant sows. From sows fed aqueous tobacco filtrate, 9.5% of the newborn pigs were deformed. From those fed tobacco stalks and related chemicals, 10.7% of the newborn pigs also showed arthrogryposis identical to the anomalies seen in field occurrences. Based on collected data, tobacco is teratogenic when consumed by swine under proper conditions.

II. INTRODUCTION

Arthrogryposis, a persistent flexure or contracture of a joint, has been described and reviewed on several occasions in humans, foals, calves, lambs, and pigs (3,4,5,9). Although the clinical and pathological findings are well documented and a large amount of historical data has been amassed, the etiology is not well defined. This report describes congenital limb deformities in newborn baby pigs born following the ingestion of tobacco by the dam during pregnancy.

III. BACKGROUND

Tobacco (*Nicotiana tabacum*) is a plant native to the North American continent. It was being cultivated by the American Indians before white men arrived, and it was one of the first plants from the American continent to be taken to Europe for cultivation. Since earliest times the toxic effect of nicotine, the principal alkaloid in tobacco, has been recognized. Prior to the development of more effective drugs, nicotine sulfate was the most effective taeniacide known. It was also a commonly used insecticide, particularly for certain poultry ectoparasites.

Except for an occasional occurrence, animal poisoning from the ingestion of tobacco is not common. In areas where tobacco is commercially produced, there is an abundance of other vegetation which is generally far more palatable to livestock.

In the spring of 1967, outbreaks of deformed newborn pigs occurred on two widely separated farms in central Kentucky (1,2). In that year, from a total of 251 pigs farrowed by 25 sows on two farms, 144 pigs were deformed at birth, showing varying degrees of arthrogryposis. In the fall and winter of that same year, an epidemic of congenital limb deformities occurred in Missouri in which 14 sows farrowed 149 pigs with 59 being abnormal (3).

In the seven years following the initial occurrence of this problem, epidemics were reported on 13 more Kentucky farms. These were investigated and histories were obtained. On the 15 Kentucky farms which experienced epidemics of arthrogryposis, there were 246 sows which farrowed 2,358 pigs with 1,148 being abnormal.

Field investigations of all outbreaks were conducted as their occurrence was learned. All of the epidemics investigated occurred during the months of January, February, and March, except on one farm on which deformed pigs were farrowed in both March and July (Table 1). In any given episode the number of deformed pigs usually approximated 50% of pigs from sows bred and managed on the same approximate schedule. The occurrence of affected pigs in litters ranged from none up to every pig in the litter being abnormal.

TABLE 1

Prevalence of Congenital Arthrogryposis Among Pigs Farrowed on 15 Farms in Kentucky, 1967-1974 (2)

Farm No.	Date of occurrence (month, year)	No. sows bred	Pigs farrowed No. normal	No. deformed	Total
1	1/67	20	107	96	203
2	3/67	5	0	48	48
3	2/68	25	116	120	236
4	2/68	9	6	72	78
5	2/69	15	101	24	125
6	3/70	10	54	50	104
7	2/70	9	52	21	73
8	2/70	15	60	75	135
	7/70	17	91	62	153
9	1/71	18	87	75	162
10	1/72	11	49	63	112
11	3/72	29	130	129	259
12	3/72	4	23	9	32
13	2/70	8	28	60	88
	2/71	12	88	41	129
	2/72	24	106	150	256
14[1]	3/73	12	94	42	136
15[1]	2/74	3	18	11	29
Total		246	1210	1148	2358

[1]Not included in cited reference.

The afflicted pigs were usually normal in size. Frequently parturition was prolonged by several hours and many pigs died from neonatal asphyxiation. Those deformed pigs born alive were unable to walk and usually died within a few hours from apparent hypoglycemia. None of the sows giving birth to deformed pigs showed any signs of clinical illness, either during gestation or following parturition. There was no evidence of diminished fertility and no apparent increase in the occurrence of abortions.

All of these epidemics in 1967 and others occurring later were found to be related to the ingestion by the pregnant sows of tobacco stalks.

IV. RELATIONSHIP TO TOBACCO

Pregnant sows had access to freshly discarded tobacco stalks on every farm where outbreaks of deformed pigs occurred. In many instances the sows had been observed eating the stalks. The handling and disposal of tobacco stalks as grown in Kentucky is conducive to the exposure of pregnant sows to them. In the early fall, the mature tobacco plant is cut off near the ground and hung in barns to cure. In November and December, the leaves are removed from the stalks by hand and the intact stalks are discarded. Since the stalks are high in nitrogen content they are frequently scattered over pasture fields to increase soil fertility. These stalks are approximately 1.5 meters long and about 5 centimeters at the base. The outside is quite woody, but the center contains a succulent pith with a consistency resembling celery. Frequently sows were observed shredding the stalks and consuming this pith. They did not consume the woody exterior. The data collected indicated that the insult to the fetuses occurred between days 10 and 35 of pregnancy.

The first known occurrence of this problem was in 1967. On every farm where the problem had occurred, the tobacco stalks to which the sows had access were very large with an abundance of succulent pith to attract the animals. The large stalks were the result of increased fertilization and irrigation. The average yield of tobacco per acre in Kentucky was 1,625 lb per acre in 1960, 2,160 lb in 1965, and 2,710 lb in 1970. More than 1,200 components of tobacco have been identified, 117 of which are alkaloids (6). As fertilization of tobacco was increased the concentration of nitrogen, total alkaloids and nitrate increased in cured tobacco leaf and presumably in the stalks (7).

There is no evidence that there is an heredity cause of these anomalies. Usually the involved animals in field outbreaks were of mixed breed with no genetic relationship. In most instances the sows had two or more normal litters sired by the same boars either before or after the affected litters were born.

The seasonal occurrence of the outbreaks indicated the presence of a teratogenic agent. As indicated above, with one exception, the malformed pigs were farrowed between January and March.

This correlated with the 114-day gestation period of the sow and the time of exposure to tobacco stalks in late fall and early winter. We have observed that when winter freezing causes deterioration of the stalk pith, sows are no longer attracted to the stalks.

V. PATHOLOGIC FINDINGS

The anomaly involves primarily the appendicular skeleton, but the spinal column and mandible have also been affected.

No abnormalities have been found in any anatomic structures other than the skeletal system except for changes in muscles and tendons related to the limb deviations. Arthrogryposis is the outstanding feature of the syndrome with any or all of the limbs involved.

The anomaly may be manifest in a number of ways (Figures 1 and 2). The limbs may be fixed in extension or extreme flexion either anteriorly or posteriorly. In some instances there is medial deviation so that the front limbs are fixed in a "self-hugging" position. Clubbing of one or more feet is the mildest form of the anomaly. In a few instances an acute kyphosis has been observed as well as occasional brachygnathia. Cleft palate, hydrocephalus, cyclopia, and other cranial anomalies have not been observed in any instance.

Maceration and examination of the limbs showed that affected bones were thickened, curved, or twisted along the long axis and sometimes shortened. There appeared to be a malalignment of joints resulting in inability of affected pigs to flex or extend limbs.

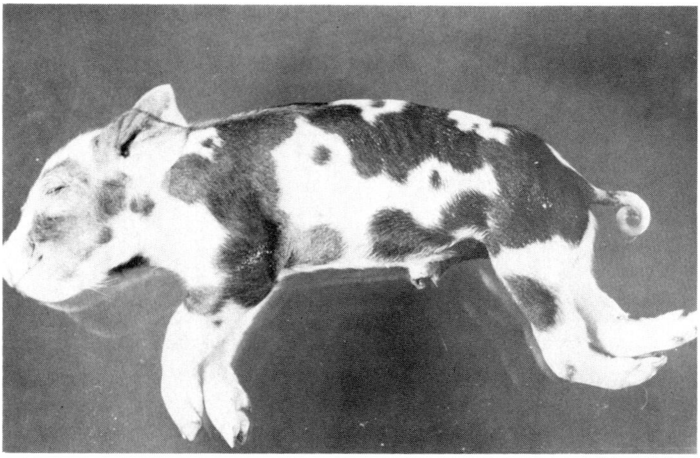

Fig. 1. *Newborn pig with arthrogryposis.*

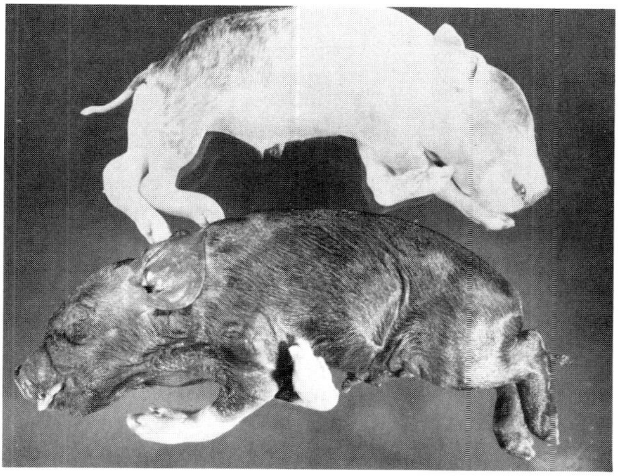

Fig. 2. *Littermates with arthrogryposis.*

VI. MATERIALS AND METHODS

Experiments involving the feeding of tobacco leaves, stalks, juice squeezed from stalks and chemicals commonly applied to tobacco were conducted. Breeding stock of known genetic origin owned by the Kentucky Agricultural Experiment Station was used with no previous occurrence of anomalies such as those described. All sows used in the trials had farrowed at least once with no deformed pigs having been born. In all experiments a balanced ration meeting the National Research Council recommendations for pregnant sows was fed to both the principle and control sows.

VII. EXPERIMENT I (TABLE 2)

Aqueous tobacco leaf filtrate was prepared from high yield burley tobacco grown on the Kentucky Agricultural Experiment Station farm. This tobacco had purposely been produced with no chemicals applied other than fertilizer to the soil. Dried tobacco leaf was finely ground in a blender with sufficient distilled water to make a slurry. This was filtered, the filtrate then added to more leaf with the process repeated until the nicotine level could not be increased. A concentration of approximately 0.50% nicotine could be attained. Freshly prepared filtrate was added to the individual ration of each sow once each day in an amount to attain the desired dosage level.

A number of commercial insecticide preparations all of which contain approximately the same ingredients are used on tobacco.

One such preparation which had been used on tobacco produced on an affected farm was selected for this trial. It contained the following active ingredients: dichlorodiphenyldichloroethane (TDE) 23.3%, dichlorodiphenyltrichloroethane (DDT) 11.6%, and dieldrin[1] 2.2%. This was added in a concentrated form directly to the sow's feed (2 ml. once daily).

Maleic hydrazide is a plant growth retardant which is sprayed on almost all tobacco produced in Kentucky. It acts to prevent "suckering" of the tobacco plant as it reaches maturity. A commercial preparation of maleic hydrazide containing diethanolamine salt of 6-hydroxy-3(2H)-pyridazinone (58%) was placed on the feed of the sows (2 ml. once a day).

A total of 12 sows (9 principals and 3 controls) were confined on a concrete floor throughout gestation. Three of the principals received aqueous leaf extract at a low level (16 mg/kg), three at a high level (32 mg/kg), and three at a low level (16 mg/kg) plus 2 ml. insecticide and 2 ml. maleic hydrazide once each day.

TABLE 2

Arthrogryposis in Pigs from Sows Fed Aqueous Leaf Extract Filtrate with or without Added Maleic Hydrazide and Insecticide (Experiment I) (8)

Sow No. (body wt/kg at start of experiment	Items added to rations (dosage per day)	Gestational period (days) for feeding additives	No. of offspring	
			Normal	Affected
5162 (96.3)	Leaf extract	10th to 48th	4	3
4033 (90.0)	(16 mg/kg)	10th to 47th	9	--
5171 (87.7)		10th to 45th	8	--
5083 (95.9)	Leaf extract	10th to 45th	12	--
5065 (88.6)	(32 mg/kg)		11	--
5073 (94.0)			5	6
5176 (92.2)	Leaf extract (16		9	--
4032 (96.8)	mg/kg) plus 2 ml			
5303 (89.0)	maleic hydrazide and 2 ml mixed insecticide	10th to 45th	10	--

VIII. RESULTS OF EXPERIMENT I

Congenital arthrogryposis was induced in pigs from two sows receiving the aqueous filtrate (Table 2). One sow receiving filtrate with a nicotine level of 16 mg/kg gave birth to four normal pigs and three which were deformed. Another sow, receiving 32 mg/kg, had five normal pigs and six which were deformed. No other

[1]Chlorinated hydrocarbon insecticides are now illegal for use on tobacco.

deformed pigs were found in those farrowed by sows used in this experiment. At no time did any sows exhibit signs of clinical illness or toxicosis.

IX. EXPERIMENT II (TABLE 3)

Twenty sows were used in this trial. A principal group of 15 sows were placed in a bluegrass sod lot and five in an adjacent bluegrass sod lot. Freshly stripped tobacco stalks collected from a farm which had experienced outbreaks of deformed pigs the previous three consecutive years were placed before the principal group as they were consumed *ad libitum*. To insure that all principal sows received tobacco stalk material, the following procedure was followed. Tobacco stalks were passed through a steel drum press, and the juice which had a nicotine content of approximately 0.12% was added to the ration of the principal group at a dosage of 0.47 L/sow/day.

TABLE 3

Arthrogryposis in Pigs from Sows Fed Tobacco Stalks and Juice (Experiment II) (8)

Sow No.	Experimental Procedure: Items fed (dosage per day)	Experimental Procedure: Gestational period (days for feeding stalks and juice)	No. of offspring: Normal	No. of offspring: Affected
1022	Tobacco stalks *ad libitum* plus 0.4 L of stalk juice	11th to 52nd	11	3
1083		Breeding day to 21st	12	--
1225		Breeding day to 21st	18	--
1898		4th to 45th	7	3
3061		10th to 44th	12	--
4462		1st to 35th	7	--
4521		26th to 34th	15	--
5061		11th to 52nd	9	4
5082		7th to 47th	12	--
5152		Breeding day to 29th	8	--
5153		5th to 45th	10	--
5162		7th to 48th	2	4
5165		Breeding day to 25th	8	--
5541		12th to 53rd	8	1
6232		15th to 49th	7	--
5054	None (controls)	---	12	--
6202		---	10	--
6233		---	7	--
5083		---	10	--
404		---	13	--

X. RESULTS OF EXPERIMENT II

Of the 161 pigs farrowed, 15 (10.7%) presented lesions of arthrogryposis (Table 3). All 15 of the deformed pigs were from five litters which contained a total of 52 pigs (Fig. 3); thus, 29% of the offspring in these litters were deformed. None of these sows presented clinical signs of toxicosis during the trial.

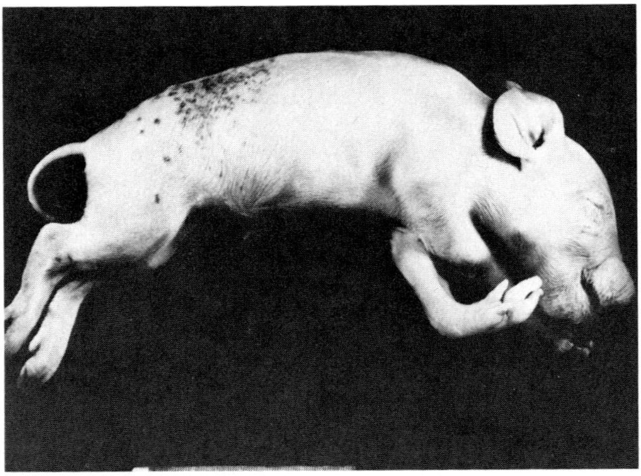

Fig. 3. *Congenital arthrogryposis in a pig from a sow (No. 5162, Experiment II) given tobacco stalks and stalk juice.*

XI. DISCUSSION

Tobacco is teratogenic when ingested by pregnant sows under certain conditions. Arthrogryposis occurring in newborn baby pigs from sows experimentally fed tobacco leaf and tobacco stalks was identical to arthrogryposis observed in more than 1200 newborn pigs farrowed in 15 separate outbreaks when sows had access to tobacco stalks.

The specific agent in tobacco responsible for these malformations is unknown. We have conducted a number of trials with specific compounds in which no deformed pigs were born. Some sows were given up to 0.3 gm nicotine, others 1 cc 40% nicotine sulfate, and others nicotine sulfate (1cc) plus mixed insecticide (2 cc) and maleic hydrazide (30 cc) between days 10 and 50 of gestation, all with no evidence of toxicity and no deformed pigs born. On the basis of these experiments, we believe that the teratogenic agent is not nicotine or any of the chemicals commonly applied to tobacco.

Several possibilities exist to account for the occurrence of this disease in the past decade. On every farm where the problem has occurred, the tobacco stalks to which the sows were exposed were from very high yield crops. It may be simply that only by exposure to very large stalks can a given sow obtain enough pith for a teratogenic effect to be manifest.

To gain a high yield, heavy fertilization practices are carried out. This may have changed the plant composition so that adequate amounts of a teratogen became present, or perhaps a change has occurred in cultured tobacco to render the stalk material more palatable to swine.

A phenomenon observed by several farmers, which we also noted, was that some sows seem to become habituated to consuming the tobacco material while others reject it. The use of swine to further understand human habituation to tobacco should be considered.

XII. ACKNOWLEDGMENTS

This investigation (No. 77-4-102) was carried out in connection with a project of the Kentucky Agricultural Experiment Station, supported by a grant from the University of Kentucky Tobacco and Health Institute, and is published with the approval of the Director of the Station.

XIII. REFERENCES

1. Crowe, M. W., *Mod. Vet. Pract.* 50, 54 (1969).
2. Crowe, M. W., and Pike, H. T., *J. Am. Vet. Med. Assoc.* 162, 453-455 (1973).
3. Menges, R. W., Selby, L. A., Marienfeld, C. J., Aue, W. A., and Greer, D. L., *Environ. Res.* 3, 285-302 (1970).
4. Leipold, H. W., Cales, W. F., Radostits, O. M., and Howell, W. E., *Am. J. Vet. Res.* 31, 1367-1374 (1970).
5. Huston, S. R., Saperstein, G., Leipold, H. W., *J. Eq. Med. Surg.* 1, 146-161 (1977).
6. Stedman, R. L., *Chem. Rev.* 68, 153-307 (1968).
7. Atkinson, W. O., Ragland, J. L., Sims, J. L., and Bloomfield, B. J., *Tobacco* 169, 21-24 (1969).
8. Crowe, M. W., Swerczek, T. W., *Am. J. Vet. Res.* 35, 1071-1073 (1974).
9. Warkany, J., "Congenital Malformations," Year Book Medical Publishers, Inc., Chicago, Illinois, 1971.

GENETIC DEFECTS AND THEIR SIMILARITIES TO BIRTH DEFECTS CAUSED BY PLANTS

H. W. Leipold
Kansas State University

I. ABSTRACT

Congenital defects are abnormalities of structure or function present at birth. Congenital defects in animals and human beings have provoked man's curiosity and fears for centuries; they now are an integral part of disease among man and animals. Though infrequent, congenital defects are important economically and biomedically. Causes of congenital defects in livestock are frequently unknown. Many environmental agents cause congenital defects in laboratory animals; however, few specific environmental agents have been identified as causing congenital defects in domestic animals. Congenital defects may be caused by genetic factors mostly by homozygosity of simple autosomal recessive genes. Congenital defects such as osteopetrosis, syndactyly, tibial hemimelia, arthrogryposis and internal hydrocephalus are used here to discuss defects in domestic animals.

II. INTRODUCTION

Many congenital defects have been identified in various species of animals throughout the world. Many more undoubtedly exist, awaiting classification and identification of their etiology. This paper discusses the nature and causes of congenital defects and genetic factors involved in their pathogenesis.

III. NATURE OF CONGENITAL DEFECTS

Congenital defects are defined as abnormalities of structure or function present at birth (1). This definition excludes causes. The term congenital is frequently considered synonymous with hereditary; however, that idea is no longer tenable, because not all congenital defects have hereditary causes. The definition also excludes structural and functional variants commonly identified by animal breeders as undesirable. Furthermore, the distinction between abnormalities and normal variants is not always obvious. In addition, many defects are present at birth but are not identifiable. Many congenital defects occur as single isolated defect of body structure or function. Others occur as syndromes consisting of several structural defects or combining structural and functional defects. Recognizing syndromes is very important in diagnosing and preventing congenital defects.

All body structures and functions are susceptible to congenital defects. Frequency of affliction of various parts vary by species, breed, sex, age of parents, geographic location, level of nutrition, and other factors (1). However, the most commonly encountered defects in all species involve those afflicting the central nervous, muscular, and skeletal systems (1-6).

It is difficult to arrive at a suitable classification system for congenital defects. Three principal systems are in use, etiologic classification, classification based on affected embryonic tissue, and classification on the basis of the principally involved body system (1).

IV. FREQUENCY OF CONGENITAL DEFECTS

The frequency of congenital defects varies by species of animal (3-8). Because congenital defects are caused by hereditary and environmental factors and their interactions, the frequency of individual defects, or defects of each body system, and the number of defects vary among breeds, among geographical areas, and among years. Frequencies are not easily obtained, as many defects are identified only on necropsy. Some go unnoticed, others are not reported for economic or other reasons, some are seen too rarely as to be accurately counted, and frequent reporting may reflect high interest of observers rather than high incidence of defects (1).

In 5,258 births reported from Kansas A. I. herds in 1954-1955, 2.1 calves (40% stillborn) in every 1,000 had serious congenital defects (9). In 4,980 births reported from Ohio herds surveyed in 1957 to 1960, 36 calves in every 1,000 had a congenital defect (10). In New Zealand the incidence of defects reported by farmers in 1957 and 1960 ranged from 3.5/1,000 in 1957 to 2.4/1,000 in 1960 (11). In English dairy herds, perinatal mortality was 4.9% with 6.8% of the dead being abnormal (12). A comprehensive study of 1,000 deformed and stillborn neonatal calves in Germany included 532 stillbirths. Eighty-four percent of the stillborn had signs only of neonatal asphyxia, 6.9% were congenitally malformed; the remaining 9.1% showed evidence of infection. The 468 malformed calves born alive died within 3 months, 2.8% had congenital malformations that caused death within 3 days and 5.1% had nonlethal malformations and died of some other cause (13). Data from 2 Angus and Hereford range herds involving 6,409 calvings during 10 years showed 4.4% stillbirths. Abnormal calves totaled 28% of the stillbirths or 1% of all calves born (3). Thus, the overall incidence of congenital malformations among calves ranged from 1/500 to 3/100, with 40-50% of the affected calves born dead and only a small fraction of the defects not externally visible. Collecting all congenitally defective calves in the German State of Hesse for nine years beginning in 1961 showed that 2,293 calves or 0.25 percent of the calf crop were defective (15). The Milk

Marketing Board of England classified 2,081 calf abnormalities as: skeletal, 56.2%; soft tissues of head, thorax, and abdomen, 27.5%; skin, hair, and muscle, 8.9%; reproductive tissue, 5.9%; and mammary gland, 1.5% (11). A total of 6,455 animals with congenital defects were among 137,717 patients in veterinary college clinics in the United States and Canada (16). A systematic collection of congenitally defective newborn calves in Kansas documented 1,275 congenital defects. Each defect was classified according to body system primarily involved: skeletal 37.3%; special senses 18.6%; muscular system 14.9%; and central nervous system 12.1% (3).

Lethal congenital defects in sheep have been estimated to be responsible for 1% of dead lambs necropsied (17). Workers in Eastern Australia reported an estimated incidence of 0.2 to 0.3% lethal defects in lambs (18). In Western Australia, the incidence of congenital defects was estimated to be 0.5 to 0.6% of lambs born (19). In the United States, the incidence was 1.4% during the first two weeks of life (20). A study of 36 birth defects in Rambouillet sheep over 15 years included higher incidence of crooked limbs, jaw anomalies, notched scrotum, and fleece color anomalies (21). Common congenital defects of lambs in a survey of 602 flock owners were, in order of frequency: bowed forelegs, micrognathia, hermaphroditism, cryptorchidism, hypospadias, proganthia, atresia ani, microtia, entropion, torticollis, polythelia, agnathia, and arthrogryposis (22). The body systems involved were: musculo-skeletal, 55.5%; digestive, 12.7%; cardiovascular, 9.7%; urogenital, 7.1%; central nervous system, 6.0%; special senses, 3.5%; integument, 3.2%; and endocrine, 1.5% (23). Although the incidence of any defect in a flock may be low and of minor importance, the cummulative effect of many may be economically significant (19).

Among a total of 6,669 dead pigs born in 2,936 litters in selected sow herds in Denmark, 410 neonatal pigs had congenital defects (24). The incidence ranges from 0.6 to 2.4 percent with a mean of 1.4 percent. The three most common congenital defects were those affecting skeletal, cardiac, and intestinal structures (24).

V. RESULTS OF CONGENITAL DEFECTS

Although economic losses due to congenital defects are less than losses due to diseases caused by nutritional or infectious agents, congenital defects may cause considerable economic loss to individual livestock owners. In addition, congenital defects due to genetic causes are particularly important because they may be repeated generation after generation. The study of congenital defects is complex and involves identification of etiologic factors before control measures are attempted. Collectively, congenital defects may comprise a small percentage of losses encountered at birth. Although such losses have been accepted as unavoidable, they are actually of considerable economic importance. Genetic problems may spread insidiously until they are economically disastrous and difficult to control. Many breed associations of livestock and pet animals have programs to control undesirable genetic traits including genetic defects. Congenital defects may be significant as a differential diagnosis, may cause obstetrical problems, and they are important as biomedical models of similar disease processes in man.

VI. CAUSES OF CONGENITAL DEFECTS

Congenital defects first seen at birth, result from disruptive events at one or more stages in the complex sequence of events of blastocyst formation and embryonic and fetal development. If such a disruptive event is not immediately lethal, it may be followed by normal development. Often that is not possible and the embryo or fetus dies and is aborted or resorbed. The result at birth serves as the diagnostic entity and it is difficult to trace the earlier events and identify causes. In general, environmentally-caused defects do not follow familial but seasonal patterns. Patterns or known stressful conditions may be linked to disease in dams.

Genetic and environmental factors may interact to manifest disease. The syndactyly gene in cattle causes fusion or non-division of functional digits; syndactylous cattle are extremely sensitive to high ambient environmental temperature and may die of hyperthermia (25). As yet little understood, complex interplay between genetic and environmental factors slowly gains in importance. Another example of such interaction between environment and genotype is photosensitivity in Southdown sheep (26). Environmental factors are becoming increasingly important as a major cause of congenital defects in livestock. Environmental factors identified in sheep include bluetongue virus, bovine virus diarrhea virus, drugs, trace elements, irradiation, plant teratogens, and others (19).

Crooked calf disease in Utah has been linked to pregnant cows eating lupine (*L. sericeus* and *L. caudatus*) during days 40-70 of gestation (27). Other plants incriminated or suspected of causing deformities in calves are *Senecio*, *Indigofera spicata*, Cycadales, *Blighia*, Loco plants, Papaveraceae, *Colchicum*, *Vinca*, and Tobacco and related plants. A long list of other plants may cause abortion and may be teratogenic (28). Recently, anagyrine was identified as the alkaloid causing crooked calf disease (29).

Viruses have been identified as teratogens in domestic animals (30). Cerebellar hypoplasia in calves is caused by prenatal infection with Bovine Diarrhea Virus (BVD) (31). Hydranencephaly may be caused by prenatal infection of Bluetongue Virus (32). Recently, the arthrogryposis-hydranencephaly syndrome was shown to be caused by prenatal Akabane virus infection (33).

Hereditary defects are defined as pathological or pathophysiological results that are determined by mutant genes or chromosomal anomalies. Chromosomal anomalies have been demonstrated in all domestic animals; however, their full role in the pathogenesis of congenital defects in domestic animals is yet to be determined (34).

Identifying genetic causes is difficult but several procedures are available. A congenitally defective offspring serves as a diagnostic entity and all genetic procedures rest on the basic assumption that genetic diseases run in families.

Hereditary congenital defects occur in typical intergenerational patterns and intragenerational familial frequencies that require enumeration of normal and abnormal offspring and identification of their familial relationships. Conformation of the genetic nature and pattern of a congenital defect should, or can be, obtained by test matings (35). Biochemical tests may be developed to detect genetic deficiencies. Such tests would be useful in selecting breeding animals, but most defects cannot yet be identified by biochemical methods (7).

VII. DIAGNOSIS OF INHERITED DEFECTS

There are only a few recent guides to the genetic diagnosis of congenital defects in domestic animals (1,34-39). Genetic analysis is based on the rule that genetic diseases run in families or that closely related animals have a greater chance of receiving the same copy of mutant and normal genes than less closely related animals do. Genetic diseases may be caused by a pair of mutant genes, by a single mutant gene, or by polygenic inheritance, and expression of genetic defects may be subject to genetic modification or may be modified by environmental causes. Genetic traits may fail to appear in the phenotype when genetic hypothesis indicates they should and thus leave incomplete penetrance.

Some diseases involve two alleles at a single locus. The simple autosomal recessive pattern requires two phenotypes of animals--normal or defective, and three genotypes (homozygote normal, heterozygote, and homozygote abnormal). However, among normal animals there are a few that can transmit the disease. Although two defective parents produce only defective calves, most defective animals do not reproduce; hence, most defective animals are born to normal parents. Each normal parent that produces a defective offspring transmits one of the two abnormal genes necessary to produce a defective animal. But most normal animals cannot transmit the disease. Mating normal homozygotes to other normal homozygotes, or even mating to heterozygotes, produce only normal animals.

When normal animals that have produced a defective offspring are mated repeatedly, 25% of their offspring will be defective and 75% will be phenotypically normal. Two of every three normal offspring from such parents are heterozygous for the abnormal gene and they will transmit it to their offspring. Thus recessive defects are "carried" in a breed generation after generation by normal animals heterozygous for the trait. The defects are exposed only when such animals are mated to others like themselves and produce a defective offspring.

Other simple inheritance patterns include dominance, incomplete dominance, and overdominance. Dominance is just the reverse of recessive. The phenotypically normal animals breed true, but the defective animals produce both normal and abnormal offspring. Diseases with dominant inheritance pattern are easily recognized because animals affected with a dominant disease produce one defective offspring in every two when mated with normal animals. The dominant defect does not skip generations as defects from simple recessive inheritance often do.

Incomplete dominance is characterized by three phenotypes--normal, slightly abnormal, and severely abnormal. The normal and severely abnormal animals breed true. Matings of slightly abnormal animals, produce 1/4 normals, 1/2 slightly abnormals, and 1/4 severely abnormals.

Overdominance is like incomplete dominance, three phenotypes are recognized--normal, superior, and abnormal. The normal and abnormal animals breed true. Superior animals mated together produce 1/4 normal, 1/2 superior, and 1/4 defective offspring.

A few reports describe diseases linked with sex (35). Streaked hairlessness is a sex-linked, incomplete dominant trait (40). Hypotrichosis associated with anodontia in Maine-Anjou cattle is a sex-linked recessive trait (40). Congenital defects may also be inherited in a polygenic manner, e.g., with many genes involved (1,37,38).

In summary, diagnosis of genetically caused congenital defects is based on the rule that genetic diseases run in families. Genes with visible or identifiable disease effects reveal typical intergenerational patterns and intragenerational segregation frequencies characteristic of certain modes of inheritance. Modes of inheritance can be analyzed according to number of phenotypes, genotypes, alleles, and loci involved. Irregularities in the phenotypic expression of the trait may result from variable expressivity of the trait and incomplete penetrance. Confirmation of the genetic nature and pattern of a congenital defect should, or can be, obtained by test matings (35).

VIII. SELECTED GENETIC DEFECTS OF CURRENT INTEREST

A. Congenital Osteopetrosis

The skeletal system accounts for one-third of all congenital defects encountered in calves, piglets, and foals which involve either the entire skeletal system or regional areas such as facial, cranial, axial and appendicular areas (1,3,42). Congenital osteopetrosis is a generalized osseous defect characterized by deposition of bone, not counterbalanced by bone absorption as has been described in foals, puppies, and calves. The most frequently involved breed of cattle is Angus. Affected Angus calves are stillborn between 250 to 260 days of gestation and the only external signs are small size and brachygnathia inferior. Their long bones are fragile and fracture easily under moderate lateral pressure. Longitudinally bones and radiographs show dense bones within bone appearance and bone marrow cavities are lacking (Fig. 1). The cerebral hemispheres of the brain are rectangular and flattened and the cerebellum is compressed. Histologic examination discloses bone in the shaft area consisting of chondroosseous tissue similar to that of early fetal stages of ossification. A preliminary breeding trial indicates osteopetrosis in Angus calves results from homozygosity of a simple autosomal recessive gene (43,44).

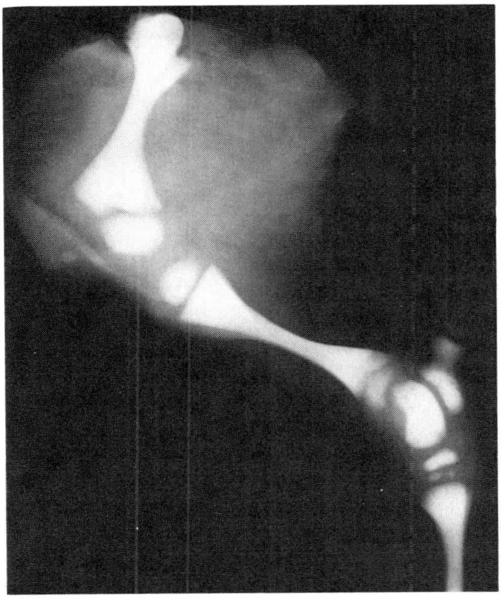

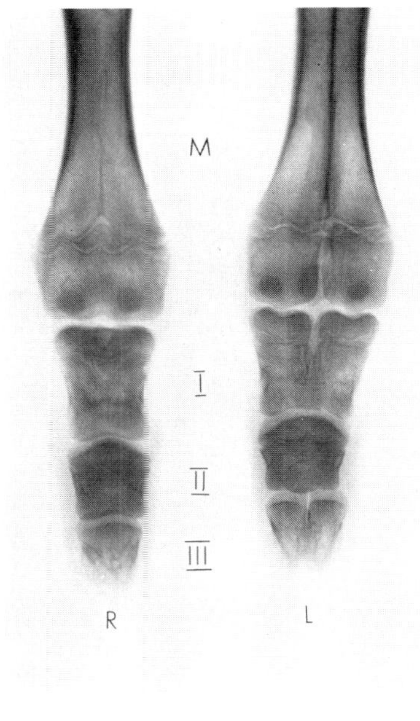

Fig. 1 (left). *Radiograph of hereditary osteopetrosis in an Angus calf. Notice lack of differentiation between bone marrow and cortex of bone. The bone is uniformly dense.*

Fig. 2 (right). *Radiograph of front legs of Holstein calf affected with hereditary syndactyly. Notice difference in synosteosis between right (R) and left (L) front leg, and changes in metacarpals (M) phalanges I, II, and III.*

B. Syndactyly

Syndactyly, defined as fusion or non-division of functional digits, occurs in cats, dogs, pigs, sheep, and cattle (4-6,42). Syndactyly, the most common single, regional skeletal defect of cattle in the United States, provides many insights into the pathogenesis of a genetic defect in cattle. It is inherited in Holstein-Friesians as a simple autosomal recessive trait with incomplete penetrance and various degrees of expressivity. Some Holstein-Friesian cattle escape their genotype syndactyly by having normal hooves; however, they will breed true if bred to a syndactylous cow or bull. Most genetically syndactylous Holstein-Friesian cattle have phenotypic expressions of the syndactylous genes. The right front foot is most frequently involved, followed in order of frequency by the left front, right rear, and left rear foot. The osteologic changes are predictable in expressivity and parallel the external pattern of right-left and front-rear gradients (Fig. 2). The synosteosis pattern of the phalanges and the number of proximal sesamoid bones are useful in the diagnosis of hereditary bovine syndactyly of Holstein-Friesian cattle. The second phalanges most frequently have horizontal synosteosis, followed by the third, and then the first. The number of proximal sesamoid bones varies from four to two with more advanced degrees of syndactyly. In addition, bovine hereditary syndactyly is a syndrome consisting of a structural defect associated with a functional defect hyperthermia, which is triggered by high environmental temperatures.

Other breeds of cattle in the United States, in foreign countries, and breeds of cattle currently being imported to the United States have similar osteologic and external changes of syndactyly, indicating the possibility of being allelic in nature in various breeds of cattle. Other structural types of syndactyly may also exist (42,45).

C. Tibial Hemimelia in Galloway Cattle

Another regional skeletal defect of hereditary nature is tibial hemimelia in Galloway cattle (46,47). It is inherited as a simple autosomal recessive trait. The defect is a syndrome consisting of changes involving the cranium, pelvic symphysis, bilateral agenesis of the tibia or reduction of its length, ventral abdominal hernia, meningocele, and reproductive system defects. The most significant pathologic change involves agenesis of the tibia (47).

D. Congenital Defects of the Muscular System

Arthrogryposis, defined as permanent joint contracture present at birth, occurs frequently in many domestic animals and may be an inherited defect in various species (48-50) (Fig. 3). Non-hereditary examples of arthrogryposis have been well studied in calves (27). Arthrogryposis neither implies a specific pathologic entity nor a specific cause. However, arthrogryposis in Charolais calves is inherited as a simple autosomal recessive trait (49). Such defective Charolais calves have been observed in Australia, Canada, France, New Zealand, and the United States (7,51). The arthrogryposis syndrome in Charolais cattle most commonly consists of tetramelic arthrogryposis and cleft palate. Hypoplasia of the patella is a useful radiographic and gross sign. Other gross or microscopic pathologic changes may include lesions in central nervous system and muscle tissue (51).

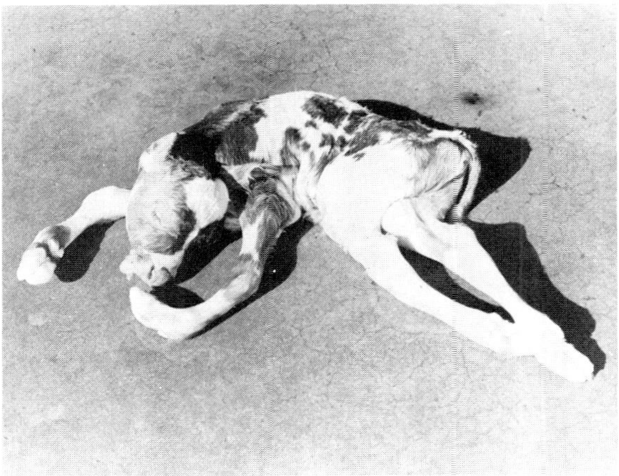

Fig. 3. *Tetramelic arthrogryposis in a Guernsey calf.*

E. Congenital Defects of the Central Nervous System

A wide variety of congenital structural and functional defects is known to afflict the central nervous system of domestic animals. Hydrocephalus, a problem in beef cattle for many years, may be difficult to recognize clinically, or it may cause death or obvious clinical signs in calves shortly after birth. A syndrome of internal hydrocephalus and associated defects in Shorthorn cattle is inherited as a simple autosomal recessive trait. In a study of 115 bovine hydrocephalus cases, 3 Hereford and 1 Shorthorn syndrome accounted for 44 of the cases, and pathogenic lesions were obstruction of the flow of cerebrospinal fluid in 30 calves. Seventy-four of the cases were classified by pathologic lesion; the remaining 41 were miscellaneous types (52). The most common lesion was stenosis of the Sylvian aqueduct seen in 30 cases, whereas meningitis accounted for only 5 cases. Hereditary influences seem to account for most of the hydrocephalus cases we encountered during our study. Recent preliminary breeding studies with horned Hereford cattle indicated an internal hydrocephalus syndrome to be inherited as a simple autosomal recessive. The syndrome consists of internal hydrocephalus, retinal dysplasia, and myopathy (Fig. 4) (53).

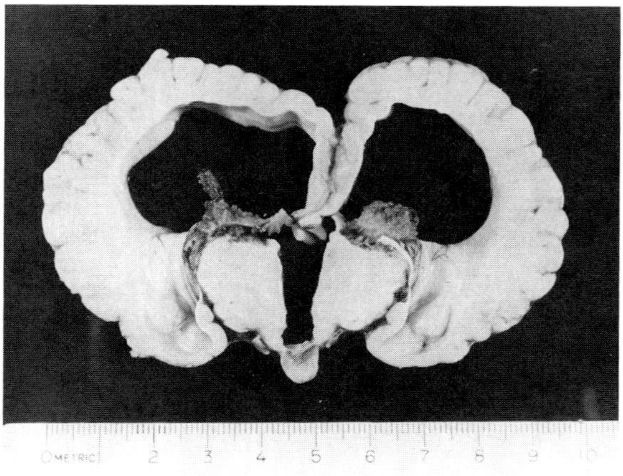

Fig. 4. *Internal hydrocephalus in a Hereford calf. Notice dilated ventricles.*

IX. REFERENCES

1. Leipold, H. W., Huston, K., and Dennis, S. M., *in* "Advances in Veterinary Science and Comparative Medicine" (C. A. Brandly and C. E. Cornelius, Eds.), Vol. 16, p. 103. Academic Press, New York, 1972.
2. Cho, D. Y., and Leipold, H. W., *Vet. Bull.* 47, 489 (1977).
3. Greene, M. J., Leipold, H. W., Huston, K., Noordsy, J. L., and Dennis, S. M., *Ir. Vet. J.* 27, 37 (1973).
4. Huston, R., Saperstein, G., and Leipold, H. W., *Equine J. Med. Surg.* 1, 146 (1977).
5. Saperstein, S., Leipold, H. W., and Dennis, S. M., *J. Am. Vet. Med. Assoc.* 167, 314 (1975).
6. Saperstein, S., Harris, S., and Leipold, H. W., *Feline Pract.* 6, 18 (1976).
7. Jolly, R., and Leipold, H. W., *N. Z. Vet. J.* 21, 147 (1973).
8. Rieck, G. W., Finger, K. M., and Herzog, A., *Giessener Beitr. Erbpathol. Zuchthyg.* 4, 29 (1972).
9. Huston, K., *Holstein-Friesian World* 54, 26 (1957).
10. Herschler, M. S., Fechheimer, N. S., and Gilmore, L. O., *J. Dairy Sci.* 45, 1493 (1962).
11. Anonymous, *in* "Report of Production, Milk Marketing Board,"

No. 10, p. 99. London, England, 1960.
12. Sellers, K. C., Smith, G. F., and Wood, P. D. P., *Br. Vet. J.* 124, 89 (1968).
13. Helmig-Schumann, H., *Zuchthygiene* 36, 217 (1964).
14. Bellows, R. A., *Agric. Res.* 19, 11 (1971).
15. Finger, K. M., Herzog, A., and Rieck, S. W., *Giessener Beitr. Erbpathol. Zuchthyg.* 112, 60 (1970).
16. Priester, W. A., Glass, G. G., and Waggoner, N. S., *Am. J. Vet. Res.* 31, 1871 (1970).
17. Hartley, W. J., and Kater, J. C., *N. Z. Vet. J.* 12, 49 (1964).
18. Hughes, K. L., Hartley, W. J., Haughey, K. G., and McFarlane, D., *Proc. Aust. Soc. Anim. Prod.* 5, 52 (1964).
19. Dennis, S. M., and Leipold, H. W., *Zuchthygiene* 11, 105 (1976).
20. Beck, C. C., Bronson, S. M., and Henneman, H. A., "Proceedings, Sheep Disease and Health Symposium, Sheep Industry Development Program," University of California, Davis, California, p. 49, 1968.
21. Ercanbrach, S. K., and Price, D. A., *J. Hered.* 62, 223 (1971).
22. Dennis, S. M., *Vet. Rec.* 95, 488 (1974).
23. Dennis, S. M., *Aust. Vet. J.* 51, 80 (1975).
24. Bille, N., and Nielsen, N. C., *Nord. Veterinaermed.* 29, 128 (1977).
25. Leipold, H. W., Dennis, S. M., and Huston, K., *Vet. Bull.* 43, 399 (1973).
26. Cornelius, C. E., and Cronwall, R. R., *Am. J. Vet. Res.* 29, 291 (1968).
27. Shupe, J. L., Binns, W., James, L. F., and Keeler, R. F., *J. Am. Vet. Med. Assoc.* 151, 198 (1967).
28. Keeler, R. F., *Clin. Toxicol.* 6, 529 (1972).
29. Keeler, R. F. *J. Toxicol. Environ. Health* 1, 887 (1976).
30. Done, J. T., *in* "Advances Veterinary Science and Comparative Medicine" (C. A. Brandly, C. E. Cornelius, and W. J. Bevridge, Eds.), Vol. 20, p. 69. Academic Press, New York, 1976.
31. Kahrs, R. F., Scott, F. W., and LaHunta, A. de, *Teratology* 3, 181 (1970).
32. Richards, W. D. C., Crenshaw, S. L., and Bushnell, R. B., *Cornell Vet.* 61, 336 (1971).
33. Kurogi, M., Inaba, Y., Goto, Y., Miura, M., Takahashi, K., Sato, T., Omori, T., and Matumoto, M., *Arch. Virol.* 47, 71 (1975).
34. Bruere, N., Proceedings, 1st World Congress Genetics Livestock Producers, Madrid, Spain, Vol 1, p. 151, 1974.
35. Leipold, H. W., and Schalles, R., *Vet. Med. SAC.* 73, 80 (1977).
36. Huston, K., *Kans. Vet.* 22, 8 (1966).
37. Hutt, F. B., "Animal Genetics," Ronald Press, New York, 1964.
38. Wiesner, E., and Willis, S., "Veterinärmedizinische Pathogenetik," S. Fischer, Jena, Germany, 1974.
39. Leipold, H. W., and Huston, K., *J. Hered.* 59, 2 (1968).

40. Eldridge, F. E., Atkseson, F. W., and Ibsen, H. L., *J. Hered.* 40, 205 (1953).
41. Drieux, H. M., Priouzeau, S., Thiery, G., and Priouzeau, M. L., *Rec. Med. Vet.* 126, 385 (1950).
42. Leipold, H. W., Adrian, R. W., Huston, K., Trotter, D. M., and Dennis, S. M., *J. Dairy Sci.* 52, 1422 (1969).
43. Leipold, H. W., Huston, K., Dennis, S. M., and Guffy, M. M., *Ann. Sel. Genet. Anim.* 3, 245 (1971).
44. Leipold, H. W., and Cook, J. E., *Am. J. Pathol.* 86, 745 (1976).
45. Leipold, H. W., Guffy, M. M., and Cook, J. E., *Comp. Pathol. Bull.* 9, 305 (1976).
46. Leipold, H. W., Guffy, M. M., and Cook, J. E., *Comp. Pathol. Bull.* 9, 1 (1977).
47. Leipold, H. W., Saperstein, J., Swanson, R. W., Schalles, R., and Guffy, M. M., *Z. Tierz. Zuechtungsbiol.* (In press).
48. Leipold, H. W., Cates, W. F., and Howell, W. E., *Can. Vet. J.* 10, 268 (1969).
49. Greene, H. J., Leipold, H. W., Huston, K., and Guffy, M. M., *Am. J. Vet. Res.* 34, 887 (1973).
50. Berg, R. T., Proceedings, 1st World Congress Genetics Livestock Producers, Madrid, Spain, 3, 1974.
51. Leipold, H. W., Greene, H. J., and Huston, K., *Vet. Med. SAC.* 68, 1139 (1973).
52. Greene, H. J., Leipold, H. W., and Hibbs, C. M., *Cornell Vet.* 64, 496 (1974).
53. Leipold, H. W., and Schalles, R., *Am. Hereford J.* 68, 14 (1977).

EPIDEMIOLOGICAL INVESTIGATIONS OF POISONOUS PLANT-INDUCED BIRTH DEFECTS

Lloyd A. Selby
University of Missouri-Columbia

I. ABSTRACT

Epidemiological studies of birth defects induced by poisonous plants have encompassed not only observational studies but also analytical and experimental studies. Epidemiologic investigative techniques have been used as a diagnostic aid to determine what agent, host and environmental factors were associated with a birth defect(s) in domestic animals. Although many of these investigations included laboratory studies, they usually began with field observations on the frequency and pattern of defects in a herd or population that had grazed either in a particular pasture or over a large, defined geographical region.

Epidemiologic field studies have suggested that not only the toxic plant but also man-made or other natural environmental factors were associated with defects in domestic animals. The mere presence of the poisonous plant alone was not enough; it must have been consumed. However, field investigations have in many instances been used to determine what poisonous plants probably induced birth defects in domestic animals.

II. INTRODUCTION

Epidemiology as a science concerns itself with the study of disease problems in human (1) or animal populations (2). A major epidemiologic concept is that disease problems are multifactorial in nature, and it is the interaction of the disease agent, the environment and host factors that determines if the disease will occur. It is through epidemiologic investigations that the ecology of the disease and its expression in a population can be defined (3). This report describes the use of epidemiologic investigations in determining the role of poisonous plants in inducing birth defects in domestic animals. Included is a discussion of those agents, hosts, and environmental factors that have been associated with plant-induced birth defects.

III. BACKGROUND FROM THE FIELD

A birth defect is the imperfect development of a body organ or structure in the embryo; it can be considered as a marked deviation from the normal. Sometimes, one may observe a spectrum of pathologic effects that suggests a number of different defects, but in reality it is a single defect with its range of deviation that has been observed (4). Yet at other times one may indeed observe a number of different defects.

The etiology of birth defects in domestic animals is complex. The disease agent may be infectious, noninfectious, genetic, environmental, or a combination of these factors. However, in a majority of defects in domestic animals the etiologic agent is unknown. Epidemiologic field investigations of reported outbreaks of defects in animals may furnish information which suggests an association between etiologic factor(s) and the defect that has been observed.

An important point to keep in mind is the stage of pregnancy during which the animal is exposed to the disease agent. Depending on the toxic dose obtained by the pregnant dam and the stage of pregnancy, one may observe a spectrum of disease from a mummified, stillborn, defective or aborted fetus to a normal, liveborn one. These categories may not be mutually exclusive. It is the first third of pregnancy which is the most "critical period" during which birth defects are generally initiated. A summary of the mean and range of the gestation period, as well as the first third or "critical period" of pregnancy, for most domestic animals is presented in Table 1.

TABLE 1

Mean, Range, and Critical Period[1] of Gestation for Domestic Animals (5)

Species	Gestation period in days		Critical period[1] in days
	Mean	Range	
Cattle *Bos taurus*	284	210-335	1-95
Dog *Canis familiaris*	63	53-71	1-21
Goat *Capra hircus*	151	135-160	1-50
Horse *Equus caballus*	336	264-420	1-112
Cat *Felis catus*	63	52-69	1-21
Sheep *Ovis aries*	151	144-152	1-50
Swine *Sus scrofa*	114	101-130	1-38

[1]Critical period for birth defects is considered to be first third of mean gestation period.

Possible exceptions to the "critical period" occur with some of the multiple defects where a defect in a vital organ or body structure produces other defects. In these instances it is difficult to determine which defect was the primary one.

It is also important to secure information from the people most involved with the production of the species being studied. It is these individuals who may be able to provide accurate, detailed observations concerning the defects under investigation. As an example, those involved in the swine industry who were most concerned with defects in swine were found to be the producers, agricultural extension agents, farm advisors, or feed salesmen. Similar data can be compiled for the other domestic animals, and such a compilation has in fact already been developed for sheep (6).

In addition, a plant may be poisonous not only because it contains a natural toxin, but because it may concentrate a trace substance(s) which in turn is toxic. On the other hand, a plant may be deficient in a particular substance, or the vegetative material may act as a growth medium for certain toxin-producing bacteria or fungi. For example, *Fusarium culmarum* has been associated with abortions, stillbirths, and non-lethal birth defects in domesticated pigs (7).

IV. EPIDEMIOLOGICAL INVESTIGATIONS

Epidemiological studies may be observational, analytical, experimental, or theoretical in nature as shown in Table 2. Most, if not all, epidemiological field investigations start with simple descriptive observations, and as the study progresses the design may become more complex. Some field investigations of plant-induced birth defects have been a combination of observational and analytical study designs. Regardless of the initial design, these studies do have some common elements: They start as field not laboratory studies; the primary objective of the study is to control or prevent defects from occurring; and the diagnostic procedure used is one of population statistics, for example, a description of the frequency and pattern of occurrence of the defect(s) being observed (9). This is as true of the follow-up investigation of an outbreak of birth defects possibly associated with poisonous plants as it is of the routine surveillance of animal intoxications with their related pathological evaluation and, in some instances, subsequent field investigations. Prior to collecting data on field observations, one needs to design and pretest a survey questionnaire on which one can record observations of those factors that might be related to plant-induced birth defects. An example of descriptive data which was collected in investigations of swine birth defects using direct interview techniques is presented in Table 3.

The overall strategy is that of using a sound "scientific method" (10). The classic four stages of modern scientific method are observation, hypothesis, deduction, and experimentation. Preliminary field observations are evaluated and one can then state a hypothesis to be tested by additional field studies. It is

TABLE 2

Epidemiological Study Designs[1] *(1,8)*

Name	Definition
Observational	
Descriptive studies	Description of diseases; e.g., malformed individuals in a population.
Intervention studies	Attempts to lower expected number of malformed offspring by selective breeding, immunization, or removal from access to toxic plants.
Analytical (natural experiments)	
Case-control studies (Retrospective)	Sample of cases (malformed individuals) and controls (non-malformed individuals) compare the rate of study characteristics in both groups.
Cross-sectional studies (Retrospective)	Sample of population containing malformed and non-malformed individuals with and without study characteristics, at one point in time.
Cohort studies (Prospective)	Sample of individuals (1) with (2) without certain characteristics. Evaluate and compare these groups to determine disease (malformation) rate in each group.
Experimental	Investigator has control over population group he is studying by deciding which groups are exposed to a possible etiologic factor or preventative measure.
Theoretical	
Models or computer simulation	Statistical model to explain different variables and their impact on the occurrence of disease in a theoretical population.

[1]Some epidemiologists and statisticians consider epidemiological studies to be only observational (observational + analytical) and experimental (experimental + theoretical).

TABLE 3

Variables about which Descriptive Data was Collected on Swine Birth Defects using Direct Interview Techniques on 334 Missouri Swine Farms

Host Factors:
Age, Sex, Breed of Defective Pig, Dam and Sire
Number and Breed of Females Bred
Number of Pigs Born Alive, Dead and Defective
Description of Defect(s)
Other Species with Defects on Farm
Agent Factors:
Poisonous Plants
Abnormal Feed
Drugs Administered, Illness, Vaccination, Pesticides Used in Feed or on Pregnant Sows during First Third of Pregnancy
Environmental Factors:
Drylot or Pasture
Feed and Minerals Fed during Gestation Cycle
Water Supply
Where Female Farrowed
Unusual Happenings

equally important to record filed observations, collect defective animals for a clinical-pathological evaluation and, if available, collect samples of plants suspected of being associated with the birth defects. Also, in the study of disease one should locate the affected herd(s) geographically by using maps (11,12). Maps may vary from simple spot maps to more detailed maps that are made with adjustments to calculate disease incidence. An example of such a map is Figure 1 where swine herds with birth defect rates in the upper and lower "octile" are shown. A comparison of groups with varying disease rates frequently will shed new light on the epidemiology of the disease (e.g., birth defects).

Although many field studies are descriptive, one should attempt to go a step further and design an analytical study. The latter studies are designed to test one or more specified "epidemiological hypotheses;" they usually have a standardized study design, record system, and analytical methods that have been chosen *a priori*. In field studies usually one deals with observations and not with variables that can be controlled. The epidemiologist may design an analytical study (e.g., case-control study) to determine the strength of association between variables, the importance of the association, as well as the statistical significance of the association. The investigator may also decide to use complex statistical techniques, such as multiple regression (9). In contrast, the experimental study involves manipulation or control of study variables. Feeding trials using poisonous plants to

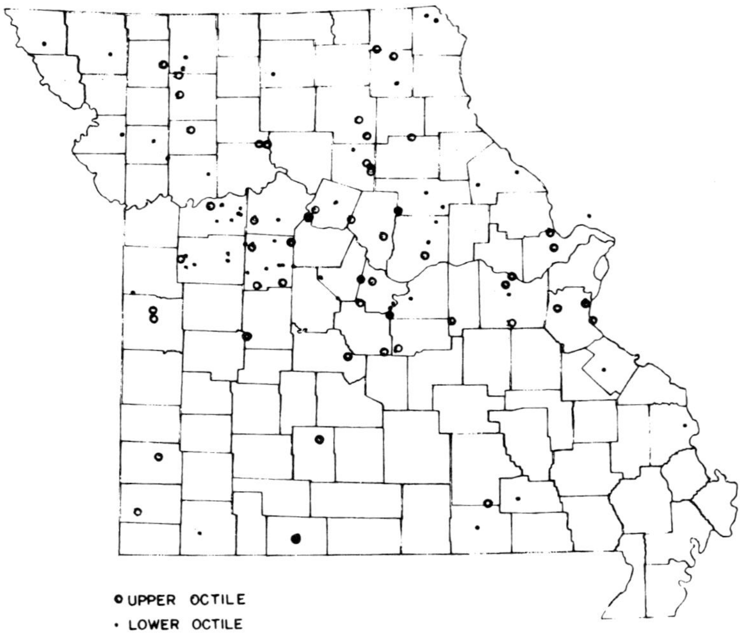

Fig. 1. *Computer plotted map showing the geographic location of swine herds, with birth defects, plotted by x, y coordinates (13). Shown is the upper and lower octile of birth defect rates per 1000 total births in 334 swine herds.*

attempt to induce birth defects in some groups of animals with non-exposed animals used as controls are experimental studies.

Observational epidemiologic studies that suggested plant-induced defects in domestic animals are presented in Table 4. Besides the studies cited, other investigators have reviewed the known or suspected teratogenic hazards associated with range plants (32,33). Not all the cited studies concerned poisonous plants or the natural toxins they contained. A number of the investigations uncovered possible deficiencies in trace elements or vitamins in the vegetation being consumed by the animals. These findings, along with other field or laboratory observations, suggest that deficiencies in essential elements and vitamins may also induce birth defects in domestic animals.

In addition to, or sometimes as a result of observational studies, experimental studies have been conducted to evaluate the association between plants and birth defects in domestic animals.

TABLE 4

Epidemiological Field Studies of Suspected Plant-Induced Birth Defects in Domestic Animals

Agent	Species	Reference
Hypothyroidism (due to iodine deficiency)	Swine	Smith, 1917 (14)
Brassica (with low vitamin A high nitrates) (*Brassica napus*)	Swine	Case, 1957 (15)
Vitamin A (deficiency)	Swine	Goodwin and Jennings, 1958 (16)
Grassland lupine (*Lupinus laxiflorus*)	Cattle	Wagnon, 1960 (17)
Manganese (deficiency)	Cattle	Dyer, 1961 (19) Dyer, *et al.*, 1964 (21)
False hellebore (*Veratrum californicum* Durand)	Sheep	Binns, *et al.*, 1962 (4)
Locoweeds (*Oxytropis sp.; Astragalus sp.*)	Cattle & Sheep	James, *et al.*, 1967 (21)
Sudan grass pasture (*Sorghum vulgare*)	Horses	Princhard and Voss, 1967 (22)
Choline (deficiency)	Swine	Cunha, 1968 (23)
Tobacco stalks (*Nicotiana tabacum*)	Swine	Crowe, 1969 (24); Menges, *et al.*, 1970 (25); Crowe and Pike, 1973 (26)
Wild black cherry (*Prunus serotina*)	Swine	Selby, *et al.*, 1971 (27)
Copper (deficiency)	Sheep	Kavanagh, *et al.*, 1972 (28)
Poison hemlock (*Conium maculatum*)	Swine	Edmonds, *et al.*, 1972 (29) Dyson, 1977 (30)
Jimson weed (*Datura stramonium*)	Swine	Leipold, *et al.*, 1973 (31)

Selected studies that represent experimental epidemiological studies are summarized in Table 5.

V. DISCUSSION

The bases for epidemiologic studies of populations of domestic animal as well as major problems encountered in surveying these populations have been documented (2). Epidemiologic field studies (i.e., observational studies) take as much careful planning, organization and design as is necessary with experimental studies in the laboratory. Because most of the variables being measured

TABLE 5

Selected Experimental Feeding Studies of Plant-Associated Birth Defects in Domestic Animals

Agent	Species	Reference
Vitamin A Deficiency, Excess	Swine	Hale, 1935 (34) Palludan, 1966 (35)
False hellebore (*Veratrum californicum*)	Sheep	Binns, *et al.*, 1963 (36)
Locoweeds (*Astragalus spp.*)	Sheep	James, *et al.*, 1967 (21) James, *et al.*, 1969 (37)
(*Lupinus caudatus*)	Cattle	Shupe, *et al.*, 1967 (18)
Leucaena (mimosine)	Swine	Wayman, *et al.*, 1970 (38)
(*Pinus ponderosa*)	Sheep	James and Call, 1971 (39)
Tobacco (Nicotine alkaloids)	Swine	Crowe and Swerczek, 1974 (40)
Alkaloid coniine (*Conium maculatum*)	Cattle	Keeler, 1974 (41)

are not under direct control, the epidemiologist must use the most sophisticated study design and statistical techniques possible. In field investigations of plant-induced birth defects in domestic animals, multiple visits and interviews are necessary before the complete picture can be defined of what environmental, host, and agent factors are related to the defects. Data on the genetic history of the herd and the role that breeding might have in producing the defects also have to be evaluated in detail. One may think that producers of purebred animals would be more uncooperative than producers of crossbred animals. In the Missouri study the converse was found to be true; and in those instances where it could be documented that poisonous plants had a major role in inducing birth defects, genetic factors were found not to be associated with the defects (25,27,29). The possibility of a genetic-environment interaction being associated with birth defects in domestic animals is always a possibility, but to the best of my knowledge this interaction has not yet been documented in the field. On the other hand, the statistical basis for such an interaction is well documented (42).

Environmental factors besides poisonous plants include natural and man-made (i.e., husbandry) factors. In the latter instance, at least in swine, studies suggest that it is natural and not man-made environmental factors that should be considered in evaluating environmental factors that might be associated with birth defects (43). Similar environmental factors exist for cattle but not for sheep that are being cared for by sheepherders. In this instance, husbandry factors may have a role in plant-induced birth defects, e.g., from false hellebore (44).

Another important consideration is the geographic distribution of affected herds with birth defects as compared with the distribution of poisonous plants. In the Missouri study we found that it was easier to determine either a genetic or plant-induced cause of birth defects in herds with "epidemics" of defects. This also appeared to be true with the outbreaks of defects associated with consumption of tobacco by pregnant sows in Kentucky (26). The same has, however, not been observed with certain specific defects seen in cattle (18) and sheep (4,44). Thus, we must continue both the routine surveillance of select defect(s) known to be induced by poisonous plants as well as the intensive follow-up of "outbreaks" of defects in domestic animals if we are to be able to control or prevent plant-induced birth defects.

VI. ACKNOWLEDGMENTS

The swine birth defect project was supported by Public Health Service Grant No. ES00082. Appreciation is expressed to Mr. Harley T. Wright, University of Missouri-Columbia for technical assistance in producing Figure 1.

VII. REFERENCES

1. MacMahon, B., and Pugh, T. F., "Epidemiology Principles and Methods," Little, Brown and Company, Boston, 1973.
2. Selby, L. A., Edmonds, L. D., and Hyde, L. D., *Can. J. Comp. Med.* 40, 135 (1976).
3. Gordon, J. E., *Am. J. Med. Sci.* 235, 337 (1958).
4. Binns, W., James, L. F., Shupe, J. L., and Thacker, E. J., *Arch. Environ. Health* 5, 106 (1962).
5. Altman, P. L., and Dittmer, D. S., "Biological Data Book," Federation of American Society for Experimental Biologists, Washington, 1964.
6. Ruppanner, R., *J. Am. Vet. Med. Assoc.* 161, 1033 (1972).
7. Miller, J. K., Hacking, A., Harrison, M. A., and Gross, V. J., *Vet. Rec.* 93, 555 (1973).
8. Lilienfeld, A. M., "Foundations of Epidemiology," Oxford University Press, New York, 1976.
9. Schwabe, C. W., Riemann, H. P., and Franti, C. E., "Epidemiology in Veterinary Practice," Lea and Febiger, Philadelphia, 1977.
10. Beveridge, W. I. B., "The Art of Scientific Investigation," Random House, New York, 1957.
11. Haggett, P., "Locational Analysis in Human Geography," St. Martin's Press, New York, 1966.
12. Hopps, H. C., *Ann. N. Y. Acad. Sci.* 199, 325 (1972).
13. Wright, H. T., Marienfeld, C. J., and Silberg, S. L., *Public Health Rep.* 83, 427 (1968).
14. Smith, G. E., *J. Biol. Chem.* 29, 215 (1917).
15. Case, A. A., *Sheep Breeder Sheepman* 77, 11 (1957).
16. Goodwin, R. F. W., and Jennings, A. R., *J. Comp. Pathol.* 68,

82 (1958).
17. Wagnon, K. A., *J. Range Manage.* 13, 89 (1960).
18. Shupe, J. L., Binns, W., James, L. F., and Keeler, R. F., *J. Am. Vet. Med. Assoc.* 151, 198 (1967).
19. Dyer, I. A., *Proc. West. Sec. Am. Soc. Anim. Prod.* 12, 67 (1961).
20. Dyer, I. A., Cossett, W. A., Jr., and Roa, R. R., *Bioscience* 14, 31 (1964).
21. James, L. F., Shupe, J. L., Binns, W., and Keeler, R. F., *Am. J. Vet. Res.* 28, 1379 (1967).
22. Prichard, J. T., and Voss, J. L., *J. Am. Vet. Med. Assoc.* 150, 871 (1967).
23. Cunha, T. J., *Feedstuff* 40, 25 (1968).
24. Crowe, M. W., *Mod. Vet. Pract.* 50, 54 (1969).
25. Menges, R. W., Selby, L. A., Marienfeld, C. J., Aue, W. A., and Greer, D. L., *Environ. Res.* 3, 285 (1970).
26. Crowe, W. M., and Pike, H. T., *J. Am. Vet. Med. Assoc.* 162, 453 (1973).
27. Selby, L. A., Menges, R. W., Houser, E. C., Flatt, R. E., and Case, A. A., *Arch. Environ. Health* 22, 496 (1971).
28. Kavanagh, P. J., Purcell, D. A., and Thompson, R. H., *Vet. Rec.* 90, 538 (1972).
29. Edmonds, L. D., Selby, L. A., and Case, A. A., *J. Am. Vet. Med. Assoc.* 160, 1319 (1972).
30. Dyson, D. A., and Wrathall, A. E., *Vet. Rec.* 100, 241 (1977).
31. Leipold, H. W., Oehme, F. W., and Cook, J. E., *J. Am. Vet. Med. Assoc.* 162, 1059 (1973).
32. Binns, W., James, L. F., Keeler, R. F., Balls, L. D., *Cancer Res.* 28, 2323 (1968).
33. Keeler, R. F., *Clin. Toxicol.* 5, 529 (1972).
34. Hale, F., *Am. J. Opthalmol.* 18, 1087 (1935).
35. Palludan, B., *in* "Biomedical Research," (L. K. Bustad and R. O. McClellan, Eds.), p. 51. Fayn Printing Company, Seattle, 1966.
36. Binns, W., James, L. F., Shupe, J. L., and Everett, G. A., *J. Vet. Res.* 24, 1164, 1963.
37. James, L. F., Keeler, R. F., and Binns, W., *Am. J. Vet. Res.* 30, 377 (1969).
38. Wayman, O., Iwanaga, I., and Hugh, W. I., *J. Anim. Sci.* 30, 583 (1970).
39. James, L. F., and Call, J. W., cited by R. F. Keeler, *Clin. Toxicol.* 5, 529 (1972).
40. Crowe, M. W., and Swerczek, T. W., *Am. J. Vet. Res.* 35, 1071 (1974).
41. Keeler, R. F., *Clin. Toxicol.* 7, 195 (1974).
42. Freeman, G. H., *Heredity* 31, 339 (1973).
43. Selby, L. A., Edmonds, L. D., Stewart, R. W., Lower, W. R., and Parke, D. W., *Environ. Res.* 6, 77 (1973).
44. Binns, W., *J. Am. Vet. Med. Assoc.* 164, 284 (1974).

PLANT ESTROGENS AFFECTING LIVESTOCK IN AUSTRALIA

R. I. Cox
CSIRO Division of Animal Production, Australia

I. ABSTRACT

The estrogenic activity of some cultivars of subterranean clover has been the cause of serious infertility of ewes in Australia. After the identification of the estrogens as isoflavones, clarification of metabolic changes and development of new cultivars of low estrogen content, the problem has been greatly reduced. Other possible control methods, including immunization of animals to phyto-estrogens, are discussed. Salient features of the estrogenic coumestans which occur in alfalfa and other medics are noted, although these are not considered a current problem of consequence.

II. INTRODUCTION

Subterranean clover (*Trifolium subterraneum* L.) has been widely sown in grazing areas of Australia over the past 50 years to improve pastures. A serious decrease in fertility in sheep grazing such pastures in Western Australia in the 1940s was described in detail and considered to be due to estrogenic substances in the clover (1). The infertility was accompanied by cystic glandular hyperplasia of the cervix and uterus and became known as "clover disease." Isolation of isoflavones with estrogenic activity from clovers followed, and marked variations in estrogenic activity of different cultivars of *T. subterraneum* was found.

Although many estrogenic substances are known to occur in plants, pasture plants which have been found to cause estrogenic effects in various countries are mainly of the species *T. subterraneum*, red clover (*T. pratense*), alfalfa (*Medicago sativa*), and barrel medic (*M. truncatula*). The estrogens in the clover species are usually isoflavones, whereas the medics contain coumestans.

A significant re-evaluation of the plant compounds which produce estrogenic effects in the sheep was necessary following observations that there is extensive metabolism of phyto-estrogens in the rumen. During such metabolism, compounds of very different estrogenicity from those in the original plant can be produced. This led to the definition of formononetin as the main compound producing biological effects in sheep, although it has little estrogenic activity in itself but, after conversion in the rumen, yields the estrogenic metabolite, equol.

Selection and breeding of strains of clovers low in estrogen, particularly formononetin, has produced a range of cultivars of

T. subterraneum for a variety of rainfall conditions and soil types.

Through management and agronomic measures, clover disease is now uncommonly seen in its severe form in Australia. However, more moderate depression of fertility of about 10-20% is still extensive and has been estimated to result in about a million ewes failing to lamb each year in Australia (2).

The use of clover cultivars of low estrogenic content is now appropriate in the improvement of new areas; the replacement of established and estrogenic clovers is a prolonged and expensive process. Thus methods of controlling clover disease by treatment of the animal may be a useful alternative to the agronomic approach in some situations. Some possible approaches to animal treatment will be considered in this review, particularly possible immunophysiological methods. Immunization to phyto-estrogens, which has shown some evidence of being able to partially block the effects of phyto-estrogens in sheep is of general interest because the principle may be applicable to various toxic substances derived from pastures.

A number of detailed reviews of plant estrogens have appeared (2,3,4,5,6). This paper will emphasize developments in the area mainly in the last seven years.

III. PATHOLOGICAL AND PHYSIOLOGICAL CHANGES ASSOCIATED WITH PHYTO-ESTROGENS

A. Permanent Infertility in Ewes

After sheep have grazed highly estrogenic pastures for several years, the fertility of that flock of ewes becomes depressed. The pathological condition, cystic glandular hyperplasia, is almost always found in the cervix and uterus of ewes affected by such clover disease (1,3,5). The infertility persists for long periods after the ewes are taken off estrogenic pastures (7,8); this situation and the term "permanent infertility" are usually associated with conditions in which mating of the sheep takes place when the clover has dried off and the pasture is of low estrogenicity; they are therefore grazing green clover later in the season and after mating. The main cause of the infertility is a failure of fertilization associated with poor sperm penetration to the oviduct (8,9). The establishment of a reservoir of sperm in the cervix immediately after mating is necessary for normal fertility in sheep (10). In sheep affected by clover disease, the number of sperm entering the cervix is considerably lower than normal and a major factor in this failure appears to be the increased amount and fluidity of the cervical mucus in affected sheep (11). There may also be a higher than normal loss of embryos in the first two months after mating in ewes affected by clover disease (8,9).

Associated pathological conditions contribute to the clover

infertility and, with very high phyto-estrogen intake, uncommonly seen now, to increased death rates in ewes. *Hydrops uteri* and uterine infections are most frequently found associated with cystic glandular hyperplasia (8,9).

Histological examination of the ovaries, pituitary gland, and adrenal cortex have not revealed abnormalities in ewes with clover disease (12) although there is some evidence that the response of the hypothalamus of such ewes to an estrogenic stimulus is subnormal (13). The estrous cycles of infertile ewes are usually of normal length (7,14) and where abnormal cycle lengths occur in some ewes they are often due to pathological conditions such as *hydrops uteri* (12). Progesterone concentrations in the plasma of infertile ewes is generally closely similar to normal ewes (11), although not always (14).

B. Temporary Infertility in Ewes

Where sheep are mated while grazing highly estrogenic clover, a decrease in fertility can occur at that mating (15). The infertility does not persist in subsequent years if the sheep are maintained on non-estrogenic pastures (15). These features are used to differentiate a "temporary infertility" from the permanent infertility noted above. There is not a unanimous agreement on these definitions amongst research workers. The evidence available suggests that this infertility may be due to a depressed fertilization rate and also to a disturbance in the rate of transport of ova through the oviducts (16,17).

Infertility caused by coumestans may be more akin to the temporary infertility situation and there is little data to suggest long-term effects from these estrogens.

C. Rams and Wethers Grazing on Estrogenic Pastures

The fertility and sperm production of rams is unaffected by grazing estrogenic pastures for several years. However, wethers develop enlarged teats and sometimes start lactating. The teat enlargement is a sensitive index of the potency of pastures (18, 19). The bulbourethral gland enlarges slowly on prolonged grazing of estrogenic pastures and may be a factor in the above normal mortality of wethers on clover. Another cause of death is urinary obstruction due to production of sediments, containing phyto-estrogens, in the kidneys (20).

IV. ESTROGENIC SUBSTANCES IN PASTURE LEGUMES

A. Compounds Isolated

The plant constituents that have been isolated and found to

have estrogenic activity include the isoflavones - formononetin, daidzein, genistein, biochanin A (3,4), largely from *Trifolium* species (Table 1); the coumestans, coumestrol and 4'-O-methylcoumestrol (4) have been isolated from the *Medicago* group (Fig. 1a).

TABLE 1

Typical Isoflavone Content of Leaves (Green)

Species	Cultivar	Isoflavone % of dry matter Formononetin	Genistein	Biochanin A
T. subteranneum L. (Subterranean clover)	Yarloop	1.5	2.8	0.5
	Dwalganup	1.3	1.6	0.8
	Dinninup	1.2	1.1	1.5
	Geraldton	0.9	0.6	0.9
	Daliak	0.2	0.4	0.15
	Woogenellup	0.15	2.0	0.6
	Clare	0.15	2.8	0.1
	Notham A	0.12	1.5	0.4
	Uniwager	0.06	0.01	0.01
	Mt Barker	0.06	0.9	2.0
	Trikkala[1]	0.15	0.9	2.0
	Nungarin[1]	0.1		
T. pratense (red clover)		1.1	0.1	1.0
T. repens (white clover)	Ladino	0.02	0.01	0.02

Above 0.3% formononetin is hazardous to fertility.

[1]Cultivars released in 1977, Trikkala being a substitute for Yarloop for high rainfall areas and Nungarin is early maturing.

Sources: Rossiter (6); Braden & McDonald (5); Francis (23).

Other minor constituents of related structure, such as angolensin and 3'-methoxycoumestrol (4,21) also occur. Of the isoflavones, formononetin is the main constituent of significance to grazing sheep because of changes that occur during rumen metabolism, as will be discussed later.

In the plant, the isoflavones occur largely as glycosides (22) which are rapidly and easily hydrolyzed by glycosidases when the leaf cell structure is ruptured. Other estrogens which occur in plants are usually of different structure from the steroid estrogens found in animals, and this wide range of molecular structures showing estrogenic activity is a distinctive feature of estrogens as a hormonal class. The isoflavones and coumestans are relatively weak estrogens, in the range of 10^{-3} and 10^{-5} as active as estradiol-17β in vaginal cornification or uterine weight bioassays.

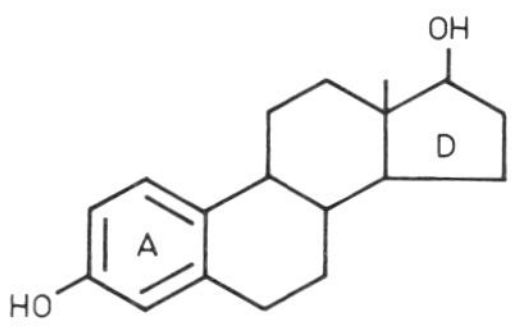

Oestradiol - 17β

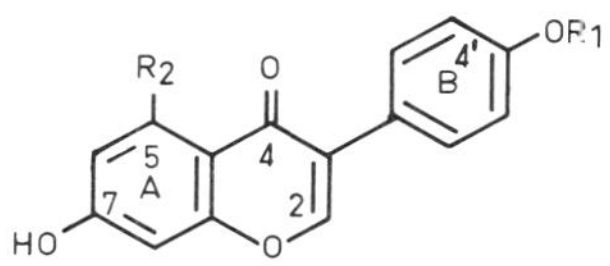

	R1	R2
Genistein	H	OH
Biochanin-A	CH3	OH
Daidzein	H	H
Formononetin	CH3	H

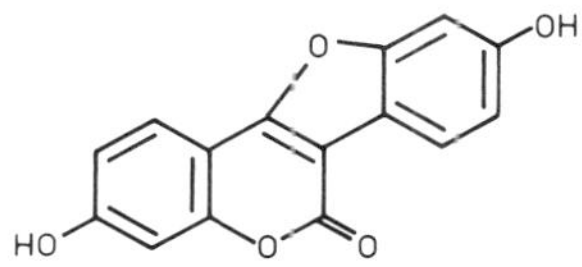

Coumestrol

Fig. 1a. *Structure of estradiol-17β and some phyto-estrogens.*

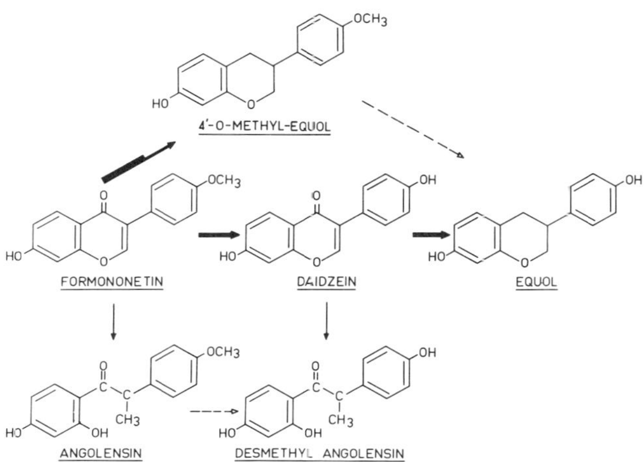

Fig. 1b. *Metabolism of formononetin in sheep. Conversions that are major:* ➞ *; minor* → *; variable* ➞ *; possible* - - → .

Thus, the estrogenicity of some leguminous pastures is usually associated with a daily intake by sheep of gram amounts of phyto-estrogens.

B. Effects of Environmental Factors on Phyto-Estrogen Levels in Legumes

The effect of environmental factors, such as temperature and light, or deficiencies in phosphate, zinc, and nitrogen on the plant content of isoflavones has been studied (reviewed 4; 6,24). Among these, of particular practical significance to estrogenicity of pastures, is the increase in isoflavone content under conditions of phosphate deficiency (24). The main factor which can increase coumestan concentrations is fungal infection (4,25,26). White clover, which normally has a negligible estrogenic content, of under 5 p.p.m., can, after fungal infection, contain over 100 p.p.m. of coumestan, sufficient to produce estrogenic effects in sheep grazing the pastures (21,27). Some of these coumestans had not been isolated previously (21). Such findings illustrate the need to be on the alert for new phyto-estrogens or situations leading to their formation.

V. ISOFLAVONOIDS WITH ESTROGENIC ACTIVITY

A. Metabolism of the Isoflavones in Sheep and the Significance of Formononetin

The metabolism of the isoflavones in the animal, especially conversions occurring in the rumen, have been found to result in products with very different degrees of estrogenic activity from the plant constituents (5). Such metabolism together with observations on the relative estrogenic potency in sheep of various cultivars of subterranean clover, led during the 1960s to a complete revision of the cultivars identified as deleterious to sheep (3,28,29). The result has been that formononetin has been implicated as the main isoflavone resulting in estrogenic effects in the sheep, and genistein is not of importance, at least in permanent infertility.

Formononetin, often present at levels of 1-2% of dry weight in a number of cultivars of subterranean and red clovers, has little or no estrogenic activity itself, but is converted in the rumen largely to equol, which is appreciably estrogenic (Fig. 1b). Indeed, equol is probably the main estrogen responsible for clover disease (5,29). In contrast, the 5-hydroxy-isoflavones genistein and biochanin A, which are themselves estrogenic when given parenterally, are metabolized almost completely to p-ethylphenol and other inactive compounds in the rumen (5). During grazing, ruminal degradation of genistein and biochanin A appears to increase markedly over the first few days of feeding until their estrogenic effects in the sheep are negligible. In contrast, the proportion of formononetin converted to equol does not change much with time and so the estrogenicity remains high (30). About 70% of the formononetin ingested by sheep was found to be converted to urinary equol (31), together with a small amount of daidzein and desmethylangolensin (32). This general pattern has been confirmed in observations on a series of over 30 wethers fed a diet of dried pelleted red clover (33).

B. 4'-O-Methylequol as a Metabolite of Formononetin

Other metabolites of formononetin have also been found, one of which has been identified as 4'-O-methylequol and small amounts of angolensin appear to be present, as well as an unidentified compound (Fig. 1b). The O-methylequol was found to be present in appreciable amounts in the urine of 9 of 30 animals, and in some, the levels found approached those of equol (33). In urine samples taken from sheep in Western Australia, all animals showed methylequol with the concentration of this compound exceeding that of equol in about half of them (Cox and Lightfoot, unpublished observations). O-Methylequol was also isolated from renal deposits, which can cause urinary tract blockage in wethers and in the urine of sheep grazing estrogenic pastures (20).

Such a metabolite is of interest in that an appreciable proportion of formononetin may be metabolized by an alternative route involving reduction without prior demethylation. This methoxy compound is likely to be less estrogenic than equol and hence the proportion of equol to methylequol could be of significance in relation to biological effects in the sheep. In the cytosol assay system (34) it is about a tenth as active as equol (unpublished observations). The factors that affect the extent to which formononetin is metabolized by this route have yet to be elucidated.

Phyto-estrogens and their metabolites are absorbed, largely from the rumen, and circulate in the blood. Conjugation with glucuronic acid and some further metabolism probably occurs in the liver. Rapid excretion occurs, mainly in the urine. In contrast, the excretion route for metabolites of the endogenous steroid estrogen is largely fecal. Phyto-estrogens and their metabolites circulating in blood plasma are preponderantly in the form of glucosiduronates and in this form are probably biologically inactive (31). Less than 1% are present as the biologically active unconjugated form and small amounts appear to be present as the sulfo-conjugates (35) which are of significance as they probably can be converted *in vivo* to the active unconjugated form. In the case of coumestrol, however, relatively high proportions are present in the unconjugated and sulfo-conjugated forms as are shown for some typical analyses in Table 2.

C. Actions of Trace Elements on Estrogenic Effects in Sheep

Investigations have been carried out on the influence of cobalt or selenium intake on clover-induced infertility. No improvement was found in the fertility of affected ewes after

TABLE 2

Phyto-Estrogen Fractions in Sheep Plasma

	Dinninup Clover Ingested				Ingested or administered Coumestrol		
Animal	1		2		3	4	5
Fraction	Formononetin (μg/100 ml plasma)	Equol	Formononetin (μg/100 ml plasma)	Equol	Coumestrol (ng/100 ml plasma)		
Unconjugated	1.61	1.1	1.4	0.8	307	95	191
Sulfate	0.87	7.3	2.8	6.9	496	190	176
Glucuronide	39.7	209	157	161	608	613	695
Sulfoglucuronide	0.99	13.2	1.2	<0.05			

treatment with cobalt or selenium (36). On the other hand, it was reported that selenium treatment prevented the depression in fertility seen in ewes grazing estrogenic pastures (37). However, the effect of selenium supplementation on reproductive performance of ewes grazing estrogenic pasture has been shown to vary with the hemoglobin type of the animals (14). Cobalt supplementation to sheep has been reported as exacerbating their infertility on estrogenic pastures (38). It is evident that trace element interactions with infertility are of considerable interest and practical significance.

D. Metabolism of Isoflavones in Species other than Sheep

Whether phyto-estrogens have deleterious effects in cattle remains equivocal. Some hyperestrogenic disturbances in cattle have been attributed to phyto-estrogens (4,39), yet there have been no reports of such effects from Western Australia. A comparative study showed that there were similar concentrations of phyto-estrogens in the plasma of sheep and cattle grazing on the same pastures (40). The metabolism of formononetin to equol was an important conversion in both species, but the evidence suggested that the rates of metabolism and conjugation might be faster in cattle than in sheep.

There has been little study of the metabolism of phyto-estrogens in non-ruminants. Caution is required in deducing estrogenicity in one species from data obtained in another species. Thus, genistein is estrogenically active when fed to laboratory test animals (41), whereas when fed to sheep it is rendered virtually inactive by ruminal degradation. In poultry, the conversion of genistein to equol has been reported, and is well supported by the data obtained (42). Any species in which effects of phyto-estrogens are being considered needs to be studied by bioassay using that species; suitable techniques for the sheep have been discussed by Braden and McDonald (5). In addition, a method using RNA:DNA ratios in uterine tissue has been proposed (43). Discrepancies in bioassay data between species may indicate metabolic differences. A useful biochemical measure of the estrogenicity of compounds *in vitro*, which may be correlated with *in vivo* findings, is the competitive binding reaction for the estrogen-specific protein in uterine cytosols (34,44).

VI. METABOLISM AND PHYSIOLOGICAL EFFECTS OF COUMESTANS

The coumestans are relatively much more estrogenic than the isoflavones, and thus the lower concentrations at which they occur are still sufficient to result in harmful effects in the animal. In addition to producing an increase in uterine weight (45) and increasing teat length in wethers (28), coumestans also suppress estrus and inhibit ovulation (46). The suppression of estrus is probably brought about through an action of the coumestans in lowering the ovarian estrogen secretion in the sheep. The isoflavones do not show this action.

Little work has been done on the metabolism of coumestans in sheep. It is known that 4'-O-methyl coumestrol is demethylated to coumestrol in the rumen (5). Using the cervical mucus response test in ovariectomized ewes there is a decline in this biological effect over a two-week period of coumestan intake, suggesting that the coumestans are inactivated or the animal becomes insensitive (45). That the mechanism of this change involves an alteration in sensitivity of the animal is supported by analyses of blood in sheep fed a diet containing coumestans. The blood content of coumestrol in both the free and conjugated forms remains high over a period of 17 days while on the estrogenic diet (47). Coumestans have been reported as producing only sporadic outbreaks of infertility (4,45). There is no evidence of permanent effects of coumestans on fertility.

Coumestans pose a relatively small problem in Australia compared with the isoflavones; smaller areas are sown to lucerne as compared with the clovers, although the area being sown is increasing. Also, it is less likely that the coumestans present a long-term danger in relation to infertility in domestic animals.

VII. POSSIBLE CONTROL OF CLOVER DISEASE THROUGH ANIMAL TREATMENT

Although agronomic methods are likely to be of increasing importance in the control of clover disease, it is pertinent to consider the ways in which prevention could operate through treatment of the animal. These include immunization against phyto-estrogens, genetic selection of sheep for resistance to clover disease, alteration of phyto-estrogen metabolism, and administration of estrogen antagonists or blocking agents.

A. Immunization of Animals to Phyto-Estrogens

The immunophysiological approach depends on raising specific antibodies in the sheep to the phyto-estrogens by active immunization. These antibodies may then bind and in effect bring about a partial neutralization of the circulating phyto-estrogens and hence reduce their biological effects. The concepts underlying such procedures were outlined for the steroids (48) and production of antibodies to phyto-estrogens has been demonstrated in rabbits (49) and sheep (50). Immunogens need to be prepared by covalent conjugation of phyto-estrogen derivatives with an antigen protein (Fig. 2). In our laboratory, such derivatives of phyto-estrogens,

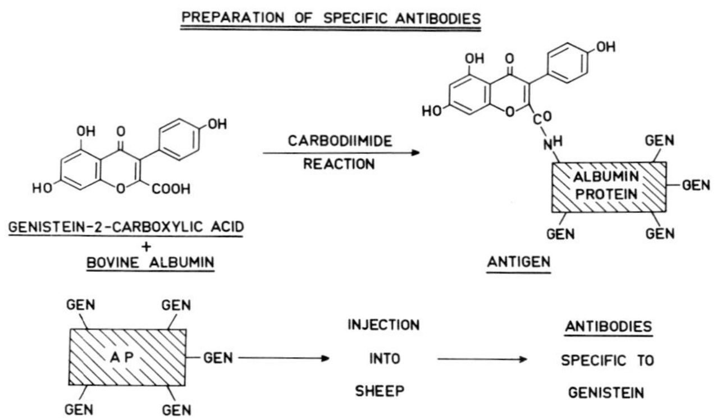

Fig. 2. *Diagramatic representation of immunization to a phyto-estrogen.*

including equol, formononetin, genistein, and daidzein, have been combined to bovine serum albumin, injected into sheep, and have resulted in the formation of specific antibodies. The sera do not show appreciable reactions with steroid estrogens and tests with small groups of sheep indicate that the normal estrous cycle and pregnancy are not affected (51). The lack of any effective uptake of steroid estrogen by antibodies to phyto-estrogen is also demonstrated by comparison with the effects of immunization of sheep to estradiol (51) where very low titers only are effective in blocking the estrous cycle. Preliminary biological tests on sheep immunized against phyto-estrogens and then injected with or fed diets containing phyto-estrogens have indicated that there has been partial success in protecting the animal from estrogenic effects. Genistein, when injected, resulted in significantly less response in uterine RNA:DNA ratio in genistein-immunized ewes compared to a control group receiving injections (Cox, Braden, and Little, unpublished). Equol-immunized wethers have shown a significant protection compared to a control group in terms of bulbourethral gland enlargement during 3 months grazing Yarloop clover (Cox, Wilson, and Obst, unpublished). Ovariectomized ewes immunized to equol and grazing clover tended ($0.2 > P < 0.1$) to a difference from control animals in uterine weights (Cox, Wilson, Lightfoot, and Marshall, unpublished).

Present immunization procedures need to be considerably improved for further experiments and it is by no means clear yet whether this approach can provide sufficient protection for the grazing animal, particularly as it is ingesting gram amounts of phyto-estrogens daily. However, this approach represents a newer technique of potential in controlling phyto-estrogens and is a model for other toxic substances. In general, it may be considered where a low molecular weight compound circulating in the blood plasma could be taken up on a selective antibody. The further metabolism, inactivation, and clearance of the compound must be possible without the opportunity for most of it to exert a biological effect. Other plant toxic agents may be more readily controlled by this approach than the phyto-estrogens, and some are currently under investigation.

B. Other Possible Methods of Animal Treatment

The genotype-pasture interaction on the fertility of ewes has been discussed in a number of studies (52). It has recently been noted that selection of animals which maintain fertility while grazing estrogenic pastures may be an approach (2). The genetic selection of resistant animals would be greatly assisted if there were some biochemical or metabolic marker for resistance. Reports have suggested that the blood hemoglobin type of the ewe is correlated with resistance to infertility on estrogenic pastures (53), although other data have not been in agreement. However, the selenium status of the flock may affect this correlation with hemoglobin type (54).

The alteration of the metabolism of phyto-estrogens in the animal is a potential method for the control of clover disease. The rumen is the most accessible site in which to accomplish this, but such changes may be difficult to maintain. Such an approach would necessitate a greater understanding of the factors affecting rumen metabolism of phyto-estrogens.

Administration of inhibitory compounds would either require a potent substance with a lower estrogenicity than the weak phyto-estrogens, yet selective enough not to interfere appreciably with endogenous estradiol action or alternatively, the use of other hormones which would exert antagonistic effects. This approach would seem difficult to achieve. The administration of androgens and progestagens to ewes has not yielded promising results (55), although this may be an approach with wethers. Data showing that ovariectomized ewes treated with progesterone still show increases in uterine weight when feeding on estrogenic forage, suggests that this hormone would not provide a blocking action (56).

VIII. PRESENT RECOMMENDATIONS FOR THE CONTROL OF CLOVER INFERTILITY

The extensive body of data and experience now available should make it possible to prevent the occurrence of estrogenic problems where land is being first sown to pastures. With existing pastures effects of estrogens can be minimized and outlines of the options have been noted (2,23). These include alterations to the farming enterprise, changes in flock husbandry, and changes in pasture management.

IX. REFERENCES

1. Bennetts, H. W., Underwood, E. J., and Shier, F. L., *Aust. Vet. J.* 22, 2 (1946).
2. Lightfoot, R. J., *Proc. Aust. Soc. Anim. Prod.* 10, 113 (1974).
3. Moule, G. R., Braden, A. W. H., and Lamond, D. R., *Anim. Breed. Abstr.* 31, 139 (1963).
4. Bickoff, E. M., *Commonw. Bur. Pastures Field Crops Rev. Ser.* No. 1, 1968.
5. Braden, A. W. H., and McDonald, I. W., *in* "Australian Grasslands" (R. Milton Moore, Ed.), p. 381. Australian National University Press, Canberra, 1970.
6. Rossiter, R. C., *Aust. Vet. J.* 46, 141 (1970).
7. Underwood, E. J., and Shier, R. L., *Aust. Vet. J.* 27, 63 (1951).
8. Turnbull, K. E., Braden, A. W. H., and George, J. M., *Aust. J. Agric. Res.* 17, 907 (1966).
9. Fels, H. E., and Neil, H. G., *Aust. J. Agric. Res.* 19, 1059 (1968).
10. Mattner, P. E., *Nature (London)* 212, 1479 (1966).
11. Smith, J. F., *J. Reprod. Fertil.* 24, 132 (1970).
12. Hearnshaw, H., Brown, J. M., Cumming, I. A., Goding, J. R., and Nairn, M., *J. Reprod. Fertil.* 28, 160 (1972).
13. Findlay, J. K., Cumming, I. A., Chamley, W. A., Buckmaster, J. M., Goding, J. R., and Hearnshaw, H., *J. Reprod. Fertil.* 32, 341 (1973).
14. Obst, J. M., Seamark, R. F., and McGowan, C. J., *Nature (London)* 232, 497 (1971).
15. Morley, F. H. W., Axelsen, A., and Bennett, D., *Proc. Aust. Soc. Anim. Prod.* 5, 58 (1964).
16. Holst, P. J., and Braden, A. W. H., *Aust. J. Biol. Sci.* 25, 167 (1972).
17. Lightfoot, R. J., and Wroth, R. H., *Proc. Aust. Soc. Anim.*

Prod. 10, 130 (1974).
18. McKeown, N. R., *Aust. J. Sci.* 24, 457 (1962).
19. Braden, A. W. H., Southcott, W. H., and Moule, G. R., *Aust. J. Agric. Res.* 15, 142 (1964).
20. Nottle, M. C., and Beck, A. B., *Aust. J. Agric. Res.* 25, 509 (1974).
21. Wong, E., and Latch, G. C. M., *N. Z. J. Agric. Res.* 14, 633 (1971).
22. Beck, A. B., and Knox, J. R., *Aust. J. Chem.* 24, 1509 (1971).
23. Francis, C. M., *J. Agric. West. Aust.* 16, 2 (1976).
24. Rossiter, R. C., and Beck, A. B., *Aust. J. Agric. Res.* 17, 447 (1966).
25. Shemesh, M., Lindner, H. R., and Ayalon, N., *Refu. Vet.* 26, 1 (1969).
26. Francis, C. M., and Millington, A. J., *Aust J. Agric. Res.* 22, 75 (1971).
27. Newton, J. E., and Betts, J. E., *J. Agric. Sci. Cambridge* 80, 323 (1973).
28. Millington, A. J., Francis, C. M., and McKeown, N. R., *Aust. J. Agric. Res.* 15, 20 (1964).
29. Shutt, D. A., and Braden, A. W. H., *Aust. J. Agric. Res.* 19, 545 (1968).
30. Lindsay, D. R., and Francis, C. M., *Aust. J. Agric. Res.* 20, 719 (1969).
31. Shutt, D. A., Weston, R. H., and Hogan, J. P., *Aust. J. Agric. Res.* 21, 713 (1970).
32. Batterham, T. J., Shutt, D. A., Hart, N. K., Braden, A. W. H., and Tweedale, H. J., *Aust. J. Agric. Res.* 22, 131 (1971).
33. Cox, R. I., and Braden, A. W. H., *J. Reprod. Fertil.* 36, 492 (1974).
34. Shutt, D. A., and Cox, R. I., *J. Endocrinol.* 52, 299 (1972).
35. Wong, M. S. F., and Cox, R. I., "Proceedings 4th Asia and Oceania Congress of Endocrinology," Abstract 53 (H. K. Ibbertson, G. C. Liggins, and I. M. Holdaway, Eds.), University of Auckland, Auckland, 1971.
36. Davies, H. L., *J. Aust. Inst. Agric. Sci.* 32, 216 (1966).
37. Godwin, K. O., Kuchel, R. E., and Buckley, R. A., *Aust. J. Exp. Agric. Anim. Husb.* 10, 672 (1971).
38. Gardiner, M. R., and Nairn, M. E., *Aust. Vet. J.* 45, 215 (1969).
39. Thain, R. I., *Aust. Vet. J.* 44, 218 (1968).
40. Braden, A. W. H., Thain, R. I., and Shutt, D. A., *Aust. J. Agric. Res.* 22, 663 (1971).
41. Biggers, J. D., and Curnow, D. H., *Biochem. J.* 58, 278 (1954).
42. Cayen, M. N., Tang, N. G., and Common, R. H., *Biochim. Biophys. Acta* 111, 349 (1965).
43. Little, D. A., and Lambourne, L. J., *Aust. J. Biol. Sci.* 27, 675 (1976).
44. Shemesh, M., Lindner, H. R., and Ayalon, N., *J. Reprod.*

Fertil. 29, 1 (1972).
45. Kelly, R. W., and Lindsay, D. R., *Aust. J. Agric. Res.* 26, 305 (1975).
46. Kelly, R. W., Adams, N. R., and Lindsay, D. R., *Aust. J. Agric. Res.* 27, 253 (1976).
47. Kelly, R. W., and Lindsay, D. R., *Aust. J. Biol. Sci.*, In press (1977).
48. Lieberman, S., Erlanger, B. F., Bieser, S. M., and Agate, F. J., *Recent Prog. Horm. Res.* 15, 165 (1959).
49. Bauminger, S., Lindner, H. R., Perel, E., and Arnon, R., *J. Endocrinol.* 44, 567 (1969).
50. Cox, R. I., Wong, M. S. F., Braden, A. W. H., Trikojus, V. M., and Lindner, H. R., *J. Reprod. Fertil.* 28, 157 (1972).
51. Cox, R. I., and Wilson, P. A., *J. Reprod. Fertil.* 46, 524 (1976).
52. Davies, H. L., Rossiter, R. C., and Maller, R., *Aust. J. Agric. Res.* 21, 359 (1970).
53. Wroth, R. H., Lightfoot, R. J., Marshall, T., and Steele, P., *J. Agric. West. Aust.* 14, 225 (1973).
54. Obst, J. M., McGowan, C. J., and Walker, S. K., *Proc. Aust. Soc. Anim. Prod.* 10, 135 (1974).
55. Davies, H. L., *Rep. Div. Plant Ind. C.S.I.R.O. Aust.* 68 (1967).
56. Kelly, R. W., Alison, A. J., and Shirley, D. K., *Aust. J. Agric Res.* 27, 101 (1976).

LOCOWEED POISONING IN THE UNITED STATES

K. R. Van Kampen, R. W. Rhees, and Lynn F. James
Utah State University; Brigham Young University; and Poisonous Plant Research Laboratory, Agricultural Research Service U.S. Department of Agriculture

I. ABSTRACT

Locoweed poisoning caused by plants of the genera Oxytropis *and* Astragalus *is devastating to livestock, resulting in multi-faceted clinical signs including emaciation, visual impairment, neurological abnormalities (including incoordination), birth defects, abortions, and habituation. All types of range livestock and some wild animals may be affected. Gross lesions of the in-toxication are not distinctive, but the neurovisceral cytoplasmic vacuolation of various body tissues observed in light and electron microscopy are characteristic. Sequential development of the lesions, their distribution and correlation with clinical signs are discussed.*

II. INTRODUCTION

Locoweed (*Astragalus* and *Oxytropis spp.*) has been characterized as one of the most destructive plants to livestock in the Western United States (1). It is distributed widely and varies greatly in toxicity from species to species (2). Its effects on livestock are multifaceted and include clinical signs of emaciation, visual impairment, functional neurological abnormalities (including incoordination), birth defects, abortions, and habituation (1). Sheep, cattle, and horses are most commonly poisoned, although there are reports of poisoning of some wild species of animals (3). Vivid descriptions of the clinical signs of locoweed poisoning were given by Matthews in Texas (4) and by Marsh (5,6) in Montana early in this century.

The toxic substance or substances in locoweed have not been isolated or characterized inspite of numerous attempts to do so. Sequential development of the lesions in animals suggests that the toxin or the toxic effects are accumulative (1). Clinical signs do not appear until the animal has eaten the plants over an extended period of time and many of the lesions in the parenchymal organs can be repaired without permanent damage if the animals are removed from locoweed infested areas before the onset of clinical signs.

III. GROSS LESIONS OF LOCOWEED INTOXICATION

Lesions found in animals poisoned by locoweed included generalized emaciation, hypertrophy of thyroid glands, pale-tan discoloration of kidneys and liver, and generalized lymphadenopathy (1). Pregnant ewes had diminished blood supply to the fetus, characterized by diminished vascularization of fetal membranes. The number and size of blood vessels in the intercodyledonary areas of the placenta were reduced (8). Normal pooling of blood, centrally, in the placentome often extended over the periphery of the placentome and spilled into the intercodyledonary area. Areas of hemorrhage were apparent through the exterior uterine wall. After fetal death, the normally concave placentome became flattened or everted. No gross changes were noted in uterine walls, cervix, vagina, or ovaries. Fetal tissues became distended by edema and contained focal cuticular hemorrhages. Abortion often followed. Musculoskeletal deformities occurred in some fetuses. Rams had hypoplastic testicles and enlarged seminal vesicles (9).

IV. SEQUENTIAL DEVELOPMENT OF THE MICROSCOPIC LESIONS

Microscopically, the principle lesion of locoweed poisoning is vacuolar degeneration of the cytoplasm of varying body cells (1). The lesions of locoweed intoxication may occur as early as the 4th day following the continuous ingestion of locoweed (7). These appear first in the epithelial cells of the proximal tubules of the kidney. After the 8th day, lesions are found in the neurons of the cerebrum, cerebellum, and the autonomic ganglia of the digestive system, the hepatocytes of the liver, the reticuloendothelial cells of the spleen and lymph nodes, and the transitional epithelium of the urinary bladder. Beyond the 12th day of initiation of the toxicoses, lesions are also found in the neurons of the spinal cord, the adrenal cortical cells, the follicular epithelium of the thyroid gland, parathyroid tissue, pancreatic ascinar cells, reproductive organs, lung, thymus, and abomasum (Table 1). At the light microscopic level, lesions were not found in the myocardium or the skeletal muscle.

In the pregnant ewe, distinct changes were noted in the chorionic epithelium characterized by vacuolation and metaplasia from cuboidal to columnar epithelium. Hemorrhages occurred in the placentome and the uterine wall. Luteal cells of the corpus luteum of the ovary were extremely vacuolated (8).

In the ram (9), the number of mature sperm in the seminiferous tubules, epididymis and the vas deferens was markedly reduced. Spermatogonia were severely vacuolated as was the cytoplasm of Sertoli cells and primary spermatocytes. Secondary spermatocytes and spermatids were less numerous. The pseudostratified epithelium of the epididymis was hypertrophied and vacuolated. The secretory epithelium of the seminal vesicles was distended by vacuolar degeneration causing an enlargement of these organs.

TABLE 1

Sequential Development of Lesions in Tissues of Sheep Fed Locoweed

Tissue	Days fed locoweed							
	4	8	12	16	20	24	28	32
Abomasum	-	-	-	-	-	+	+	+
Adrenal	-	-	-	+	+	+	+	+
Autonomic ganglia (neurons)	-	+	+	+	+	+	+	+
Basal ganglia	-	+	+	+	+	+	+	+
Cerebellum	-	+	+	+	+	+	+	+
Cerebral cortex	-	+	+	+	+	+	+	+
Duodenum	-	-	-	-	-	-	-	-
Hippocampus	-	+	+	+	-	+	+	+
Ileum	-	-	-	-	-	-	-	-
Kidneys (proximal tubules)	+	+	+	+	-	+	+	+
Liver (hepatocytes)	-	+	+	+	-	+	+	+
Lung	-	-	-	-	-	+	+	+
Lymph node	-	+	+	+	-	+	+	+
Medulla oblongata	-	-	-	+	-	+	+	+
Midbrain	-	+	+	+	-	+	+	+
Myocardium	-	-	-	-	-	-	-	-
Omasum	-	-	-	-	-	-	-	-
Ovary	-	-	+	+	+	+	+	+
Pancreas	-	-	-	+	+	+	+	+
Parathyroid	-	-	+	-	-	+	+	+
Pineal	-	-	-	+	*	*	*	*
Pituitary	-	-	-	-	-	-	+	+
Reticulum	-	-	-	-	-	-	-	-
Rumen	-	-	-	-	-	-	-	-
Skeletal muscle	-	-	-	-	-	-	-	-
Spinal cord	-	-	-	-	+	+	+	+
Spleen (R.E. cells)	-	+	+	+	+	+	+	+
Thalamus	-	+	+	+	+	+	+	+
Thymus	-	-	-	-	-	-	+	+
Thyroid	-	-	+	+	+	+	+	+
Urinary bladder	*	+	+	+	+	+	+	+

* Indicates that tissues were not taken for examination.
- No vacuoles.
+ Vacuoles in the cytoplasm

V. CLINICAL PATHOLOGY

SGOT values increased as hepatic damage progressed. Serum calcium decreased and alkaline phosphate increased. Protein bound iodine decreased. Many of the circulating lymphocytes contained large cytoplasmic vacuoles in the latter stages of the intoxication (10). Anemia, previously noted by Matthews (4), was not shown.

VI. ELECTRON MICROSCOPIC STUDIES

Electron microscopic studies by Rhees (unpublished results) have demonstrated that the vacuolar lesions within the cytoplasm resulted primarily from continued enlargement of single membrane lined structures presumed to be lysosomes. At later stages of the intoxication, mitochondrial swelling and degeneration may also be observed. In the central nervous system, cytoplasmic vacuolar degeneration was found in the neurons and glial cells. In addition, fluid accumulations separated the lamina of the myelin sheathes of the axons. Some severe axonal degeneration was observed as the intoxication progressed. Mitochondrial degeneration was most severe in the central nervous system.

VII. CORRELATION OF CLINICAL SIGNS WITH PATHOLOGIC CHANGES

Having ascertained the nature and extent of the lesions in the tissues, the explanation of the clinically observed consequences of locoweed poisoning become clear. The typical description of locoweed poisoning in cattle and horses described a highly excitable, "loco" acting animal (1,4,5,6,11,12) when in fact the large majority of poisoned cattle, sheep, and horses become extremely

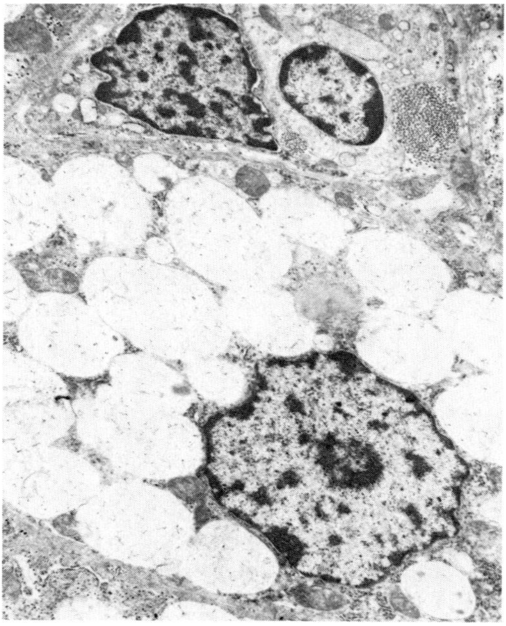

Fig. 1. *Lesions in the liver from locoweed poisoning.*

depressed and emaciated (1,11). The extensive neuronal and axonal lesions in the central nervous system accounted for the failure in coordination, prehension, and other motor functions. Lesions in the liver (Fig. 1), parathyroid, pancreas (Fig. 2), and thyroid (Fig. 3) apparently affected the assimilation and metabolism of ingesta and the degeneration of neurons in the autonomic ganglia of the gut probably impaired intestinal motility.

Observers often mentioned that vision is impaired and the eye appears dull in "locoed" sheep, cattle, and horses. Microscopically, there was cytoplasmic vacuolation of the ganglion cells and bipolar neurons in the inner ganglion layer of the retina (13). These lesions were identical to those described by Whittem and Walker in Aberdeen Angus (14). Hypertrophy and cytoplasmic vacuolation of the epithelium of the lacrimal gland was markedly vacuolated resulting in poor lacrimation and hence the "dull appearing" eye.

Changes in the vascularization of the fetus and fetal membranes and also lesions in the fetus, placenta, and ovaries seem to be related to the reproductive consequences of abortion, fetal malformation and diminution of birth size, but the exact mechanisms have not been worked out (15,16,17). Damage to the male reproductive tract was severe enough to impair reproduction, although it has not been verified by breeding studies (9,18).

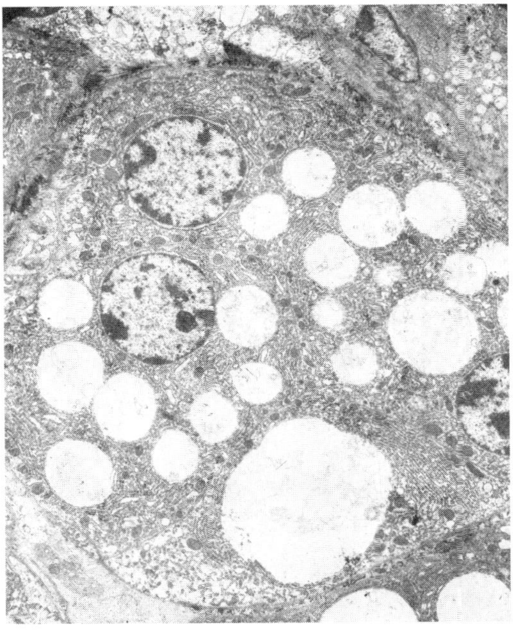

Fig. 2. *Lesions in the pancreas from locoweed poisoning.*

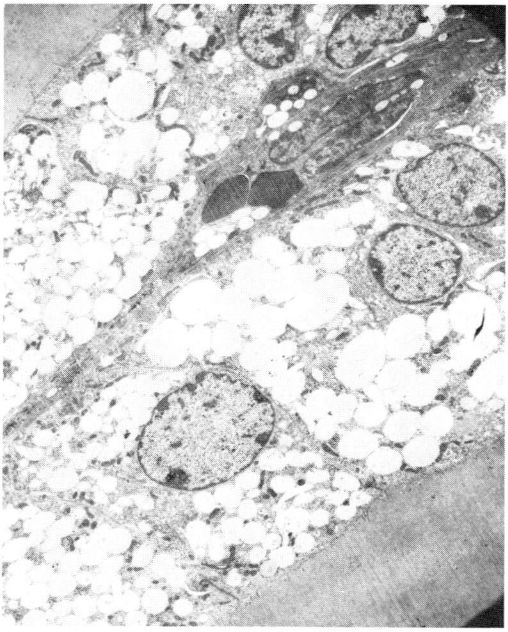

Fig. 3. *Lesions in the thyroid from locoweed poisoning.*

VIII. SIMILARITY TO OTHER DISEASES

Locoweed intoxication has been compared to *Swainsona* poisoning in Australia (19,20,21) and hereditary manosidosis in New Zealand (22). Comparative lesions were discussed by William Hartley in this symposium. Histopathologic changes are similar although there are some distinct clinical differences. The toxic agent(s) in locoweed has not been identified although water soluble extracts cause lesions in experimental rats.

IX. SUMMARY

The clinical signs, gross, light and electron microscopic lesions of locoweed intoxication have been described. Clinical signs include emaciation, visual impairment, neurological disturbances (including incoordination), birth defects, abortion, and habituation. Gross lesions are mainly discolorations and enlargements of various body organs including the thryoids, liver, and kidneys. Light microscopic lesions include neurovisceral cytoplasmic vacuolation. Electron microscopy suggests that the vacuolation results from swollen lysosomes. The toxic agent(s) from locoweed has not been isolated or characterized.

X. REFERENCES

1. Van Kampen, K. R., and James, L. F., *Pathol. Vet.* 6, 413 (1969).
2. Kingsbury, J. M., "Poisonous Plants of the United States and Canada." Prentice-Hall, Englewood Cliffs, New Jersey, 1964.
3. Adcock, J., *J. Wildl. Dis.* (1968).
4. Matthews, F. P., *Tex. Agric. Exp. Stn. Bull.* 456 (1932).
5. Marsh, C. D., *U.S. Dep. Agric. Bull.* 112 (1909).
6. Marsh, C. D., *U.S. Dep. Agric. Bull.* 1245 (1929).
7. Van Kampen, K. R., and James, L. F., *Pathol. Vet.* 7, 503 (1970).
8. Van Kampen, K. R., and James, L. F., *Vet. Pathol.* 8, 193 (1971).
9. James, L. F., and Van Kampen, K. R., *Am. J. Vet. Res.* 32, 1253 (1971).
10. James, L. F., Van Kampen, K. R., and Johnson, A. E., *Am. J. Vet. Res.* 31, 663 (1970).
11. James, L. F., Van Kampen, K. R., and Staher, G. R., *J. Am. Vet. Med. Assoc.* 155, 525 (1969).
12. Oehme, F. W., Bailie, W. E., and Hulbert, L. C., *J. Am. Vet. Med. Assoc.* 152, 271 (1968).
13. Van Kampen, K. R., and James, L. F., *Am. J. Vet. Res.* 32, 1293 (1971).
14. Whittem, J. M., and Walker, *J. Pathol. Bacteriol.* 74, 281 (1957).
15. Keeler, R. F., James, L. F., Binns, W., and Shupe, J. L., *Can. J. Comp. Med.* 31, 334 (1967).
16. James, L. F., Shupe, J. L., Binns, W., and Keeler, R. F., *Am. J. Vet. Res.* 28, 1379 (1967).
17. James, L. F., Keeler, R. F., and Binns, W., *Am. J. Vet. Res.* 30, 377 (1969).
18. Shupe, J. L., James, L. F., Hoffman, K., and Binns, W., *Cornell Vet.* 58, 59 (1968).
19. James, L. F., Van Kampen, K. R., and Hartley, W., *Pathol. Vet.* 7, 116 (1970).
20. Huxtable, C. R., *Aust. J. Exp. Biol. Med. Sci.* 48, 71 (1970).
21. Huxtable, C. R., *Aust. J. Exp. Biol. Med. Sci.* 50, 109 (1972).
22. Jolley, R. D., and Hartley, W. J., *Aust. Vet. J.* 53, 1 (1977).

VIII. OTHER TOXICITIES

Chairman: Coburn Williams

TOXICOLOGICAL SIGNIFICANCE OF PLANT FUROCOUMARINS

G. Wayne Ivie
Veterinary Toxicology and Entomology Research Laboratory, Agricultural Research Service, U.S. Department of Agriculture

I. ABSTRACT

Plants containing photosensitizing furocoumarins have been used by man for more than 3000 years in the treatment of certain skin disorders. This review considers the past and current uses of furocoumarins in medicine, their occurrence and distribution in plants, mode of photosensitizing action, and toxicological properties, with particular emphasis on their phototoxicity to livestock and poultry. Although only a few furocoumarin-containing plants have been implicated as photosensitizers of domestic animals, furocoumarins occur in a large number of plant species in several families, and it is likely that these compounds are involved in a significant number of the photosensitization cases observed in domestic animals.

II. INTRODUCTION

For more than 3000 years, Indian and Egyptian civilizations have used preparations from certain plants to treat skin depigmentation (leukoderma, vitiligo), by application to skin that is subsequently exposed to sunlight (1). Only in the late 1940's was it established that the photosensitizing and pigment-stimulating agents in these plants were a group of compounds known as furocoumarins. From an Egyptian laboratory it was reported that several furocoumarins were present in bishop's weed (*Ammi majus*), and that certain of these purified compounds were effective in treating leukoderma (2). Crude preparations from *A. majus* have been used for centuries in Egypt in the treatment of this disorder.

Since the Egyptian report of the photosensitizing action of plant furocoumarins, extensive research has been conducted to determine the distribution of these compounds in plants, their biochemical mechanism of action, clinical applications in leukoderma and other disorders, and toxicological properties. It is also becoming increasingly apparent that ingestion of furocoumarin-containing plants is a significant cause of photosensitization in domestic animals. This report considers the toxicological significance of naturally-occurring furocoumarins, and reviews the known information on their interactions of a photosensitizing nature with livestock and poultry.

III. CHEMISTRY, DISTRIBUTION, AND BIOLOGICAL ACTION OF FUROCOUMARINS

A. Chemistry and Nomenclature

The furocoumarins are a group of heterocyclic compounds that are considered to be derivatives of coumarin. The furan ring may be fused with coumarin in several different ways, but most of the naturally occurring furocoumarins with photosensitizing activity are derivatives of the linear compound, psoralen (Fig. 1). Isopsoralens also occur in plants, but are not as widely distributed as psoralens.

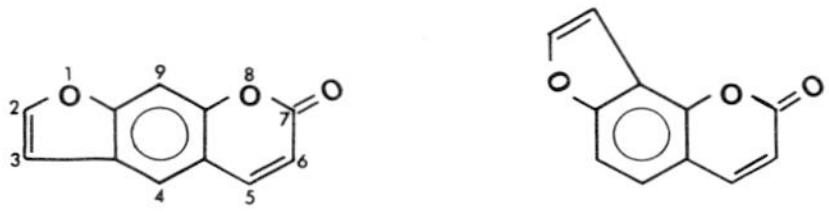

Fig. 1. *Structures of psoralen and isopsoralen.*

Several systems of nomenclature have been used to describe the furocoumarins, but the currently most acceptable would appear to be that used by *Chemical Abstracts* for the past 10 years. Thus, psoralen is named as 7*H*-furo[3,2-*g*][1]benzopyran-7-one, with the positions numbered as indicated above.

Although unsubstituted furocoumarins (such as psoralen) are found in many plant species, numerous derivatives of these compounds have been isolated from plants. A review published in 1962 (3) lists 27 furocoumarins that occur in plants, but a cursory examination of the more recent literature indicates that many more such compounds are now known from plants. Most of the derivatives arise through addition of alkyl or alkoxy groups at (in the case of psoralen) positions 2,3,4,5,6, or 9 often accompanied by reduction of the 2,3-double bond. Structures of some of the more common or clinically important psoralens isolated from plants are shown in Fig. 2.

B. Distribution in Plants

Most of the natural furocoumarins isolated have been from five major plant families: Umbelliferae, Rutaceae, Leguminosae, Moraceae, and Orchidaceae (4). The seeds (5,6) and roots (7) are major sources of furocoumarins in some of the more clinically important plant species that are cultivated solely to obtain these

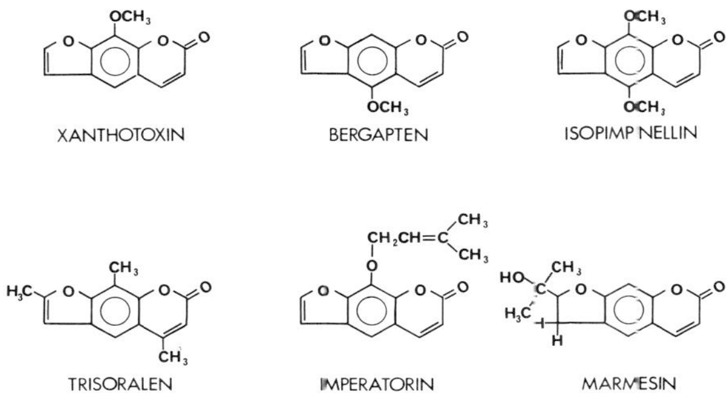

Fig. 2. *Structures of some substituted psoralens.*

photosensitizers.

Furocoumarins also appear to be generated as phytoalexins in some plants. Parsnip infected experimentally with *Ceratocystis fimbriata* accumulates xanthoxin, which is a growth inhibitor of the fungus (8), and celery infected with *Sclerotinia sclerotiorum* produces furocoumarins that are not produced by the fungus in culture, or by healthy celery (9,10). Although some (9,10) originally believed that these furocoumarins were generated as fungal metabolites, more recent evidence (11) indicates that the compounds likely are produced by the plants as phytoalexins.

C. Structure-Activity Relationships in Photosensitizing Action

Extensive testing of both naturally occurring and synthetic furocoumarins has revealed rather rigid structural requirements for high photosensitizing activity (4,11). Generally, linear furocoumarins (e.g. psoralens) are much more active than furocoumarins with angular structures, and substitutions that increase the polarity of the molecule usually decrease its activity. The introduction of electron donating groups such as methyl at positions 2 or 9 enhances photosensitizing activity, while the introduction of electron-withdrawing groups such as hydroxyl or nitro at the same positions has the opposite effect. Although the addition of methoxy group at position 4 (bergapten) or 9 (xanthotoxin) only partially reduces the photosensitizing activity of psoralen, the addition of longer alkoxy groups in these positions greatly reduces or eliminates activity (4,12).

D. Clinical Application

Xanthotoxin has been used extensively in the past as the drug of choice for treatment of leukoderma, but it is being replaced by the considerably more active trimethyl derivative, trisoralen (Fig. 2). Trisoralen occurs in plants (9,11), but is prepared synthetically for drug use. Xanthotoxin is effective in the promotion of suntanning while minimizing sunburn (13), and is also very effective in the treatment of psoriasis when used in conjunction with longwave UV light (14).

E. Mode of Photosensitizing Action

Furocoumarins are primary photosensitizers; i.e. they interact directly with cellular constituents and light to produce cellular damage. The initiation of the photosensitization reaction by furocoumarins is dependent upon the absorption by the compounds of longwave UV light (optimum wavelength, 340-360 nm). Furocoumarins effectively absorb shortwave UV radiation, but these wavelengths apparently do not initiate significant photosensitization reaction in skin (4).

Considerable research has been directed toward determining the mechanisms by which furocoumarins and light interact to initiate skin pigmentation and other photosensitizing effects. Probably the most important discovery in this regard was the observation in the mid-1960's (12) that furocoumarins form photoadducts with pyrimidine bases when exposed to longwave UV and thus inhibit DNA synthesis. Furocoumarins have been shown to photobind to pyrimidine bases and nucleic acids in the skin, but the photobiological effects produced by furocoumarin photoreactions with the skin (erythema followed by skin pigmentation) are not immediately observed. Erythema develops on the skin only after a sufficient degree of damage has been produced to the cellular components (12).

The sequence of events involved in furocoumarin-induced melanization of skin has been considered by Pathak (15), who suggested that the mechanism of action may involve photoinduced gene derepression, resulting in increased melanocyte production, or alternatively, induction of a somatic mutation due to photobinding of the furocoumarin to DNA.

More details on the chemistry, biological properties, pharmacological applications, and mode of action of photoactive furocoumarins can be obtained from several recent, extensive reviews (4,12,15-19).

IV. TOXICOLOGICAL PROPERTIES OF PLANT FUROCOUMARINS

A. Toxicity to Mammals

Some furocoumarins are moderately toxic to mammals and, as expected, the toxicity syndrome does not include symptoms of photosensitization unless the treated animals are exposed to longwave UV light. In the absence of light, the acute LD_{50} values (oral or intraperitoneal) for xanthotoxin and imperatorin (Fig. 2) range between 300-600 mg/kg body weight in the rat and mouse (4, 20). Rats fed psoralen or imperatorin at 30 mg/kg/day for 60 days in the absence of UV light showed no overt toxicity symptoms, and at necropsy the only significant pathological finding was slight hypertrophy of the liver (19).

In the presence of activating UV light, furocoumarins may induce phototoxicity at very low concentrations. The recommended oral dose of xanthotoxin for treatment of leukoderma in humans is 20-60 mg, followed by no more than one hour of exposure to long-wave UV (22). However, an oral dose of 75-100 mg of xanthotoxin, which corresponds to only about 1 mg/kg of body weight, can be dangerous with as little as one hour of subsequent sunlight exposure (23). Phototoxicity symptoms include severe erythema followed by blistering and peeling of the skin. Susceptibility to the phototoxic actions of furocoumarins is to a great extent dependent on the degree of skin pigmentation already present. Fair-skinned individuals are much more likely to suffer sunburn or blistering reactions from furocoumarin exposure than are more pigmented individuals (4).

Many cases of contact photodermatitis have been reported in humans who have had dermal contact with furocoumarin-containing plants, including figs, carrots, parsley, and several others (3). One of the more serious such problems has been periodic outbreaks of "celery dermatitis" occurring among workers who handle this plant (17). Symptoms of the dermatitis include erythema and blistering on the hands and forearms. The causative agents of this disorder were identified in 1963 by Scheel and co-workers (9) as the furocoumarins xanthotoxin and trisoralen (Fig. 2), which celery produces as phytoalexins in response to "pink rot" infection with *Sclerotinia sclerotiorum*.

B. Mutagenicity and Carcinogenicity

Because furocoumarins photobind to DNA, it is not surprising that numerous reports have appeared regarding their mutagenicity (4). Some furocoumarins are highly effective inducers of chromosome aberrations; however, with very few exceptions, furocoumarins do not show any detectable mutagenic activity in the absence of radiation (4).

Excessive exposure to shortwave UV light has long been known to increase the incidence of skin tumors; thus, definition of the skin photosensitizing and photomutagenic actions of furocoumarins quickly made them suspect photocarcinogens. However, the first report on the photocarcinogenic effects of furocoumarins in mammals indicated that albino mice fed xanthotoxin and exposed to shortwave UV light experienced considerably *lower* incidence of ear tumors than did control mice receiving radiation only (24). The degree of protection provided by the dietary xanthotoxin was proportional to its concentration up to 500 ppm in the diet (24). In contrast, other studies have shown that oral or intraperitoneal treatment of mice with xanthotoxin does increase the incidence of skin tumors after exposure to fluorescent lighting (25) or combined short- and longwave UV light (26).

Furocoumarins have been clinically tested as a prophylactic agent against skin cancer in human patients (27). Subjects given daily 20-mg oral doses of xanthotoxin during a 2-year total trial period did not show significant differences in the incidence of skin tumors over patients receiving placebos. Photocarcinogenic studies with furocoumarins to date thus indicate that different wavelengths of UV radiation may result in protection from, induction of, or no effects on skin cancer. With regard to the possible genetic and carcinogenic hazards of these compounds to man, Scott and co-authors (4) suggest that because furocoumarins apparently are not mutagenic in the absence of UV radiation, it is not likely that genetic alterations in human germinal cells will occur due to the inability of radiation to penetrate to these cells. These authors also state that years of clinical experience in the treatment of leukoderma has given no indication of the development of skin cancer in humans continuously treated with furocoumarins and deliberately exposed to UV radiation. They further note that at some concentrations, furocoumarins may in fact be effective prophylactics against skin cancer by promoting melanogenesis and thickening of the epidermis (4).

C. Toxicity to Other Organisms

Limited studies have shown that furocoumarins are toxic to some aquatic organisms. Xanthotoxin at about 15 ppm in the water was lethal to the fish *Lebistes reticulatus*, and several other furocoumarins tested were only slightly less active (28). These studies predate knowledge of the photosensitizing properties of furocoumarins and were apparently conducted in the absence of UV light. Bergapten and isopimpinellin (Fig. 2) at 2-5 ppm in the water under outdoor conditions, are lethal to the snail *Biomphalaria boissi*, and have been proposed as control agents for the snail vectors of schistosomiasis (29).

Furocoumarins also show antimicrobial activity, both in the absence of activating UV light (30,31) and in its presence (32, 33). There seems to be little doubt that photoinduced lethal mutations account for the high phototoxicity of furocoumarins to microorganisms (4), but the mechanisms involved in the toxicity of furocoumarins to microbes in the absence of UV radiation are less understood.

D. Furocoumarin Photosensitization of Livestock and Poultry

Apparently the first report of photosensitization of domestic animals that can be attributed to a furocoumarin-containing plant came from Uruguay in 1946; confirmatory studies were published in 1960 (34). These studies showed that consumption of the seed of *Ammi visnaga* followed by exposure to sunlight caused vesicular dermatitis in chickens and ducks. In later work in Israel, *A. visnaga* failed to photosensitize goslings (35), ducklings, and turkey poults (36), but it did induce mild signs of photosensitization in chickens (36). *Ammi visnaga* produces primarily nonsensitizing furochromones rather than furocoumarins, but xanthotoxin and isopimpinellin (Fig. 2) have been isolated from the plant (37). Differences in the furocoumarin content of the Israeli and Uruguay collections probably account for the observed differences in photosensitizing activity. Although *A. visnaga* has been considered a close relative of the potent photosensitizing plant *A. majus* (discussed below), it has recently been concluded on the basis of morphological, anatomical, and chemical differences that *A. visnaga* should be placed in a separate genus *Visnaga*, and that the two plants cannot be considered closely related (38).

The first furocoumarin-containing plant identified in the United States as a problem to domestic animals was spring parsley (*Cymopterus watsoni*). Binns and co-workers (39) reported that sheep grazing on the plant suffered a severe photosensitization syndrome, with the udders and teats of photosensitized ewes being so sensitive from erythema and blistering that the ewes refused to let their lambs nurse. Loss of lambs from starvation and dehydration was as high as 25% in some flocks in Utah and Nevada. Laboratory studies confirmed that the photosensitization syndrome in sheep was indeed caused by *C. watsoni* (39). The plant is also highly phototoxic to sunlight-exposed chicks (40). Force-feeding the plant to chicks induced erythema and edema of the unfeathered and undowned portions of the skin, followed about 2 months after exposure by sloughing of the comb and wattles, deformation of the upper beak, legs, and feet, and scarring of the ocular opening (41). Linear furocoumarins, including the potent photosensitizers xanthotoxin and bergapten, were subsequently isolated from *C. watsoni* (42,43). A related plant, *C. longipes*, is also a strong photosensitizer in ducks, chickens, and turkeys (43), and has recently been shown to contain phototoxic furocoumarins (44).

Bishops weed (*Ammi majus*), used for centuries in Egypt in the treatment of leukoderma (2), was first implicated in the photosensitization of domestic animals by Israeli workers in 1974 (46-48). A field outbreak of photosensitization in goslings was traced to the ingestion of *A. majus* growing abundantly in the open rearing pastures (46). The condition was reproduced experimentally in young geese (47-49) and ducklings (50). As little as 0.5 g of *A. majus* seeds/bird/day induced severe sunlight photosensitization in the young birds, with subsequent deformation of the beak, feet, wings, and ocular areas that persisted as permanent structures (49,50).

Photosensitization of dairy cattle by *A. majus* has also been reported from Israel (51). Cattle that were confined outdoors ingested feed "extensively" contaminated with *A. majus* for about

1 week, and experienced blistering and peeling on the unpigmented areas of the muzzle, udder, teats, and vulva. Milk production was reduced by about 20%. Two weeks after feeding of the *A. majus*-contaminated ration was discontinued, the cattle had almost completely recovered and milk production was back to normal. A group of heifers that received the same *A. majus* contaminated ration, but were housed under a covered shed, showed no symptoms of photosensitization (49).

Ammi majus also is found in the coastal regions of the southern United States, and as far as 150 miles inland. In Texas, periodic severe outbreaks of photosensitization, affecting thousands of animals, have been observed in cattle for many years. The distribution of these outbreaks coincides with the distribution of *A. majus* (52). The photosensitization syndrome in cattle involves severe blistering and peeling in light-skinned animals, and cloudy corneas which can lead to blindness. Apparently blind white-tail deer have been observed in areas where the photosensitization of cattle is a problem (52). Although it is not certain that the causative agent in these field outbreaks of photosensitization is *A. majus*, recent studies in our laboratory have shown that experimental feeding of *A. majus* to cattle and sheep, followed by exposure to sunlight, induces a photosensitization syndrome very similar to that seen in the field (52,53). Cattle fed whole *A. majus* plant (in various stages of maturity but containing little seed) at levels as high as 10 g/kg/day experienced blistering and subsequent necrosis and peeling of the skin of the muzzle (52). Sheep fed the whole plant (52) or mature seed (53) suffered more seriously from photosensitization, with symptoms including severe erythema, blistering, and necrosis of the ears, vulva, and muzzle. Sheep given a single oral dose of mature *A. majus* seed at levels as low as 2 g/kg showed within 4 days cloudy corneas, corneal edema, and keratoconjunctivitis. The eye lesions were of such severity that it was concluded that permanent blindness could be expected in some cases (53).

Analysis of the furocoumarins in the mature seed of the Texas *A. majus* has revealed twelve 4- and/or 9-alkoxy substituted psoralens, including xanthotoxin and bergapten as major components, but also including several furocoumarins that have not previously been reported from this plant (54). Assay of these compounds for photosensitizing activity is underway (55).

V. CONCLUSIONS

A cursory review of the recent literature indicates that potentially photoactive furocoumarins have been isolated from at least a hundred plant species. To date, however, only 4 furocoumarin-containing plants have been shown to cause photosensitization in domestic animals: *Ammi visnaga* in Uruguay and Israel; *A. majus* in Israel and the United States; and *Cymopterus watsoni* and *C. longipes* in the United States. The photosensitization syndrome produced by each of these plants is similar and can be summarized as follows: In young birds, the acute effects are inflammatory in nature and include erythema and blistering on the beak, feet, and exposed skin which subsequently forms a thick crust or scab. Keratoconjunctivitis is usually observed and is often followed by closure of the eyes with serous fluid that dries and seals the eyelids together. Chronically, young birds experience deformation of the upper beak, feet, and legs, sloughing of the comb and wattles in chickens, and scarring of the ocular opening. More serious ocular lesions are seen in ducks and geese (49,50). In cattle and sheep, acute effects of erythema and blistering on the non-pigmented areas of the muzzle, ears, vulva, and mammary glands are often accompanied by keratoconjunctivitis and cloudy cornea, which may lead to blindness in some cases. The only other apparent chronic effect in cattle and sheep is occasional permanent damage to the tips of the ears (41).

Although documented cases of furocoumarin photosensitization in domestic animals are few, the occurrence of these compounds in a large number of plant species suggests that furocoumarins may be involved in a significant portion of the photosensitization cases observed in domestic animals. Furocoumarins should certainly be suspected where animals experience photosensitization syndromes similar to those described above. Because furocoumarin-containing plants are known to cause contact photodermatitis in man (3), the possibility that certain of these plants may evoke similar responses in domestic animals merits consideration.

VI. REFERENCES

1. Fitzpatrick, T. B., and Pathak, M. A., *J. Invest. Dermatol.* 32, 229 (1959).
2. Fahmy, I. R., and Abu-Shady, H., *Q. J. Pharm. Pharmacol.* 21, 499 (1948).
3. Pathak, M. A., Daniels, F., and Fitzpatrick, T. B., *J. Invest. Dermatol.* 39, 225 (1962).
4. Scott, B. R., Pathak, M. A., and Mohn, G. R., *Mutat. Res.* 39, 29 (1976).
5. Balbaa, S. I., Hilal, S. H., and Haggay, M. Y., *Egypt J. Pharm. Sci.* 16, 351 (1956).
6. Bradu, B. L., and Atal, C. K., *Indian J. Pharm.* 32, 165 (1970).
7. Sarin, Y. K., and Jamwal, P. S., *Indian J. Pharm.* 37, 145 (1975).
8. Johnson, C., Brannon, D. R., and Kuc, J., *Phytochemistry* 12, 2961 (1973).
9. Scheel, L. D., Perone, V. B., Larkin, R. L., and Kupel, R. E., *Biochemistry* 2, 1127 (1963).
10. Wu, C. M., Koehler, P. E., and Ayres, J. C., *Appl. Microbiol.* 23, 852 (1972).
11. Yu, H., *Kuo Li Tai-wan Ta Hsueh Chih Wu Ping Ch'ung Hai Huseh*

Kan 4, 133 (1975) (*Chem. Abs.* 84:176825W, 1976).
12. Musajo, L., and Rodighiero, G., *Photophysiology* 7, 115 (1972).
13. Stegmaier, O. C., *J. Invest. Dermatol.* 32, 345 (1959).
14. Van Scott, E. J., *J. Am. Med. Assoc.* 235, 197 (1976).
15. Pathak, M. A., Kramer, D. M., Fitzpatrick, T. B., *in* "Sunlight and Man" (M. A. Pathak, Ed.), p. 335. University of Tokyo Press, 1974.
16. Feuer, G., *Prog. Med. Chem.* 10, 85 (1974).
17. Richards, D. E., *Microb. Toxins* 8, 3 (1972).
18. Scheel, L. D., *Microb. Toxins* 8, 47 (1972).
19. Perone, V. B., *Microb. Toxins* 8, 67 (1972).
20. El Mofty, A. M., *J. Egypt. Med. Assoc.* 31, 651 (1948).
21. Mukherji, A., *J. Sci. Ind. Res.* 19, 223 (1960).
22. Klingman, A. M., and Goldstein, F. P., *Arch. Dermatol.* 107, 548 (1973).
23. Daniels, F., Hopkins, C. E., Imbrie, D. J., Bergerson, L., Miller, O., Crowe, F., and Fitzpatrick, P. B., *J. Invest. Dermatol.* 32, 321 (1959).
24. O'Neal, M. A., and Griffin, A. C., *Cancer Res.* 17, 911 (1957).
25. Hakim, R. E., Griffin, A. C., and Knox, M., *Arch. Dermatol.* 82, 522 (1960).
26. Forbes, P. D., Davies, R. E., and Urback, F., *Food Cosmet. Toxicol.* 14, 303 (1976).
27. MacDonald, E. J., Griffin, A. C., Hopkins, C. E., Smith, L., Garrett, H., and Black, G. I., *J. Invest. Dermatol.* 41, 213 (1963).
28. Spath, E., and Kuffner, F., *Monatschrift* 69, 75 (1936).
29. Schonberg, A., and Latif, N., *J. Am. Chem. Soc.* 76, 6208 (1954).
30. Dadak, V., and Hodak, K., *Experientia* 22, 38 (1966).
31. Vichkonova, S. A., Rubinchik, M. A., Adgina, V. V., Izosimova, S. B., Makarova, L. V., Shipuliana, L. D., and Goryunova, L. V., *Rastit. Resur.*9, 370 (1973) (Chem. Abs. 79:111980V, 1973).
32. Fowlks, W. L., Griffith, D. G., and Oginsky, E. L., *Nature* 181, 571 (1958).
33. Mikkelson, V. E., Fowlks, E. W., and Griffith, D. G., *Arch. Phys. Med. Rehabil.* 42, 609 (1961).
34. Trenchi, M., *Avian Dis.* 4, 275 (1960).
35. Shlosberg, A., Egyed, M. N., and Eilat, A., *Avian Dis.* 18, 544 (1974).
36. Egyed, M. N., Shlosberg, A., and Eilat, A., *Avian Dis.* 19, 831 (1975).
37. Harrison, P. G., Bailey, B. K., and Steck, W., *Can. J. Biochem.* 49, 964 (1971).
38. Pimenov, M. G., and Pogorecova, O. U., *Rastit. Resur.* 10, 216 (1974).
39. Binns, W., James, L. F., and Brooksby, W., *Vet. Med. Small Anim. Clin.* 59, 375 (1964).

40. Williams, M. C., and Binns, W., *Am. J. Vet. Res.* 29, 111 (1968).
41. Van Kampen, K. R., Williams, M. C., and Binns, W., *Am. J. Vet. Res.* 30, 1663 (1969).
42. Williams, M. C., *Weed Sci.* 18, 479 (1970).
43. Stermitz, F. R., Thomas, R. D., and Williams, M. C., *Phytochemistry* 14, 1681 (1975).
44. Yost, G. S., Stermitz, F. R., and Williams, M. C., *Phytochemistry* 16, 1097 (1977).
45. Egyed, M. W., Shlosberg, A., and Eilat, A., *Vet. Human Toxicol.* 19, 11 (1977).
46. Eilat, A., Malkinson, M., Shlosberg, A., and Egyed, M. N., *Refu. Vet.* 31, 83 (1974).
47. Egyed, M. N., Malkinson, M., and Shlosberg, A., *Avian Pathol.* 3, 79 (1974).
48. Shlosberg, A., Egyed, M. N., and Eilat, A., *Avian Dis.* 18, 544 (1974).
49. Egyed, M. N., Shlosberg, A., Eilat, A., and Malkinson, M., *Avian Dis.* 19, 822 (1975).
50. Egyed, M. N., Shlosberg, A., Eilat, A., and Malkinson, M., *Vet. Rec.* 97, 198 (1975).
51. Egyed, M. N., Shlosberg, A., Cohen, U., and Beemek, A., *Refu. Vet.* 31, 128 (1974).
52. Dollahite, J. W., Younger, R. L., and Hoffman, G. O., *Am. J. Vet. Res.* In press (1977).
53. Witzel, D. A., Dollahite, J. W., and Jones, L. P., *J. Am. Vet. Med. Assoc.* In press (1977).
54. Ivie, G. W., Unpublished data (1977).
55. Witzel, D. A., and Ivie, G. W., Unpublished data (1977).

SESQUITERPENE LACTONES FROM LIVESTOCK POISONS

Werner Herz
Department of Chemistry, The Florida State University

I. ABSTRACT

The different classes of naturally-occurring sesquiterpene lactones are described briefly. Certain sesquiterpene lactones are responsible for the toxicity of several livestock poisons in the U.S., such as Helenium autumnale, microcephalum *and* tenuifolium, Hymenoxys odorata *and* richardsonii, *and* Dugaldia hoopesii. *Sesquiterpene lactones may also be responsible for the toxicity of some other livestock poisons belonging to the Compositae. Possible reasons for the toxic effects of the lactones involved in livestock poisoning are suggested.*

II. INTRODUCTION

Sesquiterpene lactones are characteristic constituents of Compositae or certain subdivisions thereof although instances of their occurrence in other plant families are coming to light (for recent reviews see refs. 1 and 2). In the present contribution, the occurrence and toxicity of sesquiterpene lactones in some well-known stock poisons of the Compositae family will be discussed.

In Fig. 1, various classes of known sesquiterpene lactones are arranged in order of what might be called "increasing biogenetic complexity." Such a scheme is useful for systematizing the nearly 700 sesquiterpene lactones that are now known, as well as for illuminating phylogenetic relationships among plants, as has been done at various levels of the Compositae (1-5). The reader is referred to these references and to an article now in press (Herz, W., Israel Journal of Chemistry) for a discussion of the various classes of sesquiterpene lactones, their distribution within Compositae and possible biogenetic routes leading to them. For the purpose of this article, it is sufficient to state that germacranolides of various types and guaianolides are most widely distributed in the various tribes and represent about 35% and 20% of the total number of lactones known so far, that eudesmanolides (~15%) are mainly, but not exclusively, concentrated in the Anthemidae, that helenanolides and secohelenanolides (~12%) are so far primarily restricted to subtribe Gaillardinae of Heleniantheae (for at least one signficant exception see later) whereas ambrosanolides and secoambrosanolides (about 8%) are found in subtribe Ambrosiinae which also encompasses most of the xanthanolides (~5%). Representatives of the remaining classes comprise the rest of the total.

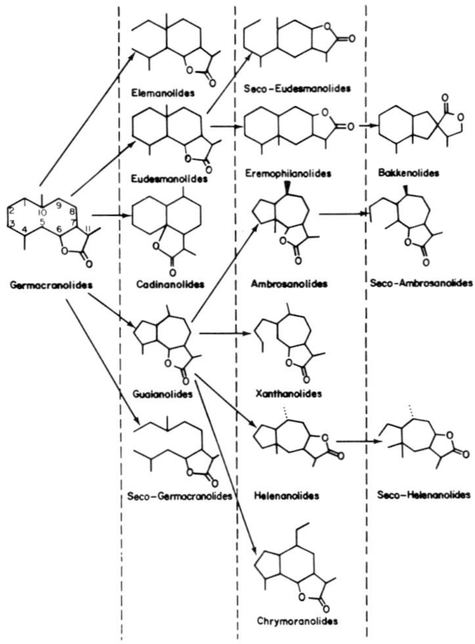

Fig. 1. *Classes of sesquiterpene lactones in Compositae. Arrangement illustrates presumed biogenetic relationships.*

III. *HELENIUM* SPECIES (SNEEZE WEEDS)

Historically, the first sesquiterpene lactones isolated and characterized from stock poisons were those from sneeze weeds (*Helenium sp.*), several of which are known to be toxic when eaten by livestock (6). Helenalin, the main constituent (7,8) of *H. autumnale* L. which is widely distributed through the southeastern U.S., was shown to be highly irritating to the nose, eyes, and stomach (9) and toxic to dogs (9,10). Its structure was shown to be 1, a helenanolide, then representing a novel sesquiterpene lactone skeleton, as the result of an extensive series of studies due mainly to Herz and coworkers (11). A number of minor constituents of *H. autumnale*, all chemically closely related to helenalin, have since been characterized (12-15); in addition the discovery of chemovars of *H. autumnale* (13,16-18) has highlighted the well-known variability of the species which is now being restudied (private communication from Dr. M. W. Bierner).

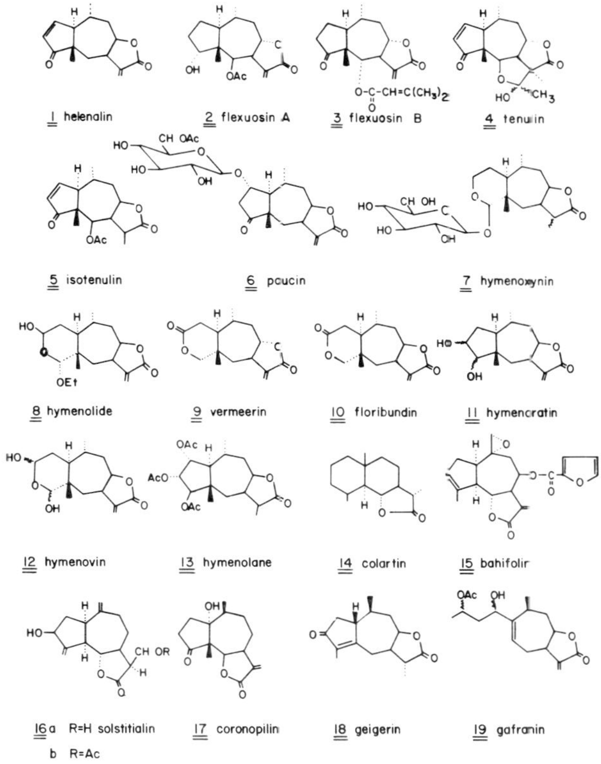

Fig. 2. *Individual sesquiterpene lactones.*

Helenalin is also the main constituent of *H. microcephalum* DC (small head sneeze weed) (1,19,20), apparently one of the most toxic plants of this group [as little as 2.5 g of green plant/kg of body weight causes acute poisoning and death in cattle (21)] (for some minor constituents see 22).

That helenalin is the only significant toxic constituent of *H. microcephalum* has been confirmed by an extensive study (23) of its mammalian toxicity (sheep, mice, rabbit, and hamsters), its oral median lethal dose being between 85 and 150 mg/kg. Since helenalin is found not only in *H. microcephalum* and *H. autumnale*, but in a number of other *Helenium* (2,24) as well as in one Western and two South American *Gaillardia* species, it may contribute to the toxicity of a number of species whose distribution is such that it has not made them known as livestock poisons. *H. flexuosum*

Raf. (=*H. nudiflorum* Nutt.) which is reported to be a livestock poison (6) yielded two helenanolides 2 and 3 closely related to helenalin (2) which may account for the toxicity of this plant.

H. amarum (Raf.) Rock (=*H. tenuifolium* Nutt., Southeastern bitterweed) is widely distributed in the southeastern U.S. and is of economic importance to the dairy industry, because its ingestion imparts a bitter taste to milk and renders it impalatable. It is also a livestock poison (6), but seems to affect horses and mules to greater extent than other species (25,26). As the result of work mainly by Herz and coworkers (11,27), tenulin, the very bitter principle (28-30) whose presence in milk at levels as low as 1 ppm renders it unsalable, was shown to to a mixture of two epimers 4, also belonging to the helenanolide series. When treated with weak base, tenulin is isomerized to isotenulin (5) which itself may be a minor constituent of *H. amarum* and other *Helenium* species (2). Some minor constituents of *H. amarum* closely related to isotenulin have also been identified (30). A recent thorough study of the toxicity of tenulin (31) showed that while it was by far the most poisonous constituent present, its toxicity was low and that human consumption of milk resulting from dairy animals grazing on *H. amarum* did not constitute a significant health hazard. The distribution of tenulin, isotenulin and related compounds in other *Helenium* and *Gaillardia* species has been summarized (2).

IV. *HYMENOXYS* SPECIES

Hymenoxys odorata DC (western bitterweed) is an important livestock poison in its range (Southwestern U.S.) which causes considerable loss of sheep (6) and occasionally cattle (32). Another species, *Hymenoxys richardsonii* (Hook.) Ckll. var. *floribunda* (pingue) causes extensive loss of sheep in Colorado, New Mexico, and Arizona, although cattle and goats may also be affected (6). The symptoms of Western Bitterweed and pingue poisoning have been described (6) and appear to be similar.

In the course of their phytochemical studies of *Hymenoxys* species (33-36), Herz and coworkers (33) isolated the helenanolides and modified helenanolides paucin (6), hymenoxynin (7), and hymenolide (8) from *H. odorata* and vermeerin (9) and floribundin (psilostrophin, 10) from *H. richardsonii*, established their structure and suggested that one or more of these substances might be responsible for the toxicity because they and related lactones exhibited cytotoxicity and antileukemic activity *in vivo*. Somewhat earlier, the helenanolide hymenoratin (11) which can be looked upon as a biological precursor of 8 had been isolated from a more Southern collection of *H. odorata* (37). Subsequent thorough studies (38,39) resulted in isolation and identification of hymenovin (12),[1] a mixture of two hemiacetals epimeric at C-2

[1]It is most likely that hymenolide (8) isolated earlier (33) is an artifact which results from reaction of one of the isomers of hymenovin with ethyl alcohol during one stage of purification.

or C-4, as the principle responsible for most, if not all, of the toxicity of *H. odorata* and *H. richardsonii*; it was lethal to sheep when given orally at levels as low as 100 mg/kg. Necropsy of sheep poisoned with hymenovin revealed severe congestion and areas of mucosal surface on the rumen, reticulum and abomasum. Severe toxic nephrosis with heavy proteinaceous casts and tubular degeneration was noted, primarily at the cortico-medullary junction, as well as toxic hepatosis. Partial characterization of hymenovin was also achieved by another group (40); more recently X-ray analysis of one of the two hymenovin epimers (named hymenoxon) whose stereochemistry corresponds to that of 8 and that of a minor substance 13 (hymenolane) found in *H. odorata* has confirmed the earlier findings (41).

In view of the fact that 6, 9, 10, and a variety of other helenanolides have been isolated from other *Hymenoxys* species which apparently do not serve as forage plants, it is likely that the reported toxicity of *H. lemmoni* (Greene) CK11, (6) may also be attributed to hymenovin or a varient thereof.

V. MISCELLANEOUS SPECIES

A. *Dugaldia hoopesii* Rydb. (=*Helenium hoopesii* Gray) (Orange Sneezeweed)

The poisonous properties of this species which is a major economic problem for sheep raisers on the summer ranges of the central Rocky Mountains (6) and which result in what is called "spewing sickness" have long been ascribed to a glycoside "dugaldin" (6); however, recent work (39) has shown that hymenovin (12) is the major toxic principle of this plant as well. Whether "dugaldin" is involved at all is problematical (12). The symptoms associated with "spewing sickness" are also those produced by administration of hymenovin (12).

B. *Psilostrophe* Species (Paperflowers)

P. gnaphalodes DC, *P. tagetinae* (Nutt). Greene and *P. sparsiflora* (Gray) A. Nels. have caused important loss of life of sheep on southwestern ranges, with *P. gnaphalodes* being restricted to Texas (6). Although these three species have not been investigated chemically, chemical study of a related species, *P. cooperi* (Gray) Greene, yielded (42) floribundin (psilostrophin, 10). Since the symptoms of *Psilostrophe* poisoning are similar to those reported for *Hymenoxys* and *Dugaldia* poisoning (6), the notion that hymenovin or one of its variants may be responsible for its toxicity seems plausible and warrants further investigation.

C. *Artemisia filifolia* Torr. (Sand Sage Brush)

This plant is credited with causing a disease of horses known as "sage sickness." Chemical investigation has led to the isolation of a eudesmanolide colartin (14), but nothing is known about the toxicity of this substance. Since almost all *Artemisia* species elaborate sesquiterpene lactones (1), the fact that *A. spinescens* DC Eat. has come under suspicion (6) may conceivably be traceable to a sesquiterpene lactone.

D. *Bahia oppositifolia* (Nutt.) DC

The toxicity of this species is said to be due to a cyanogenetic glycoside (6). However, all *Bahia* species investigated so far elaborate cytotoxic sesquiterpene lactones (44,45). From the above species, the guaianolide bahifolin (15) was isolated (44) which might conceivably be responsible for the toxicity.

E. *Baileya multiradiata* Harv. Gray (Desert Baileya)

Poisoning by Desert Baileya results typically from ingestion of relatively large amounts of the green plant by sheep on the range, with mortality reaching as high as 25% in bands of sheep in certain areas of Texas (6). The symptoms have been described (6). At least six sesquiterpene lactones of different types (germacranolides, guaianolides, helenanolides), several of which exhibit cytotoxicity and antitumor activity, have been isolated from this species (47,48); hence the poisoning effect might well be due to one or more of these constituents, although no feeding experiments have been carried out.

F. *Centaurea solstitialis* L. (Yellow Star Thistle)

This plant is responsible for "chewing disease" or nigropallidal encephalomalacia, a disease apparently restricted to saddle and light horses of California (6), although the plant is of mediterranean origin and of wide distribution. Production of germacranolides and guaianolides is characteristic of *Centaurea* species (1); two of them, solstitialin (16a) and solstitialin acetate (16b), have been isolated from California collections of this species (49) but nothing is known of their toxicity.

G. *Iva acerosa* (Nutt.) Jackson (=*Oxytenia acerosa* Nutt., Copperweed)

The toxicity of this species for cattle and sheep has been well established and the symptoms have been described (6).

Copperweed elaborates (50) the cytotoxic ambrosanolide coronopilin (17) which is also found in some other *Iva* species as well as in many representatives of *Ambrosia*, *Hymenoclea*, and *Parthenium* (2). Whether the substance is responsible for the toxicity of this species to stock has not been established.

H. *Viguiera annua* (Jones) Blake (Annual Goldeneye)

Cattle losses in New Mexico have been associated with ingestion of large amounts of this plant (6). Since Mexican species of this genus have been shown to contain sesquiterpene lactones (51), it is possible that the toxicity of *V. annua* is due to a substance of this type.

I. *Geigeria* Species

"Vermeerbos" (vomiting bush) represents various *Geigeria* species which cause heavy annual loss of sheep in South Africa through "vermeersiekte" (vomiting disease). The symptoms which are very similar to those produced by *Hymenoxys* and *Dugaldia* poisoning have been ascribed to a substance "vermeeric acid" (52), supposedly the acid corresponding to a dilactone vermeerin isolated originally from *G. aspera* Harv. (53), but later found in *G. africana* Gries (54), the species mainly responsible for "vermeersiekte." In the more recent work (54), "vermeeric acid" could not be isolated from *G. africana*; but neither vermeerin (9) whose structure has already been discussed, geigerin (18), the main lactone constituent of *G. aspera* (53,55,56) also found in *G. africana* (57), nor the minor sesquiterpene lactones geigerinin (a helenanolide) in *G. aspera* (57) and *africana* (54), or gafranin (58), griesenin and dihydrogriesenin (59), three xanthanolides from *G. africana*, were responsible for the toxic effects. Because of the association of vermeerin (9) and floribundin (10) with the toxic principle hymenovin (12) in *Hymenoxys* species, it is quite possible that "vermeeric acid" is either identical with hymenovin or is related to vermeerin as hymenovin is to floribundin (38).

VI. TOXICITY OF SESQUITERPENE LACTONES

The cytotoxic and antitumor activity of many sesquiterpene lactones has been linked to the presence of the α,β-unsaturated γ-lactone function found, for example, in 1,2,6,9,12, and 17, as well as to the presence of other functions potentially able to alkylate sulfhydryl groups of key enzymes (60). The circumstance that the mercaptan cysteine is antidotal to hymenovin poisoning in hamsters (38, see also 32) suggests that mercaptans may be useful antidotes for poisoning by western bitterweed and related plants by inactivating the toxin within the intestinal tract or bloodstream. They cannot be expected to reverse the biochemical lesions produced if alkylation is indeed a major mechanism of action. Since many sesquiterpene lactones are also antimicrobial agents (61), it is possible that sesquiterpene lactone toxins also exert their action by altering the microbial composition of rumen and thus affecting its vital metabolic function. Hence dysfunction may contribute to the toxicity caused by sesquiterpene lactones in stock poisons.

VII. ACKNOWLEDGMENTS

Financial support from the United States Public Health Service (CA-13121) through the National Cancer Service and the Hoffman-La Roche Foundation is gratefully acknowledged.

VIII. REFERENCES

1. Herz, W., *in* "Chemistry and Biology of the Compositae (V. Heywood, B. L. Turner, and J. B. Harborne, Eds.), p. 320. Academic Press, London, 1977.
2. Herz, W., *in* "Chemistry in Botanical Classification (G. Bendz and J. Santesson, Eds.), Nobel Symposium 25, p. 153. Nobel Foundation, Stockholm, and Academic Press, New York and London, 1973.
3. Geissman, T. A., and Irwin, M. A., *in* "Chemistry in Botanical Classification (G. Bendz and J. Santesson, Eds.), Nobel Symposium 25, p. 135. Nobel Foundation, Stockholm, and Academic Press, New York and London, 1973.
4. Mabry, T. J., *in* "Phytochemical Phylogeny," (J. B. Harborne, Ed.), p. 269. Academic Press, London, 1970.
5. Yoshioka, H., Mabry, T. J., and Timmermann, B. N., "Sesquiterpene Lactones," University of Tokyo Press, 1973.
6. Kingsbury, J. M., "Poisonous Plants of the United States and Canada," Prentice-Hall, Englewood Cliffs, N. J., 1964.
7. Reeb, E., *J. Pharm. Elsass-Lothringen* 37, 149 (1910).
8. Clark, E. P., *J. Am. Chem. Soc.* 58, 1982 (1936).
9. Lamson, P. D., *J. Pharmacol. Exp. Ther.* 4, 471 (1973).
10. Szabuniewicz, M., and Kim, H. L., *Southwest Vet.* 25, 305 (1972).
11. Romo, J., and Romo de Vivar, A., *in* "Progress in the Chemistry of Natural Products," (L. Zechmeister, Ed.), Vol. 25, p. 90. Springer Verlag, Vienna and New York, 1967.
12. Lucas, R. A., Smith, R. G., and Dorfman, L., *J. Org. Chem.* 29, 2101 (1964).
13. Herz, W., Subramaniam, P. S., and Dennis, N., *J. Org. Chem.* 34, 2915 (1969).
14. Lee, K. H., Ibuka, T., McPhail, A. T., Onan, K. A., Geissman and Waddell, T. G., *Tetrahedron Lett.* 1149 (1974); Lee, K. H., Ibuka, T., Kozuka, M., McPhail, A. T., and Onan,

K. D., *Tetrahedron Lett.* 2287 (1974); Kozuka, M., Lee, K. H., McPhail, A. T., and Onan, K. D., *Chem. Pharm. Bull.* 23, 1895 (1975).

15. Pettit, G. R., Budzinski, J. C., Cragg, G. M., Brown, P., and Johnston, L. D., *J. Med. Chem.* 17, 1013 (1974); von Dreele, R. B., Pettit, G. R., Cragg, G. M., and Ode, R. H., *J. Am. Chem. Soc.* 97, 5256 (1975).
16. Herz, W., and Subramaniam, P. S., *Phytochemistry* 11, 1101 (1972).
17. Hikino, H., Kuwano, D., and Takemoto, T., *Chem. Pharm. Bull.* 16, 1601 (1968).
18. Furukawa, H., Lee, K. H., Shingu, T., Meck, R., and Piantadosi, C., *J. Org. Chem.* 38, 1722 (1973); McPhail, A. T., Luhan, P. A., Lee, K. H., Furukawa, H., Meck, R., Piantadosi, C., and Shingu, T., *Tetrahedron Lett.* 4087 (1973); McPhail, A. T., Onan, K. D., Furukawa, H., and Lee, K. H., *Tetrahedron Lett.* 1229 (1975).
19. Clark, E. P., *J. Am. Chem. Soc.* 61, 1836 (1940); 62, 597 (1940).
20. Adams, R., and Herz, W., *J. Am. Chem. Soc.* 71, 2546, 2551, 2554 (1949).
21. Dollahite, J. W., Hardy, W. T., and Henson, J. B., *J. Am. Vet. Med. Assoc.* 145, 694 (1964).
22. Lee, K. H., Imakura, Y., and Sims, D., *J. Pharm. Sci.* 65, 1410 (1976); Lee, K. H., Imakura, Y., Sims, D., McPhail, A. T., and Onan, K. D., *J. Chem. Soc. Chem. Commun.* 341 (1976).
23. Witzel, D. A., Ivie, G. W., and Dollahite, J. W., *Am. J. Vet. Res.* 37, 859 (1976).
24. Bierner, M. W., *Biochem. Syst.* 1, 95 (1973).
25. West, E., and Emmel, M. W., *Univ. Fla. Agric. Exp. Stn. Bull.* 510, 25 (1952).

26a. Dollahite, J. W., Rowe, L. D., Kim, H. L., and Camp, B. J., *Southwest Vet.* 26, 135 (1972).

26b. McDonald, M. B., and Glaser, A., *Tenn. Agric. Exp. Stn. Cir.* 26, 19 (1929).

27. Herz, W., and Sharma, R. P., *J. Org. Chem.* 40, 2557 (1975).
28. Buehler, C. A., Whitehead, F., and Goodge, B. D., *J. Am. Chem. Soc.* 59, 2299 (1937).
29. Clark, E. P., *J. Am. Chem. Soc.* 61, 1836 (1939).
30. Lucas, R. A., Rovinski, S., Kiesel, R. J., Dorfman, L., and McPhillamy, H. B., *J. Org. Chem.* 29, 1549 (1964).
31. Ivie, G. W., Witzel, D. A., and Rushing, D. D., *J. Agric. Food Chem.* 23, 845 (1975).
32. Kim, H. L., Rowe, L. D., Szabuniewicz, M., Dollahite, J. W., and Camp, *Southwest Vet.* 28, 84 (1974).
33. Herz, W., Aota, K., Holub, M., and Samek, Z., *J. Org. Chem.* 35, 3338 (1970).
34. Herz, W., Aota, K., and Hall, A. L., *J. Org. Chem.* 35, 4117 (1970).

35. Wagner, H., Iyengar, M. A., Hörhammer, L., and Herz, W., *Phytochemistry* 11, 3087 (1972).
36. Herz, W., Aota, K., Hall, A. L., and Srinivasan, A., *J. Org. Chem.* 39, 2013 (1974).
37. Ortega, A., Romo de Vivar, A., and Romo, J., *Can. J. Chem.* 46, 1538 (1968).
38. Ivie, G. W., Witzel, D. A., Herz, W., Kannan, R., Norman, J. O., Rushing, D. D., Johnson, J. H., Rowe, L. D., and Veech, J. A., *J. Agric. Food Chem.* 23, 814 (1975).
39. Ivie, G. W., Witzel, D. A., Herz, W., Sharma, R. P., and Johnson, A. E., *J. Agric. Food Chem.* 23, 681 (1976).
40. Kim, H. L., Szabuniewicz, M., Rowe, L. D., Camp, B. J., Dollahite, J. W., and Bridges, C. H., *Res. Commun. Chem. Pathol. Pharmacol.* 8, 381 (1974).
41. Kim, H. L., Rowe, L. D., and Camp, B. J., *Res. Commun. Chem. Pathol. Pharmacol.* 11, 647 (1975); Pettersen, R. C., and Kim, H. L., *J. C. S. Perkin II* 1399 (1976).
42. de Silva, L. B., and Geissman, T. A., *Phytochemistry* 9, 59 (1970).
43. Torrance, S. J., and Steelink, C., *J. Org. Chem.* 39, 1068 (1974).
44. Herz, W., Bhat, S. V., Crawford, H., Wagner, H., Maurer, G., and Farkas, L., *Phytochemistry* 11, 371 (1972).
45. Romo de Vivar, A., and Ortega, A., *Can. J. Chem.* 47, 2849 (1969).
46. Herz, W., and Bhat, S. V., *J. Org. Chem.* 37, 906 (1972).
47. Waddell, T. G., and Geissman, T. A., *Phytochemistry* 8, 2371 (1969).
48. Pettit, G. R., Herald, C. L., Judd, G. F., Bollinger, G., and Thayer, P. S., *J. Pharm. Sci.* 64, 2023 (1975).
49. Thiessen, W. E., Hope, H., Zarghani, Heinz, E., Deuel, P., and Hahn, E. A., *Chem. Ind.* 460 (1969); Zarghani, N., and Heinz, D. E., *Chem. Ind.* 1557 (1969).
50. Farkas, L., Nogradi, M., Sudarsanam, V., and Herz, W., *J. Org. Chem.* 31, 3228 (1966).
51. Cuevas, L. A., Garcia Jiminez, F., and Romo de Vivar, *Rev. Latino-am. Quim.* 3, 22 (1972); Guerrero, C., Ortega, A., Diaz, E., and Romo de Vivar, A., *Rev. Latino-am. Quim.* 4, 118 (1973); Guerrero, C., Santana, M., and Romo, J., *Rev. Latino-am. Quim.* 7, 41 (1976); Romo de Vivar, Guerrero, C., Diaz, E., Bratoeff, E. A., and Jimenez, L., *Phytochemistry* 15, 525 (1976).
52. Rimington, C., Roets, G. C. S., and Steyn, D. G., *Onderstepoort J. Vet. Sci.* 7, 507 (1936); de Waal, *Onderstepoort J. Vet. Sci.* 10, 395 (1938).
53. Rimington, C., and Roets, G. C. S., *Onderstepoort J. Vet. Sci.* 17, 485 (1936).
54. Anderson, L. A. P., de Kock, W. T., Pachler, K. G. R., and v. d. M. Brink, C., *Tetrahedron* 23, 4153 (1967).
55. Perold, G. W., *J. S. Afr. Chem. Inst.* 8, 12 (1955); *J. Chem. Soc.* 47 (1957).

56. Barton, D. H. R., and Levisalles, J. E. D., *J. Chem. Soc.* 4518 (1958); Barton, D. H. R., and Pinhey, J. T., *Proc. Chem. Soc.* 279 (1960); Barton, D. H. R., Pinhey, J. T., and Wells, R. J., *J. Chem. Soc.* 2518 (1964).
57. de Villiers, J. P., *J. Chem. Soc* 2412 (1959); de Villiers, J. P., and Pachler, K. G. R., *J. Chem. Soc.* 4989 (1969).
58. de Villiers, J. P., *J. Chem. Soc.* 2048 (1961); Anderson, L. A. P., de Kock, W. F., Nel, W., and Pachler, K. G. R., *Tetrahedron* 24, 1687 (1968); de Kock, W. T., and Pachler, K. G. R., *Tetrahedron* 24, 1701 (1960).
59. de Kock, W. T., Pachler, K. G. R., Ross, W. F., Wessels, P. L., and DuPreez, I. C., *Tetrahedron* 24, 6037 (1968); de Kock, W. T., Pachler, K. G. R., and Wessels, P. L., *Tetrahedron* 24, 6045 (1968).
60. Hanson, R. L., Lardy, H. A., and Kupchan, S. M., *Science* 168, 378 (1970); Kupchan, S. M., *Trans. N. Y. Acad. Sci.* 32, 85 (1970); Kupchan, S. M., Fesster, D. C., Eakin, M. A., and Giacobbe, T. J., *Science* 168, 376 (1970); Kupchan, S. M., Eakin, M. A., and Thomas, A. M., *J. Med. Chem.* 14, 1147 (1971).
61. For a review of biological activities of sesquiterpene lactones in general, see Rodriguez, E., Towers, G. H. N., and Mitchell, J. C., *Phytochemistry* 15, 1537 (1976).

OAK POISONING IN CATTLE

R. J. Panciera
College of Veterinary Medicine, Oklahoma State University

I. ABSTRACT

Oak poisoning of cattle occurs in sporadic or minor epidemic proportion in many parts of the world. The buds, leaves, twigs, and seeds of many species are toxic. Tannins or their metabolites are thought to be the poisonous principle. Signs of alimentary and renal dysfunction are prominent features of disease. Renal functional deficit, the result of toxic renal tubular necrosis is a fundamental process. All diseased animals have elevated levels of blood urea nitrogen; many are hypoproteinemic, hypoalbuminemic, hyponatremic, hyperkalemic, hypochloremic, hypocalcemic, and hyperphostatemic. Therapy is largely symptomatic and of questionable efficacy. Control measures involve management of animals to avoid exposure to toxic quantities of the plant during seasons of high risk.

II. INTRODUCTION

Poisoning of cattle by ingestion of oak buds, leaves, twigs, and acorns occurs in many parts of the world. The disease has been reported from widespread regions of the U.S.A. (1-15) and from Europe (16-26).

There are more than 60 species of oak in North America (6). Several species are known to be toxic; Kingsbury suggests that all should be regarded as potentially toxic (6). Species identified as common causes of toxicity in U.S.A. are *Quercus havardii*, *Q. breviloba*, and *Q. gambelii* (2,3,6,9). The species most commonly mentioned in European literature is *Q. robur* (16,17,18,23,24). Reported with less frequency is poisoning by *Q. marilandica*, *Q. velutina*, *Q. rubra* var. *borealis*, *Q. prinus*, *Q. stellata*, *Q. coccinea*, *Q. lobata*, and *Q. incana* (5,6,32). Many reports of poisoning do not identify the responsible species.

Disease may occur sporadically or in epidemic proportion (2, 17) and appears to be identical regardless of the part of the plant consumed (6). Disease occurs seasonally, bud and leaf poisoning in the spring and acorn poisoning in the fall. I have, however, seen disease in mid and late summer due to consumption of leaves under extreme drouth conditions when normal herbage was not available.

Seasonal incidence may be related not only to seasonal availability of the various parts of the plant but also to variances in toxicity at different times of the year. Young leaves and recently fallen green acorns are thought to be more toxic than mature leaves and dry acorns (16,23). Pigeon *et al.* (28) demonstrated marked reduction in tannin content of oak leaves as they matured. Further, young leaves are considerably more palatable than mature leaves (3,9). Many episodes of poisoning in Oklahoma occur when cattle graze recently cleared pastures containing young oak sprouts and seedlings. Poisoning by acorns usually occurs shortly after they have fallen (5,16,17,23). Many outbreaks of acorn poisoning occur in Oklahoma; most affected animals are calves rather than mature cattle even though cows and calves have access to the same pastures.

Experimental feeding of the plant has repeatedly resulted in poisoning of cattle and sheep (3,5,23). Experimental feeding of fresh, frozen, or dried blossoms, buds, leaves, and twigs of *Q. havardii* caused disease in cattle, sheep, goats, rabbits, and guinea pigs. The experimental disease in ruminants and the rabbit closely resembled natural disease (7,9).

Evidence indicates that tannins or their metabolites are most likely the toxic principle (27,28). Tannins are present in highest concentration in the various parts of the plants during seasons when poisoning is prevalent; they are absorbed into the circulation, and they are toxic when administered parenterally (16,18,23,27,28,29). Householder and Dollahite (30) obtained a positive correlation between severity of illness and levels of serum tannic acid in calves experimentally poisoned with *Q. havardii*.

Tannic acid, pyrogallol, and gallic acid administered by stomach tube produced disease in rabbits resembling that produced by *Q. havardii* (27). Tannin derived from *Q. havardii* and administered by stomach tube was toxic to rabbits. The LD50 was 6.9 gm/kg per day for 5 days (28). The same workers showed that gallic acid was the only polyhydroxyphenolic derivative of acid hydrolysis of tannin from *Q. havardii*. The histopathology of oak poisoning in the rabbit has not been reported leaving some question whether experimental disease in the rabbit is comparable to disease in cattle. While cattle have repeatedly been poisoned by feeding the plant, studies of orally administered oak tannins in cattle are limited and have not clearly demonstrated toxicity (9, 18). In summary, evidence infers but does not firmly establish that tannic acid or its derivatives are the toxic principle of oak poisoning in cattle.

III. CLINICAL SIGNS

Initial signs of disease include anorexia, depression, clear watery nasal discharge, dry and thinly crusted nose, and rumen atony. Body temperature is usually normal or subnormal. Slight elevation of the tail head often accompanies initial constipation, the latter is followed in 2-10 days by voidance of dark, thin, mucoid, and often bloody feces. Stools are not usually voluminous.

Fragments of acorns may be present in feces. Dehydration occurs; scleral vessels may become markedly congested. Subcutaneous edema of the neck, brisket abdomen, and perineum is frequent. Abdominal distention due to ascites and rapid shallow breathing due to hydrothorax occur occasionally.

While malaise and alimentary disorder are major presenting signs, evidences of renal disease are consistent features of oak poisoning. Clear, nearly colorless urine is voided with increased frequency. Polyuria is reported but I have not seen data on total daily urine output. Hemoglobinuria has been reported; I have not seen it, nor has it been reported in recent publications. The specific gravity of urine is always low, usually in the range of 1.008 to 1.014. Mild to moderate proteinuria and granular and cellular casts are usually present; occasionally there are mild glycosuria and occult blood.

Blood urea nitrogen and creatinine are consistently elevated. Data obtained in our laboratory from random field cases have shown the following abnormalities: marked elevation of blood urea nitrogen in 15 of 15 cases, hypoproteinemia in 10 of 15, hypoalbuminemia in 7 of 11, hypoanatremia in 8 of 11; hyperkalemia in 4 of 10; hypochloremia in 12 of 13, hypocalcemia in 2 of 2, and hyperphosphatemia in 2 of 3. Householder *et al.* (30) assayed several serum constituents in calves experimentally poisoned with *Q. havardii*. The calves had significant elevations of blood urea nitrogen. Fowler and Richards (5) reported markedly diminished renal clearance of sodium sulfanilate in one cow.

The course of acute and subacute illness from onset to death may be from 1 day to 3 or 4 weeks. Chronic disease results in protracted delibitating illness due to decompensating renal function over a period of weeks. Mortality rates as high as 85% have been reported (2).

IV. PATHOLOGIC FINDINGS

The constant and essential lesion of the disease is renal tubular necrosis. Affected kidneys in the acute state are generally pale and swollen and have a smooth surface. The parenchyma often possesses a barely perceptible spongy or fine honeycomb appearance and tiny opaque angular whitish flecks when viewed from the surface. Petechiae are sometimes scattered throughout the cortex (Fig. 1). The cut surface is moist, the cortex pale, cortical striations are often accentuated and contain barely perceptible white flecks and streaks. In more chronic cases the kidney is pale, slightly and irregularly dimpled or roughened due to tubular degeneration and atrophy.

Whereas renal lesions are always present; lesions in other tissues are not. Edema, generalized or localized, often occurs. The perirenal connective tissue is often markedly edematous, especially in acute cases. Occasionally following subacute or chronic course there are streaks of hemorrhage or brown hemosiderin

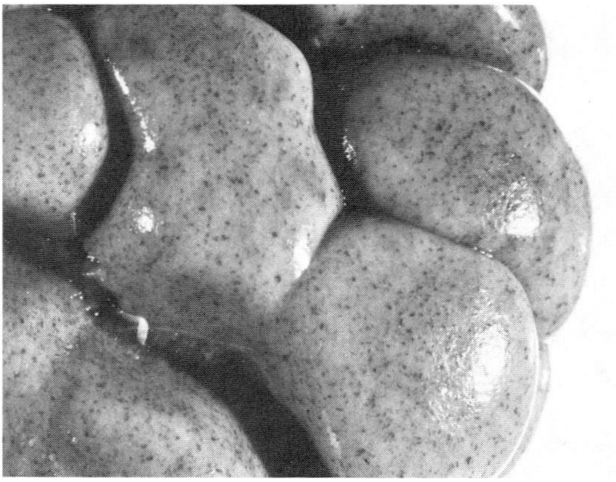

Fig. 1. *Kidney - Pale granular cortical surface with numerous petechiae.*

deposits in the region reflecting resolved perirenal edema. There may be ascites, hydrothorax, hydropericardium, mesenteric, abomasal and intestinal edema, and extensive edema of subcutaneous tissues ventrally and elsewhere. Varying degrees of mucosal congestion, hemorrhage, erosion, and ulceration may be present in the gastrointestinal tract (Fig. 2). The colonic mucosa is often congested at the apex of its rugae and sometimes diffusely petechiate. Accompanying the advanced uremic state may be extensive focal or or diffuse ulceration of the mucosa of the pharynx, esophagus, and

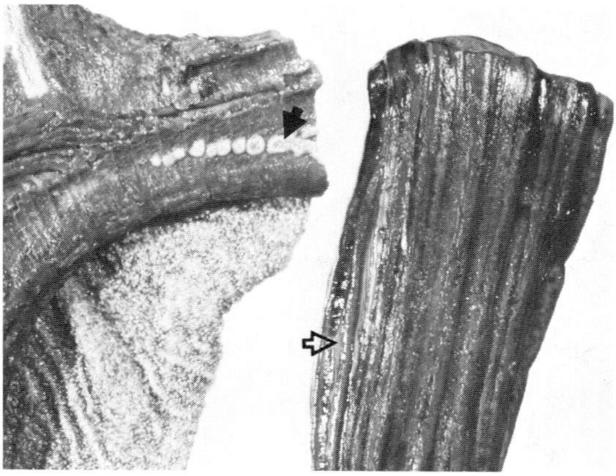

Fig. 2. *Rumen (left) and esophagus. Extensive ulceration of mucosa. Remaining intact epithelium on rumen pillar and esophagus (arrows).*

rumen, particularly the rumen pillars. Hydrothorax results in degrees of pulmonary atelectasis. We have occasionally seen widespread petechial and ecchymotic hemorrhages or serous membranes in conjunction with the above described lesions.

The histologic changes in oak poisoning of cattle have been described by several workers (5,12,17,23). The basic microscopic lesion is renal tubular necrosis. Most characteristic in the acute stage are groups of necrotic proximal tubules devoid of epithelial cells, instead consisting of a space limited by the basement membrane and completely filled with an acidophilic granular coagulum containing bits of pale basophilic nuclear debris (Fig. 3 and 4). Other tubules are lined by swollen or flattened degenerate epithelial cells occasionally containing hyaline cytoplasmic droplets. Widespread dilation of cortical tubules often containing hyaline, granular, or cellular casts is common. Medullary tubules likewise are often distended and contain casts. Glomeruli are often slightly hypercellular and have swelling of the capsular and glomerular epithelium. In the acute stage the cortical interstitium is edematous and occasionally contains focal hemorrhages. Later stages are represented by cortical tubular dilation, degeneration, regeneration, and cast formation. The cortical interstitium has a moderate increase in fibrous connective tissue and contains small aggregates of lymphocytes and plasma cells (5,12, 17,23) (Fig. 5). Ultrastructural alterations in the kidney of rabbits resulting from administration of tannic acid have been reported by Boler *et al.* (29).

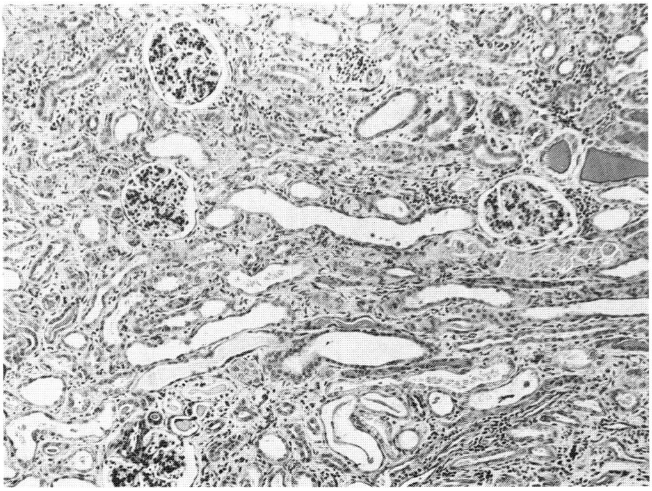

Fig. 3. *Kidney - Tubular dilatation, granular and lyaline casts, mild hypercellularity of glomeruli.*

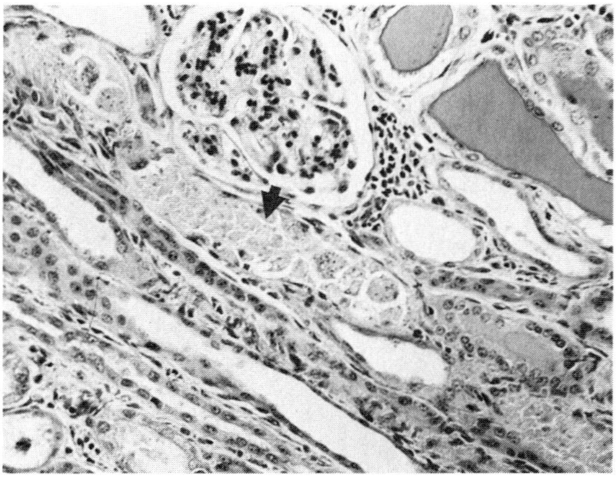

Fig. 4. *Kidney - Necrotic tubule (arrow) devoid of epithelial cells and filled with eosinophilic debris and bits of pale basophilic nuclear debris. Other tubules have dense hyaline casts and flattened epithelium.*

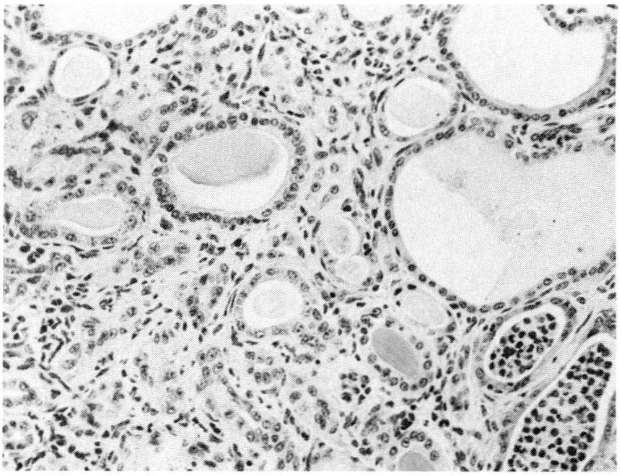

Fig. 5. *Kidney, chronic illness. Edematous, hypercellular interstitium separating dilated tubules that contain hyaline and cellular casts.*

V. THERAPY AND CONTROL

Apparently there have been no controlled studies on the therapy of oak poisoning. Treatment is largely symptomatic. Attempts to restore fluid and electrolyte balance seem indicated. Adrenal mineralocorticoids may aid in excretion of potassium and retention of sodium. Thoracentesis to remove pleural fluid has provided relief to severely dyspneic calves.

Prevention of poisoning may be accomplished by avoiding exposure to vegetation or acorns when they are especially toxic or highly palatable. Supplemental feeding of pastured animals during periods of hazard reduces the probability of disease (2,32). Some observations, however, indicate that certain animals consume oak by choice (2,16,23). Dollahite *et al.* (31,32) showed that calcium hydroxide incorporated in supplemental feed was effective in preventing illness in cattle fed toxic quantities of oak.

VI. DISCUSSION

Good clinical and pathologic criteria exist by which oak poisoning may be recognized. Presumptive clinical diagnosis requires awareness that the disease exists, consideration of environmental and seasonal factors, and knowledge of the variety of clinical manifestations that lead the diagnostician to conduct the special examinations that identify renal tubular necrosis. Histopathologic changes in the kidney of acutely or subacutely fatal cases have reasonable diagnostic specificity in the context of diseases in Oklahoma. However, the renal lesions of *Amaranthus retroflexus* poisoning, in my limited experience, are very similar to those of oak poisoning.

Additional studies are required to identify the toxic principle and to further characterize the pathophysiology of the disease in cattle. Such studies might provide a more rational basis for therapy and control.

VII. REFERENCES

1. Beck, J. S., and Beck, C. C., *Vet. Med.* 67, 1003-1006 (1972).
2. Boughton, T. R., and Hardy, W. T., *J. Am. Vet. Med. Assoc.* 89, 157-162 (1936).
3. Dollahite, J. W., *Southwest. Vet.* 14, 198-201 (1961).
4. Foley, O. F., *Am. J. Vet. Med.* 12, 244 (1917).
5. Fowler, M. E., and Richards, W. P. C., *J. Am. Vet. Med. Assoc.* 147, 1215-1220 (1965).
6. Kingsbury, J. M., "Poisonous Plants of the United States and Canada," pp. 444-446. Prentice-Hall, Englewood Cliffs, New Jersey, 1964.
7. Kingery, B. W., Richter, W. R., and Dingel, R. M., *Iowa State Univ. Vet.* 22, 30-31 (1960).
8. Kinsley, A. T., *Vet. Med.* 20, 354-355 (1925).
9. Marsh, D., Clawson, A. B., and Marsh, H., "Oak Leaf Poisoning of Domestic Animals," *U. S. Dep. Agric. Bull.* 767, 1919.
10. Palmer, R. L., *Mod. Vet. Pract.* 43, No. 10, 72 (1962).
11. Pammel, L. H., *Am. J. Vet. Med.* 12, 323 (1917).
12. Smith, H. A., *Southwest. Vet.* 13, 34-36 (1959).

13. McGowen, B. A., *Southwest. Vet.* 24, 68 (1970).
14. Peet, R. L., *Mod. Vet. Pract.* 52, No. 10, 54 (1970).
15. Slaughter, T. S., *Vet. Med. Small Anim. Clin.* 59, 227-230 (1964).
16. Blin, P. C., and Cuq, P., *Rec. Med. Vet.* 132, 674-687 (1956).
17. Cedarvall, A., Johansson, H. E., and Jonsson, L., *Nord. Veterinaermed.* 25, 639-644 (1973).
18. Clarke, E. G. C., and Cotchin, E., *Br. Vet. J.* 112, 135-139 (1956).
19. Gould, G. N., and Morgan, K. G., *Vet. Rec.* 14, 33-35 (1934).
20. Jones, L. L., *Vet. Rec.* 14, 329-330 (1934).
21. Llewellyn, C. A., *Vet. Rec.* 74, 1238 (1962).
22. Sodermark, N., *North Am. Vet.* 6, 31 (1935).
23. Stober, M., and VonBenton, K., *Dtsch. Tieraerztl. Wochenschr.* 81, 153-176 (1974).
24. Tailhardat, B., *Rev. Med. Vet.* 103, 853 (1952).
25. Towers, K. G., *Vet. Rec.* 62, 74-75 (1950).
26. Wolter, R., *Rev. Med. Vet.* 125, 1481-1485 (1974).
27. Dollahite, J. W., Pigeon, R. F., and Camp, B. J., *Am. J. Vet. Res.* 23, 1264-1267 (1962).
28. Pigeon, R. F., Camp, B. J., and Dollahite, J. W., *Am. J. Vet. Res.* 23, 1268-1270 (1962).
29. Boler, R. K., Brown, J. S., and Arkegler, R. B., *Am. J. Pathol.* 49, 15-32 (1966).
30. Householder, G. T., and Dollahite, J. W., *Southwest. Vet.* 16, 107 (1963).
31. Dollahite, J. W., Householder, G. T., and Camp, B. J., *Southwest. Vet.* 16, 115-117 (1963).
32. Dollahite, J. W., Householder, G. T., and Camp, B. J., *J. Am. Vet. Med. Assoc.* 148, 908-912 (1966).

GLUCOSINOLATES IN CRUCIFEROUS PLANTS

Cecil H. VanEtten and Harvey L. Tookey
Northern Regional Research Center, Agricultural Research Service,
U.S. Department of Agriculture

I. ABSTRACT

Vegetables, forage plants, and oilseeds from the Cruciferae are of considerable economic importance as food or feed. Examples are cabbage, forage kale, and rapeseed. Glucosinolates, a group of compounds found in these plants, are the source of substances that may be deleterious if consumed under certain conditions. These substances are organic nitriles and isothiocyanates or products derived from them. The compounds found in a particular plant material depend on the specific glucosinolates in the plant, the genetic source, the treatment of the plant material prior to the hydrolysis of the glucosinolates, and the conditions during that hydrolysis. Biological responses caused by the products from the glucosinolates thus depend on subtle differences in the treatment of the plant material.

II. INTRODUCTION

Glucosinolates, formerly called thioglucosides, are found for the most part in Cruciferae and related families Capparaceae, Limnanthaceae, and Resedaceae. Of 1500 species of Cruciferae, the 300 species tested all contain glucosinolates (1). Over 70 naturally occurring glucosinolates have now been discovered (2). The glucosinolates sinigrin and sinalbin were identified in the Cruciferae by 1840 and were shown to yield products by action of thioglucosidase,[1] an enzyme which is also present in the plant. This presentation describes recent methods of analyses for the glucosinolates and their enzymic hydrolysis products. These methods, in conjunction with small animal tests, may be used to show the biological effects of specific compounds from the glucosinolates.

Available reviews include those concerning the biological effects of ingestion of crucifers (4-7), the chemistry of the glucosinolates (2,8,9), the problems in the use of oilseed meals in animal feeds (10,11), the transfer of deleterious substances into milk from animals fed crucifers (12,13), and the taxonomy of the cultivated crucifers (14,15). General reviews include a book on rapeseed (16) and a book on the chemistry and biology of the

---

[1]Myrosinase has been used as a name for the enzyme hydrolyzing the glucosinolates; thioglucoside glucohydrolase (EC 3.2.3.1), or thioglucosidase is recommended by the International Union of Biochemistry (3).

Cruciferae (17).

III. GLUCOSINOLATE CHEMISTRY

A. Formulas and Nomenclature

Glucosinolates are anions usually found in nature as their potassium salts. The glucosinolates differ from each other in the organic aglucon part of the molecule (R group in Scheme I). They

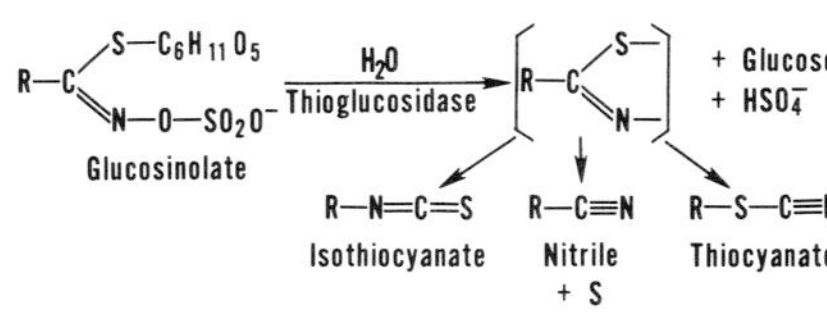

SCHEME 1

are hydrolyzed by the accompanying thioglucosidase when wet plant material is crushed. During hydrolysis, β-D-glucose and HSO_4 ion are always released; the organic aglucon portion may hydrolyze to give organic isothiocyanates, nitriles, or thiocyanates.

Sinigrin, sinalbin, progoitrin, and *epi*-progoitrin are trivial names for individual glucosinolates. Others have been named by prefixing "gluco" to the botanical name of the plant from which they were first isolated, e.g., gluconapin and glucobrassicin. The chemical name glucosinolate (GS) has now been adopted to which a prefix is added that describes the organic structure of the aglucon (18). For example, sinigrin is allyl-GS, sinalbin is *p*-hydroxybenzyl-GS, progoitrin, and *epi*-progoitrin are (*R*)- and (*S*)-2-hydroxy-3-butenyl-GS, respectively.

B. Glucosinolates Found in Cultivated Plants

Cruciferous plants are cultivated for vegetables, condiments, oilseeds, and forage. From 1 to 12 glucosinolates are found in each plant, but usually from 1 to 4 predominate.

Although cabbage contains many different glucosinolates, the amount present in the part eaten is only about 1% of that found in seed meals from the Cruciferae (Table 1). Rapeseed meals from *Brassica napus* except the Bronowski varieties are much higher in (*R*)-2-hydroxy-3-butenyl-GS, the source of goitrin or 5-vinyl-oxazolidine-2-thione (5-vinyl-OZT), than are varieties from *B. campestris*. These differences are one of the factors that contribute to the diversity of feeding results reported in the literature before the glucosinolate composition of the many varieties

TABLE 1

Glucosinolates in Selected Vegetables and Oilseeds[1]

Name and plant part	R-Group of glucosinolate[2]	Amount, ppm	
		Mean	Range
Brassica oleracea L.[3] Cabbage; head	Allyl-	156	15-525
	3-Butenyl-	17	1-74
	3-Methylsulfinylpropyl-	160	36-425
	(*R*)-2-Hydroxy-3- butenyl-	24	4-77
	4-Methylsulfinylbutyl-	53	<1-225
	2-Phenylethyl-	6	2-15
	3-Indolylmethyl's-	233	64-500
	Total glucosinolates	709	300-1290
Broccoli, Brussels sprouts, cauliflower, collards, kale, kohlrabi	Similar to cabbage		
B. campestris L.[4] Rape, turnip rape, Polish rape; seed meals	3-Butenyl-	28,000	18,000-44,000
	(*R*)-2-Hydroxy-3-butenyl-	8,000	2,000-20,000
	Total glucosinolates	37,000	30,000-48,000
B. napus L. Rape, winter rape, Argentine rape; seed meals	3-Butenyl-	14,000	10,000-23,000
	(*R*)-2-Hydroxy-3-butenyl-	41,000	18,000-50,000
	Total glucosinolates	55,000	34,000-78,000
Bronowski varieties	Total glucosinolates	14,000	2,000-36,000
Crambe abyssinica,[5] Hochst ex. R.E. Fries Seed meal	(*S*)-2-Hydroxy-3-butenyl-	91,000	80,000-97,000
	Total glucosinolates	101,000	92,000-110,000

[1]Amount for vegetables reported on a fresh weight basis and for the oilseeds on the defatted meal.

[2]Under the conditions of the assay 2-hydroxy-3-butenyl-GS is the source of 5-vinyl-OZT, indolylmethyl-GS's are the source of thiocyanate ion, and the remaining GS's form isothiocyanates.

[3]Source of data for cabbage (19); other *B. oleracea* (20). Cabbage also may contain small amounts of 3-methylthiopropyl-, 4-methylthiobutyl-, 4-methylsulfonylbutyl-, and benzyl-GS's.

[4]Data for rapeseed (21).

[5]Data for crambe (22,23).

was known.

Other horticultural crops such as radish (*Raphanus sativus*), Chinese cabbage and turnip (*B. campestris*), and rutabaga (*B. napus*) contain similar but yet different glucosinolates from those found in cabbage. The condiments from *Armoracia* (horseradish), *B. carinata* (Ethiopian rapeseed), *B. juncea* (brown mustard), and *B. nigra* (black mustard) contain allyl-GS, the source of allyl isothiocyanate (allyl-NCS), the pungent substance that contributes to their characteristic flavor. *B. hirta* (white mustard seed) contains *p*-hydroxybenzyl-GS, the source of the isothiocyanate that provides its flavor.

C. Thioglucosidase Hydrolysis

Specific enzymic hydrolysis products from the aglucon designated by R in Scheme I include stable isothiocyanates and nitriles of allyl-, 3-butenyl-, 3-methylsulfinylpropyl-, 4-methylsulfinylbutyl-, and phenylethyl-GS's listed in Table 1. When the aglucon is (*R*)- or (*S*)-2-hydroxy-3-butenyl-, a ring compound 5-vinyl-OZT may be formed from the postulated isothiocyanate intermediate (Scheme II). When the aglucons contain a terminal unsaturation,

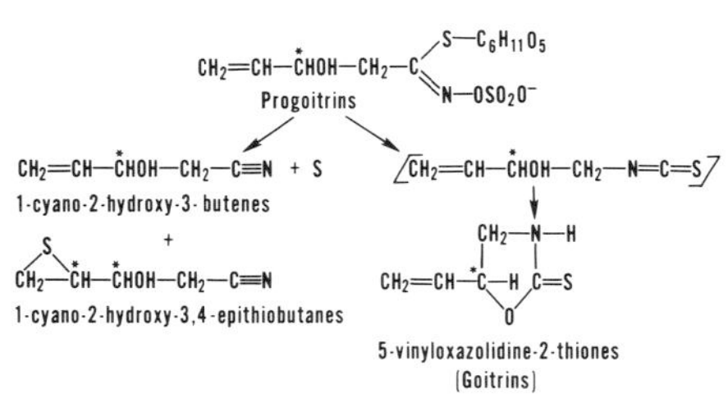

SCHEME 2

enzymic hydrolysis of the glucosinolates may yield a mixture of the unsaturated nitriles and nitriles containing an episulfide group at the terminal carbons (24). The indolylmethyl-GS's (glucobrassicins) (25,26) form thiocyanate ion which is estimated as a means of determining these two glucosinolates.

The course of hydrolysis to form nitriles or isothiocyanates depends on the prior treatment of the plant material and the conditions under which the hydrolysis is carried out (Table 2). These observations indicate nitrile formation is more apt to occur during autolysis of the natural plant before it has received any treatment except crushing when wet. Hydrolysis to form nitriles in crambe seed is more rapid than when vinyl-OZT is formed (27). The only clear-cut demonstration of the formation of epithionitriles other than by autolysis has been shown recently. An isolated proteinaceous factor from crambe seed was required to be

TABLE 2

Factors Affecting the Course of Glucosinolate Hydrolysis[1]

Plant part	Products favored by prior plant treatment	
	Nitriles	Isothiocyanates
Seed	Fresh	Long storage
	Low temperature storage	High temperature storage
Leaves	Undried	Air dried
Seed	Air dried	Dried with heat
Defatted seed meal	Room temperature dried	Dried with heat
	Products favored by conditions of hydrolysis	
Defatted seed meal	Autolysis of fresh material	Hydrolysis with prepared thioglucosidase
	Low pH	High pH
	Low temperature (0 to 25° C)	High temperature (up to 75° C)
	Low moisture	High dilution with water

[1]Conditions observed by study of crambe and rapeseed, defatted seed, leaves (27,28), and cabbage leaves (29).

added back to a thioglucosidase fraction to give epithio nitriles from the (*S*)-2-hydroxy-3-butenyl-GS substrate (30).

Another element not as extensively studied is the genetic source of the plant. Some are more apt to form isothiocyanates under most conditions than are others (27). The part of the plant is also involved. For example, rutabaga and horseradish roots yield only vinyl-OZT and allyl-NCS, respectively, when they are crushed and autolyzed.

Enzymic activity, regardless of the aglucon hydrolysis product, is ascribed to a single enzyme. However, several isozymes (proteins that vary in size but have the same enzyme activity) have been isolated as glycoproteins (31,32) and have sulfhydryl groups essential to their activity (33).

Thioglucosidases are not limited to plants. Intestinal bacteria (34,35) and certain fungi (36) also form such an enzyme. The part that ruminal and intestinal bacteria play in ruminant and nonruminant digestion has not been extensively studied. However, goitrin is formed from progoitrin by *in vivo* and *in vitro* action of the microflora of the nonruminant (6).

IV. METHODS OF ANALYSIS

A. Total Glucosinolates

Glucose and HSO_4 ion are always released by thioglucosidase hydrolysis of glucosinolates. The amount of either resulting from the hydrolysis provides a measure of total glucosinolate (37,38). With the availability of sensitive and specific methods for the colorimetric determination of *D*-glucose, rapid microanalytical methods were developed (39-42). These methods are useful in plant breeding programs to develop varieties low in glucosinolate content. In order to apply these methods to plants that contain large amounts of free glucose, the plant extract is first passed through an anion exchange resin in the chloride form which adsorbs the glucosinolates. The glucosinolates, now free of glucose, are hydrolyzed by adding thioglucosidase while still retained on the washed resin. The glucose remains in the buffered water phase, and the neutral aglucon hydrolysis products are quantitatively extracted into dichloromethane for their individual separation and analysis by gas-liquid chromatography (GLC) (43,44).

B. Aglucon Products of Glucosinolate Hydrolysis

In early methods, volatile isothiocyanates were steam-distilled into aqueous ammonia to form thioureas, which reacted with standard silver nitrate (45). Goitrin was estimated from its ultraviolet absorption (46). Development of GLC gave quantitative methods (47,48) which were modified to include nitriles and 5-vinyl-OZT (49,50).

In early work, lack of knowledge concerning the conditions required for quantitative hydrolysis to isothiocyanate and vinyl-OZT often gave low analytical results. The native sample should be carefully treated with wet heat to inactivate the endogenous thioglucosidase without any hydrolysis of the glucosinolates. If this procedure is followed by addition of thioglucosidase and incubation at pH 5 to 7, isothiocyanates and 5-vinyl-OZT are formed to the exclusion of nitriles (23,47,51).

The indolylmethyl-GS's are estimated from the thiocyanate ion they form by hydrolysis at pH 7. The *p*-hydroxybenzyl-GS, found only in white mustard seed (*B. hirta*), also forms thiocyanate ion by decomposition.

C. Problems of Analysis

The previous discussion covered the procedures to be applied to natural products which have not been modified so that the thioglucosidase and its substrate have interacted. However, any treatment such as chopping, shredding, cooking, or drying of vegetables or forages, or heating during processing of oilseeds may bring about hydrolysis to give different products depending on conditions (Table 2). At least three tests are required on such samples. They are: (a) test for thioglucosidase activity, (b) analysis for free 5-vinyl-OZT, isothiocyanates, and nitriles, and (c) analysis for unhydrolyzed glucosinolate.

V. BIOLOGICAL EFFECTS

A. Action of Specific Compounds from the Glucosinolates

1. (R)- *and* (S)-*5-vinyl-OZT (Goitrin)*

When (*R*)- or (*S*)-5-vinyl-OZT is fed to rats or man, radioactive iodine uptake by the thyroid is suppressed (6,46). Hyperplasia of the thyroid develops after the compounds are fed to rats (52). The (*R*) and (*S*) isomers are equivalent in antithyroid activity (6). Feeding 5-vinyl-OZT to chicks as 0.15% of the ration depresses growth rate and causes hyperplasia and hypertrophy of the thyroids. Radioactive iodine uptake is depressed during initial feeding but later the uptake returns to normal (53). Naturally occurring oxazolidine-2-thiones other than 5-vinyl-OZT also are goitrogens (6). Presumably, these compounds affect the thyroid as do the substituted thiourea drugs used in the treatment of hyperthyroidism. In contrast to thiocyanate ion, the antithyroid effect is not counteracted by excess amounts of iodine.

2. *Thiocyanate Ion*

In the treatment of hypertension in humans with thiocyanate ion, it was observed that the patients developed enlarged thyroids (54). Similar thyroid enlargement in animals is prevented by increasing the iodine content of the ration (55) unless the thiocyanate ion is fed at high levels (56). Thiocyanate ion from indolylmethyl-GS's in cabbage (Table 1) causes thyroid enlargement in rats provided that the ration contains iodine in the low range of the amount considered to be adequate (57).

3. *Organic Isothiocyanates*

The organic isothiocyanates are irritating to tissues and are vesicants at high concentrations. It would be surprising if large enough amounts could be eaten *per se* to cause malfunction of the thyroid. However, if glucosinolates are consumed with food, it is conceivable they might hydrolyze to give isothiocyanates in sufficient amounts to be goitrogenic. When allyl-NCS was fed by stomach tube to rats at a dosage equivalent to that available in 40 g of cabbage daily, the thyroids showed histological changes indicative of goiter (58). Daily doses of 2 to 4 mg of allyl-NCS force-fed to rats inhibited thyroid uptake of radioactive iodine and increased the thiocyanate ion concentration of the blood plasma (59). Iodine uptake by the rat thyroid is also inhibited by 3-methylsulfonylpropyl-NCS which comes from a pasture weed *Rapistrum rugosum* (60). It appears that metabolic detoxification of organic-NCS as well as organic nitriles includes conversion to thiocyanate ion (61).

4. *Organic Nitriles*

Many feeding tests with crucifer seeds resulted in poor growth and in pathologic changes in the liver, kidney, and other body organs without major pathologic changes in the thyroid. It was not until 1969 that feeding experiments clearly showed the role of nitriles in such pathological changes. Crambe seed meal autolyzed to contain nitriles (62) or an isolated nitrile fraction from the meal (Table 3), caused poor growth in rats, early death, major changes in the liver, and some changes in the kidney (62). In contrast, feeding of the same meal autolyzed under conditions to contain mostly 5-vinyl-OZT instead of the nitriles or the feeding of pure 5-vinyl-OZT, gave growth 85% of that of the controls with enlargement of the thyroid, but normal kidneys and livers (62). LD_{50} tests showed the nitriles to have acute toxicities ranging from 170 to 240 mg/kg whereas the LD_{50} of 5-vinyl-OZT was 1260-1400 mg/kg (63). Recently other workers have reported similar evidence for the toxic nature of the nitriles in rapeseed (64-66).

TABLE 3

Rat Feeding of Isolated epi-*Progoitrin, 5-Vinyl-OZT, and Nitriles*[1]

Compound	Amount in ration, percent	Weight, percent of control	Organ Wt. per 100 g body Wt.		
			Liver g	Kidney g	Thyroid mg
(*S*)-2-Hydroxy-3-butenyl-GS, (*epi*-Progoitrin)	0.5	92	4.1[2]	0.6	11.2
(*S*)-2-Hydroxy-3-butenyl-GS, (*epi*-Progoitrin)	0.85	85[2]	4.7[2]	0.8[2]	9.0
(*S*)-2-Hydroxy-3-butenyl-GS, (*epi*-Progoitrin)	1.50	71[2]	4.1[2]	0.8[2]	13.9[2]
(*R*)-5-Vinyl-OZT (goitrin)	0.23	85[2]	4.0[2]	0.6	14.7[2]
Nitrile mixture	0.10	17[2,3]	5.6[2]	1.5[2]	6.1
Nitrile mixture	0.20	--[3]			

[1]Five rats on each ration fed for 90 days. Nitrile mixture contained some dichloromethane solubles from autolyzed crambe seed meal.

[2]Differs from control value ($P < 0.01$).

[3]Two animals fed 0.1% nitrile died within 84 days; the remaining 3 were autopsied. All animals fed 0.2% nitrile fraction died within 14 days.

5. *Unhydrolyzed Glucosinolates*

Following the feeding of 2-hydroxy-3-butenyl-GS (progoitrin) to man and to rats, the radioactive iodine uptake of the thyroid is inhibited. 5-Vinyl-OZT appears in the blood and in the urine. Thioglucosidase activity of microorganisms found in the gut probably forms 5-vinyl-OZT from the 2-hydroxy-3-butenyl-GS (6). Pathologic changes observed in the liver of rats fed isolated 2-hydroxy-3-butenyl-GS (Table 3) suggests that progoitrin may be hydrolyzed in the gut to yield nitriles as well as 5-vinyl-OZT.

B. Glucosinolates and Human Goiter

The literature on endemic goiter includes references to the consumption of large amounts of cabbage and related plants as a contributing factor to goiter (67,68). About 96% of human hypothyroid goiter is probably due to iodine deficiency (6).

After feeding high levels of moistened rapeseed and of *Brassica* forage to cows, Finnish investigators found no significant increase of goitrogens in the milk (69). Only about 0.05% of the amount of crystalline 5-vinyl-OZT fed was found in the milk. Concentrations were no higher than 100 μg/L (70). Consumption in excessive amounts by adults of milk from cows fed high levels of *Brassica* forage did not cause depression of iodine uptake in the thyroid (71).

Milk from cattle in an area in Finland where endemic goiter is present contained 50 to 100 μg/L of 5-vinyl-OZT. Rats fed the milk over long periods developed enlarged thyroids (72). It appears from work done by these investigators that *Brassica* vegetables may contribute to endemic goiter, but the problem appears not to be a serious one.

Tests for thiocyanate ion in milk showed an increase from 2 mg/L to 5 to 8 mg/L when animals were fed a high level of *Brassica* forage. Feeding cows thiocyanate ion equal to that found in 30 to 60 kg *Brassica* forage per day gave concentrations in the milk up to 18 mg/L. No evidence for this milk being goitrogenic was found. Further studies did show that as the thiocyanate ion increased in the milk, the iodine content decreased. When thiocynate feeding was stopped and the ion fell to normal levels, the iodine content of the milk increased (73). This work has been confirmed by others. The results indicate iodine deficiency could develop in the young if such milk was the only source of nourishment.

C. Feeding Studies with Cruciferae Oil Seed Meals

Except for breeding stock, rapeseed meal may be fed safely at no more than 10% of the ration to cattle, sheep, swine, and poultry. Meals carefully processed have been used successfully as 15% of the ration for broilers (10). Selections from Bronowski varieties containing less than 1% total glucosinolate have been developed.

In recent years, many papers have appeared on the detoxification of various crucifer oilseed and meals by extraction, steam stripping, and empirical treatment with inorganic chemicals. Various methods of water extraction have provided feeding meals and protein isolates of high quality protein - free of glucosinolates and their aglucon hydrolysis products. However, the meals may cause adverse effects because of phytates that are not extracted from the meal. This effect can be overcome by added zinc (74). With these precautions, the meals appear satisfactory for animal feed but the cost of extraction prevents their practical use. Feed meals prepared by chemical treatment have not given as satisfactory a response in feeding trials.

Ruminants are less susceptible than monogastric animals to the toxic effects of crucifer plants (75). Crambe meal containing 1.1 to 3.7% 2-hydroxy-3-butenyl-GS, 0.6 to 1.5% derived nitriles, but little 5-vinyl-OZT and no thioglucosidase, have been fed to cattle in finishing trials. Weight gains and feed efficiency were satisfactory (76). Cattle were fed these rations through finishing periods of over 90 days. Meat, fat, kidneys, and livers were analyzed at slaughter for glucosinolates and their hydrolysis products. With a method sensitive to 1 ppm, none of these substances were found (50).

VI. AREAS OF FUTURE WORK

The Food and Drug Administration of the United States has proposed regulations prohibiting new varieties of vegetables that are significantly higher in natural toxicants than those that are currently in use (77). Implementation requires extensive research in methods of analysis accompanied by biological testing of suspected toxicants. If the tests include those for chronic toxicity, much time and effort will be required. It is believed that adequate methods of analysis have been developed for assay of the *Brassica* crops. Application of the methods to cabbage (20,29) and to oilseeds (4) shows there is an array of compounds formed which by their structure indicate they may be harmful if consumed in large amounts.

Current work in United States Department of Agriculture with the cooperation of the Agricultural Experiment Stations includes analyses of crucifer vegetable crops and isolation of aglucon hydrolysis products in sufficient quantity for biological testing. Plant breeding to select new crucifer vegetables low in glucosinolate content, as has been done with the rape oilseeds, is to be expected. The glucosinolates in crucifer forages and their aglucon hydrolysis products have not been thoroughly investigated. Knowledge of the glucosinolates applied to new food processing methods should prevent food products from appearing on the market in which the glucosinolates or their aglucons are concentrated.

Basic information on the thioglucosidase enzyme system is needed to relate it to the course the hydrolysis follows and to why the hydrolysis products are different with different species.

By further study of the enzyme system, insight and control of the hydrolysis to give either nitriles or isothiocyanates may be found.

VII. REFERENCES

1. Kjaer, A., *in* "The Biology and Chemistry of the Cruciferae" (J. G. Vaughan, A. J. MacLeod, and B. M. G. Jones, Eds.), p. 207. Academic Press, New York, 1976.
2. Ettlinger, M. G., and Kjaer, A., *in* "Recent Advances in Phytochemistry" (T. J. Mabry, Ed.), Vol. I, p. 59. Appleton-Century-Crofts, New York, 1968.
3. Florkin, M., and Stotz, E. H., *in* "Comprehensive Biochemistry" (M. Florkin and E. H. Stotz, Eds.), Vol. 13, p. 142. Elsevier, Amsterdam, 1965.
4. VanEtten, C. H., and Wolff, I. A., *in* "Toxicants Occurring Naturally in Foods," 2nd Ed. (Committee on Food Protection, Food and Nutrition Board National Council), p. 210. National Academy of Sciences, Washington, D.C., 1973.
5. Tookey, H. L., VanEtten, C. H., and Daxenbichler, M. E., *in* "Toxic Constituents of Plant Foodstuffs" (I. E. Liener, Ed.), 2nd Ed., in press, 1978.
6. Greer, M. A., *Recent Prog. Horm. Res.* 18, 187-219 (1962).
7. Greer, M. A., Kendall, J. W., and Smith, M., *in* "The Thyroid Gland" (R. Pitt-Rivers and W. R. Trotter, Eds.), p. 357. Butterworth, London and Washington, D.C., 1964.
8. Kjaer, A., *in* "The Chemistry of Organic Natural Products" (L. Zechmeister, Ed.), p. 122. Springer-Verlag, Vienna, 1960.
9. Kjaer, A., and Larsen, P., *Biosynthesis* 2, 71 (1973).
10. Bowland, J. P., Clandinin, D. R., and Wetter, L. R. (Eds.) "Rapeseed Meal for Livestock and Poultry--A Review," Canada Department of Agriculture Publication 1257, 1965.
11. Rutkowski, A., *J. Am. Oil Chem. Soc.* 48, 863 (1971).
12. Virtanen, A. I., *Experientia* 17, 241 (1961).
13. Walker, N. J., and Gray, I. K., *J. Agric. Food Chem.* 18, 346 (1970).
14. Downey, R. K., *in* "Rapeseed Meal for Livestock and Poultry--A Review" (J. P. Bowland, D. R. Clandinin, and L. R. Wetter, Eds.), p. 7. Canada Department of Agriculture Publication 1257, 1965.
15. Vaughan, J. G., *Bioscience* 27, 35 (1977).
16. Appleqvist, L. A., and Ohlson, R. (Eds.), *in* "Rapeseed," Elsevier Publishing Company, Amsterdam, 1972.
17. Vaughan, J. G., MacLeod, A. J., and Jones, B. M. (Eds.), *in* "The Biology and Chemistry of the Cruciferae," Academic Press, New York, 1976.
18. Ettlinger, M. G., and Dateo, J. P., Jr., Department of Chemistry, Rice Institute, Houston, Texas. Final report on Contract DA-19-129-QM-1059 to Quartermaster Research and Engineering Command, Natick, Massachusetts, 1961.
19. VanEtten, C. H., Daxenbichler, M. E., Williams, P. H., and

Kwolek, W. F., *J. Agric. Food Chem.* 24, 452 (1976).
20. Josefsson, E., *Phytochemistry* 6, 1617 (1967).
21. Josefsson, E., and Appelqvist, L. A., *J. Sci. Food Agric.* 19, 564 (1968).
22. Daxenbichler, M. E., VanEtten, C. H., Brown, F. S., and Jones, Q., *J. Agric. Food Chem.* 12, 127 (1964).
23. VanEtten, C. H., Daxenbichler, M. E., Peters, J. E., Wolff, I. A., and Booth, A. N., *J. Agric. Food Chem.* 13, 24 (1965).
24. Daxenbichler, M. E., VanEtten, C. H., and Wolff, I. A., *Phytochemistry* 7, 989 (1968).
25. Gmelin, R., and Virtanen, A. I., *Ann. Acad. Sci. Fenn. Ser. A2.* 107, 1 (1961).
26. Gmelin, R., and Virtanen, A. I., *Acta Chem. Scand.* 16, 1378 (1962).
27. VanEtten, C. H., Daxenbichler, M. E., Peter, J. E., and Tookey, H. L., *J. Agric. Food Chem.* 14, 426 (1966).
28. VanEtten, C. H., and Daxenbichler, M. E., *J. Agric. Food Chem.* 19, 194 (1971).
29. Daxenbichler, M. E., VanEtten, C. H., and Spencer, G. F., *J. Agric. Food Chem.* 25, 121 (1977).
30. Tookey, H. L., *Can. J. Biochem.* 51, 1654 (1973).
31. Lönnerdal, B., and Janson, J.-C., *Biochim. Biophys. Acta* 315, 421 (1973).
32. Henderson, H. M., and McEwan, T. J., *Phytochemistry* 11, 3127 (1972).
33. Tookey, H. L., *Can. J. Biochem.* 51, 1305 (1973).
34. Oginsky, E. L., Stein, A. E., and Greer, M. A., *Proc. Soc. Exp. Biol. Med.* 119, 360 (1965).
35. Tani, N., Ohtsuru, M., and Hata, T., *Agric. Biol. Chem.* 38, 1623 (1974).
36. Reese, E. T., Clapp, R. C., and Mandels, M., *Arch. Biochem. Biophys.* 75, 228 (1958).
37. Sandberg, M., and Holly, O. N., *J. Biol. Chem.* 96, 443 (1932).
38. Schultz, O. E., and Gmelin, R., *Z. Naturforscher.* 7b, 500 (1952).
39. Lein, K.-A., *Angew. Bot.* 46, 263 (1972).
40. Bjorkman, R., *Acta Chem. Scand.* 26, 1111 (1972).
41. VanEtten, C. H., McGrew, C. E., and Daxenbichler, M. E., *J. Agric. Food Chem.* 22, 483 (1974).
42. McGregor, D. I., and Downey, R. K., *Can. J. Plant Sci.* 55, 191 (1975).
43. VanEtten, C. H., and Daxenbichler, M. E., *J. Assoc. Off. Anal. Chem.*, 60, 946 (1977).
44. Daxenbichler, M. E., and VanEtten, C. H., *J. Assoc. Off. Anal. Chem.*, 60, 950 (1977).
45. Wetter, L. R., *Can. J. Biochem. Physiol.* 33, 980 (1955).
46. Astwood, E. B., Greer, M. A., and Ettlinger, M. G., *J. Biol. Chem.* 181, 121 (1949).
47. Youngs, C. G., and Wetter, L. R., *J. Am. Oil Chem. Soc.* 44, 551 (1967).

48. Anderson, D. L., *J. Assoc. Off. Anal. Chem.* 53, 1 (1970).
49. Daxenbichler, M. E., Spencer, G. F., Kleiman, R., VanEtten, C.H., and Wolff, I. A., *Anal. Biochem.* 38, 374 (1970).
50. VanEtten, C. H., Daxenbichler, M. E., Schroeder, W., Princen, L. H., and Perry, T. W., *Can. J. Anim. Sci.* 57, 75 (1977).
51. Appelqvist, L. A., and Josefsson, E., *J. Sci. Food Agric.* 18, 510 (1967).
52. Carroll, K. K., *Proc. Soc. Exp. Biol. Med.* 71, 622 (1949).
53. Clandinin, D. R., Bayly, L., and Caballero, A., *Poult. Sci.* 45, 833 (1966).
54. Barker, M. H., *J. Am. Med. Assoc.* 106, 762 (1936).
55. Astwood, E. B., *J. Pharmacol. Exp. Ther.* 78, 79 (1943).
56. Greer, M. A., Stott, A. K., and Milne, K. A., *Endocrinology* 79, 237 (1966).
57. Michajlovskij, N., and Langer, P., Hoppe-Seyler's *Z. Physiol. Chem.* 312, 26 (1958).
58. Langer, P., and Stolc, V., *Endocrinology* 76, 151 (1965).
59. Langer, P., Hoppe-Seyler's *Z. Physiol. Chem.* 339, 33 (1964).
60. Bachelard, H. S., and Trikojus, V. M., *Nature* 185, 80 (1960).
61. Greer, M. A., *Physiol. Rev.* 30, 513 (1950).
62. VanEtten, C. H., Gagne, W. E., Robbins, D. J., Booth, A. N., Daxenbichler, M. E., and Wolff, I. A., *Cereal Chem.* 46, 145 (1969).
63. VanEtten, C. H., Daxenbichler, M. E., and Wolff, I. A., *J. Agric. Food Chem.* 17, 483 (1969).
64. Lo, M. T., and Hill, D. C., *Can. J. Physiol. Pharmacol.* 50, 962 (1972).
65. Josefsson, E., *J. Sci. Food Agric.* 26, 1299 (1975).
66. Srivastava, V. K., Philbrick, D. J., and Hill, D. C., *Can. J. Anim. Sci.* 55, 331 (1975).
67. Kelly, F. C., and Snedden, W. W., *in* "Endemic Goitre," p. 91. World Health Organization Monog. Ser. No. 44, World Health Organization, Geneva 1960.
68. Michajlovskij, N., Sedlak, J., Jusic, M., and Buzina, R., *Endocrinol. Exp.* 3, 65 (1969); *Chem. Abstr.* 73, 118299q.
69. Kreula, M., and Kiesvaara, M., *Acta Chem. Scand.* 13, 1375 (1959).
70. Virtanen, A. I., Kreula, M., and Kiesvaara, M., *Acta Chem. Scand.* 12, 580 (1958).
71. Vilkki, P., Kreula, M., and Piironen, E., *Ann. Acad. Sci. Fenn. Ser. A2.* 110, 1 (1962).
72. Peltola, P., *in* "Current Topics in Thyroid Research" (C. Cassano and M. Andreoli, Eds.), p. 872. Academic Press, New York, 1965.
73. Piironen, E., and Virtanen, A. I., *Z. Ernaehrungswiss* 3, 140 (1963).
74. Shah, B. G., Jones, J. D., McLaughlin, J. M., and Bear-Rogers, J. L., *Nutr. Rep. Int.* 13, 1 (1976).
75. Josefsson, E., *in* "Rapeseed: Cultivation, Composition, Processing, and Utilization" (L. A. Appelqvist and R. Ohlson, Eds.), p. 354. Elsevier Publishing, Amsterdam, 1972.

76. Perry, T. W., Beeson, W. M., Tallent, W. H., and Mohler, M. T., *J. Anim. Sci.* 39, 248 (1974) (abstract).
77. Hanson, C. H., Ed., *in* "The Effect of FDA Regulations (GRAS) on Plant Breeding and Processing," CSSA Special Publication No. 5, Crop Science Society of America, 677 S. Segor Road, Madison, Wisconsin, 1974.

TALL LARKSPUR AND CATTLE ON HIGH MOUNTAIN RANGES

E. H. Cronin and D. B. Nielsen
Poisonous Plant Research Laboratory, Agricultural Research Service
U.S. Department of Agriculture and
Department of Economics, Utah State University

I. ABSTRACT

*This report presents information and data to illustrate the impact of larkspur on the livestock industry from the pioneer period to the present period. Results of grazing management, grubbing, and chemical control are discussed. Data are presented demonstrating advances and environmental safety of containing barbey larkspur (*Delphinium barbeyi *Huth) with herbicides.*

II. INTRODUCTION

Species of the genus *Delphinium* L., commonly known as larkspurs, are native on every continent in the Northern Hemisphere, but only in western North America are they considered a problem on grazing lands. The genus is also the source of many popular perennials found in the flower gardens of the world. Its popularity as a garden plant may eventually provide an opportunity for some horticultural varieties to become naturalized in the Southern Hemisphere. Three species have escaped from flower gardens to become naturalized in North America (1).

Ewan (1) defined 79 species that occur in North America; only 4 occur east of the Mississippi River. California contains the most species, including 22 endemic species. More than 231 binomials have been applied to the 79 species, creating an almost impenetrable morass of synonymy.

The poisonous properties of larkspur were recognized by the ancient herbalists of Greece and Rome (2). Early colonists arriving in North America were, therefore, already aware of the poisonous properties of these plants. During colonial times the eastern species were known as "stagger weed" because of their effects on cattle, but livestock deaths in the East, as in Europe, were rare.

Westward migration of the livestock industry brought reports of catastrophic losses from poisoning with species of larkspur, particularly in the short-grass prairie, the Rocky Mountain, and the Intermountain Region. Losses were sustained as these pioneer livestockmen entered new areas, where the larkspur were components of the pristine vegetation. To the cattle industry the larkspur remain the most important poisonous plants on our grazing lands--more important than all other poisonous plants combined. Each

Western State and Canadian province lists one of more larkspur species as one of its important poisonous plants.

Traditionally, two types of larkspur are recognized in North America: the low larkspur and the tall larkspurs. Low larkspurs, usually less than 75 cm tall, inhabit the drier low-elevation range-lands used for spring or fall grazing. They are among the first plants to produce green herbage in the spring, complete their annual reproductive cycle, and enter dormancy in early summer as the soil moisture is depleted. The tall larkspurs grow on sites with deep soils where soil moisture seldom limits plant growth, on high mountain ranges used for summer grazing. The tall larkspurs remain green throughout the growing season.

The toxic substances in the larkspurs are diterpenoid alkaloids; a single species may contain a dozen or more such compounds. Many species are known to be poisonous but many have never been evaluated through feeding trials or chemical analyses. Little information is available on the toxicity or the dynamics of concentration of the individual alkaloids.

New growth, or young portions of larkspur, are more toxic than the mature portions of the plant. Concentrations of alkaloids are lowest in the stems and highest in the flowering raceme. In general, the plants are most toxic in the spring and lose toxicity throughout the growing season, especially after flowering. Management of livestock on ranges infested with larkspur has been based on the relative toxicity of the whole plant. Cattle are not allowed to graze areas where larkspurs are abundant until the flowers start to open. This practice reduces losses by preventing consumption while the plants are most toxic, but it does not prevent losses.

Managing livestock to minimize losses, long an accepted practice on land infested with poisonous plants, is effective where alternative grazing areas are available. This option, however, is rapidly being eliminated by the loss of grazing lands to other uses and by the increasing demand for meat by a growing human population. The rancher's grazing resources are now restricted. Meat production depends on maintenance or improvement of existing grazing lands.

Management of livestock to minimize losses from poisoning thus limits the use of a grazing area to a period when the poisonous plants are unpalatable or dormant, or when the level of toxic substances in the plant is at a minimum. Grazing pressure may then endanger the species that are most palatable during the period in which grazing can be permitted. Limitation to the same grazing period year after year does not maintain or improve forage production.

Federal land management agencies, eager to improve the forage production and quality of the watershed, are turning to a rest-rotation system for management of livestock on Federal lands. In the rest-rotation system, each unit in the system is grazed during a different period in each of the years required to complete a full rotation within the system. Livestock may thus be required to graze a unit while its poisonous plants are most toxic. Under these conditions, an unacceptable burden is placed on the rancher because of potential livestock losses.

We know of no evidence that any grazing management system has controlled or reduced the population of a poisonous plant. Nor should grazing management be expected to control the population of poisonous plants when they are components of the climax vegetation or a disclimax community. Either livestock must be immunized against the toxic substances in the plant or the plant population must be reduced to a level where losses do not occur in order to implement a grazing system designed to improve forage production.

III. THE MANTI CANYON CATTLE ALLOTMENT

A cattle allotment with an average annual loss of 36 head was selected to study the relationships between larkspur and cattle. Objectives of the study included determination of: (a) ecological factors that permit larkspur to become established and to maintain its population, (b) time of grazing, (c) reasons cattle graze larkspur, (d) feasibility of controlling larkspur with herbicides without adverse impacts on the resource or the environment, and (e) economic feasibility of controlling larkspur to reduce cattle losses.

The Manti Canyon Cattle Allotment, an 8,000 ha summer grazing allotment on U.S. Forest Service land in central Utah, was selected for the study. It is grazed by 800 to 850 cows and their calves from June until October. The allotment ranges in elevation from 1,740 m on the west at the mouth of the canyon to over 3,120 m on the east at the summit of the Wasatch Plateau.

The allotment contains three main divisions. The lower division contains 3,000 ha dominated by Utah juniper [*Juniperus osteosperma* (Torr.) Little] and scrub gambel oak (*Quercus gambelii* Nutt.). The middle 1,800 ha division is dominated by quaking aspen (*Populus tremuloides* Michx.) except at its upper boundary where Engleman spruce (*Picea engelmanii* Parry ex Engelm.) and the subalpine fir [*Abies lasiocarpa* (Hook.) Nutt.] become dominant. Forage production on the lower two division furnishes about 1,300 animal unit months each summer. The upper 3,200 ha division, in the subalpine zone, supplies about 2,100 AUMs from about the middle of July until the first of October. It is the most productive division of the allotment. It is also the division where an average of 4% of the total permitted cattle are lost each year. The source of the losses is barbey larkspur (*Delphinium barbeyi* Huth), one of the tall larkspurs and the most toxic species of *Delphinium* known. Only 137.6 ha, about 4.3% of the division, were infested with larkspur. However, these few hectares of larkspur limit the profit of the permittees grazing cattle on the allotment and dictates the grazing practices used on the allotment.

The vegetation on the Subalpine Division is dominated by extensive herbaceous communities with small scattered groves of

Engleman spruce and subalpine fir. Quaking aspen also form groves on south- and west-facing slopes.

Precipation in the subalpine zone averages about 72 cm annually, with about two-thirds falling as snow (3). This heavy snowfall is an important factor in the distribution of barbey larkspur and exerts a considerable influence on the grazing pattern of the cattle.

Barbey larkspur grows in small patches in groves of trees, scattered along the permanent streams, and around the many springs and seeps. It thrives on sites where winter winds accumulate deep snowdrifts that persist for 3 to 6 weeks after the snow has melted from the surrounding areas. These late-melting drifts form in the lee of any obstruction to the prevailing winds, such as groves of trees, or ridges, and in depressions in the terrain.

The average frost-free period for the subalpine zone of the Wasatch Plateau is about 80 days (3). The growing season is much shorter for the vegetation under the late-melting snowdrifts. The crest of a drift may exceed 4.5 m at its maximum development. Although the short growing season may reduce the number of species that can survive and reproduce on these sites; the environmental conditions are relatively mild compared with the remainder of the subalpine zone. The snow cover insulates the vegetation from the extreme cold of the winter and the heavy frosts of the spring. In the summer the melting snow produces a plentiful supply of soil moisture for the normally frost-free period of July and August. Only during September and sometimes into October is the vegetation subjected to freezing temperatures until the insulating snow cover is renewed.

The losses are caused more by the distribution of the larkspur than by its abundance. Barbey larkspur is the most conspicuous and abundant species found on the snowdrift sites. These sites are seldom extensive individually but they occur frequently. Because of the abundance of moisture from melting snow, their vegetation is lush, including many highly palatable forage species and it is also more succulent than the surrounding vegetation. Therefore, cattle find the vegetation attractive and graze it heavily while abundant other forage remains available on the surrounding areas.

Domestic livestock have grazed the Wasatch Plateau since 1875. During the first 28 years grazing was unrestricted. Livestock from local farms and ranches along with numerous transient herds of sheep destroyed much of the vegetation on the plateau. Violent floods of mud, water, and rocks resulted, damaging the towns and cultivated land in the valleys below (4). The creation of the Manti National Forest in 1903 brought regulations for grazing but did not stop the floods. About 1911 the Forest Service initiated the first studies of the effects of watershed vegetation on erosion and floods. Many of the vegetation plots and the paddocks for studying the effects of grazing still exist today over 60 years after the studies were begun.

Ellison's 1954 report (3) is most helpful in understanding the role of barbey larkspur in the vegetation of the plateau. The objectives of his studies were the reconstruction of the character of the original vegetation and evaluation of the changes in the vegetation and soil since pioneer days. He reported that on relic sites, protected by natural barriers from grazing by domestic livestock, barbey larkspur constituted from less than 1% to over 50% of the vegetation. On sites where overgrazing had been most destructive he found larkspur plants growing on soil pedicles. Only the soil held by the larkspur clumps was not lost to erosion. He concluded that barbey larkspur was a component of the climax vegetation and was the most tenacious species where overgrazing had precipitated drastic erosion.

IV. LIFE HISTORY OF BARBEY LARKSPUR

Barbey larkspur, a hemicrypthophyte, begins its annual growth while under snow. Shoots as long as 10 cm have been measured as the snow melted from over them. After snowmelt, shoots grow very rapidly, reaching heights of 45 to 60 cm in the first 2 weeks. Elongation of the racemes adds height to the plant during the 3rd week. The lower flowers on the raceme open about the 3rd week and flowering continues acropetally for another 3 weeks or longer. Seed are dispersed in September.

Most seed fall at the base of the parent plant (5). Seed are shaken from the partially open follicles by wind and animals shaking the stems. Seed may be catapulated as much as 5 m from the parent plant when large animals pass over it forcing the stem nearly horizontal and then suddenly releasing it which causes it to whip violently (6). Seed falling on a crusted snow surface may be transported long distances by the wind. Seed transported by wind would probably be carried to another snowdrift site where the seed, like snow particles, would be deposited.

Seed germination may begin as early as January and continue until after snowmelt. Most seed either germinates or disintegrates within a year. Germination studies indicate that between 70 and 90% germinate (5,7). Less than 28% of established seedlings survive through the fourth year (5).

The energy budget of seedlings is devoted to root development until the receding snow exposes them to the stimulation of the sun. The first foliage leaf is produced about 7 to 10 days after snowmelt. By the end of the first summer the plant will have produced from one to four foliage leaves, and the root will have developed into a distinct taproot. The plant may be less than 3 cm tall but the root will have extended as deep as 10 cm below the soil surface. By the end of the second summer the plant may have produced as many as six leaves, reaching a height of 6 cm, and the taproot may extend as much as 20 cm below the soil surface. Below 20 cm the seasonal maximum water potential of the soil seldom, if ever, drops to -13 bars so the plant has adequate water. Reproductive maturity may not be reached until the fourth year and is probably much later for most juveniles competing for space with mature plants.

Once barbey larkspur reaches its reproductive stage of growth it may survive 75 years or more as indicated by surviving pedicellated plants on the Wasatch Plateau. Seed are produced almost every year. Holman (5) estimated that a large plant (20 "stalks") may produce over 37,000 seed each year. Few seedlings or juveniles survive in a stable population of mature plants; but because mature plants are long-lived, only a few juveniles need survive to maintain a stable population.

V. CATTLE LOSSES

The factors that influence the utilization of larkspur by cattle and the reasons that an animal may ingest lethal levels have not been determined. Among the factors that have been suggested are the weather, lack of available forage, and annual variation in toxicity of the plants.

To determine whether losses were correlated with some of these factors, we collected records of losses on three contiguous cattle allotments that share the same weather and support the same plant communities: Manti Canyon, Six Mile Canyon, and Twelve Mile Canyon cattle allotments. The three allotments differ in size, carrying capacity, and proportions of the various plant communities represented. Annual losses on the three allotments should be correlated between allotments if the losses are influenced by factors common to all, such as weather; but, this was not the case (Fig. 1). Losses varied greatly both between allotments and years on the same allotment. The coefficient of determination between allotments for years did not exceed 0.36. In as much as the variation in losses between years on one allotment cannot be explained by the variation on another allotment, it appears that the factors influencing losses must vary within each allotment.

To learn when and why cattle grazed the poisonous larkspur, we observed cattle for 3 summers during the morning and evening feeding period. They were observed for 2 weeks after being turned into the subalpine division of the Manti Canyon Cattle Allotment. This period normally accounts for most of the early losses on the subalpine grazing units.

When cattle first entered the subalpine zone, they appeared to graze only grasses, but within 4 to 8 days their diet changed dramatically to include many forbs. As they began to utilize forbs, the cattle moved into the patches of larkspur on the snowdrift sites for the first time. But they did not utilize the larkspur until they had utilized, or trampled most of the tall bluebell (*Mertensia arizonica* Greene). Cattle began to utilize the tips of larkspur stems when the tall bluebell was no longer available or acceptable, which coincided with the time that the larkspur flowers were opening. The first dead cattle were found 7 to 10 days after they entered the subalpine division.

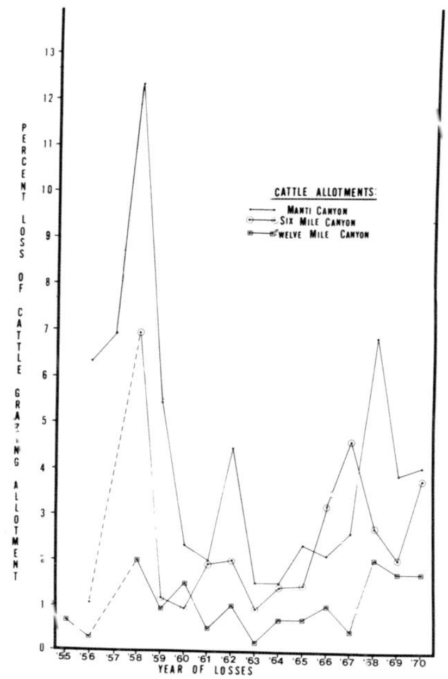

Fig. 1. *Tall larkspur and cattle on high mountain ranges.*

Rumens of 11 cows were examined; all but one contained many nodes of larkspur. Some were large nodes that could have been obtained only by grazing the large, coarse stems. Normally, cattle select the young leaves, the stem tips and flower buds, or the seed pod.

Cattle whose rumens contained nodes of larkspur became severely bloated before body heat was lost or joints stiffened. The dead cows ranged in age from yearlings to cows at least 6 years old. The older cows had grazed on the Manti Canyon many seasons before their death.

Backtracking from dead cows led to large patches of larkspur. Many larkspur plants in these patches had been utilized to within 15 cm of the soil surface. Although other cattle had grazed these patches, the tracks of the cows that had died led past the severely grazed plants, suggesting that just before death they had ingested massive amounts of the poisonous plants.

Losses of calves have been attributed to starvation or disease due to poor nutrition after the death of their mothers. Observation of the grazing behavior of calves and examination of their rumen contents suggested that they died from ingestion of barbey larkspur.

Calves weigh between 135 and 180 kg on entering the subalpine zone. They are still nursing three to four times daily, but they also utilize a surprising amount of forage. Their grazing appears to be a random selection of plant species rather than the highly selective grazing behavior of mature animals. Calves appear to utilize any plant that is close and convenient, wherever they happen to stop.

On steep terrain cows usually leave their calves resting in groves of trees during a grazing period, especially in the morning. After grazing the cows return to the groves to nurse their calves. Toward the end of the grazing period, while waiting to nurse, hungry calves may become restless and move about or around the grove. The calves may then ingest leaves and sometimes stem tips of barbey larkspur. Because of their small size, calves could easily ingest a lethal amount of larkspur by selecting only leaves and small stem tips.

The rumen contents of six calves were examined. Larkspur nodes were found in their rumens and the dead calves bloated rapidly, suggesting that they died of larkspur poisoning. During the 3 summers that cattle were observed, all the calves of dead cows are believed to have survived. Thus, the earlier assumption that losses of calves are a direct result of the loss of the mother, was not corroborated by our observations.

VI. CONTROL OF BARBEY LARKSPUR

Forcing sheep to graze patches of larkspur before allowing cattle to graze the area has been suggested as a method of reducing cattle losses. Available evidence (3) and our observations suggests that this method would not be effective. Sheep normally utilize larkspur late in the season, select portions of the plant that are seldom grazed by cattle, and would not reduce the larkspur population without depleting the associated vegetation.

On Cedar Mountain in southern Utah, barbey larkspur is so abundant that cattle cannot be used to harvest the forage. Sheep are turned into the heavily infested pastures and allowed to graze freely within fenced pastures. Sheep usually select the basal leaves and lower leaves on the stem while ignoring the flowers and seed pods. They utilize larkspur lightly until fall when most of their diet consist of larkspur herbage. Ranchers in the area report deaths of sheep when the animals are stressed by herding during this period of heavy larkspur utilization.

Under this management system sheep select permanent bedgrounds. Around the bedgrounds, sheep keep the larkspur plants stripped of leaves throughout the grazing period. However, the leafless green stems can apparently supply the photosynthetic products necessary to maintain the plant and its seed production. On one bedground used every year for the past 15 years, larkspur plants are stripped of their leaves every year throughout the growing season and continues to survive and produce seed each year.

Grubbing has been used successfully for control of larkspur. The top 25 to 30 cm of the root must be grubbed and dried if the method is to be effective. It is an expensive practice and many (8,9,10,11) have judged it impractical due to the shortage of available labor.

Of many herbicide treatments evaluated, two treatments that are effective are less expensive than most of the others (12,13): two applications of 4.5 kg/ha of either 2,4,5-T [(2,4,5-trichlorophenoxy) acetic acid] or silvex [2-(2,4,5-trichlorophenoxy) propionic acid] applied 1 or 2 years apart. Failure to make the second application allows almost complete recovery of most of the plants within 2 or 3 years, apparently because of inadequate translocation of herbicides within the plant. Herbicide applied to a single stem does not injure either stems or stem buds on the caudex surrounding the point of origin of the treated stem. Similar results were observed with fluorescent dyes (6). The second (and, rarely, a third) application is required to destroy all regenerative tissue in the caudex and root.

Applications of herbicides to control larkspur produce a plant community dominated by grass species (14). The response of the associated forbs species varied with their susceptibility to herbicide injury and their capacity to reinvade the treated area.

Western yarrow (*Achillia lanulosa* Nutt.) increases under heavy grazing and lacks palatability (3). It was resistant to 2,4,5-T and silvex. Its density remained stable following treatment.

Michaux sage (*Artemisia michauxiana* Bess), another rhizomatous increaser which tends to maintain its dominance on invaded sites was susceptible to the herbicides, and its density is significantly reduced by the double herbicide treatments. On plots treated with a single application of herbicide, michaux sage invaded the space formerly occupied by susceptible species of forbs.

Porter ligusticum (*Ligusticum porteri* Coult. & Rose) was destroyed by a single application of 2,4,5-T or silvex but its re-establishment on treated areas was rapid. It is palatable and is utilized, especially the large flower buds, by both domestic and game animals.

Tall bluebell, one of the preferred forage species was very susceptible to 2,4,5-T and silvex. High mortality of seedlings and a 2- to 3-year juvenile stage (15) probably also contributed to its absense from treated areas.

Many annual species, dandelion (*Taraxacum officinale* Weber), and nuttal viola (*Viola nuttallii* Pursh) increased after applications of herbicides but seldom persisted after the grass seedlings matured and gained vigor.

The dominant grasses on treated sites depended as much on the grazing regime imposed after treatments as on the treatments themselves. Where treated areas were grazed prior to maturity of the grass seed, letterman needle-and-thread grass (*Stipa lettermani* Vassey) became dominant. Annuals, dandelion, and nuttal viola also invaded these sites. Only slender wheatgrass [*Agropyron trachycaulum* (Link) Malte] increased under early grazing but never became a dominant species under early or late grazing.

Mountain brome (*Bromus carinatus* Hook., & Arn.) disappeared from treated areas which were grazed before seed maturation. It increased and dominated treated areas that were protected from grazing. Its greatest increase occurred on treated areas grazed after seed maturation. Mountain brome is a short-lived grass but is one of the most productive and palatable species found on the snowdrift sites. It is a key species for managing the forage on the subalpine zone.

VII. CONTROL OF CATTLE LOSSES

The North Fork Grazing Unit of the subalpine division of the Manti Canyon Allotment was selected for evaluation of the effects of larkspur control on cattle losses. The ranchers considered it the most dangerous grazing unit on the allotment. The 818.4-ha unit consists of the subalpine portions of the North Fork and Jolley Hole drainages. Of the 42.3 ha of barbey larkspur scattered in patches over the unit, approximately 28 ha were treated. Started in 1969 and completed in 1975 the larger, dense patches of larkspur were sprayed with 4.5 kg/ha of 2,4,5-T and resprayed within the 2-year limit required for control of larkspur. The spraying did not contaminate the streams; the maximum acceptable level of 2,4,5-T in culinary water is 2.0 ppb, and the highest level measured during the control program was 1.69 ppb (16).

The average annual loss on this grazing unit from the period 1956 through 1970 was 13 cattle. About two-thirds of the annual loss occurred when this unit was grazed early in the subalpine grazing season, and about one-third of the losses occurred when it was used at the end of the season.

Evaluation of the effects of controlling larkspur on cattle losses requires an estimate of the losses that would have occurred if larkspur had not been controlled. Two methods of estimating losses were considered. The long-term average annual loss of 13 cattle for the North Fork Grazing Unit could be used but the large variation in losses from year to year renders this figure inaccurate as an estimate of losses during any specific year. It would probably be the most accurate estimate of losses over a 10-year period or longer. The second method uses the relative number of losses on the North Fork unit compared with losses on the other (untreated) subalpine units, depending on the grazing period. When the North Fork unit was used early, its losses were estimated as twice the number lost on the remainder of the subalpine units. When grazed late, its losses were estimated as half of those on the remaining untreated grazing units. This method is more accurate for a single year and compensates for the variation between years (16).

The estimated cost of the two applications of 2,4,5-T for control of larkspur is $2,050, including herbicide, equipment, and labor (17). Estimates of cattle saved as a direct result of controlling barbey larkspur vary from 62 to 78 cattle, depending on the method used to estimate losses expected in the unit if larkspur had not been controlled (Table 1). The long-term average cost of replacing a cow is $250 per head (17). Therefore, the estimated savings from control of larkspur on the North Fork Grazing Unit to date ranges from $14,750 to $18,750, depending on the method used to estimate expected losses. The North Fork Grazing Unit can now be used safely and in its turn in the regular rest-rotation grazing system, an additional benefit. Its regular use is reducing the grazing pressure on the other subalpine grazing units. The ranchers now consider it to be the safest grazing unit on the allotment. With proper grazing management the forage production, the carrying capacity, and the quality of the watershed should all increase.

Table 1. Actual and Estimated Cattle Losses on the Subalpine Grazing Units of Manti Canyon Allotment from 1971 through 1976 when Selected Patches of Barbey Larkspur Were Controlled in the North Fork Grazing Unit.

	Losses by year						
	1971	1972	1973	1974	1975	1976	Total
Total losses for all subalpine grazing units.	14	14	2	6	32	21	89
Losses on all grazing units except the North Fork Grazing Unit.	14	11	2	6	32	21	86
Losses on the North Fork Grazing Unit.	0	3	0	0	0	0	3
Grazing period on the North Fork Grazing Unit.	Sept. 1 to Oct. 1	July 15 to Aug. 10	Aug. 10 to Oct. 1	Sept. 1 to Oct. 1	Sept. 1 to Oct. 1	Sept. 1 to Sept. 20	
Estimate of losses expected on the North Fork Grazing Unit based on losses occurring on the remaining subalpine units.	7	25	1	3	16	10	62[1/]
Estimate of losses expected on the North Fork Grazing Unit based on the average annual losses for the preceding 15 years	13	13	13	13	13	13	78[2/]

1/ Replacement cost of 62 cows equals $15,500.
2/ Replacement cost of 78 cows equals $19,500.

VIII. SUMMARY

Larkspurs are distributed throughout the Northern Hemisphere and have the potential to become naturalized in the Southern Hemisphere. Their toxic properties have been recognized for centuries. Numerous alkaloids are responsible for their toxicity. In western North America the larkspurs are the source of more cattle losses than all the other poisonous plants combined.

Two types of larkspurs are recognized: the low larkspur and the tall larkspurs. The low larkspurs, growing on low-elevation spring ranges, are utilized because they produce the first green herbage in the spring. The tall larkspurs are utilized throughout the growing season on summer ranges of the high mountains.

In the past, losses have been minimized by allowing cattle to graze ranges infested with tall larkspur only after the plants have flowered and when the concentrations of alkaloids are lowest. New grazing regulations and the need to improve forage production on infested grazing lands are removing this option for managing livestock on larkspur-infested ranges.

The Manti Canyon Cattle Allotment on the Wasatch Plateau in central Utah has had an average annual loss of 36 cattle since 1956. Barbey larkspur, one of the tall larkspurs, is responsible for these death losses. It grows only in the subalpine zone of the allotment, infesting only about 4.3% of the area in the zone. Barbey larkspur is a climax species, dominating sites where winter winds accumulate hugh snowdrifts that persist 3 to 6 weeks after snow has melted from surrounding areas. Moisture from the melting snowdrifts produces lush vegetation that is more attractive to cattle than the drier and more mature forage surrounding the snowdrift sites.

Studies of the life history of barbey larkspur indicate its capacity to maintain dominance on the snowdrift sites. It produces an abundant supply of seed which germinate or disintegrate within a year. Germination of seed is high, but mortality of seedlings is also high. The juvenile stage persists for 3 years or more and few plants survive to maturity. Reaching reproductive maturity, the plant may survive 75 years or more, negating the need for survival of many immature plants.

Livestock losses vary substantially from year to year. On three continuous allotments, losses within years were not significantly correlated, indicating that conditions common to all allotments either do not influence losses or are only minor components of the factors that influence losses.

Mature cattle appear to ingest lethal amounts of larkspur while grazing large dense patches of plants on sites where late-melting snowdrifts produce lush growth. Calves appear to ingest lethal amounts in small patches associated with groves of trees, while waiting to nurse when their mothers return from grazing.

The high mortality of seedlings and juveniles and the prolonged juvenile stage indicate that a reduction of the mature population would require many years to replace. Applications of selective herbicides appear to be the most efficient and effective method of reducing the larkspur population. Two applications of 4.5 kg/ha of either 2,4,5-T or silvex applied 1 or 2 years apart were the most effective and most economical treatment evaluated. Both applications must be completed within 2 years if larkspur is to be controlled.

Applications of the herbicides converted the larkspur-dominated community to a grass-dominated community. Early grazing of treated areas produced communities dominated by letterman needle-and-thread grass, a grass of low palatability and productivity. Grazing of treated areas after seed of mountain brome had matured and was readily shattered from the spike produced a community dominated by this short-lived species but produces abundant forage and is one of the species preferred by cattle. Grass communities, especially those dominated by mountain brome improve the quality of the watershed in comparison with the pretreatment barbey larkspur-dominated community.

Control of the large, dense patches of barbey larkspur on about 66% of the area supporting larkspur in one subalpine grazing unit has drastically reduced cattle losses on the unit. About $2,050 were expended for the larkspur control, including the herbicide, equipment, and labor. Losses were reduced from an expected 62 to 78 cows down to three cows. Replacement for a dead cow would have been about $250 so the saving as a direct result of controlling larkspur amounts to $14,750 to $18,750. Larkspur production has not increased since the treatments were completed and the benefits should continue to accrue. Additional benefits include improving grazing management, which should in turn improve forage production and increase carrying capacity.

IX. ACKNOWLEDGMENTS

The authors wish to express their appreciation to the U.S. Forest Service and its personnel at Ephraim District Office, Manti-LaSal National Forest for their cooperation throughout this study.

X. REFERENCES

1. Ewan, J. A., *Univ. Colo. Stud. Ser. D* 2, 55 (1945).
2. Kingsbury, J. M., "Poisonous Plants of the United States and Canada," Prentice-Hall, Englewood Cliffs, New Jersey, 1964.
3. Ellison, Lincoln, *Ecol. Monogr.* 24, 89 (1954).
4. Reynolds, R. V. R., *U.S. For. Serv. Bull.* 91 (1911).
5. Holman, J. R., Ph.D. Dissertation, Utah State University, 1973.
6. Cronin, E. H., *J. Range Manage.* 24, 258 (1971).
7. Williams, M. C., and Cronin, E. H., *Weed Sci.* 16, 381 (1968).
8. Aldous, A. E., *U.S. Dep. Agric. Farmers' Bull.* 826 (1917).
9. Durrel, L. W., Jensen, R., and Dlinger, B., *Colo. Agric. Ext. Serv. Bull.* 412A (1952).
10. Marsh, C. D., and Clawson, A. B., *U.S. Dep. Agric. Bull.* 34 (1918).
11. Welsh, H., and Morris, H. E., *Mont. Agric. Exp. Stn. Circ.* 197 (1956).

12. Cronin, E. H., and Nielsen, D. B., *J. Range Manage.* 25, 213 (1972).
13. Cronin, E. H., *J. Range Manage.* 27, 219 (1974).
14. Cronin, E. H., *J. Range Manage.* 29, 202 (1976).
15. Matthews, V. B., and Conrad, P. W., *Ecology* 49, 1113 (1968).
16. Cronin, E. H., Nielsen, D. B., and Madsen, N., *J. Range Manage.* 29, 364 (1976).
17. Nielsen, D. B., and Cronin, E. H., *J. Range Manage.* 30 (1977) (In press).

LARKSPUR TOXICOSIS: A REVIEW OF CURRENT RESEARCH

John D. Olsen
Poisonous Plant Research Laboratory, Agricultural Research Service
U.S. Department of Agriculture

I. ABSTRACT

*The factors influencing the toxicity of larkspur plants (*Delphinium spp.*) and the effect of larkspur toxicosis on animals are reviewed. The changes in total alkaloid concentration in various parts of the plant are discussed in relation to stage and year of growth. A bioassay to estimate and compare relative toxicity of larkspur plants showed considerable promise. The toxicity of an extract from larkspur was similar to that of the original ground plant when given to sheep and cattle. Any stage of toxicosis can now be induced by controlled infusion of larkspur extract into the rumen of cattle. This laboratory model will be very useful for studying pathophysiological effects produced by larkspur and also for testing methods of alleviating the toxicosis.*

II. INTRODUCTION

Larkspur toxicosis frequently affects cattle on mountain pastures of the western United States. Deaths are common; annual mortality losses on certain cattle allotments are as high as 12% (1). Cattle readily eat larkspur flowering stems and leaves (2) as well as the dry tops of the plant in the seed stage (3). Cattle deaths have also been reported from consumption of leaves and stems of both low and tall larkspur before flowering (4,5). The high mortality of livestock attributed to larkspur toxicosis stimulated the U.S. Department of Agriculture to begin experimental investigations of poisonous plants (3,6,7). In extensive experiments cattle, sheep, and horses were fed fresh green larkspur plants. Estimation of the lethal dose for the various species was difficult, and experimental results were quite variable; however, the clinical signs of larkspur toxicosis were documented (7). These signs, in order of appearance, include uneasiness, stiff gait, and a characteristic straddled stance with the hind legs held far apart. The animal may collapse suddenly, usually forelegs first. After a varying period of quiet, the animal usually regains the ability to stand, but signs of weakness may return quickly, accompanied by involuntary muscle twitches. Nausea and abdominal pain are commonly observed. If vomition occurs, death usually results from asphyxiation caused by inhalation of vomitus. Otherwise, death results from respiratory paralysis. Constipation is nearly always observed (8).

The toxic dose of larkspur depends upon variables such as animal species, individual animal susceptibility, growth stage of the plant, amount ingested, and the time over which the plant is ingested.

Extracts from larkspur have been used with varying success to poison animals under laboratory conditions. Materials such as chloroform and benzene extracts of dried leaves (9), alcohol and water extracts of roots or of fresh plant material (3,6), and crude alkaloid extracts (10,11) have been used, but the data reported were insufficient to establish the relationship between toxicity and the amount of plant material originally used for extraction.

A number of alkaloids have been extracted from *Delphinium spp.* (12), but studies characterizing their individual pathophysiologic effects are scarce. Most information listing pathophysiologic effects of larkspur alkaloids on livestock has been extrapolated from earlier studies with delphinine and is presumed to be accurate for the other alkaloids from *Delphinium spp.* However, reservation in the use of such information is warranted because "related alkaloids frequently form mixtures that are not readily separable... For this reason much of the early work, some of which dates back to the first half of the nineteenth century, is now of historical rather than chemical interest" (13). The pathophysiology of larkspur toxicosis needs to be studied with alkaloid preparations purified by appropriate, recently developed techniques. It should be recognized, however, that the predominant clinical signs of larkspur toxicosis might be induced by "common" metabolic products of the alkaloid mixture present in the particular *Delphinium sp.* of concern; and the "historical" studies of the pathophysiologic effects of delphinine may adequately explain the toxicosis syndrome. Future studies of the relative toxicity and pathophysiologic effects of individual alkaloids, as well as appropriate mixtures of alkaloids, should improve our understanding of this phenomenon.

Current investigations at our laboratory have been designed to: (a) study the factors that influence toxicity of larkspur, thereby establishing guidelines for laboratory and field investigations and for potential range-management practices; and (b) study the pathophysiologic effects of larkspur toxicosis to gain knowledge for evaluation of diagnostic techniques and alleviator or antidotal substances.

III. TOXICITY

The toxicity of larkspur varies, and the variation can potentially be due to plant as well as animal differences. Some of these factors, e.g., the decline in toxicity of the plant as it matures, have been studied (3,6,7,10,14) but rigorous scientific comparisons have been sparse. Therefore, the assumptions about differences in toxicity are not well documented by controlled studies. Confusion pertaining to relative toxicity also can arise from statements such as "larkspur is not poisonous to sheep because clinical signs of poisoning are seldom seen on larkspur-infested range;" in fact, larkspur is definitely toxic to sheep, although they do not often eat enough to cause clinical signs of poisoning.

Estimating larkspur toxicity is difficult. At present, there is no generally accepted laboratory method that establishes a standard for quantitation of larkspur toxicity.

The lethal property of an extract containing larkspur alkaloids is well known. Total alkaloid content might, therefore, indicate toxicity, but several factors need to be considered before this assumption is made.

Heyl *et al.* (15) apparently were the first to measure the content of total alkaloids in various parts of three species of larkspur native to the rangeland of the western United States. They analyzed mature plants of *Delphinium nelsonii* and reported the total alkaloid content for seeds, flowers, seed pods, roots, and leaves (listed in descending order of alkaloid concentration). Beath (10,11) isolated the crude alkaloid fraction of several species of larkspur at vegetative, mature-flowered, and seed stages of growth. He observed that the mature-flowered stage contained the least amount of alkaloid, and the relative amount (g of alkaloid/g of plant) in the seed was about equal to that in the vegetative stage. Significant differences in total alkaloid content of *Delphinium spp.* also were apparent in Beath's data.

Extensive determinations of total alkaloid in various parts of larkspur plants throughout the growing season have been reported more recently. Williams and Cronin (16,17) studied total alkaloid content of leaves and stems from *Delphinium barbeyi* over 2 years of growth. Significant differences in total alkaloid content occurred between years when compared on a calendar-day basis, presumably because the plant matured later in 1965 than in 1963. If total alkaloid content accurately represents stage of growth, the relative development of the plant generally differed by about 20 days between those years (Fig. 1). It is likely that total alkaloid content of larkspur can be affected by factors influencing the vigor of the plant because Laycock (18) observed that clipping larkspur in the vegetative growth stage for two consecutive years produced smaller plants that did not flower, and that contained a lower total alkaloid concentration. Total alkaloid content in the apex, leaf, and stem of *Delphinium occidentale* has also been measured throughout the growing season (17,18,19). Apexes and upper leaves and stems often are the plant parts initially selected by grazing cattle (20), and these parts contain relatively high amounts of total alkaloid (Fig. 2).

Total alkaloid concentration *per se* may or may not be the most suitable indicator of toxicity. Each species of larkspur usually contains a mixture of alkaloids (12), e.g., *D. occidentale*, which causes significant death loss of cattle, contains at least 12 known alkaloids (21). But the relative concentration (and in many

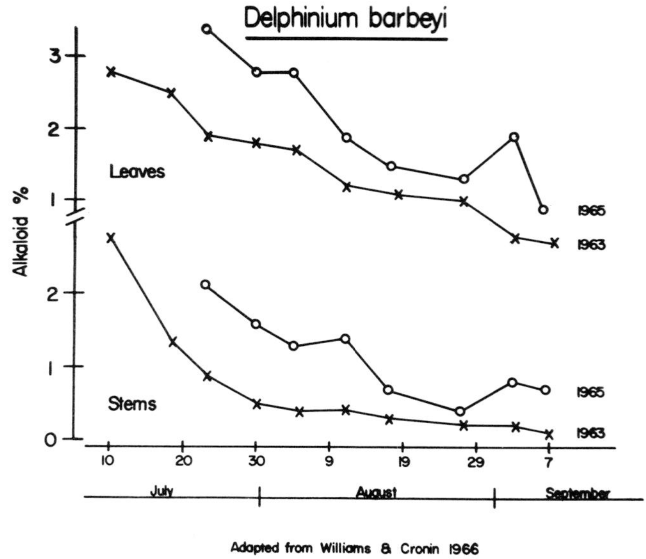

Fig. 1. *Total alkaloid content of* D. barbeyi *collected throughout two growing seasons at Hougaard Fork of Manti Canyon in central Utah.*

cases, the identity) of the alkaloids in most species is unknown. Furthermore, the relative concentration of a particular alkaloid may change with the stage of growth (19). Since it seems likely that the toxicity of the predominant individual alkaloids can vary (10,11), the relative toxicity of a species (and possibly a particular growth stage) of larkspur may be better correlated with the content of certain individual alkaloids, than with the total alkaloid content. Such a correlation between individual alkaloid content and toxicity must await future chemical analysis of important species of larkspur and determination of the relative toxicity of the individual alkaloids of each.

A suitable method for comparison of toxicity of species of larkspur is needed to provide a common base for the design of experiments and to assess factors that may influence the toxicity of larkspur on the range. The usefulness of such a method depends ultimately upon the accuracy of the correlation between the calculated toxicity and the measured toxicity of the plant for cattle. The determination of the median lethal dose (LD_{50}) of a toxic substance for the animal at risk has provided a common and useful reference point in toxicology, but it would be unrealistic to try to establish the LD_{50} for cattle of each plant preparation of

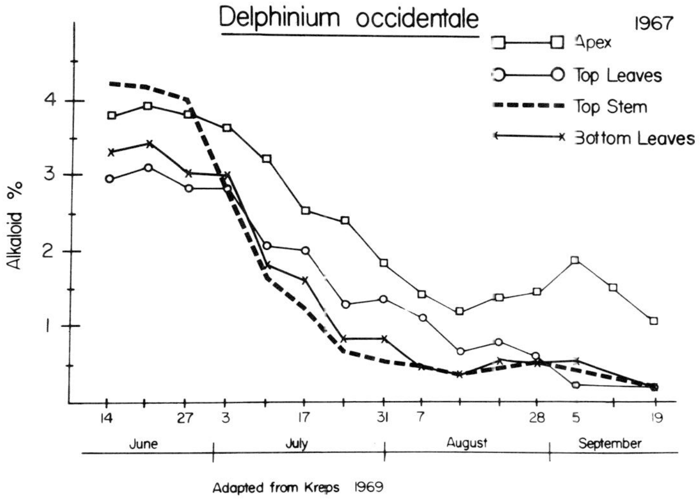

Fig. 2. *Total alkaloid content of plant parts from* D. occidentale *collected throughout the growing season on the Utah-Idaho border in Franklin Basin, Cache National Forest.*

interest; hence the need for a suitable reference measurement.

A bioassay technique has been developed for estimation of the toxicity for rats of an alcoholic extraction product from larkspur (22). A weighed amount of air-dried, ground plant material is treated with 95% ethanol (volume = 10 times the weight of the plant) for 72 hours at room temperature. The resulting alcoholic extract is filtered, and the plant residue is washed with a volume of alcohol equal to that used for extraction. The two alcoholic extracts are combined and evaporated to dryness. Then the dried residue from the alcohol solution is extracted with buffered saline and the resulting saline suspension is filtered. Each 1 ml of final saline extract is obtained from 1 gm of original plant material and contains all of the alkaloidal material not lost during purification. Therefore, the toxicity can be expressed in terms of the equivalent amount of dried plant material. The saline extract is subcutaneously injected into rats. The LD_{50} is calculated from the mortality rate at 24 hours after injection, according to the method of Weil (23).

In repeated bioassays for toxicity of a uniformly mixed sample of *D. barbeyi* (collected during prebloom and early flowerbud stages of growth) LD_{50}'s for rats ranged from 5.0 to 6.7 mg of dried plant equivalent per g of body weight (22).

The rat bioassay was used in a preliminary study to determine the feasibility of measuring differences in toxicity between larkspurs from different locales (24). The above-ground parts of

Delphinium barbeyi, D. glaucescens, and *D. occidentale* were collected during the early flowerbud stage; however, the plant samples were heterogeneous in that stalks without flower buds were included. Therefore, variability in the toxicity reflected the additive effects of stage of growth, plant species, growth site, and environmental factors. *Delphinium barbeyi* was the most toxic and *D. occidentale* the least toxic, as measured by the bioassay (Table 1). The predominant alkaloid or the chemical form in which it existed may have varied among the three species, so the efficiency of the extraction of toxic material may also have varied. Also, the correlation between the toxicity measured by the bioassay of the LD_{50} for cattle remains to be established for plant material of different toxicity. In one study with *D. barbeyi* (25) the toxicity to cattle of an alcoholic extract like that used in the bioassay was the same as the toxicity of original plant material, when the two were compared on the basis of total alkaloid content.

TABLE 1

Medial Lethal Dose (LD_{50}) for Rats of Alcoholic Extracts from Delphinium barbeyi, Delphinium glaucescens, *and* Delphinium occidentale

Plant species	LD_{50}[1] (mg/g)	Confidence[2] interval
D. barbeyi	4.5	4.0 - 5.1
D. glaucescens	16.2	12.3 - 21.4
D. occidentale	40.4	37.6 - 43.5

[1]Calculated by method of Weil (22) and expressed as milligrams of dried plant material (equivalent to extract subcutaneously injected) per gram of body weight.

[2]Estimate of an interval that will encompass the LD_{50} in 95 of 100 tests.

The bioassay method is being used to estimate differences in toxicity of larkspurs during various stages of plant growth and among different years of growth, and to determine the effects on toxicity of geographical site of growth and other environmental factors.

IV. PATHOPHYSIOLOGIC EFFECTS

The effect of larkspur poisoning on animals can vary with species, individual characteristics, and the manner in which toxicosis is induced.

In the past, several genera and species of laboratory animals have been given various extracts from larkspur (3,6,10), but until recently no standardized comparison of the response of the different species had been made. An extract of uniformly mixed collections of *D. barbeyi* was prepared in a manner similar to that previously described (22), and the final saline extract was injected subcutaneously into rats, mice, hamsters, and sheep. Sensitivity was highest for sheep and lower for mice, hamsters, and rats (listed in descending order of sensitivity) (26).

Tolerance for larkspur is higher in sheep than in cattle (7, 14,27), and it has been suggested (27) that grazing sheep before cattle may remove enough larkspur to make the range safe for the cattle grazing it later. The toxic dose for sheep was estimated to be about six times that for cattle (27); however, no data were published to support that conclusion.

The comparative toxicity for cattle and sheep of *D. barbeyi* ground plant material and extract was tested recently (25). Aboveground parts of larkspur plants were collected in central Utah in 1975. The stage of growth varied from plants with no conspicuous flowerbuds to those with well-formed buds and occasionally flowers. These growth stages are representative of those available to cattle when deaths from larkspur poisoning are commonly observed. All the plant material was air dried, ground, and thoroughly mixed before storage. Some of this material was weighed, rehydrated to 80% water content and put directly into the rumen; some was treated with 95% ethanol and the dried residue from this alcohol extraction was extracted with buffered saline. This final saline extract was injected directly into the rumen. Total dose of either ground plant or extract was given within 30 minutes. The LD_{50} was calculated for each group of animals on the basis of mortality by 48 hours after the dose was given. The clinical signs of larkspur poisoning, whether produced by ground plant or extract, were similar in cattle and sheep, with only minor exception. The cattle died faster than sheep given similar toxic materials and relative doses. Relative toxicity for both ground plant and extract, expressed as milligrams of total alkaloid per kilogram of body weight, was similar for the two animal species, although the extract seemed to be slightly more toxic. When an extract containing 1.1% total alkaloid was administered to sheep the LD_{50} was 175 mg total alkaloid/kg body weight (139-219 = confidence interval) and when administered to cattle 43 mg total alkaloid/kg body weight (35-53 = confidence interval). When ground plant material containing 2.2% total alkaloid was administered either to sheep or cattle, the LD_{50}'s were slightly larger than the corresponding LD_{50}'s using extract [sheep - 198 (162-242 = confidence interval), cattle - 55 (46-64 = confidence interval)]. The confidence intervals take into account the potential variation (estimated at ± 0.1%) in determination of the percentage total alkaloid in ground plant and extract. The data indicate that sheep can tolerate about 3.5 to 4 times as much larkspur alkaloid than can cattle. Because ground plant and extract produced the same clinical syndrome, we can reasonably assume that the major types of plant alkaloids (or their chemical product with an equivalent effect) that cause larkspur poisoning were present in the extract. This conclusion is further supported by the similarity in relative toxicity of ground plant and extract for cattle and sheep.

The effects of prolonged controlled infusion of larkspur extract into the rumen of cattle were studied (28). By use of this procedure, larkspur poisoning could be produced in the laboratory in a highly controlled and reproducible manner. The desired stage of toxicosis was repeatedly induced when the extract was infused at a given rate long enough to produce a steady-state condition. Individual animals varied significantly in their ability to tolerate infusion of the extract. This laboratory model should be very useful for study of the pathophysiological effects of larkspur poisoning and also for evaluation of potential methods of alleviating the toxicosis.

V. REFERENCES

1. Cronin, E. H., Nielsen, D. B., and Madson, N., *J. Range Manage.* 29, 364-367 (1976).
2. Wilcox, E. V., *Mont. Agric. Exp. Stn. Bull.* 22, 45-47 (1899).
3. Chestnut, V. K., and Wilcox, E. V., *U.S. Dep. Agric. Div. Bot. Bull.* 26, 65-80 (1901).
4. Glover, G. H., *Colo. Agric. Exp. Stn. Bull.* 113, 1-19 (1906).
5. Marsh, C. D., Clawson, A. B., and Marsh, H., *U.S. Dep. Agric. Farmers' Bull.* 531, 1-15 (1913).
6. Crawford, A. C., *U.S. Dep. Agric. Bur. Plant Ind. Bull.* 111, 5-12 (1907).
7. Marsh, C. D., Clawson, A. B., and Marsh, H., *U.S. Dep. Agric. Bull.* 365, 1-91 (1916).
8. Kingsbury, J. M., "Poisonous Plants of the United States and Canada," Prentice-Hall, Englewood Cliffs, New Jersey, 1964.
9. Wilcox, E. V., *Mont. Agric. Exp. Stn. Bull.* 15, 37-51 (1897).
10. Beath, O. A., *Wyo. Agric. Exp. Stn. Bull.* 120, 55-88 (1919).
11. Beath, O. A., *Wyo. Agric. Exp. Stn. Bull.* 143, 51-70 (1925).
12. Keith, L. H., and Pelletier, S. W., *in* "Chemistry of the Alkaloids," (S. W. Pelletier, Ed.), Chap. 19. Van Nostrand Reinhold Co., New York, 1970.
13. Stern, E. S., *in* "The Alkaloids," (R. H. F. Manske and H. L. Holmes, Eds.), Vol. IV, p. 275-333. Academic Press, New York, 1954.
14. Fleming, C. E., Miller, M. R., and Vawter, L. R., *Nev. Agric. Exp. Stn. Bull.* 105, 1-22 (1923).
15. Heyl, F. W., Hepner, F. E., and Loy, S. K., *Am. Chem. Soc. J.* 35, 880-885 (1913).
16. Williams, M. C., and Cronin, E. H., *Weeds* 11, 317-319 (1963).
17. Williams, M. C., and Cronin, E. H., *J. Range Manage.* 19, 274-279 (1966).
18. Laycock, W. A., *J. Range Manage.* 28, 257-259 (1975).

19. Kreps, L. B., Ph.D. Dissertation, Utah State University, 1969.
20. Knowles, K., Masters Thesis, University of Idaho, 1974.
21. Mayo, D. W., Ph.D. Dissertation, Indiana University, 1959.
22. Olsen, J. D., *Am. J. Vet. Res.* 38, 277-279 (1977).
23. Weil, C. S., *Biometrics* 8, 249-263 (1952).
24. Olsen, J. D., *J. Range Manage.* 30, 237-238 (1977).
25. Olsen, J. D., *J. Am. Vet. Med. Assoc.* (In press).
26. Olsen, J. D., Progress Report, Project No. 5702-11960-006, Current Information Retrieval Service, U.S. Department of Agriculture, 1975.
27. Marsh, C. D., Clawson, A. B., and Marsh, H., *U.S. Dep. Agric. Farmers' Bull.* 988, 1-12 (revised) (1934).
28. Olsen, J. D., "Dose-Response Characteristics for Larkspur Poisoning Determined by Controlled Infusion of Extract into the Rumen of Cattle," Am. Vet. Med. Assoc. 114th Annual Meeting Proc. Atlanta, Georgia, July 1977. (Abs.), *Vet. Human Toxicol.* (In press).

THE NATURE AND MECHANISM OF ACTION OF THE CALCINOGENIC PRINCIPLE OF *Solanum malacoxylon* AND *Cestrum diurnum*, AND A COMMENT ON *Trisetum flavescens*

R. H. Wasserman
New York State College of Veterinary Medicine, Cornell University

I. ABSTRACT

Calcinosis in grazing animals has been described in various parts of the world and the cause has been attributed to the ingestion of certain plant species. In Argentina and Brazil, the plant involved is Solanum malacoxylon; *in Miami, Florida,* Cestrum diurnum; *and in Austria and Germany,* Trisetum flavescens. *Glycosides of the active metabolite of vitamin D_3, i.e., 1,25-dihydroxycholecalciferol, have been identified in* S. malacoxylon *and* C. diurnum, *and are undoubtedly the calcinogenic principles in these plants. The calcinogenic principle in* T. flavescens *has not been identified.*

II. INTRODUCTION

Calcinosis can be defined simply as the deposition of calcium salts in soft tissues. This disease occurs in hypervitaminosis D, and as a consequence of the ingestion of calcinogenic plants, such as *Solanum malacoxylon* (syn. *S. glaucophyllum*), *Cestrum diurnum*, and *Trisetum flavescens*. The symptoms and signs of the disease vary with animal species and the extent of the intoxication. In "Enteque seco," the name given to the *S. malacoxylon*-related disease in Argentina, the affected animals show loss of weight, stiffness of forelimbs, arching of back, emaciation, and possibly death (1,2). At autopsy, there is extensive soft tissue calcification, particularly of the cardiovascular system, tendon, ligaments, lungs, diaphragm, and kidney. Another frequent sign is hypercalcemia and hyperphosphatemia. Similar symptoms are associated with "Espichamento," the calcinotic disease of Brazil caused by *S. malacoxylon* (3).

We had recently shown that *Cestrum diurnum* is the causative agent of calcinosis in the Miami, Florida area. In horses, there is progressive weight loss, lameness of increasing severity, calcium deposits in elastic tissues, and osteopetrosis (4). Similar symptoms were noted in affected cattle (5).

In the alpine region of Germany and Austria, the calcinosis of grazing animals is termed "enzootic calcinosis" and is due to the ingestion of *Trisetum flavescens* (6).

III. VITAMIN D METABOLISM

Understanding the nature of the aforementioned calcinotic diseases requires an appreciation of current views on the metabolism of vitamin D. Recent reviews (7-9) on this aspect should be consulted for details.

Vitamin D_3, acquired from the diet or produced in the skin by a reaction dependent on ultra-violet light, is further metabolized to more active derivatives. In the liver, vitamin D_3 is hydroxylated in the 25-position, yielding 25-hydroxycholecalciferol [25(OH)D_3]. The kidney is capable of producing at least two products from the 25(OH)D_3 precursor, the 1,25-dihydroxycholecalciferol [1,25(OH)$_2D_3$] or the 24,25-dihydroxycholecalciferol [24,25-(OH)$_2D_3$]. The 1,25(OH)$_2D_3$ is the most active form of the vitamin and is considered to be a hormone. The biological activity of 24,25(OH)$_2D_3$ is substantially less than that of 1,25(OH)$_2D_3$.

The concept that 1,25(OH)$_2D_3$ functions hormonally comes from the fact that it is produced at one site (kidney) and acts elsewhere (intestine, bone). Further, the rate of production of 1,25(OH)$_2D_3$ is feed-back regulated by the calcium and phosphorus status of the animal (Fig. 1). Under conditions of calcium or

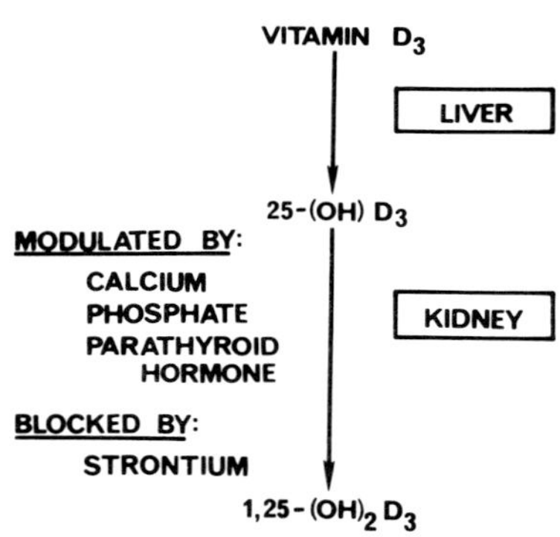

Fig. 1. *Factors that affect the hydroxylation of 25-hydroxycholecalciferol by the kidney.*

phosphate deprivation, the rate of formation of 1,25(OH)$_2D_3$ is accelerated and that for 24,25(OH)$_2D_3$ is decreased and, under conditions of calcium or phosphate adequacy, a reversal in the comparative rate of production of these derivatives occurs. Parathyroid hormone, according to some, also stimulates the formation of 1,25(OH)$_2D_3$.

The formation of 1,25(OH)$_2D_3$ can be blocked by a diet containing a high content of stable strontium (Fig. 1) (10,11). This situation has provided a useful model for studying the calcinogenic plants and other substances thought to contain 1,25(OH)$_2D_3$-like bioactivity.

Although vitamin D and its metabolites exert manifold effects in animals, a prominent response pertinent to the present discussion is that of the intestine. When vitamin D_3 is administered to a vitamin D-deficient rachitic animal, there is an increase in calcium absorption and the induction of a specific calcium-binding protein (CaBP) (7). CaBP, at least in the chick, is a sensitive indicator of its vitamin D status. In strontium-fed chicks, vitamin D_3 in physiological concentrations is biologically ineffective because the kidney 1-hydroxylase reaction is suppressed and, as a consequence, calcium absorption and CaBP synthesis are inhibited. As would be predicted, the administration of $1,25(OH)_2D_3$ to strontium-inhibited chicks stimulates the formation of CaBP and increases the degree of calcium absorption.

IV SOLANUM MALACOXYLON

Dried leaves of *S. malacoxylon* (from several sources but primarily from Dr. H. R. Camberos, Ministry of Agriculture, Argentina and Dr. G. K. Davis, University of Florida), in the initial studies, were first extracted with methanol:chloroform mixture (2:1, v/v); this inactive extract was discarded. An aqueous extract was then produced from the dried residue and, in one of several experiments, given by gavage to rachitic chicks. Duodenal ^{47}Ca absorption was determined by the ligated loop technique and CaBP levels assessed by radial immunoassay as a function of time after dose (12). The results of this experiment (Fig. 2) showed

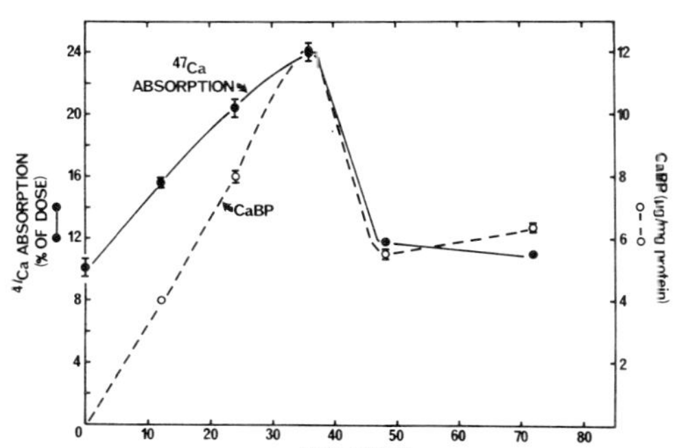

Fig. 2. *Time response of rachitic chicks to* S. malacoxylon *extract. Rachitic chicks, maintained on a rachitogenic diet during experiment, were given per os 2 ml of a partially purified aqueous extract of* S. malacoxylon. *At various times thereafter, the degree of duodenal* ^{47}Ca *absorption in situ and duodenal CaBP levels were measured in different groups of chicks, 6 chicks per group. The values are given as the mean ± SEM. The SEM is contained within the diameters of the mean points when no range lines are present. From Wasserman* et al. *(12).*

that the aqueous extract of *S. malacoxylon* contained vitamin D-like activity since both ^{47}Ca absorption and CaBP synthesis were stimulated. A bioassay of *S. malacoxylon* suggested that the plant contains about 1.3 x 10^5 I.U. vitamin D_3 equivalents per kg dried leaf (12).

TABLE 1

Effect of Partially Purified Aqueous Extract of Solanum malacoxylon *on ^{47}Ca Absorption and Duodenal CaBP in Stable Strontium-Inhibited Chicks*[1]

Group	Type of diet[2]	Addition to diet	Solanum extract given per os[3]	Duodenal ^{47}Ca absorption (% dose)	Duodenal CaBP (µg/mg protein)
1	Normal Ca	1200 IU vit. D_3/kg	-	26.4 ± 2.1	16.4 ± 1.2
2	High Sr	1200 IU vit. D_3/kg	-	9.8 ± 1.4	1.5 ± 0.1
3	High Sr	-	+	29.6 ± 6.4	36.0 ± 2.6

[1]Chicks fed a commercial chick starter diet for 3 weeks and then placed on experimental diets. One group was given the normal Ca diet for 9 days and another the high Sr diet for the same period. The third group was fed the high Sr diet for 5 days and then fed the high Sr diet minus vit. D_3 plus given the Solanum extract per os for an additional 4 days. At this time, the degree of duodenal absorption of ^{47}Ca in situ and duodenal CaBP levels were determined.

[2]The basal diet was the Cornell rachitogenic diet.

[3]The extract was prepared as follows: The Solanum leaf was extensively extracted with methanol:chloroform mixture and then the residue was extracted with water. The water extract was lyophilized and the active principle dissolved in 75% ethanol. The ethanolic extract was dried under N_2 at 60° C and redissolved in water. The dose given was equivalent to 100 mg of the original leaf.

Values represent the mean ± SEM of 5 chicks per group.

From Wasserman *et al.* (12).

Partially purified *S. malacoxylon* extract was next given to strontium-inhibited chicks (12). From Table 1, it can be seen that the strontium diet considerably depressed ^{47}Ca absorption and CaBP synthesis (Group 2), and that the *Solanum* extract essentially reversed the inhibitory effect (Group 3). These data provided the first direct evidence that the plant contained a substance or substances that exerted a biological response similar to $1,25(OH)_2D_3$.

Walling and Kimberg (13) demonstrated that *S. malacoxylon*

stimulated calcium transport in vitamin D-deficient, nephrectomized rats, and Schneider *et al.* (14) obtained similar responses in alloxan- and streptozotocin diabetic rats. In these conditions the formation of 1,25$(OH)_2D_3$ is either absent (anephric) or suppressed (diabetic). These findings are consistent with the presence of a 1,25$(OH)_2D_3$-like substance in the *Solanum* plant.

Despite the near biological equivalence between the *Solanum* factor and 1,25$(OH)_2D_3$, the solubility properties of the *Solanum* factor indicated it to be chemically distinct from 1,25$(OH)_2D_3$. However, it soon became apparent that the *Solanum* factor was a steroidal glycoside and that the active steroid was most likely generated *in vivo* by the cleavage of glycosidic linkage by endogenous or bacterial enzymes, releasing a functionally active steroid (15,16).

Purification of the factor was achieved by a multi-step procedure that included hydrolysis of the glycoside by a source of mixed hydrolases and the chromatographic separation of the steroid from related substances on silicic acid, micro-celite, and macro-celite columns. The final product yielded a u.v. spectrum identical to that of 1,25$(OH)_2D_3$, and showed a maximum at 264 nm and a minimum at 228 nm, characteristic of the 5,6-*cis*-triene system (17). Mass spectrometry of the purified product (18) was done by direct probe analysis (Fig. 3A) or in combination with gas chromatography (Fig. 3C). The direct probe spectrum is very similar to authentic 1,25$(OH)_2D_3$, yielding the parent molecular ion at m/e 416 and peaks at m/e 398, 380, and 362. The latter peaks represent the parent molecule minus 1,2 and 3 H_2O, respectively. The other fragments are also characteristic of 1,25$(OH)_2D_3$.

The g.c.-mass spectrum (Fig. 3C) nicely coincided with that of authentic 1,25$(OH)_2D_3$ (Fig. 3B). Cyclization of the steroids during the course of the gas chromatographic separation accounts for the difference between that spectrum and that produced by direct probe analysis (8).

V. CESTRUM DIURNUM

Leaves of *C. diurnum* were dried at room temperature and ground to a fine powder. The ground leaf was extracted with chloroform (inactive, discarded) and the residue extracted with methanol: chloroform (2:1, v/v). The methanol:chloroform extract contained vitamin D-like activity, unlike a comparable extract from *S. malacoxylon* (19). Bioassay of the plant leaf in rachitic chicks indicated it to contain about 3 x 10^3 I.U. vitamin D_3 equivalents per kg dried leaf or about one-tenth that of the South American plant (19).

The possible presence of 1,25$(OH)_2D_3$ activity in *C. diurnum* was tested by the use of the strontium-inhibited chick model (19, 20). As shown in Fig. 4, the stable strontium diet depressed calcium absorption and inhibited CaBP synthesis, even in the presence of vitamin D_3. Inclusion of *C. diurnum* leaf powder at

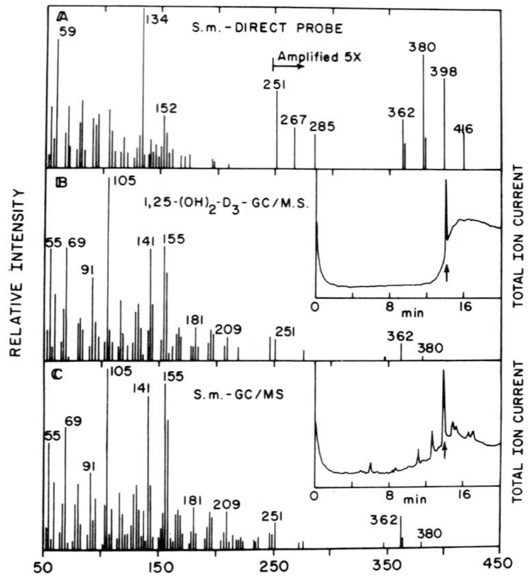

Fig. 3. *Analysis of the lipophilic fragment of* S. malacoxylon *by gas chromatography and mass spectrometry. (A) Direct probe mass spectrum of 1 μg of purified hydrolyzed* S. malacoxylon. *(B) Gas chromatogram-mass of 1 μg of synthetic 1,25-(OH)$_2$D$_3$. The inset shows the gas chromatographic trace; the arrow shows the peak fraction which was characterized by mass spectrometry. (C) Gas chromatogram-mass spectrum of 2 μg of purified hydrolyzed* S. malacoxylon. *The inset shows the gas chromatographic tract; the arrow shows the peak fraction which was characterized by mass spectrometry. From Wasserman* et al. *(18).*

levels of 1.5% or 3.0% in the diet reversed the inhibition in a dose-related fashion. This provided evidence that the Miami plant also contained a substance that mimicked the action of 1,25(OH)$_2$D$_3$. *C. diurnum* extract was also able to stimulate calcium and phosphate absorption in the anephric rat (21).

The purification of the factor in *C. diurnum* was recently achieved, using methodology similar to that for the *S. malacoxylon* factor (22). The *C. diurnum* factor also occurs as a steroidal glycoside in the plant and, after hydrolysis, acts biologically and chromatographically like authentic 1,25(OH)$_2$D$_3$. A preliminary mass spectrum in combination with gas chromatography has been obtained, and the spectral pattern is similar to that of authentic 1,25(OH)$_2$D$_3$ analyzed under the same conditions.

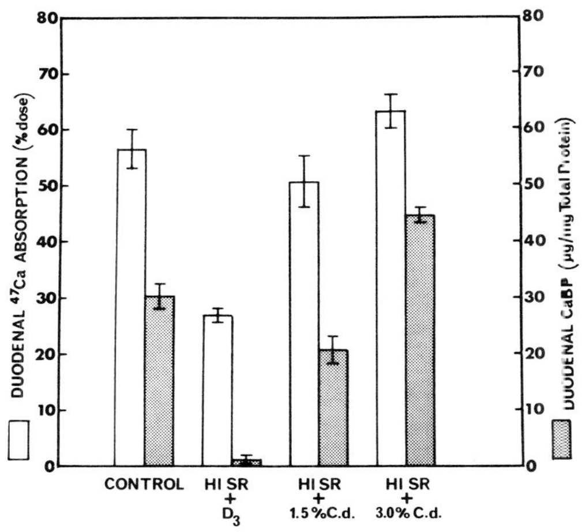

Fig. 4. *Prevention by* C. diurnum *of the inhibitory effect of dietary stable strontium on calcium absorption and the synthesis of the vitamin D-induced calcium-binding protein. Values represent the mean ± SEM of 6 chicks per group. Modified from Wasserman* et al. *(20).*

VI MECHANISM OF CALCINOSIS PRODUCTION

From the foregoing, it is evident that *S. malacoxylon* and *C. diurnum* contain substances that appear to be glycosides of 1,25-$(OH)_2D_3$. With this information, an explanation of the cause of the disease can be offered. In the previous brief discourse on vitamin D metabolism, it was mentioned that the renal formation of the active metabolite of vitamin D, i.e., 1,25$(OH)_2D_3$, was subjected to negative feed-back regulation. If, however, a source of 1,25$(OH)_2D_3$ is supplied exogenously, it is evident that the regulatory step is by-passed. As a consequence, excess intestinal CaBP is synthesized, and excessive amounts of calcium and phosphate are absorbed. This over-abundant absorption of mineral apparently cannot be physiologically accommodated and deposition of mineral into soft tissues (calcinosis) and osteopetrosis occur. These and accessory events associated with calcinosis are summarized graphically in Fig. 5. The possibility that the soft tissues are directly and adversely affected by excess 1,25$(OH)_2D_3$ should also be considered.

VII. COMMENT ON TRISETUM FLAVESCENS

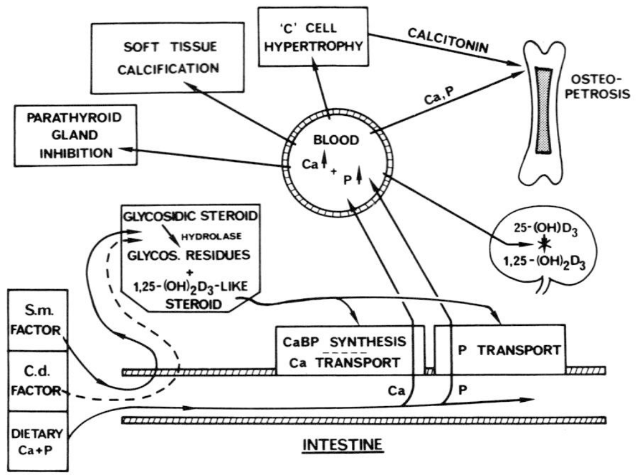

Fig. 5. *Proposed scheme by which calcinosis is produced in grazing animals due to the ingestion of the calcinogenic plants,* Solanum malacoxylon *(S.m.) and* Cestrum diurnum *(C.d.). From Wasserman (24).*

Specimens of *T. flavescens* obtained from Germany were dried and their biological properties investigated by a similar protocol as used with *S. malacoxylon* and *C. diurnum* (23). It was disclosed that *T. flavescens* contained only about 600-800 vitamin D_3 equivalents per kg dried plant. One of the three batches tested was able to cause a minimal induction of CaBP in strontium-inhibited chicks. The data therefore indicated that most or all of the vitamin D activity in *T. flavescens* is not equivalent to $1,25(OH)_2D_3$. From this, it was concluded that either the mechanism by which *T. flavescens* causes calcinosis differs from that of the other two calcinogenic plants, or that the $1,25(OH)_2D_3$ activity in *T. flavescens* is very labile and/or present in very low concentrations.

VIII. REFERENCES

1. Worker, N. A., and Carrillo, B. J., *Nature (London)* 215, 72 (1967).
2. Carrillo, B. J., and Worker, N. A., *Rev. Invest. Agropecu. INTA* 4, 9 (1967).
3. Döbereiner, J., Tokarnia, C. H., DeCosta, J. B. D., Campos, J. L. E., and Dayrell, M. D., *Pesqui. Agropecu. Bras. Ser. Vet.* 6, 91 (1971).
4. Krook, L., Wasserman, R. H., Shively, J. N., Tashjian, A. H., Jr., Brokken, T. D., and Morton, J. F., *Cornell Vet.* 65, 26 (1975).

5. Krook, L., Wasserman, R. H., McEntee, K., Brokken, T. D., and Teigland, M. B., *Cornell Vet.* 65, 557 (1975).
6. Dirksen, G., Plank, P., Simon, U., Hänichen, T., Daniel, P., Spiess, A., *Dtsch. Tieraertztl. Wochenschr.* 81, 1 (1974).
7. Wasserman, R. H., and Corradino, R. A., *Vitam. Horm.* 31, 43 (1973).
8. Haussler, M., *Nutr. Rev.* 32, 257 (1974).
9. DeLuca, H. F., and Schnoes, H. K., *Annu. Rev. Biochem.* 45, 631 (1976).
10. Omdahl, J. L., and DeLuca, H. F., *J. Biol. Chem.* 247, 5520 (1972).
11. Corradino, R. A., Ebel, J. G., Craig, P. H., Taylor, A. N., and Wasserman, R. H., *Calcif. Tissue Res.* 7, 81 (1971).
12. Wasserman, R. H., Bar, A., Corradino, R. A., Taylor, A. N., and Peterlik, M., *in* "Calcium-Regulating Hormones" (R. V. Talmage, M. Owens, and J. A. Parson, Eds.), pp. 318-329. Excerpta Medica, Amsterdam, 1975.
13. Walling, M. W., and Kimberg, D. V., *Gastroenterology* 69, 200 (1975).
14. Schneider, L. E., Wasserman, R. H., and Schedl, H. P., *Endocrinology* 97, 649 (1975).
15. Peterlik, M., and Wasserman, R. H., *FEBS Lett.* 56, 16 (1975).
16. Peterlik, M., Bursac, K., Haussler, M. R., Hughes, M. R., and Wasserman, R. H., *Biochem. Biophys. Res. Commun.* 70, 797 (1976).
17. Haussler, M. R., Wasserman, R. H., McCain, T. A., Peterlik, M., Bursac, K. M., Hughes, M. R., and Haussler, M. R., *J. Nutr.* 106, 457 (1976).
18. Wasserman, R. H., Henion, J. D., Haussler, M. R., and McCain, T. A., *Science* 194, 853 (1976).
19. Wasserman, R. H., Corradino, R. A., Krook, L., Hughes, M. R., and Haussler, M. R., *J. Nutr.* 106, 457 (1976).
20. Wasserman, R. H., Corradino, R. A., and Krook, L., *Biochem. Biophys. Res. Commun.* 62, 85 (1975).
21. Walling, M. W., Kimberg, D. V., Wasserman, R. H., and Feinberg, R. R., *Endocrinology* 98, 1130 (1976).
22. Hughes, M. R., Haussler, M. R., McCain, T. A., Villareale, M., and Wasserman, R. H., *Nature* 268, 347 (1977).
23. Wasserman, R. H., Krook, L., and Dirksen, G., *Cornell Vet.* 67, 333 (1977).
24. Wasserman, R. H., *in* "Dukes' Physiology of Domestic Animals," 9th Edition (M. J. Swenson, Ed.), Chap. 34. Cornell University Press, Ithaca, 1977.

HAIRY VETCH (*Vicia villosa* ROTH) POISONING IN CATTLE

R. J. Panciera
College of Veterinary Medicine, Oklahoma State University

I. ABSTRACT

*A disease of cattle, apparently associated with the ingestion of hairy vetch (*Vicia villosa *Roth), was observed in 23 herds. Clinically, the disease was characterized by dermatitis, conjunctivitis, diarrhea, and other less prominent signs. The morbidity was 6 to 8%, and the mortality approached 50% of clinically affected animals. Pathologic changes consisted basically of extensive infiltration of many organs by lymphoreticular cells, plasma cells, multinucleated giant cells, and eosinophils.*

II. INTRODUCTION

Hairy vetch, *Vicia villosa* Roth, is a legume adapted to growth throughout much of the USA and temperate climates of the world. It is perhaps the most widely cultivated vetch in the USA where it is used as pasturage, harvested as hay and silage, and utilized as a cover crop (1). In Oklahoma it is often seeded in the fall with small grains or drilled into established sod to provide winter and spring pasture. Major growth occurs in April, May, and June; maturation and seed production in mid June and July. In more northern climates maturity is reached later in the summer.

Several species of the genus, *Vicia* are reported to be toxic (2,3,4), but none of the reported syndromes resemble the disease I will describe.

Poisoning from consumption of the seed of hairy vetch results in growth depression and death in chicks and turkey poults (5,6, 7). Arscott and Harper (8) were not able to determine whether mortality was due to a toxic principle or to unpalatability and malnutrition.

Three apparently different syndromes in cattle have been reported due to consumption of hairy vetch. In the first syndrome illness and death were recorded in a group of cattle after eating seed (9). There was acute onset of nervous derangement including bellowing, sexual excitement, locomotor difficulty, and convulsions. I have seen this syndrome and death in four of five mature dairy cattle within several hours after consumption of a mixture of rye and hairy vetch seed. A second syndrome, associated with consumption of hairy vetch pasture resulted in death of 6 of 36 cattle (10). Signs included subcutaneous swellings of the head, neck, and body and herpetiform eruptions in the oral mucous membranes, purulent nasal discharge, rales, cough, congestion, and cyanosis of mucous membranes, alopecia, weakness, and loss of appetite. Death occurred after 12 to 15 days illness. Necropsy revealed serohemorrhagic effusions in the subcutis, inflammation of the stomach, severe bronchitis and incipient pneumonia, edema of the glottis, yellowish liver, and punctiform myocardial hemorrhages. Peritonitis and nephritis were seen in some cattle. The third syndrome, reported in 1966 (11), is the major topic of this presentation.

Since October, 1955, I have seen a disease in cattle that occurred only when the cattle had access to pastures containing hairy vetch (*V. Villosa* Roth). The clinical and pathologic details of the disease based on observations made in the study of cases from outbreaks of the disease will be presented.

III. CLINICAL SIGNS

Prominent among the clinical signs were dermatitis which varied in character according to the stage of illness. Initially, the coat became roughened, and small (2 to 5 mm.) papular swellings and larger plaques developed in the skin. These sometimes became confluent giving rise to diffuse lesions. Exudation of clear to slightly yellow fluid occurred through the epithelial surface, and the exudate dried with the formation of yellow-brown, crusty material. Removal of the crusts exposed an underlying erythematous or blanched epithelial surface or erosion. There was usually pruritus, sometimes intense. The skin became obviously thickened, less pliable, and often assumed a somewhat folded or fissured appearance (Fig. 1). Alopecia involving the affected

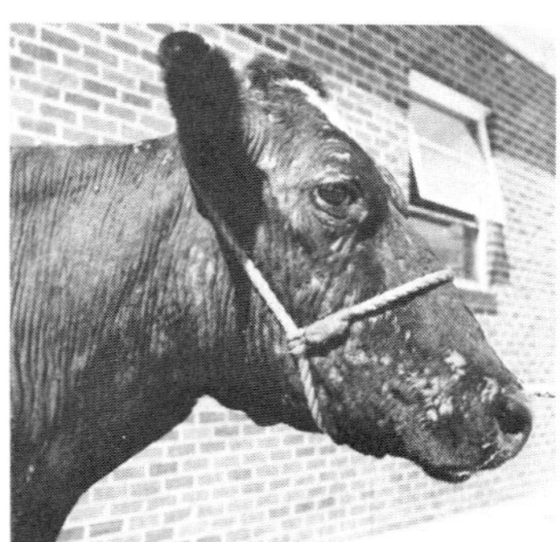

Fig. 1. *Thickening and folding of skin of neck and face of cow. Notice hairless plaquelike lesions in skin of face.*

areas occurred as a late stage in the cutaneous lesion. Ulceration occasionally ensued and was attributed, in part, to self-mutilation. The skin of the escutcheon, perineum, udder and teats, tailhead, and neck was generally involved at the onset of disease. Later, and less consistently, lesions appeared in the skin of the face, trunk, and limbs. Cutaneous lesions were distributed without regard to pigmentation.

Conjunctivitis, manifested by congestion and edema of the conjunctiva and lids, and a serous, mucous or cloudy ocular discharge was seen in some cattle. Occasionally, cattle had serous or mucous discharge and salivation. Severe diarrhea, sometimes bloody, was a relatively frequent sign in advanced cases. Labored respiratory movements and cough also occurred but not consistently. Body temperatures were variable; temperatures as high as 106° F (41.1° C) were recorded in some animals, but many did not have elevated body temperatures. The temperature of the individual animal sometimes fluctuated between normal and elevated.

Loss of appetite and considerable loss of body weight frequently accompanied the cases of disease that were more than mild. A few affected cattle were reported to have voided red urine; I saw this in one animal. The source and nature of the pigment(s) were not determined.

Abortion occurred in two of the 30 fatal cases. One rancher reported three abortions in a group of 90 cattle, seven of which had obvious signs of the disease. The cause(s) of abortion were not determined. The evidence available was considered inadequate to assume a relationship between the discoloration of urine, abortion, and this syndrome.

Most outbreaks of the disease occurred in cattle pastured on mixtures of hairy vetch and small grains including rye, wheat, or oats, but two herds were pastured on Bermuda grass overseeded with vetch. Twenty-two of the twenty-three outbreaks occurred between April and July. One occurred in December. With the exception of three years, sporadic cases or outbreaks have come to our attention annually since 1959.

The disease was most prevalent and severe in cattle three years or older. Younger cattle usually had mild disease but two are known to have died.

Eleven of the 23 herds involved consisted of Holstein-Friesians and 12 of Aberdeen Angus. Disease did not develop until at least two weeks after cattle had access to pastures containing vetch. In most instances six or more weeks transpired before signs of illness were recognized in one or more animals. Illness was not noticed in one cow that eventually died of the disease until about two weeks after she was removed from the pasture containing vetch; however, the first sign in this cow was alopecia, which suggested that she had been ill at least one or two weeks earlier. The morbidity rate, somewhat inaccurate because of difficulties in recognition of mildly affected animals, ranged from one cow to as high as 35 percent (mean 6 to 8 percent). Mortality usually approached 50 percent of those cattle recognized as ill, but varied from 0 to 100 percent. The interval between observed onset of illness and death varied between three days and five weeks, most cattle having died after a course of illness of about 10 to 20 days. The reported three-day interval is believed to have resulted from an error in observation.

There have been no consistent aberrations in the limited hematologic and clinical chemical data obtained.

IV. PATHOLOGIC FINDINGS

The basic lesion of the disease is cellular infiltration occurring in relatively discrete multifocal distribution or more diffuse pattern resulting in disruption of the architecture and often enlargement of the infiltrated organ. This lesion exists in many organs. The lesions were gray to gray-yellow, moderately firm and, when not extensive, fairly sharply demarcated from adjacent normal tissue. The renal cortex usually contained multiple 2-4 mm foci on the surface and extending into the cortical parenchyma as nodular foci or gray streaks (Fig. 2). Myocardial

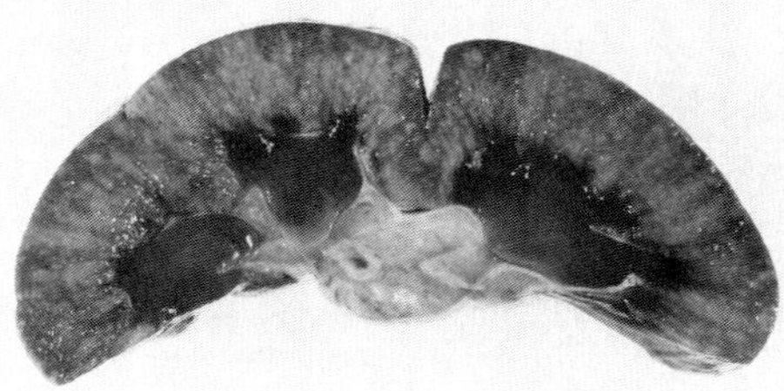

Fig. 2. *Multiple grayish foci representing cellular infiltrations in the renal cortical parenchyma.*

infiltrate existed as yellow-gray foci or streaks most evident in the ventricles.

The adrenal glands were often markedly enlarged because of diffuse and extensive cellular infiltration of both the cortex and medulla, occasionally to a degree that they were grossly unrecognizable as adrenal glands. Radial gray streaks were present in the cortex of less severely affected adrenals; diffuse medullary infiltration existed in some (Fig. 3). Lymph nodes ranged from normal to markedly enlarged with either obliteration of cortical architecture by rather homogenous gray infiltrate or gray nodular formations up to 8 mm diameter in the cortex. Occasionally the spleen was moderately enlarged, sometimes with enlargement of splenic follicles. Thyroid glands were sometimes enlarged and diffusely pale or mottled gray.

Histologic lesions in the various organs were similar, consisting of focal or widespread infiltration by macrophages, lymphocytes, plasma cells, multinucleated giant cells, and often

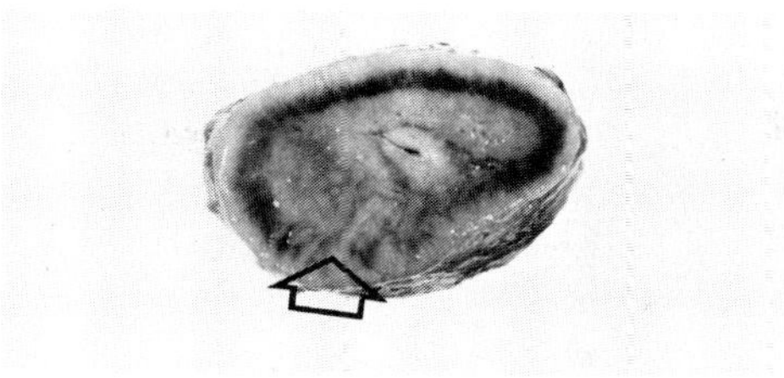

Fig. 3. *Adrenal gland- Cortical and medullary architecture disrupted (arrow) by cellular infiltration.*

numerous eosinophils. Cellular infiltrates were most prevalent in the renal cortical interstitium, myocardium, adrenal medulla and cortex, and the dermis. They occurred less frequently in the thyroids, the mandibular, parotid and pharyngeal salivary glands, pancreas, spleen, lymph nodes, and portal areas of the liver. Occasionally other organs including the trachea, bronchi, gall bladder, intestine, ovary, and endometrium contained cellular infiltrate. Neither were all the listed organs nor those not listed examined in each case of the disease; therefore, the stated incidence of lesions is incomplete and of limited accuracy.

Myocardial fibers within and immediately adjacent to infiltrated areas were degenerate or necrotic and occasionally mineralized (Fig. 4). Atrophy of renal tubules and glandular elements

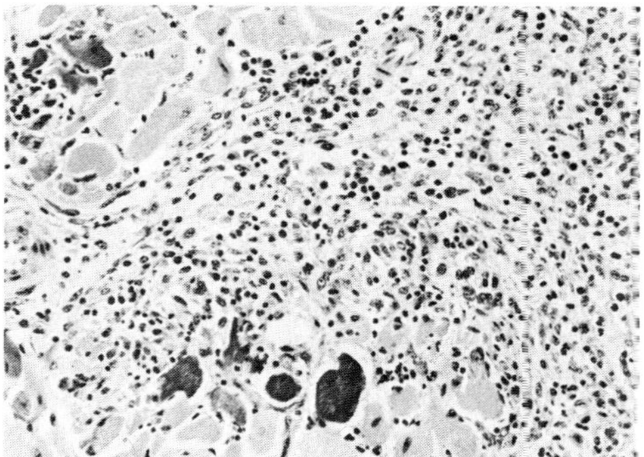

Fig. 4. *Myocardium- Cellular infiltration, myonecrosis, and mineralization.*

occurred in organs where cellular infiltration was marked (Fig. 5). Infiltration of the adrenal was occasionally so extensive that adrenal cortical and medullary architecture was not perceptible. Cellular infiltration of lymph nodes was predominately cortical where cellular infiltration occurred within hyperplastic follicles or diffusely throughout the cortex causing effacement of

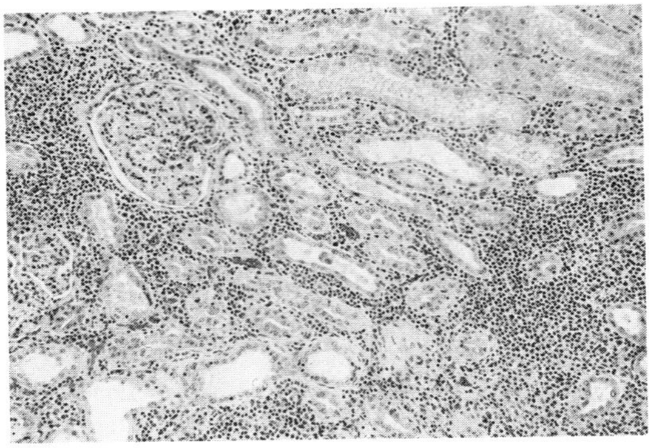

Fig. 5. *Cellular infiltrate in renal cortical interstitium.*

cortical architecture. Cellular infiltration of the spleen was usually in splenic follicles. Granulomatous foci composed of groups of multinucleated giant cells, large mononuclear cells and marginal eosinophils commonly constituted the reaction within the spleen (Fig. 6). Affected thyroids had cellular infiltrates

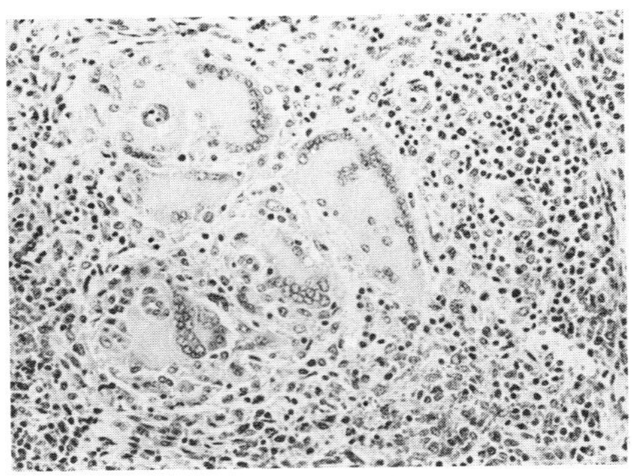

Fig. 6. *Multinucleated giant cells in splenic granuloma.*

dispersed diffusely or in irregular nodules within the interfollicular stroma (Fig. 7). Displacement or atrophy and replacement of follicles were present in areas of intense cellular infiltration. Infiltrating cells sometimes transmigrated follicular epithelium and were distributed within colloid.

The cutaneous lesion was an exudative dermatitis which, in mild cases, was characterized by mild hyperkeratosis and infiltration by lymphocytes, plasma cells, eosinophils, and a few histocytes about dermal blood vessels. More severe lesions contained more intense and diffuse cellular infiltrates, particularly dense

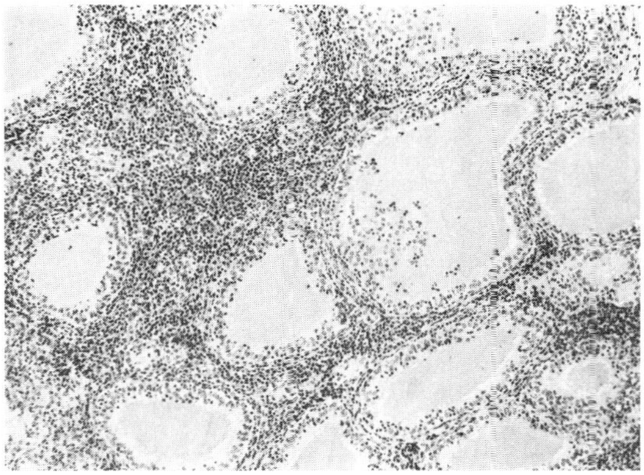

Fig. 7. *Thyroid- Cellular infiltration of interfollicular stroma.*

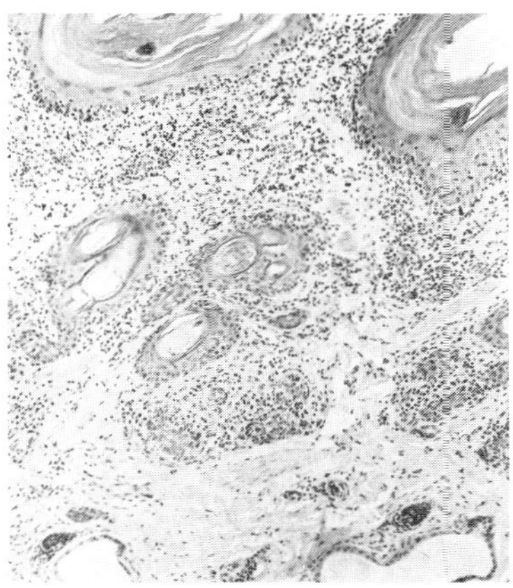

Fig 8. *Skin- Hyperkeratosis of epidermis, edema, and cellular infiltration of basal epithelium and dermis.*

about vessels and adnexal structures (Fig. 8). Edema of the dermis and basal layers of the epidermis and invasion of the epidermis by dermal cellular infiltrate often existed, occasionally with focal ulceration of the epidermis. The walls of many dermal arterioles were moderately thickened and hyalinized, and endothelial nuclei were swollen.

V. DISCUSSION

I am not aware of attempts to isolate and identify a toxic principle responsible for this syndrome. Our attempts to reproduce disease have been limited to enforced grazing of three cattle for 28 days in a stand of pure vetch. Disease did not develop. This result is not particularly surprising since thousands of cattle each year are pastured in hairy vetch usually without incident. The cause and effect relationship between hairy vetch and disease remains only circumstantial; there is clearly an association, one strengthened by the occurrence of the disease in widespread regions of this country only in cattle with access of hairy vetch pasture. I have reviewed cases from Georgia, Missouri, New York, and Texas.

There are implications in the literature that insects that parasitize vetch might be responsible for "vetch toxicosis" syndromes (10). While some of the pastures in which the cases of this series occurred were heavily infested with aphids, others were either free or nearly free of infestation. It is perhaps significant that the majority of cases of the disease occur in Oklahoma during May and June, a season when hairy vetch is at the zenith of its growth and, concomitantly, the small grains with which vetch is usually seeded become mature and unpalatable. It is likely that the absolute and relative intake of vetch is greatest during this period. It may also be significant that severe disease has occurred mainly in adult cows; younger animals usually are mildly or not at all affected. The reason for this is not apparent but may be related to the amount of the plant consumed or possibly to repeated exposure to the plant.

Also notable is the breed incidence of disease. Each of the 12 beef cattle represented in this series of necropsies was Angus, yet Hereford cattle are the predominant beef breed in the State. The obvious inference of this observation is that Angus cattle are more susceptible to the syndrome than are Hereford cattle.

Differentiation between this disease and the cutaneous arthropod infestations, allergic urticarias, cutaneous mycoses, photosensitization, highly chlorinated naphthalene poisoning, and pox and other viral dermatoses should be relatively simple through consideration of the herd history, distribution and character of the lesions, course of disease, and presence or absence of other signs.

There is some similarity between the grossly visible, visceral lesions of this disease and those of malignant lymphoma, but distinct differences exist in the homogeneity of the infiltrating cell populations, in the organs affected and in the pattern of invasion of the individual organ. Invasion in the vetch related syndrome can generally be recognized to consist of multiple focal lesions with or without confluence rather than the relatively diffuse infiltration that characterizes lymphomatous involvement. Distinction between the vetch syndrome and the various granulomatous diseases and diseases with a pronounced lymphoreticular response is possible by consideration of the herd history, distribution of lesions, and other factors.

VI. REFERENCES

1. Henson, P. R., and Schotch, H. A., *U. S. Dep. Agric. Farmers' Bull.* 1740, 1968.
2. Kingsbury, J. M., "Poisonous Plants of the United States and Canada," p. 362-364. Prentice-Hall, Englewood Cliffs, New Jersey, 1964.
3. Steyn, D. G., "The Toxicology of Plants in South Africa," pp. 103-109. Central News Agency Ltd., Johannesburg, Union of South Africa, 1934.
4. Watt, J. M., and Breyer-Brandwijk, M. G., "The Medicinal and Poisonous Plants of Southern and Eastern Africa," p. 667. E & S Livingstone, Edinburgh and London, 1962.
5. Thayer, R. H., and Heller, V. G., *Proc. Okla. Acad. Sci.* pp. 40-43 (1945).
6. Arscott, G. H., and Harper, J. A., *Poult. Sci.* 43, 271-273 (1964).
7. Keinholz, E. W., Jensen, L. S., and McGinnis, J., *Poult. Sci.* 41, 367-371 (1962).
8. Harper, J. A., and Arscott, G. H., *Poult. Sci.* 41, 1968-1974 (1962).
9. Claughton, W. P., and Claughton, *Auburn Vet.* 10, 125-126 (1955).
10. Volker, R., and Frohner, E., "Lehrbuch der Toxikologie fur Tierarzte," 6th Ed., pp. 272-273. Ferdinand Enke, Stuttgart, Germany, 1950.
11. Panciera, R. J., Johnson, L., and Osburn, B. I., *J. Am. Vet. Med. Assoc.* 148, 804-808 (1966).

LUPINOSIS: CHEMICAL PROPERTIES OF PHOMOPSIN A, THE MAIN TOXIC METABOLITE OF *Phomopsis leptostromiformis*

C. C. J. Culvenor, L. W. Smith, J. L. Frahn, and P. A. Cockrum
CSIRO Division of Animal Health

I. ABSTRACT

Phomopsin A, the main toxic metabolite of Phomopsis leptostromiformis *responsible for lupinosis, has an empirical formula approximately* $C_{33}H_{44}N_5O_{13}Cl$. *There are 3 acidic centers per molecule which are probably phenolic, β-diketone or ββ-triketone in nature. Ultraviolet, infrared, and nuclear magnetic resonance spectra are described. These and the mild acid hydrolysis of phomopsin A to oxalacetic acid and an amine suggest that the metabolite is related to tenuazonic acid.*

II. INTRODUCTION

Lupinosis is a disease with a long history, having first appeared in Europe over 100 years ago after lupin species came into use there as a fodder crop (1). It has become an important problem in the sheep industry in Western Australia where lupins were initially used as a valuable crop in coastal areas. They are now increasingly grown in other areas for their high-protein seed, including the eastern states where lupinosis has also appeared.

Lupinosis occurs when sheep graze post-harvest roughage which, through humid or wet weather, has become infested with the fungus *Phomopsis leptostromiformis*. Affected sheep lose appetite and eventually collapse. The main lesions are in the liver which is bright yellow or orange and fatty in acute cases and tan colored, small, distorted, and cirrhotic in chronic cases (1,2).

Investigations in the Division of Animal Health have been centered on the isolation of the toxic metabolite(s) of *P. leptostromiformis* responsible for the disease and determination of their chemical structure.

III. ISOLATION

Initial fractionation studies were carried out in Western Australia by Petterson and Beck who used a bioassay based on the mitosis-arresting effect of the toxin on mouse liver cells (3). They established methods for extracting the toxin from lupin roughage with aqueous methanol and for its further concentration by extraction from aqueous solution with butanol at pH 3.5 and re-extraction back into water at pH 8. They concluded that the toxin had phenolic or acidic properties.

Our fractionations were conducted on extracts of a *P. leptostromiformis* culture grown on lupin seeds, with a cell culture assay for routine assessment and an *in vivo* young rat assay developed from the mouse assay for critical checking. In the young rat assay, abnormal mitotic figures were counted in liver sections 18 hours after injection of toxin (4). After more than the usual problems and difficulties, occasioned by a relatively unstable toxin and unexplained losses of toxicity during fractionations, the preparation of a crystalline mixture of two active metabolites, phomopsins A and B, was accomplished (5). Two key steps were partitioning into aqueous tetrahydrofuran and chromatography on macroreticular polystyrene resin.

The crystalline mixture, resolvable into its two components by electrophoresis, was highly active in the young rat assay and produced typical signs of lupinosis in a sheep when given intraperitoneally. Phomopsins A and B, after electrophoretic separation, were each active in the young rat.

IV. PHOMOPSINS A AND B

The crystalline product obtained from the initial fractionation experiments was approximately 80% phomopsin A, 20% phomopsin B, but it contained also small amounts of other apparently related compounds, detectable by electrophoresis and tentatively named phomopsins C, D, and E. The series of metabolites produce spots on pherograms which absorb strongly under UV light and also form yellow spots changing to white on a brown background when sprayed with a $KMnO_4$ - CrO_3 - H_2SO_4 reagent. The formation of this family of metabolites has hindered structural studies because of the need for resolution into pure components. The only satisfactory method available so far is electrophoresis on 1 mg batches. A recent repeat isolation from a new lupin seed culture overcame the problem when the product was found to be 99% phomopsin A. Some of the metabolites are apparently formed by slow hydrolysis or other reactions during the course of isolation.

Phomopsin A like the mixture of phomopsins A and B, crystallizes most readily from aqueous tetrahydrofuran, forming colorless prisms, which effloresce rapidly in the air and decompose above 205° without melting. Phomopsin A also crystallizes from mixtures of methanol, ethanol and water. Microanalysis of crystals dried at 60° *in vacuo* gave the following results: C, 51.7; H, 5.8; N, 9.4; O, 27.4; Cl, 4.6; S, 0.0; P, 0.0%. The presence of chlorine was confirmed by qualitative test and an X-ray emission spectrum, the latter also demonstrating absence of metals. On this basis the empirical formula of phomopsin A is approximately $C_{33}H_{44}N_5O_{13}Cl$ which requires C, 52.5; H, 5.9; N, 9.3; O, 27.6; Cl, 4.7%; mol. wt. 754.2. Allowing for ± 0.3% error in the chlorine analysis, the empirical formula might be in the range

C_{31}-C_{35} and the formula weight 710-810.

Although some evidence pointed to the molecular weight being double the formula weight - elution volume from Sephadex G25, failure to give a mass spectrum with a molecular ion, size of the unit cell in two different crystals as determined by X-ray diffraction measurements (B. J. Poppleton, unpublished results) - there is a firm indication from ^{13}C nuclear magnetic resonance (nmr) spectra that the molecular formula is the same as the empirical formula. A proton-decoupled ^{13}C nmr spectrum contains strong peaks (I, 30-100% of the highest peak) for 30 carbon atoms, 6 weaker peaks (I, 20-30%) which are visibly separate and 9 other weak peaks which are close to strong peaks and may possibly be instrumental artifacts. Some of the low-intensity peaks may represent carbon atoms of long relaxation time or the presence of a tautomer or geometric isomer (e.g. *cis-trans* amide isomerism), but the total number of carbons is unlikely to exceed 36. An approximately C_{70} formula is possible only if the molecule is made up of two equal halves.

Paper electrophoresis has provided evidence on the equivalent weight and the type of acidic grouping. Phomopsin A forms a sharply defined spot with anionic mobility 5.7 cm/hr/kv at pH 9.2. If size and charge are the main factors involved, comparison with other compounds suggests an equivalent weight of 220-280. Thus there are probably 3 anionic centers per molecule. The change of mobility with pH indicates that ionization is complete at pH 9 and fully suppressed at pH 4, with half-ionization at pH 7. Thus phomopsin A has an acidity between those of simple phenols and carboxylic acids and similar to that of phenols with a ring-activating group (e.g. p-nitrophenol, pK 7.1) or tetramic acids [e.g. pyrrolidine-2,4-dione, pK_a 6.4; N-methylpyrrolidine-2,4-dione, pK_a 7.05 (6)]. Carboxylic acids or 3-acyltetramic acids such as tenuazonic acid [pK_a 3.4 (7)] are unlikely unless subject to a strong deactivating effect. The electrophoresis evidence on ionization is in accord with solubility in water at pH 7.5 and above, but sparing solubility at pH 3. Phomopsin A also has weakly basic groupings since it is soluble in dilute hydrochloric acid.

Phomopsin B has an anionic mobility of 4.5 cm/hr/kv at pH 9.2, but has not yet been studied in detail.

V. ULTRAVIOLET AND INFRARED SPECTRA

The ultraviolet absorption of phomopsin A (Fig. 1) is closely similar to that of the mixed crystals of phomopsins A and B (5) making allowance for the calculation of molar extinction coefficients on the present basis of molecular weight, 754; λ_{max} (log ε) values: in methanol 210 (4.73), 227 (sh), 290 (4.20) nm; in dilute HCl 210 (4.71), 227 (sh), 286 (4.24) nm; in dilute NaOH 221 (4.58), 254 (4.30), 280 (4.14) nm. It approximates the absorption of certain simple aromatic and heteroaromatic nuclei, including

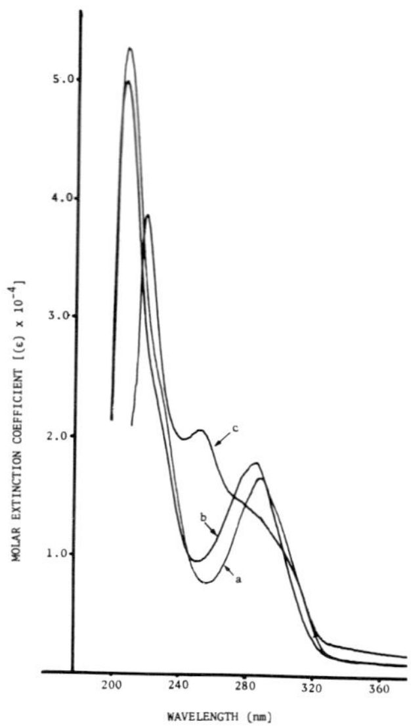

Fig. 1. *Ultraviolet spectrum of phomopsin A: (a) in methanol, (b) in dilute HCl, (c) in dilute NaOH.*

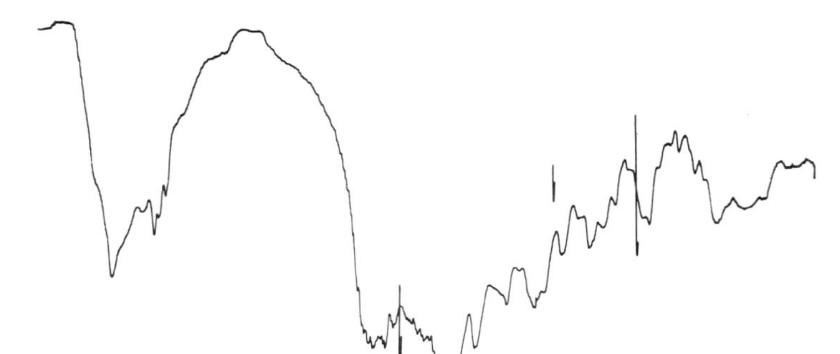

Fig. 2. *Infra-red spectrum of phomopsin A (KBr disc).*

phenols, without showing in alkali the typical shift to higher wavelength and increased intensity exhibited by phenols. However the peak at 254 nm in dilute NaOH might represent the shoulder at 227 nm in acid or alcohol solution. There are also resemblances to, and differences from, the spectra of 3-acyltetramic acids. Thus tenuazonic acid has peaks at 217, 277 in ethanol, 220, 277 nm in dilute HCl and 240, 279 nm in dilute NaOH(6) but the absorption is weaker in the 210-220 nm region than for phomopsin A.

The infrared spectrum measured as a KBr disc (Fig. 2) shows strong and broad absorption at 3300-3500 cm^{-1}, corresponding to hydrogen-bonded OH or NH and strong peaks at 1600- 1700 cm^{-1} appropriate to amide carbonyls or hydrogen-bonded aromatic or enolic carbonyls. Ester groupings of the latter type are not excluded (e.g. salicylic acid, ν_{CO} 1684 cm^{-1}) nor are carbamates.

VI. NUCLEAR MAGNETIC RESONANCE SPECTRA

Proton nmr spectra of phomopsin A were of disappointing quality apparently because of isomerism or restricted freedom of movement due to large molecular size. The 60 MHz spectrum shown in Fig. 3 is of fully ionized phomposin A in D_2O at pH 9-10 with dioxan as internal reference and lock. There appear to be 6 methyl peaks (chemical shifts relative to dioxan, δ3.70): a triplet and singlet, δ1.07 due to CH_3-CH_2 and CH_3-C; 3 singlets, δ1.54, 1.63, 1.77, due to CH_3-C-OCOR, CH_3-C-NHCOR, or CH_3-C=C; and a singlet, δ2.36, probably due to NCH_3 or CH_3-C=C. A small multiplet, δ3.53, possibly due to CH-O or CH-N, is obscured by the lock

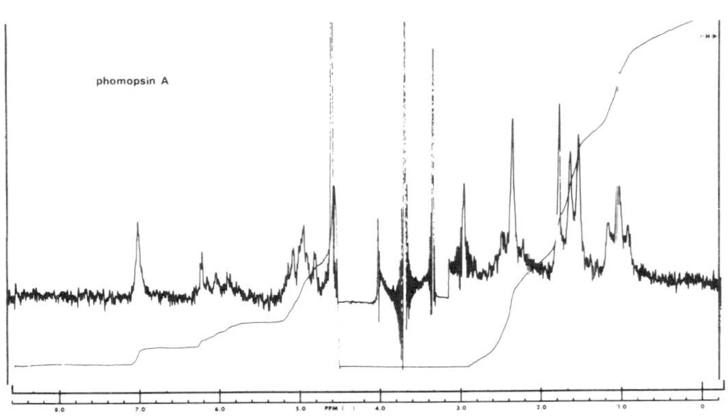

Fig. 3. *Proton nmr spectrum of phomopsin A, measured at 60 MHz in D_2O, pH 9-10, with dioxan as internal reference, δ3.7.*

signal. An approximately 6-proton multiplet centered on δ4.95 may be due to CH-O-acyl, CH-N-acyl or protons adjacent to two deshielding groups. Of the remaining multiplets in the C=C or aromatic region, the lines centered on δ5.96 could possibly be an AB system with further splitting, and those at δ6.24, 7.02 are approximate singlets representing 1 and 2 protons, respectively. With additional background signals in the high-field region, there are at least 32-36 H-atoms not subject to D_2O exchange. In d_5-pyridine, the low-field protons undergo further massive deshielding appearing at δ9.30, 10.00, 10.63 (relative to internal trimethylsilane). This indicates a specific, "face-to-face" binding of pyridine to an unsaturated and probably acidic system in phomopsin A.

A well-resolved, proton-decoupled ^{13}C-resonance spectrum was obtained on phomopsin A in D_2O at pH 9-10 (Fig. 4). It shows 30 main peaks made up of 8 aliphatic carbons, 7.9 - 33.2 ppm.; 7 aliphatic carbons bearing O- or N- substituents, 55.8 - 86.7 ppm.; 11 aromatic or similar carbons, 113.8 - 150.3 ppm.; and 4 carbonyl or similar carbons, 169.5 - 171.5 ppm.

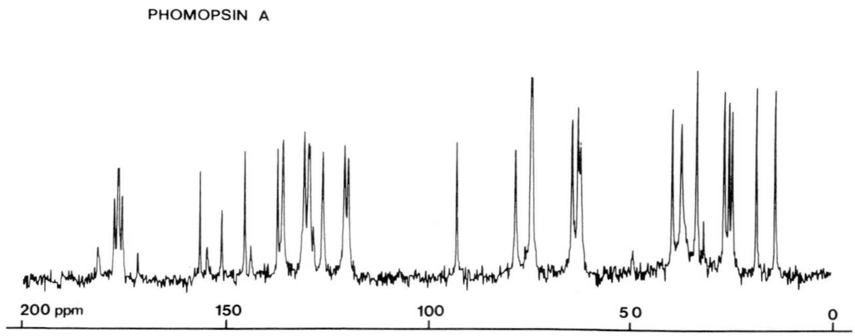

Fig. 4. *Noise-decoupled* ^{13}C*-nmr spectrum of phomopsin A in* D_2O*, pH 9-10, relative to methanol, 49.3 ppm.*

Off-resonance spectra are not yet available to aid interpretation but the carbon at 7.9 ppm. can be matched with the CH_3-CH_2 protons and the carbon at 12.6 ppm. with the singlet methyl, δ1.07. The carbon atoms at 18.5, 19.3, and 20.5 ppm. are probably the methyls δ1.54 - 1.77 in the proton spectrum but further correlation of the C and H resonances are at present too speculative.

The number of peaks in the aromatic region is surprisingly high compared with the few protons in the proton spectrum which could be regarded as aromatic. The unsaturated system present is apparently fairly heavily substituted.

The carbonyl peaks have shifts appropriate to amides, the adjacent low-intensity peaks possibly indicating the existence of tautomers or *cis-trans* isomers. The minor peaks, being one at higher field and one at lower field, suggest tautomers in which two carbonyls are alternative sites for hydrogen-bonding as in 3-acetyl-5-benzyltetramic acid (7).

VII. MASS SPECTRA

Phomopsin A has been examined in Varian MAT-111, Varian MAT-311A, and Finnegan 3300 mass spectrometers, operating under electron impact, field desorption, and chemical ionization conditions, respectively. Failure to obtain a molecular ion or even a recognizable spectrum for phomopsin A under these conditions is indicative of a highly involatile substance. Under chemical ionization conditions, a spectrum was obtained of an apparent, chlorine-containing, decomposition product. Peaks of m/e 434 and 436 (intensity ratio 3:1) in this spectrum are believed to represent M+1 ions for the decomposition product (M.N. Galbraith, unpublished results).

Derivatization has also failed to give other than small fragments. Methylation of phomopsin A with diazomethane in aqueous ether-tetrahydrofuran and examination of the project by gc-ms gave a spectrum with a clearly defined apparent molecular ion, m/e 159.

VIII. HYDROLYSIS

In 0.1N HCl at room temperature, phomopsin A is converted over a period of several days into a product which has similar UV absorption and color reactions, greatly reduced anionic mobility at pH 9.2 and cationic mobility at pH 4.6. The other product is oxalacetic acid, identified by electrophoretic comparison with authentic material and by its rapid change during the period of hydrolysis into pyruvic acid. Phomopsin B is also hydrolyzed in 0.1N HCl to oxalacetic acid and a product which does not move at pH 9.2 but has cationic mobility at pH 4.6. The main hydrolysis product of phomopsin A develops blue and purple colors when the electrophoresis sheet is sprayed with ninhydrin and nitrous acid, respectively. Although this was initially taken as evidence for a primary aromatic amino group in the hydrolysis product, the nitrous acid reaction being regarded as diazotization and self-coupling, the development of similar colors from phomopsin A with other reagents suggests that a different origin is possible.

Phomopsin A does not give a purple color when sprayed with nitrous acid on an electrophoresis sheet but it does when dissolved in 2N H_2SO_4 and treated with sodium nitrite. It gives the same color, verified by measurement of UV and visible absorption with a broad maximum at 520 nm, when dissolved in 2N HNO_3 or when treated in dil. H_2SO_4 with periodic acid. Strong acidity (mineral acid stronger than 1N) appears to be necessary for color development, suggesting that hydrolysis may be a necessary first step. The color may be due to oxidation but it is also consistent with charge-transfer complex formation which is known to lead to broad absorption bands in the visible region. We have also shown that the purple color obtained by treating 5-*sec*-butyltetramic acid, a hydrolysis product of tenuazonic acid, with sodium nitrite (8) has a similar broad absorption band near 500 nm.

Oxalacetic acid is formed with surprising ease in view of the probable lack of carboxyl and ester groupings in phomopsin A. The relevant carbonyls are apparently present in the form of readily hydrolyzed amide or tricarbonyl systems.

IX. DISCUSSION

Of the many metabolites which have been isolated from species of *Phomopsis* and related genera, the cytochalasins and tenuazonic acid are probably of greatest interest in the present context. Both types of metabolite occur in *Phomopsis* and/or *Phoma spp.* (9-14). The cytochalasins have high mammalian toxicity and exert unique effects on cell division but chemically they appear to be unrelated to phomopsin A. Tenuazonic acid is an inhibitor of protein synthesis rather than a nucleotoxic agent but there are distinct possibilities that its main structural feature, a 3-acyltetramic acid grouping, may be present in phomopsin A. As indicated above, the UV spectrum of tenuazonic acid is not dissimilar to that of phomopsin A and a structure of this type could account for the OH, NH, and carbonyl absorption in the IR spectrum of phomopsin A. Like phomopsin A, tenuazonic acid has a substantial nitrogen content and it gives a spot on pherograms which shows the same dark color under UV light and the same colors (yellow → white) with the $KMnO_4$ reagent.

Tenuazonic acid is also reported to give a yellow color, and the de-acyl compound formed from it by hydrolysis in dilute acid a pink-purple color with nitrous acid (8). Attempts to reproduce these colors for comparison have not been fully successful, but the faint colors obtained were the same as those formed by phomopsin A and its hydrolysis product. The hydrolysis of tenuazonic acid and phomopsin A in dilute HCl, with fission of a simple acid from the main chromophore in each instance, is itself a strong parallel feature. However we refrain from suggesting a partial structure until more evidence has been obtained.

X. REFERENCES

1. Gardiner, M. R., *Adv. Vet. Sci.* 11, 85 (1967).
2. Gardiner, M. R., *J. Agric. West Aust.* 16, 26 (1975).
3. Gardiner, M. R., and Petterson, D. S., *J. Comp. Pathol.* 82, 5 (1972).
4. Peterson, J. E., *J. Comp. Pathol.* in press.
5. Culvenor, C. C. J., Beck, A. B., Clarke, M., Cockrum, P. A., Edgar, J. A., Frahn, J. L., Jago, M. V., Lanigan, G. W., Payne, A. L., Peterson, J. E., Petterson, D. S., Smith,

L. W., and White, R. R., *Aust. J. Biol. Sci.*, in press (1977).
6. Mulholland, T. P. C., Foster, R., and Haydock, D. B., *J. Chem. Soc. Perkin Trans.* 2121 (1972).
7. Yamaguchi, T., Saito, K., Tsujimoto, T., and Yuki, H., *J. Heterocycl. Chem.* 13, 533 (1976).
8. Stickings, C. E., *Biochem. J.* 72, 332 (1959).
9. Patwardhan, S. A., Pandey, R. C., Sukh Dev, and Pendse, G. S., *Phytochemistry* 13, 1985 (1974).
10. Wells, J. M., Cutler, H. G., and Cole, R. J., *Can. J. Microbiol.* 22, 1137 (1976).
11. Beno, M. A., and Cristoph, G. G., *J. Chem. Soc. D.* 344 (1976).
12. Rothweiler, W., and Tamm, Ch., *Helv. Chim. Acta* 53, 696 (1970).
13. Anon, S. Afr, *CSIR special report CHEM 250.* 76 (1976).
14. Steyn, P. S., and Rabie, C. J., *Phytochemistry* 15, 1 (1976).

TOXIC AMINO ACIDS OF PLANT ORIGIN

M. P. Hegarty
C.S.I.R.O., Division of Tropical Crops and Pastures

I. ABSTRACT

The chemical and physiological properties of some non-protein amino acids found in plants which have been shown to be toxic to man, livestock, and domestic animals are reviewed. Compounds discussed include hypoglycin A, the lathyrogenic amino acids, mimosine, indospicine, and canavanine. Most of these compounds have low general toxicities but prolonged administration of them can result in toxic effects in various mammalian tissues. Some features of the deleterious effects of these compounds are interference with the metabolism of the normal protein amino acids and involvement of specific tissues such as the skin and the thyroid (mimosine and its metabolite in ruminants), the liver (indospicine and canavanine), and the brain (some of the lathyrogenic amino acids).

II. INTRODUCTION

Almost 300 non-protein amino acids have been isolated from or identified in higher plants. While some of them have a wide distribution the occurrence of many is restricted to a particular plant family, genus, or even to a limited number of species. Plants which synthesize these amino acids often accumulate the free compounds in high concentrations in the seeds and sometimes in the leaves but do not incorporate them into protein.

These "unusual" amino or imino acids have a wide range of chemical structures. Some of them are close chemical analogs of the protein amino acids and it is therefore not surprising to find that certain of them can act as antimetabolites when introduced into organisms in which they do not normally occur. The occurrence and biological properties of the non-protein amino acids have been the subject of a number of recent reviews (1,2,3,4).

Much of the information about adverse effects of excessive intakes of individual protein amino acids by animals and humans has been recently reviewed (5,6) as has the pharmacology of many of them (7). No comprehensive studies have been made of the physiological properties of the non-protein amino acids of plants, and most attention has been devoted to those, less than 20 in number, which have been implicated as toxic in man or livestock. With increasing use of plants as sources of protein, future investigations are likely to reveal more toxic amino acids.

The deleterious amino acids in plants do not show marked general toxicity; the single dose oral toxicity is usually low and the development of the most serious effects requires repeated dosage. Microorganisms may not only modify the structure of the compounds but may even destroy them completely. The microflora in the gastrointestinal tract may greatly reduce the apparent toxicity of ingested amino acids. The rumen microflora is well adapted to metabolizing the amino acids of plants (8) and may protect the animals from the effects of toxic compounds in their diet. However, it cannot always be assumed that the transformation product will be non-toxic as is well illustrated by the work on mimosine which is described later. While some amino acids are toxic because they can act as antagonists of protein amino acids and interfere with protein synthesis, others owe their toxicity to inhibition of enzymes not directly involved in protein synthesis or to some other chemical property. Chronic ingestion of a number of these amino acids can lead to some dramatic toxic effects on specific mammalian tissues.

This article will review information on a number of amino acids toxic in man and livestock and then consider some recent investigations on the biological properties of mimosine, indospicine, and canavanine. Emphasis is placed on results which concern the relation between the chemistry and metabolism of these compounds and their toxicity in mammals. The seleno-amino acids are involved in the toxicity of selenium-containing plants to livestock and the reader is referred to the paper by O. E. Olson (this symposium) for further information on these compounds.

III. AMINO ACIDS TOXIC IN MAN

A. Hypoglycin A

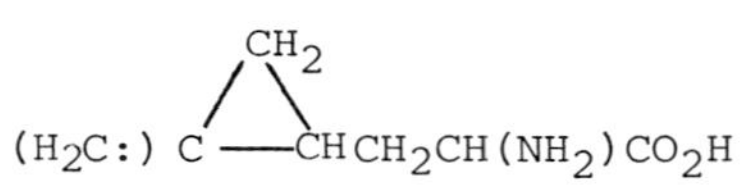

The fruit of *Blighia sapida* ("ackee") (Sapindaceae), a tree which grows in Jamaica and in parts of Africa contains the amino acid hypoglycin A, a chemical analogue of leucine, which can cause hypoglycaemia and may be responsible for the "vomiting sickness" reported in Jamaica. The fruit is sometimes eaten when food is scarce [for recent review see Van Veen (9)]. The mechanism of this sometimes fatal disease has been attributed to the profound fall in blood sugar caused by hypoglycin A. The amino acid can also cause a marked increase in the levels of unesterified fatty acids in the plasma in rats (10) and the accumulation of these may be involved in its toxic effects. In adult laboratory animals it has caused a decrease in liver glycogen and the development of fatty livers (11) and is teratogenic in rats but not in chickens (12). The plant is apparently not eaten by livestock.

B. The Lathyrogenic Amino Acids

Seeds of several species of *Lathyrus* have been implicated as the active agents in the disease complex called lathyrism. The complex has been separated into two diseases, osteolathyrism, which is characterized by severe skeletal abnormalities, and neurolathyrism, a neurological disease affecting humans, horses, and cattle living on the sub-continent of India. Neurolathyrism is caused by eating seeds of *L. sativus* and less frequently those of *L. cicera* and *L. clymenum*. As pointed out by Bell (13) outbreaks of the disease usually occur in times of famine when large quantities of *Lathyrus* meal are eaten and form a major part of the diet. This is not intended to be a comprehensive review of the lathyrogenic amino acids but to illustrate the types of amino acids involved and their likely contribution to the overall problem. Further information can be found in several recent reviews (13,14).

1. *β-N-(γ-L-Glutamyl) Aminopropionitrile*

$NCCH_2CH_2NHOCCH_2CH_2CH(NH_2)CO_2H$

This substance was isolated from *L. odoratus* (sweet pea) and produced severe skeletal abnormalities when fed to young rats (15). β-Aminopropionitrile, the active part of the molecule appears to exert its toxic action by interfering with the formation of cross-links in the chains of collagen and elastin, resulting in a weakening of blood vessels and bones. The substance is present in the seeds and leaves of *L. sylvestris* but not in *L. sativus* (16). Osteolathyrism from the consumption of *Lathyrus* species does not seem to be a major problem in man or livestock.

2. *L-α,γ-Diaminobutyric Acid*

Several *Lathyrus* species which have been tested as forage plants have been found to contain L-α,γ-diaminobutyric acid, $H_2NCH_2CH_2CH(NH_2)CO_2H$. It is present in *L. sylvestris* (flat pea) in all parts of the plant and at all stages of growth (16) and concentrations as high as 1.5% have been reported in the seed (17). It probably accounts for the reported toxicity of this species to some classes of livestock but in other species it occurs in low concentration. It acts by interfering with the urea cycle in mammals and by causing ammonia toxicity but the symptoms differ from those of classical lathyrism.

3. *α-Amino-β-oxalylaminopropionic Acid*

Although conclusive proof is lacking that human lathyrism is solely due to α-amino-β-oxalylaminopropionic acid (β-oxalyl-L-diaminopropionic acid), $HO_2CCONHCH_2CH(NH_2)CO_2H$, this compound is neurotoxic and occurs in concentrations as high as 2.5% in

L. sativus seed together with small amounts of the α-oxalyl isomer. It has caused neurological symptoms in young rats, guinea pigs, and dogs (18). It has been suggested (19) that its toxicity may result from lysosomal damage in the brain, while recent research suggests that when injected into immature animals it acts as a powerful excitant as does glutamic acid (20). No evidence is available on the effects of oral administration in this context. It accumulates in concentrations > 0.25% in the seeds of some species of *Crotalaria* and *Acacia* (21) a fact which needs to be considered in determining the potential use of these seeds for human and animal nutrition.

IV. AMINO ACIDS TOXIC IN LIVESTOCK

A. Mimosine

Mimosine occurs in *Mimosa pudica* (Leguminosae) and in large amounts in the leaves (8-10% of the dry weight of young leaves) and seeds (3-5%) of *Leucaena leucocephala* a pan-tropical shrub legume which has potential as a pasture legume in the tropics and sub-tropics. It has not been detected in other genera. Mimosine has a range of physiological properties, causing loss of hair in horses, cattle, and laboratory animals and shedding of the fleece in sheep. It can cause eye-cataracts in rats and problems in reproduction in rodents. A number of reviews have been published (1,2,4,7) summarizing information on its physiological properties and on the many chemical and biochemical studies made to determine its mode of action. The reader is referred to these reviews for references to the original literature.

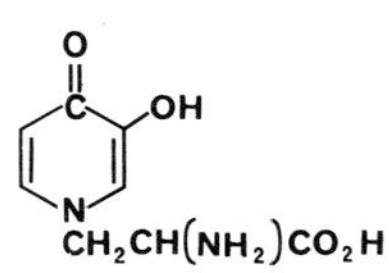

Mimosine

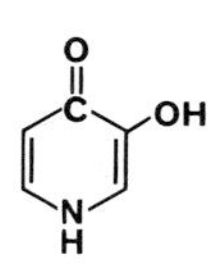

3-hydroxy-4(IH)-pyridone

Recent research on mimosine has been concerned with the observation that it is inhibitory to certain tumors, with its potential use as a chemical defleecing agent in sheep, and with problems which have arisen with the use of *L. leucocephala* as a pasture legume for cattle in northern Australia. These investigations have provided new information on its physiological properties and mechanisms of action.

Mimosine suppressed the formation of tumors in mice inoculated with Harding-Passey melanoma but did not cause regression of established tumors (22). It has been suggested that it had a specific inhibitory effect on the phenoloxidase activity of the melanocyte cells. Chemically, mimosine is an analogue of 3, 4-dihydroxyphenylalanine (DOPA) and has an X-ray crystal structure very similar to that of DOPA (23). It was shown to be weakly inhibitory to other types of tumors (24). It is therefore potentially useful as a model compound in the study of these tumors.

As part of a search for chemicals suitable for (25,26,27) defleecing sheep, Reis and co-workers followed up the original observations (28) that administration of mimosine to sheep caused shedding of the fleece which could be readily removed by hand (Fig. 1a). Intravenous infusion of mimosine at a rate of 80 mg/kg body weight a day for 1 1/2 - 2 days caused an abrupt cessation of wool growth within 2 days and the fleece could be removed in about 14 days (26). For defleecing, a plasma concentration of mimosine of 0.1-0.2 mM for 30-36 hours was necessary (25). The concurrent infusion of tyrosine, phenylalanine, or cystine with mimosine failed to prevent any of the effects of mimosine on wool growth (26) suggesting that it was not acting as an antagonist to any of these amino acids, a possibility suggested by various authors. A single oral dose of mimosine of 450-600 mg/kg either as the pure compound or in the pelleted foliage of *L. leucocephala* was effective for defleecing sheep (27) as was a daily dose of 300 mg/kg if given on two successive days.

Most of the mimosine given intravenously was rapidly excreted unchanged. When given orally the excretion products were mimosine, dominant on the day after dosing, and 3-hydroxy-4(IH)-pyridone (DHP), the transformation product of mimosine in the rumen (28), an important component during the second and third days. Mimosinamine (decarboxylated mimosine) was a minor excretion product.

To determine the parts of the mimosine molecule essential for its inhibitory properties several structure-activity studies have been made. Mimosine was a potent inhibitor of incorporation of [^{3}H] thymidine into DNA in sheep skin slices at a concentration of 2×10^{-4}M (29). The 3-hydroxy-4-oxo function of the pyridone ring was essential for activity while the amino acid side chain was not a toxiphoric center, but changes in its polarity affected the inhibitory activity. For inhibitory activity in mouse bone marrow cells in liquid culture (Hegarty, Lee, Christie, and Court submitted for publication) both the 3-hydroxy-4-oxo function and an amino acid or amine side chain were necessary. DHP was active in the sheep skin slice system (epidermoid cells) but inactive in the mouse bone marrow system (mesenchymal cells), while the reverse was the case with mimosinamine. It seems likely that different cells may vary in their susceptibility to the various compounds. Mimosine affects a number of biochemical constituents and biochemical processes in mammalian cells and the effects may be complex. A number of mechanisms of action have been proposed mainly on the basis of studies *in vitro* [for further information see (1) and (2)]. These are: it could act as an amino acid antagonist interfering with the metabolism of phenylalanine, tyrosine, DOPA, or cystine, or by complexing with pyridoxal phosphate and affecting enzymes which require this substance, or by chelating heavy metals and so inhibiting enzymes containing or requiring these metals. It has recently been shown to inhibit collagen synthesis *in vitro* (30). It seems clear that different mechanisms may operate in different cells.

Prolonged ingestion of *L. leucocephala* by cattle in northern Australia has caused low weight gains, hair loss, and goiter in adult cattle (31,32) even when the animals received iodine supplementation. Goitrous offspring have been produced by sheep and cattle fed during pregnancy on diets containing a high proportion of *L. leucocephala* leaves (33,34). The cause of the goiters is not mimosine but DHP to which the major part of the ingested mimosine is converted in the rumen (35). Mice on normal diets low in iodine containing 0.5% mimosine did not develop goiters and there were no histological changes in the thyroids. Mice fed similar diets into which 1% DHP had been incorporated developed hyperplastic goiters, histologically similar to those in goitrous cattle grazing *L. leucocephala* (Fig. 1b). DHP depressed the uptake of [^{125}I] by the thyroid in rats, (35) being intermediate in activity between the known goitrogens resorcinol and methyl thiouracil. The action of DHP, like that of these known goitrogens, is on the organic binding of iodine in the thyroid gland not on the iodide trapping and concentrating mechanism. Thiocyanate released the trapped but unbound iodide from the rat thyroid which had been inhibited with DHP but DHP did not release iodide from the methyl thiouracil inhibited thyroid gland (Hegarty, Lee, Christie, and Court, in preparation). These results explain the failure to overcome the problem in the field with iodine supplementation. A plant breeding program to develop mimosine-low or mimosine-free varieties of *L. leucocephala* is in progress in the C.S.I.R.O., Division of Tropical Crops and Pastures and some success has been achieved in reducing the mimosine content (E. M. Hutton, personal communication).

Hyperactivity or excitability in cattle grazing the legume in the Northern Territory, Australia is a problem when the stock are handled (36). The cause has not been established. Although the general toxicity of DHP is low it has been shown to be an inhibitor of catechol-O-methyl transferase, one of the enzymes responsible for the inactivation of adrenalin and non-adrenalin (37). Inhibitors of this enzyme are known to potentiate the action of these amines (38) and the possibility that the hyperactivity may be associated with the prolonged absorption of large amounts of DHP needs to be investigated.

B. Indospicine

Indospicine, $H_2NC(:NH)CH_2CH_2CH_2CH_2CH(NH_2)CO_2H$, which is a chemical analog of arginine, occurs in the leaves (0.1-0.5% of the dry weight) and seeds (0.1-2%) of *Indigofera spicata* (creeping indigo) a potentially useful tropical pasture legume (39). It has not been detected outside the genus *Indigofera*. A recent survey of the seeds of 32 species showed that indospicine was present in high concentrations (0.5-1%) in 4 species and in trace amounts in another 8 species (Charlwood, Bell, Ryan, and Hegarty, in preparation). High concentrations of canavanine were present in a number of the species (40).

Indospicine caused characteristic liver damage in rats and mice similar to that observed in cattle grazing the plant. The pattern of liver damage consisted of enlargement of hepatocyte nuclei and nucleoli, proliferation of duct epithelial and ovoid cells and a slight degree of necrosis, and could be differentiated from that produced by the typically necrotizing hepatotoxins such as carbon tetrachloride, the nitrosamines, and the pyrrolizidine alkaloids (41). A single dose of indospicine monohydrochloride (2 g/kg body wt) given by stomach tube produced a marked rise in liver triglycerides and a 48% increase in liver wet weight in 24 hr, water being the main contributor to the increase in wet weight (42). The similarity of the histological changes produced by the purified amino acid to those produced by feeding diets of *I. spicata* seed indicated that the indospicine content of the seed was the major factor contributing to its hepatotoxic effect. Chronic feeding of these diets to rats produced greatly enlarged, coarsely nodular livers (Fig. 1c) but no hepatomas were observed (41). Indospicine caused infertility and teratogenic effects in rats and mice. In rats, a dose of 2 g/kg on day 13 of gestation caused an 80% incidence of cleft palates (43).

Indospicine is an arginine antagonist, inhibiting rat liver arginase (44) and arginine decarboxylase from *Escherichia coli* (Dr. W. V. Groman, personal communication). The major biochemical action of indospicine is a primary blockage of arginine incorporation into liver protein resulting in a secondary depression of incorporation of other amino acids (45). Indospicine can competitively inhibit arginine metabolism in various mammalian cells grown in liquid culture (46,47). The degree of inhibition was related to the concentration of indospicine and the inhibition could be reversed by the addition of arginine. Synthesis of DNA is eventually inhibited in these systems but it is doubtful if this could occur at the concentrations of indospicine attained in the liver in feeding experiments. The liver lesion was interpreted as a restricted hepatic response to a growth stimulus, possibly the mobilization of tissue amino acids. Indospicine causes a severe aminoaciduria which could be associated with its toxicity.

The general toxicity of indospicine is low. Rats given 5 g/kg by stomach tube survived and apart from the livers, the organs of rats from chronic feeding experiments showed no abnormalities (41,

42). Indospicine is not appreciably metabolized in the rat and is excreted unchanged (Hegarty, Court, and Christie, unpublished

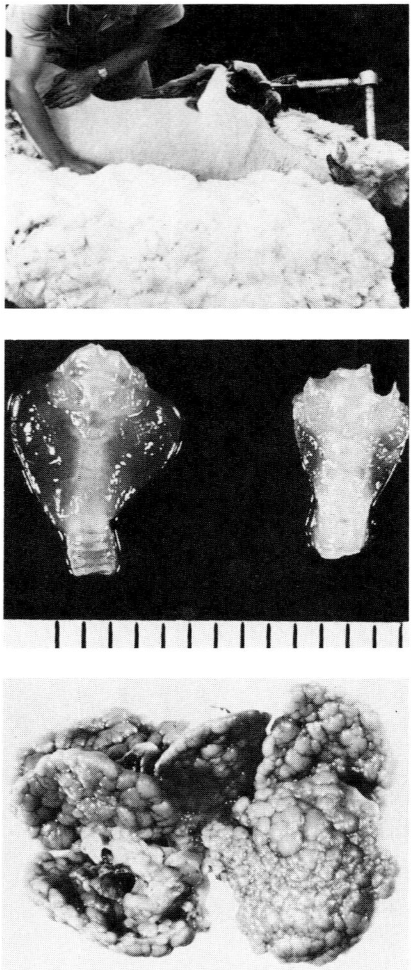

Fig. 1a (top). *Removal of fleece by hand from a sheep which had eaten a sole diet of* Leucaena leucocephala *leaves for 14 days.* Fig. 1b (middle). *Thyroid glands of adult Swiss mice which had been fed a low-iodine diet containing 1% 3-hydroxy-4-(1H) pyridone (left) and low-iodine diet alone (right) for 12 weeks. Scale shows mm divisions.* Fig. 1c (bottom). *Liver from rat fed 24%* Indigofera spicata *seed diet for 18 weeks showing nodular cirrhosis. Liver weight 8.2 g; body weight 194 g. Reproduced by permission of Longman Group LTD.*

results).

The growth of various microorganisms is inhibited by indospicine (48). The marked growth inhibition by indospicine in *Pseudomonas aeruginosa* is interesting because this organism has proven resistant to most amino acid analogues tested.

C. Canavanine

Canavanine, $H_2NC(:NH)NHOCH_2CH_2CH(NH_2)CO_2H$, a chemical analog of arginine, occurs in the seeds of some leguminous plants often in high concentrations, e.g. up to 5% of the dry weight of seeds of *Canavalia ensiformis* (jack bean). It occurs only in the subfamily Papilionoidae and has been detected in the seeds of 60% of the species and 35% of the genera which have been examined (49). These include many species of potential importance as sources of protein (50). When seeds containing canavanine germinate the canavanine is metabolized and the mature plants contain only small amounts (39).

Canavanine acts as an arginine antagonist in many microorganisms but evidence of toxic effects in mammals is conflicting. Mice fed on diets containing up to 0.1 g/kg/day showed no toxic symptoms (54), but a single oral dose of 2 g/kg of canavanine sulphate killed mice in 24 hr (52). To investigate the toxicity of canavanine Hegarty, Schepisi, and Christie (submitted for publication) administered canavanine hydrochloride (400 mg/kg body weight) to rats by stomach tube every 3 days for 6 weeks and as a single dose of 2.5 g/kg body weight. No evidence of general toxicity was observed and no histological changes detected in any organs except the liver. Similar histological changes were observed in the livers in both chronic and acute experiments. These consisted of fatty change, enlargement of the hepatocytes especially affecting the nuclei, portal tract cellularity and occasional focal necrosis. The changes were qualitatively similar to those produced by indospicine but were mild in view of the high dose needed to produce them. Canavanine is therefore a weak hepatotoxin in the rat when given orally. As canavanine is known to be degraded by bacteria it is possible that some destruction takes place in the gastrointestinal tract and this may explain its low apparent toxicity.

V. REFERENCES

1. Thompson, J. F., Morris, C. J., and Smith, I. K., *Annu. Rev. Biochem.* 38, 137 (1969).
2. Hegarty, M. P., and Peterson, P. J., *in* "Chemistry and Biochemistry of Herbage" (G. W. Butler and R. W. Bailey, Eds.), Vol. 1, p. 1. Academic Press, London, 1973.
3. Fowden, L., *in* "Recent Advances in Phytochemistry" (V. C. Runeckles, and E. E. Conn, Eds.), Vol. 8, p. 95. Academic

Press, New York, 1974.
4. Bell, E. A., *FEBS Lett.* 64, 29 (1976).
5. Harper, A. E., Benevenga, N. J., and Wohlhueter, R. M., *Physiol. Rev.* 50, 428 (1970).
6. Harper, A. E., *in* "Toxicants Occurring Naturally in Foods" (Committee on Food Protection, Food and Nutrition Board, National Research Council), 2nd Ed., p. 130. National Academy of Sciences, Washington, 1973.
7. Milne, M. D., *Clin. Pharmacol. Ther.* 9, 484 (1968).
8. McDonald, I. W., *in* "International Encyclopedia of Food and Nutrition" (D. Cuthbertson, Ed.), Vol. 17, Part I, p. 87. Pergamon Press, Oxford, 1969.
9. Van Veen, A. G., *in* "Toxicants Occurring Naturally in Foods" (Committee on Food Protection, Food and Nutrition Board, National Research Council), 2nd Ed., p. 464. National Academy of Sciences, Washington, 1973.
10. Tanaka, K., Isselbacher, K. J., and Shih, V., *Science* 175, 69 (1972).
11. Chen, K. K., Anderson, R. C., McCowen, M. C., and Harris, P. N., *J. Pharmacol. Exp. Ther.* 121, 272 (1957).
12. Persaud, T. V. N., and Kaplan, S., *Life Sci.* 9, 1305 (1970).
13. Bell, E. A., *in* "Toxicants Occurring Naturally in Foods" (Committee on Food Protection, Food and Nutrition Board, National Research Council), 2nd Ed., p. 153. National Academy of Sciences, Washington, 1973.
14. Sarma, P. S., and Padmanaban, G., *in* "Toxic Constituents of Plant Foodstuffs" (I. E. Liener, Ed.), p. 267. Academic Press, New York, 1969.
15. McKay, G. F., Lalich, J. J., Schilling, E. D., and Strong, F. M., *Arch. Biochem. Biophys.* 52, 313 (1954).
16. Simola, L. K., *Acta Bot. Fenn.* 81, 1 (1968).
17. Ressler, C., Redstone, P. A., and Erenberg, R. H., *Science* 134, 188 (1961).
18. Rao, S. L. N., and Sarma, P. S., *Biochem. Pharmacol.* 16, 218 (1967).
19. Lakshmanan, J., Cheema, P. S., and Padmanaban, G., *Nature (London) New Biol.* 234, 156 (1971).
20. Olney, J. W., Misra, C. H., and Rhee, V., *Nature (London)* 264, 659 (1976).
21. Qureshi, M. Y., Pilbeam, D. J., Evans, C. S., and Bell, E. A., *Phytochemistry* 16, 477 (1977).
22. Prabhakaran, K., Harris, E., and Kirchheimer, W. F., *Cytobios* 7, 245 (1973).
23. Mostad, A., Romming, C., and Rosenqvist, E., *Acta Chem. Scand.* 27, 164 (1973).
24. De Wys, W. D., and Hall, T. C., *Cancer Chemother. Rep.* 57, 41 (1973).
25. Reis, P. J., Tunks, D. A., and Chapman, R. E., *Aust. J. Biol. Sci.* 28, 69 (1975).
26. Reis, P. J., *Aust. J. Biol. Sci.* 28, 483 (1975).
27. Reis, P. J., Tunks, D. A., and Hegarty, M. P., *Aust. J.*

Biol. Sci. 28, 495 (1975).
28. Hegarty, M. P., Schinckel, P. G., and Court, R. D., *Aust. J. Agric. Res.* 15, 153 (1964).
29. Ward, K. A., and Harris, R. L. N., *Aust. J. Biol. Sci.* 29, 189 (1976).
30. Tang, S. Y., and Ling, K. H., *Toxicon* 13, 339 (1975).
31. Holmes, J. H., *Proc. Aust. Soc. Anim. Prod.* 11, 453 (1976).
32. Jones, R. J., Blunt, C., and Holmes, J. H., *Trop. Grassl.* 10, 113 (1976).
33. Bindon, B. M., and Lamond, D. R., *Proc. Aust. Soc. Anim. Prod.* 6, 109 (1966).
34. Hamilton, R. I., Donaldson, L. E., and Lambourne, L. J., *Aust. Vet. J.* 44, 484 (1968).
35. Hegarty, M. P., Court, R. D., Christie, G. S., and Lee, C. P., *Aust. Vet. J.* 52, 490 (1976).
36. Falvey, L., *Aust. Vet. J.* 52, 343 (1976).
37. Borchardt, R. T., *J. Med. Chem.* 16, 531 (1973).
38. Flohé, L., *Int. Pharmacopsychiatry* 9, 52 (1974).
39. Hegarty, M. P., and Pound, A. W., *Aust. J. Biol. Sci.* 23, 831 (1970).
40. Charlwood, B. V., and Bell, E. A., *J. Chromatogr.* 135, 377 (1977).
41. Christie, G. S., Wilson, M., and Hegarty, M. P., *J. Pathol.* 117, 195 (1975).
42. Christie, G. S., Madsen, N. P., and Hegarty, M. P., *Biochem. Pharmacol.* 18, 693 (1969).
43. Pearn, J. H., and Hegarty, M. P., *Br. J. Exp. Pathol.* 51, 34 (1970).
44. Madsen, N. P., and Hegarty, M. P., *Biochem. Pharmacol.* 19, 2391 (1970).
45. Madsen, N. P., Christie, G. S., and Hegarty, M. P., *Biochem. Pharmacol.* 19, 853 (1970).
46. Christie, G. S., DeMunk, F. G., Madsen, N. P., and Hegarty, M. P., *Pathology* 3, 139 (1971).
47. DeMunk, F. G., Christie, G. S., and Hegarty, M. P., *Pathology* 4, 133 (1972).
48. Leisinger, T., Haas, D., and Hegarty, M. P., *Biochim. Biophys. Acta* 262, 214 (1972).
49. Turner, B. L., and Harborne, J. B., *Phytochemistry* 6, 863 (1967).
50. Van Etten, C. H., Kwolek, W. F., Peters, J. E., and Barclay, A. S., *J. Agric. Food Chem.* 15, 1077 (1967).
51. Ogawa, M., *J. Agric. Chem. Soc. Jpn.* 10, 224 (1934).
52. Tschiersch, B., *Pharmazie* 17, 621 (1962).

PINE NEEDLE ABORTION IN CATTLE

J. W. Call and L. F. James
Utah State University and Poisonous Plant Research Laboratory, Agricultural Research Service, U.S. Department of Agriculture

I. ABSTRACT

A review of the literature and from these experimental data, it is evident that several factors are associated with pine needle abortion. The more apparent of these factors are: (a) stage of gestation; (b) stress; (c) animal condition; (d) physiology of the animal; and (e) pine needles. In this experiment pine needles induced abortion more consistently near the end of gestation. In addition, it was apparent that animals are depressed and develop signs of impending abortion very rapidly.

II. INTRODUCTION

Consumption of the needles of *Pinus ponderosa* (yellow or ponderosa pine) was suspected as a cause of abortion in cattle as early as 1920 (1). In 1952, the needles were shown experimentally to cause abortion in cattle (2). Reports were published in 1961 of anti-estrogenic properties of pine needle extract fed to mice (3). Chow *et al.*, suggested in 1974 that the abortifacient in pine needles might be a mycotoxin (4). Folklore has it that Indian women prepared and drank a water extract of ponderosa pine needles to cause abortion (5). Other reports indicate that sheep and deer may abort as a result of consuming pine needles (5).

Pine needle abortion in range cattle is a problem frequently observed in western Canada and the United States (6) and, in fact, in areas wherever ponderosa pine trees grow. Although the extent of pine needle abortion in cattle is not known, it is probably a more serious problem than has been suspected based on interviews with ranchers. In addition to the abortion loss, there is also a high incidence of retained placenta and impaired breeding performance.

There are also considerable amounts of forage not utilized because ranchers cannot graze pregnant animals safely on ranges and pastures on which ponderosa pine is found unless the areas are fenced or cleared of slash and fallen trees.

Ponderosa pine grows in every state west of the Great Plains and in Western Canada (7,8). Animals have year-round access to pine needles; however, the consumption of pine needles by cattle does not appear to be a problem during the warm months. The toxic principle is present year-round in the needles. Field observations indicate that cows abort after eating either green needles,

needles of slash, or dried needles that have fallen from the trees (5).

Pine needle-induced abortions usually occur during the last trimester of pregnancy (6). Most abortions are reported during late fall, winter, or early spring, coinciding with the period that most range cows are in the last trimester of pregnancy.

Most affected cows become depressed and dull in appearance prior to aborting, thereby providing premonitory signs (6). Abortions usually commence about two days after pine needles have been fed and continue for as long as two weeks after. Cows may have a toxemia prior to and following abortion. Additional symptoms of impending abortions are edema of the vulva and udder (6). Retained placenta is a common sequel (6). In field cases the cows often have a bloody discharge from the vulva, probably of uterine origin. These cows may or may not abort (6).

Histological examination of the tissues from the aborted fetus reveals pronounced necrosis of the proximal tubule of the kidneys, moderate thickening of the interlobular space in the lungs, and pulmonary congestion. Excessive hemoglobin breakdown products were found in all tissues examined. Most tissues were also autolyzed indicating fetal death intrautero (6).

Although consumption of pine needles has been known to cause abortion in sheep, the results of a study in which cycling ewes consumed a 37 percent pine needle diet demonstrated no toxic effects (9).

Reports suggest that the environmental stress of weather, body condition, disease, and biological differences influences the effect of pine needles in the individual animal. Abortions are most likely to occur when cattle are under stress (6). This is in agreement with observations of most livestockmen and veterinarians (5). In addition, cows from pine-free areas tend to be more predisposed to pine needle abortion than native cattle (5).

It has been reported by researchers that a major problem in inducing abortion under experimental conditions is getting the animals to eat the pine needles. However, under field conditions several factors apparently cause cattle to eat pine needles: (a) sudden weather changes such as cold winds or snow storms when cattle seek shelter under trees and eat the needles; (b) when feed becomes scarce near the end of the grazing season before cattle are moved from the range; (c) changes in feed, especially to unfamiliar or poor-quality feed; (d) sudden access to pine needles; (e) boredom; and (f) accidental ingestion with other feed. In some cases under apparently normal conditions, cattle will eat sufficient pine needles to cause abortion (5).

This report deals with experimentally induced abortion in beef cattle. The objective of the experiment was to determine the various factors that may influence incidence of pine needle abortion; for instance, approximate stage of gestation, hunger, and the amount of pine needles consumed. Pathological changes early in the abortion were studied.

TABLE 1

Pine Needle Feeding Schedule[1] and Results in Beef Cattle

Animal identification:	2986	2898	2987	2988	2989	2990
Ground and via stomach pump:	Pine needles per day (kg)					
Day 1[2]	1.82	1.82	1.82	--	--	--
Day 2	--	1.82	1.82	--	--	--
Day 3	--	--	1.82	--	--	--
Mixed with alfalfa (1:2) free choice:						
Day 3	--	--	--	3.5	3.5	3.5
Days 4-6	1.6	1.6	1.6	1.6	1.6	1.6
Days 16-18	1.9	1.9	1.9	--	--	--
Day 19	--	4.5	4.5	--	--	--
Days 40-42	--	--	5.2	--	--	--
Influence on pregnancy:						
Aborted	19th day			7th day	8th day	
Live calf			58th day			
Other		Mummified fetus[3]				Did not abort

[1]All animals were fed straw free choice for 13 days prior to pine needle treatment.
[2]Starting with first day of feeding pine needles.
[3]Apparently present prior to treatment.

III. MATERIALS AND METHODS

Five Hereford and one Hereford-Angus females in the last trimester of pregnancy were restricted to a straw diet for 13 days. The animals were then given pine needles by stomach pump or chopped pine needles and alfalfa free choice, or both (see Table 1). Three animals were offered whole pine needles in addition to straw free choice three days prior to gavaging the animals with ground pine needles. These animals initially refused to eat the needles; however, all the animals eventually did eat the chopped pine needles and alfalfa mixture.

All animals were determined to be in at least the fifth month of gestation by rectal palpation.

IV. RESULTS AND DISCUSSION

Three cows aborted. First to abort was one of the cows given pine needles free choice for three days (Table 1). She aborted on the fifth day after starting on pine needles (seventh day after the first group was treated with pine needles). A second cow administered no needles by stomach pump, but having free access to pine needles, aborted on the sixth day. The third cow in this group did not abort and, when removed from the project because she had squamous cell carcinoma, was still with calf.

One of the cows that received pine needles by stomach pump, then free choice, and again a second time free choice, aborted on the fourth day after starting on the second free choice treatment. Cows that were administered needles by stomach pump did not respond as quickly as the animals that were fed straw and then given the pine needles free choice (Table 1).

All animals aborted at about the same stage of gestation (near term). It appears in this research that abortions were not related to animal condition, the amount of pine needles consumed at a given time, nor the length of time that the animals had been eating the needles. Abortions appeared to be closely related to the stage of gestation. One animal gave birth to a normal live calf 15 days after receiving the largest number of treatments and highest total amount of pine needles; another cow did not abort even though she was in very poor condition. She was removed from the project because of squamous cell carcinoma as mentioned above. Prior to abortion, animals became dull, showed edema and swelling of the vulva and udder; these symptoms progressed very rapidly in comparison to a normal cow approaching parturition.

V. REFERENCES

1. Bruce, E. A., "*Astragalus serotinus* and other Stock-poisoning Plants of British Columbia, Dominion of Canada," Department of Agriculture Bulletin No. 88, p. 44, 1922.
2. McDonald, M. A., *J. Range Manage*. 5, 150-155 (1952).
3. Allen, M. R., and Kitts, W. D., *Can. J. Anim. Sci*. 41,1 (1961).
4. Chow, F. H., Hamar, D. W., and Udall, R. W., *J. Reprod. Fertil*. 40, 203-204 (1974).
5. Stevenson, A. H., James, L. F., and Call, J. W., *Cornell Vet*. 62, 519-524 (1972).
6. James, L. F., Call, J. W., and Stevenson, A. H., *Cornell Vet*., In press (1977).
7. Kingsbury, J. M., "Poisonous Plants of the United States and Canada," p. 119. Prentice-Hall, Englewood Cliffs, New Jersey, 1964.
8. Yearbook of Agriculture, "Trees," p. 71. U.S. Government Printing Office, Washington, D.C., 1949.
9. Call, J. W., and James, L. F., *J. Am. Vet. Med. Assoc*. 169, 1301-1302 (1976).

Index

S

T

A B C 8 D 9 E 0 F 1 G 2 H 3 I 4 J 5